2 second edition

A TEXTBOOK OF
MODERN
TOXICOLOGY

Ernest Hodgson, PhD • Patricia E. Levi, PhD
Toxicology Program
North Carolina State University
Raleigh, North Carolina

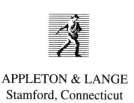

APPLETON & LANGE
Stamford, Connecticut

97 98 99 00 01 / 10 9 8 7 6 5 4 3 2 1

Prentice Hall International (UK) Limited, *London*
Prentice Hall of Australia Pty. Limited, *Sydney*
Prentice Hall Canada, Inc., *Toronto*
Prentice Hall Hispanoamericana, S.A., *Mexico*
Prentice Hall of India Private Limited, *New Delhi*
Prentice Hall of Japan, Inc., *Tokyo*
Simon & Schuster Asia Pte. Ltd., *Singapore*
Editora Prentice Hall do Brasil Ltda., *Rio de Janeiro*
Prentice Hall, *Upper Saddle River, New Jersey*

Library of Congress Cataloging-in-Publication Data

Hodgson, Ernest, 1932–
    Textbook of modern toxicology / Ernest Hodgson & Patricia E. Levi.
    —2nd ed.
        p.   cm.
    Includes bibliographical references and index.
    ISBN 0-8385-8887-5
    1. Toxicology.   I. Levi, Patricia E.   II. Title.
RA1211.H62   1997
615.9—dc21   97–78
                                                                        CIP

0-8385-8887-5

Acquisitions Editor: Linda Marshall
Production Editor: Karen Waigand Davis
Designer: Janice Barsevich Bielawa

9 780838 588871   90000

CONTENTS

....

4. REACTIVE METABOLITES — 95

Patricia E. Levi

5. ELIMINATION OF TOXICANTS — 107

Patricia E. Levi • Ernest Hodgson • Gerald A. LeBlanc

6. MODIFICATION OF XENOBIOTIC METABOLISM — 119

Ernest Hodgson

14 DIAGNOSIS AND TREATMENT OF TOXICITY — 373

Ernest Hodgson

15. BASICS OF ENVIRONMENTAL TOXICOLOGY — 389

Gerald A. LeBlanc

16. TRANSPORT AND FATE OF TOXICANTS IN THE ENVIRONMENT 407

Damian Shea

PREFACE

There are some excellent reference works in general toxicology, such as *Casarett and Doull's Toxicology* (5th edition, edited by Klaassen) and a 13-volume *Comprehensive Toxicology,* edited by Sipes, Gandolfi, and McQueen. However, the scarcity of textbooks designed for teacher and student to use in the classroom setting that caused us to write the first edition is still apparent. The first edition represented our first attempt to fill that particular niche. To the second edition we bring new material, additional experience, and continuing input from students and other teachers. Moreover, we have made important additions in environmental toxicology and we are grateful to Drs. LeBlanc and Shea for the preparation of these chapters. Our continued thanks go to Dr. Leidy for his contributions in analytical toxicology.

At North Carolina State University, we continue to teach a course in general toxicology that is open to graduate students and undergraduates at the senior level. Our experience leads us to believe that this text is suitable, in the junior or senior year, for undergraduates with some background in chemistry, biochemistry, and animal physiology. For graduate students it is intended to lay the foundation for subsequent, specialized courses in toxicology such as those in biochemical toxicology, chemical carcinogenesis, regulatory toxicology, and so forth.

We share the view that an introductory text must present all of the necessary fundamental information, but in as uncomplicated a manner as possible. To enhance readability, references have been deleted from the text. Although this may result in a text which appears simple to an advanced student, or one which is unsuitable as a reference work, a list of suggested further reading at the end of each chapter will permit students to extend their knowledge in any area of interest.

Clearly the amount of material, and the detail with which some of it is presented, is more than is needed for the average general toxicology course. This is done, however, to permit each instructor the opportunity to select and emphasize those areas of toxicology that they feel need particular emphasis. The obvious bio-chemical bias of some sections is deliberate and based on the philosophy that progress in toxicology continues to depend on further understanding of the fundamental basis of toxic action at the cellular and molecular levels.

Thanks to Ardy Hanson, whose help with the mysteries of word processing was indispensible to at least one of us, and to Linda Marshall, of Appleton & Lange, whose role as official conscience to the authors was filled with charm and grace. Thanks also to the students and faculty of the Department of Toxicology at North Carolina State University and to all of those whose comments on the first edition helped bring about the second.

Ernest Hodgson
Patricia E. Levi

Raleigh, North Carolina

INTRODUCTION TO TOXICOLOGY

ERNEST HODGSON

1.1

DEFINITION AND SCOPE, RELATIONSHIP TO OTHER SCIENCES, AND HISTORY

1.1.1 Definition and Scope

Toxicology can be defined as that branch of science that deals with poisons, and a poison can be defined as any substance that causes a harmful effect when administered, either by accident or design, to a living organism. By convention, toxicology also includes the study of harmful effects caused by physical phenomena, such as radiation of various kinds, noise, and so on. In practice, however, many complications exist beyond these simple definitions, both in bringing more precise definition to the meaning of poison and in the measurement of toxic effects. Broader definitions of toxicology, such as "the study of the detection, occurrence, properties, effects, and regulation of toxic substances," although more descriptive, do not resolve the difficulties. It is to the complications, and to the basic science behind them and their resolution, that this textbook is devoted, most particularly to the mechanisms involved, the *how* and *why* certain substances cause disruptions of biologic systems that result in toxic effects. Taken together, these difficulties and their resolution circumscribe the perimeter of the science of toxicology.

Toxicology exists in the service of society, not only in the sense of protecting humans and other organisms from the deleterious effects of toxicants, but also to serve directly by developing better selective toxicants. Thus, the study of comparative toxicology and selective toxicity contributes to the development of better and more selective anticancer drugs, pesticides, and so forth.

1

It must be emphasized at the outset that poison is a quantitative concept. Almost any substance is harmful at some dose and, at the same time, is harmless at a very low dose. Between these two limits there is a range of possible effects, from subtle long-term chronic toxicity to immediate lethality. Vinyl chloride may be taken as an example; it is a potent hepatotoxicant at high doses, a carcinogen with a long latent period at lower doses, and is apparently without effect at very low doses. Clinical drugs are even more poignant examples because, although therapeutic and highly beneficial at some doses, they are not without deleterious side effects and are frequently lethal at higher doses. Aspirin (acetylsalicylic acid), for example, is a relatively safe drug at recommended doses and is taken by millions of people. At the same time, chronic use can cause deleterious effects on the gastric mucosa, and it is fatal at a dose of about 0.2–0.5 g/kg. Some 15% of reported accidental deaths from poisoning in children are due to salicylates, particularly aspirin.

The importance of dose is seen clearly with metals that are dietary essentials but are toxic at higher doses. Thus, iron, copper, magnesium, cobalt, manganese, and zinc can be present at too low a level in the diet (deficiency), at an appropriate level (maintenance), or at too high a level (toxic). The question of dose–response relationships is fundamental to toxicology and is discussed in more detail later (Section 1.2).

The definition of a poison, or toxicant, also involves a qualitative biologic aspect because a compound, highly toxic to one species or genetic strain, may be relatively harmless to another. For example, carbon tetrachloride, a potent hepatotoxicant in many species, is relatively harmless to the chicken. Certain strains of rabbit can eat *Belladonna* with impunity while others cannot. Compounds may also be toxic under some circumstances but not others or, perhaps, toxic in combination with another compound but nontoxic alone. The methylenedioxyphenyl insecticide synergists, such as piperonyl butoxide, are of low toxicity to both mammals and insects when administered alone, but are, by virtue of their ability to block xenobiotic-metabolizing enzymes, capable of causing dramatic increases in the toxicity of other compounds.

The measurement of toxicity is also complex. Toxicity may be acute or chronic, and may vary from one organ to another as well as with the age, sex, diet, physiological condition, or health status of the organism. Even the simplest measure of toxicity, the LD50 (the dose required to kill 50% of a population of an organism under stated conditions), is highly dependent on the extent to which many of the previously mentioned variables are controlled, and LD50 values, as a result, vary markedly from one laboratory to another.

Exposure of humans and other organisms to toxicants may result from many activities; intentional ingestion, occupational exposure, environmental exposure, as well as accidental and intentional (suicidal or homicidal) poisoning. The toxicity of a particular compound may vary with the portal of entry into the body, whether through the alimentary canal, the lungs, or the skin. Even experimental methods such as injection may give rise to highly variable results; thus, the toxicity from intravenous (IV), intraperitoneal (IP), intramuscular (IM), or subcutaneous (SC) injection of a given compound may be quite different. Toxicity may vary as much as tenfold with the route of administration. Following exposure (Fig. 1.1) there are multiple possible routes of metabolism, both detoxifying and activating, and multiple possible toxic endpoints.

The scope of toxicology can be described in a number of ways. Loomis and Hayes (1996) divide the subject into environmental, economic, and forensic toxicology. The first is concerned with residues, pollution, and industrial hygiene; the second is concerned with the development of chemicals such as drugs, pesticides, and food additives; and the third deals with diagnosis, treatment, and medicolegal aspects. Although this classification is useful, it does not give adequate weight to the mechanistic approach concerned with events at the fundamental level that occur during metabolism, mode of toxic action, and so on, nor does it do justice to the wide scope of the subject.

Any attempt to define the scope of toxicology, including that which follows, must take into account the fact that the various subdisciplines are not mutually ex-

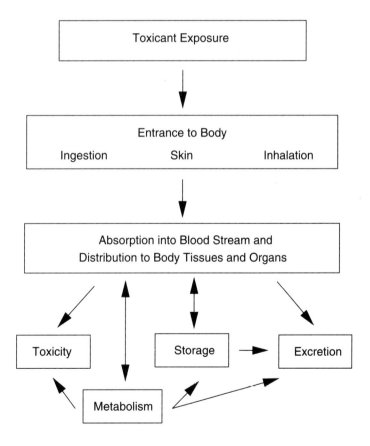

Figure 1.1. Entry and fate of toxicants in the body.

clusive and frequently are heavily interdependent. Due to overlapping of mechanisms, chemical classes, use classes and effects, clear division into subjects of equal importance is not possible. Although many specialized terms are used in the various subdisciplines of toxicology, there are some terms of importance to toxicology in general; they are defined in the glossary to be found at the end of this volume.

A. Mechanisms of Toxic Action. This includes the consideration—at the fundamental level of organ, cell, and molecular function—of all events leading to toxicity in vivo: uptake, distribution, metabolism, mode of action, and excretion. Important aspects include the following:

   1. *Biochemical toxicology* considers events at the biochemical and molecular level, including enzymes that metabolize xenobiotics, generation of reactive intermediates, interaction of xenobiotics or their metabolites with macromolecules, molecular biology of gene expression in metabolism or in modes of toxic action, and so on.

   2. *Behavioral toxicology* deals with the effect of toxicants on animal and human behavior, which is the final integrated expression of nervous function at the intact animal level. This involves both the peripheral and the central nervous systems, as well as the effects mediated by other organ systems such as the endocrine glands.

   3. *Nutritional toxicology* deals with the effects of diet on the expression of toxicity and the mechanisms for these effects.

   4. *Carcinogenesis* is of tremendous current interest and includes the chemical and biochemical events that lead to the large number of effects on cell growth collectively known as cancer.

   5. *Teratogenesis* is also of much current interest and includes the chemical and biochemical events that lead to deleterious effects on the developmental process.

   6. *Mutagenesis* is concerned with toxic effects on the genetic material and the inheritance of these defects.

   7. *Organ toxicity* considers effects at the level of organ function (eg, neurotoxicity, hepatotoxicity, and nephrotoxicity).

B. Measurement of Toxicants and Toxicity. These important aspects deal primarily with analytical chemistry, bioassay, and applied mathematics, and are designed to provide the methodology to answer certain critically important questions. Is the substance likely to be toxic? What is its chemical identity? How much of it is present? How can we assay its toxic effect and what is the minimum level at which this toxic effect can be detected? This aspect of toxicology includes a number of important fields:

   1. *Analytic toxicology* is a branch of analytic chemistry that is concerned with methods for the identification and assay of toxic chemicals and their metabolites in biologic and environmental materials.

   2. *Toxicity testing* involves the use of living systems to estimate toxic effects. It covers the entire gamut from short-term tests for genotoxicity such as the

Ames test and cell culture techniques to the use of intact animals for acute toxicity tests and for lifetime or multigeneration chronic toxicity tests. Athough the term "bioassay" is used properly only to describe the use of living organisms to quantitate the amount of a particular toxicant present, it is often used improperly to describe in vivo toxicity testing.

3. *Toxicologic pathology* is that branch of pathology which deals with the effects of toxic agents as manifested by changes in subcellular, cellular, tissue, or organ morphology.

4. *Structure-activity study* is a subdiscipline of toxicology that deals with the relationship between chemical and physical properties of xenobiotics and toxicity and, particularly, the use of such relationships for the prediction of toxicity.

5. *Biomathematics and statistics* are important subjects, related to a number of areas of toxicology. They deal with data analysis, the determination of significance, and the formulation of risk estimates and predictive models. This is particularly important in epidemiology and environmental toxicology.

6. *Epidemiology* as it applies to toxicology, is closely related to the previous subject and is of great importance because it deals with the study of toxicity as it actually occurs, rather than in an experimental setting.

C. Applied Toxicology. This includes the various aspects of toxicology as they occur in the field.

1. *Clinical toxicology* is the diagnosis and treatment of human poisoning.

2. *Veterinary toxicology* is the diagnosis and treatment of the poisoning of animals other than humans, particularly livestock and companion animals but not excluding feral species. An important concern of veterinary toxicology is the possible transmission of toxins to the human population in meat, fish, milk, and other foodstuffs.

3. *Forensic toxicology* concerns medicolegal aspects, including the detection of poisons in clinical and other samples.

4. *Environmental toxicology* is concerned with the movement of toxicants and their metabolites in the environment and in food chains and the effect of such toxicants on individuals and populations.

5. *Industrial toxicology* is a specific area of environmental toxicology that deals with the work environment. Because of the large number of industrial chemicals and possibilities for exposure as well as a number of specific laws that govern such situations, this subject is well developed.

D. Chemical Use Classes. This includes the toxicological aspects of the development of new chemicals for commercial use. In some of these use classes, toxicity, at least to some organisms, is a desirable trait; in others, it is an undesirable side effect. Use classes are not composed entirely of synthetic chemicals; many natural products are isolated and used for commercial and other uses and must be subjected to the same toxicity testing as synthetic compounds. Examples include the insecticide pyrethrin, the clinical drug digitalis, and psilocibin, a drug of abuse.

1. *Agricultural chemicals* include many compounds, such as insecticides, herbicides, fungicides, and rodenticides, in which toxicity to the target organism is a desired quality, whereas toxicity to "nontarget" species is to be avoided. Development of such selectively toxic chemicals is one of the applied roles of comparative toxicology.
2. *Clinical drugs* are properly the province of pharmaceutical chemistry and pharmacology. Only toxic side effects and testing for them fall within the science of toxicology.
3. *Drugs of abuse* are chemicals taken for psychological or other effects and may cause dependence and toxicity. Many of these are illegal, but some are of clinical significance when used correctly.
4. *Food additives* are of concern to toxicologists only when toxic or when being tested for possible toxicity.
5. *Industrial chemicals* are so numerous that testing for toxicity and controlling exposure to chemicals known to be toxic is a large field of toxicology.
6. *Naturally occurring substances* include many phytotoxins, mycotoxins, and inorganic minerals, all occurring naturally in the environment.
7. *Combustion products* are not properly a use class but are a large and important class of toxicants, generated primarily from fuels and other industrial chemicals.

E. Regulatory Toxicology. These aspects, concerned with the formulation of laws, and regulations authorized by laws, are intended to minimize the effect of toxic chemicals on human health and the environment.
1. *Legal aspects* are concerned with the formulation of laws and regulations and their enforcement. In the United States, enforcement generally falls under such government agencies as the Environmental Protection Agency (EPA), the Food and Drug Administration (FDA), and the Occupational Safety and Health Administration (OSHA). Similar government departments exist in many other countries.
2. *Risk assessment* is the definition of risks, potential risks, and the risk–benefit equations necessary for the regulation of toxic substances.

1.1.2   Relationship to Other Sciences

Toxicology should be viewed as a science and human activity in a spectrum of sciences and human activities. At one end of this spectrum are those sciences that contribute their methods and philosophical concepts to serve the needs of toxicologists, either in research or in the application of toxicology to human affairs. At the other end of the spectrum are those sciences and human activities to which toxicology contributes.

Most important in the first group are chemistry, biochemistry, pathology, physiology, and epidemiology, but such sciences as immunology, biomathematics, and ecology may also be important.

In the group to which toxicology contributes heavily are such aspects of medicine as forensic medicine, clinical toxicology, pharmacy and pharmacology, public health, and industrial hygiene. Toxicology also contributes in an important way to veterinary medicine and to such aspects of agriculture as the development and safe use of agricultural chemicals. The contributions of toxicology to environmental studies is one of the most rapidly expanding areas of the subject.

Clearly, toxicology is preeminently an applied science, dedicated to the enhancement of the quality of life and the protection of the environment. It is also much more. Frequently, the perturbation of normal life processes by toxic chemicals enables us to learn more about the life processes themselves. The use of uncoupling agents such as dinitrophenol to study oxidative phosphorylation or the use of α-amanitin to study RNA polymerases are but two of many examples of this principle. The field of toxicology has expanded enormously in recent years, both in the numbers of toxicologists and in the amount of accumulated knowledge. This expansion has been accompanied by a change from a purely descriptive science to one that uses the whole range of methodology of experimental science to investigate the mechanisms behind toxic events. Many investigators have finally realized that only through the latter method will further real progress be made.

1.1.3   History of Toxicology

Much of the early history of toxicology has doubtless been lost, like all early history. Much that has survived is of almost incidental importance in manuscripts dealing primarily with medicine. Some, however, was more specifically concerned with toxic action, and many records deal with the use of poisons either for judicial execution, political assassination, or suicide. It is also no doubt true that toxicology must rank as one of the oldest practical sciences because humans, from the very beginning, needed to avoid the numerous toxic plants and animals in their environment.

The Egyptian papyrus *Ebers,* dating from about 1500 BC, must rank as the earliest surviving pharmacopeia and is the surviving medical works of Hippocrates, Aristotle, and Theophrastus. It was published during the period 400–250 BC and included some mention of poisons. The early Greek poet Nicander treats, in two poetic works, animal toxins (Therica) and antidotes to plant and animal toxins (Alexipharmica). The earliest surviving attempt to classify plants according to their toxic and therapeutic effects is that of Dioscorides, a Greek employed by the Roman Emperor Nero about AD 50.

There appear to have been few advances in either medicine or toxicology between the time of Galen (AD 131–200) and Paracelsus (1493–1541). It was the latter who, in spite of frequent confusion between fact and mysticism, laid the groundwork for the later development of modern toxicology by recognizing the importance of the dose–response relationship. His famous statement, "All substances are poisons; there is none that is not a poison. The right dose differentiates a poison and a remedy," succinctly summarizes that concept. His belief in the value of experimentation also represented a break with much earlier tradition.

There were some important developments in the eighteenth century. Probably the best known is the publication of Ramazzini's *Diseases of Workers* in 1700, which has led to his recognition as the father of occupational medicine. The correlation between the occupation of chimney sweeps and scrotal cancer by Percival Pott in 1775 is also noteworthy.

Orfila, a Spaniard working at the University of Paris in the early nineteenth century, is generally regarded as the father of modern toxicology. He clearly identified toxicology as a separate science and in 1815 wrote the first book devoted exclusively to toxicology. (An English translation, published in 1817, was entitled *A General System of Toxicology or, a Treatise on Poisons, Found in the Mineral, Vegetable and Animal Kingdoms, Considered in Their Relations with Physiology, Pathology and Medical Jurisprudence.*) Workers of the later nineteenth century who produced treatises on toxicology include Christison, Kobert, and Lewin. The recognition of the site of action of curare by Claude Bernard (1813–1878) began the modern study of mechanisms of toxic action. Since then, advances have been numerous—too numerous to list. They have increased our knowledge of the chemistry of poisons, the treatment of poisoning, the analysis both of toxicants and toxicity, as well as mode of action and detoxication. Many of them are outlined in the pages to follow.

With the publication of her controversial book *The Silent Spring* in 1962, Rachel Carson ushered in the modern era of environmental toxicology. Her book, emphasizing stopping the widespread, indiscriminate use of pesticides and other chemicals and advocating a use pattern based on sound ecology, is often credited as the catalyst leading to the formation of the US Environmental Protection Agency, and she is regarded by many as the mother of the environmental movement. Her views are well summarized in the following, taken from Earth's Green Mantle in *The Silent Spring:*

> The earth's vegetation is a part of a web of life in which there are intimate and essential relations between plants and the earth, between plants and other plants, between plants and animals. Sometimes we have no other choice but to disturb these relationships, but we should do so thoughtfully, with full awareness that what we do may have consequences remote in time and place.

It is clear, however, that since the 1960s–1970s, toxicology has entered a phase of rapid development and has changed from a science that was almost entirely descriptive to one in which the study of mechanisms enjoys a considerable vogue. There are many reasons for this, including the development of new analytical methods since 1945, the emphasis on drug testing following the thalidomide tragedy, the emphasis on pesticide testing following the publication of

Rachel Carson's *The Silent Spring,* and public concerns with hazardous waste disposal.

DOSE–RESPONSE RELATIONSHIPS

As mentioned previously, toxicity is a relative event that depends on both the toxic properties of the chemical and the dose of the compound administered. The first recognition of the relationship between the dose of a compound and the response elicited has been attributed to Paracelsus (Section 1.1.3). It is worth noting that his statement includes not just that all substances can be toxic at some concentration, but that "the right dose differentiates a poison from a remedy," a concept that is the basis for pharmaceutical therapy.

A typical dose–response curve is shown in Fig. 1.2, in which the percentage of organisms or systems responding to a chemical is plotted against the dose. For many chemicals and effects there will be a dose below which no effect or response is observed. This is known as the *threshold dose*. This concept is of significance because it implies that there is a *no observed effect level* (NOEL) and this value can be used to determine the safe intake for food additives and contaminants such as pesticides. Although this is generally accepted for most types of chemicals and toxic effects, for chemical carcinogens acting by a genotoxic mechanism, the shape of the curve is controversial. Dose–response relationships are discussed in more detail in Chapter 11, Toxicity Testing and Risk Assessment.

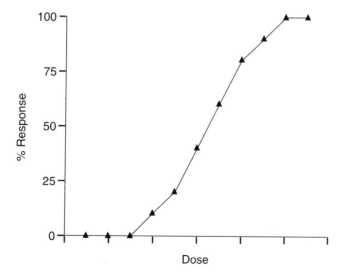

Figure 1.2. Illustration of typical dose–response curve.

1.3

SOURCES OF TOXIC COMPOUNDS

1.3.1   Synthetic Organic Compounds

Some of the compounds mentioned are natural products and are included in this section in cases in which they are closely related, by use or chemistry, to a large class of synthetic chemicals. Otherwise, they may appear in Section 1.3.7.

1.3.1.1   Air, Water, and Food Pollutants

Both the nature and the source of air pollutants vary with the location; open country remote from industry or heavy traffic will clearly differ from the center of a large city or an area downwind from a coal-fired power plant or other industry. In general, however, the principal air pollutants are CO, oxides of nitrogen, oxides of sulfur, hydrocarbons, and particulates. The principal sources are transportation, industrial processes, electric power generation, and the heating of homes and buildings.

Of the organic constituents, hydrocarbons such as benzo(a)pyrene are produced by incomplete combustion and are probably associated primarily with the automobile. The hydrocarbons are usually not present at levels high enough to cause a directly measurable toxic effect but are important in the formation of photochemical air pollution. This pollution is formed as a result of interactions between oxides of nitrogen and hydrocarbons in the presence of ultraviolet (UV) light, the resultant reactions giving rise to such lung irritants as peroxyacetyl nitrate, acrolein, and formaldehyde.

Particulates are heterogeneous mixtures, often in the form of smoke. They are important as carriers of adsorbed hydrocarbons as well as being irritants to the respiratory system. The distribution of such particles in the atmosphere, as well as in the respiratory tract, is largely a function of their size.

Water pollution by toxic chemicals comes from run-off from urban streets or from agricultural chemicals from cultivated fields, from sewage, or from specific industrial sources such as refineries, smelters, or chemical plants. Although some sources are diffuse and difficult to control, others are from specific point sources and can be controlled at the point of origin.

Agricultural chemicals found in water may include insecticides such as chlorinated hydrocarbons, organophosphates, and carbamates (see Section 1.3.1.6). The chlorinated hydrocarbons such as DDT, chlordane, and dieldrin, previously of most concern because of their persistence, are now less important because of curtailed use in the United States and some other countries. Other pesticides include herbicides, fungicides, nematocides, and rodenticides. Fertilizers, although less of a toxic hazard, contribute to such environmental problems as eutrophication. In some cases, the point source for agricultural chemicals is the manufacturing operation. The contamination of the James River in Virginia with Kepone (chlordecone) is a case in point.

Low molecular weight halogenated hydrocarbons such as chloroform, dichloroethane, and carbon tetrachloride may enter water directly or may be formed as a result of the chlorination of precursors during water purification. Chlorinated aromatics such as the polychlorinated biphenyls (PCBs), chlorophenols, and even the highly toxic 2,3,7,8-tetrachlorodibenzo-*p*-dioxin (TCDD) are found commonly in water, as are the phthalate ester plasticizers, such as di-2-ethylhexylphthalate and di-*n*-butylphthalate. Detergents, such as the alkyl benzene sulfonates, are common contaminants of water that arise from domestic effluent. Since the discovery of insecticides such as aldicarb or soil fumigants such as ethylene dibromide in ground water drawn from wells, this form of water pollution has become a new concern. A number of toxic inorganics, mentioned in Section 1.3.3, have also been found in water.

Food contaminants, as opposed to food additives, are those compounds included inadvertently in foods, either raw, cooked, or processed. They include a wide variety of products ranging from bacterial toxins such as the exotoxin of *Clostridium botulinum,* mycotoxins such as aflatoxins from *Aspergillus flavus,* plant alkaloids, animal toxins, pesticide residues, and residues of animal food additives such as diethylstilbestrol and antibiotics, to a variety of industrial chemicals such as PCBs and polybrominated biphenyls.

1.3.1.2   Chemical Additives in Food

Chemicals are added to food for a number of reasons: as preservatives, either antibacterial, antifungal, or antioxidants; to change physical characteristics, particularly for processing; to change taste; to change color; and to change odor. In general, food additives have proved to be safe and without chronic toxicity. Many were introduced when toxicity testing was relatively unsophisticated, however, and some of these have been subsequently shown to be toxic. Table 1.1 gives examples of different types of organic food additives. Inorganics, the most important of which are nitrate and nitrite, are discussed later. Certainly hundreds, and possibly thousands, of food additives are in use worldwide, many with inadequate testing. The question of synergistic interactions between these compounds has not been explored adequately. Not all toxicants in food are synthetic; many examples of naturally occurring toxicants in the human diet are known, including carcinogens and mutagens (see Section 1.3.2.3).

1.3.1.3   Chemicals in the Workplace

In an industrial society, the number of possible chemicals in the workplace is extremely high, and many of these chemicals are known to have deleterious biologic effects. Among the inorganics are metals such as lead, copper, mercury, zinc, cadmium, and beryllium, as well as fluorides, carbon monoxide, and so on. The organic compounds include aliphatic hydrocarbons (eg, hexane), aromatic hydrocarbons (eg, benzene, toluene, xylene), halogenated hydrocarbons (eg, dichloromethane, trichloroethane, trichloroethylene, vinyl chloride), alcohols (eg, methanol, ethylene

TABLE 1.1. EXAMPLES OF ORGANIC CHEMICALS USED AS FOOD ADDITIVES

Function	Class	Example
Preservatives	Antioxidants	Butylatedhydroxyanisole
		Ascorbic acid
	Fungistatic agents	Methyl p-benzoic acid
		Propionates
	Bactericides	Sodium nitrite
Processing aids	Anticaking agents	Calcium silicate
		Sodium aluminosilicate
	Emulsifiers	Propylene glycol
		Monoglycerides
	Chelating agents	EDTA
		Sodium tartrate
	Stabilizers	Gum ghatti
		Sodium alginate
	Humectants	Propylene glycol
		Glycerol
Flavor and taste modification	Synthetic sweeteners	Saccharin
		Mannitol
		Aspartame
	Synthetic flavors	Piperonal
		Vanillin
Color modification	Synthetic dyes	Tartrazine (FD&C yellow 5)
		Sunset yellow
Nutritional supplements	Vitamins	Thiamin
		Vitamin D_3
	Amino acids	Alanine
		Aspartic acid
	Inorganics	Manganese sulfate
		Zinc sulfate

glycol), esters (eg, methylmethacrylate, di-[2-ethylhexyl]phthalate), organometallics (eg, tributyltin acetate), amino compounds (eg, aniline), nitro derivatives (eg, nitrobenzene), and many others. In addition, there are many manufactured products, such as the pesticides summarized in Section 1.3.1.6 and the intermediates that occur in their synthesis.

1.3.1.4   Drugs of Abuse

All drugs are toxic at some dose and at such doses have deleterious effects on humans. Drugs of abuse either have no medicinal function or are taken at dose levels higher than would be required for therapy. Many, when properly prescribed and taken, are of clinical importance. In the latter case, the benefits, in the opinion of the physician, outweigh the risks. Although some drugs of abuse may affect only higher nervous functions—mood, reaction time, and coordination—many produce physical dependence and have serious physical effects, with fatal overdoses being a common occurrence.

The drugs of abuse include central nervous system (CNS) depressants such as ethanol, methaqualone (quaalude), and secobarbital; CNS stimulants such as cocaine, methamphetamine (speed), caffeine, and nicotine; opioids such as heroin, morphine, and mependine (demerol); and hallucinogens such as lysergic acid diethylamide (LSD), phencyclidine (PCP), and tetrahydrocannabinol (THC), the most important active principle of marijuana. A further complication of toxicological significance is that many drugs of abuse are synthesized in illegal and inadequately equipped laboratories with little or no quality control. The resultant products are therefore often contaminated with compounds of unknown, but conceivably dangerous, toxicity. The structures of some of these compounds are shown in Fig. 1.3.

1.3.1.5   Therapeutic Drugs

Essentially all therapeutic drugs can be toxic, producing deleterious effects at some dose. The danger to the individual depends on several factors, including the nature of the toxic response, the dose necessary to produce the toxic response, and the relationship between the therapeutic dose and the toxic dose. Drug toxicity is affected by all factors that affect the toxicity of other xenobiotics, including individual (genetic) variation, diet, age, and the presence of other exogenous chemicals.

Even when the risk of toxic side effects from a particular drug has been evaluated, it must be weighed against the expected benefits. The use of a very dangerous drug with only a narrow tolerance between the therapeutic and toxic doses may still be justified if it is the sole treatment for an otherwise fatal disease. However, a relatively safe drug may be inappropriate if safer compounds are available or if the condition being treated is trivial. One must also keep in mind that the dramatic expansion of the pharmaceutical industry between 1935 and 1965 placed a large number of drugs in use, many of which have not been tested for toxicity by methods now considered adequate.

The three principal classes of cytotoxic agents used in the treatment of cancer all contain known carcinogens, for example, Melphalen, a nitrogen mustard, adriamycin, an antitumor antibiotic, and methotrexate, an antimetabolite. Diethylstilbestrol (DES), a drug formerly widely used, has been associated with cancer of the cervix and vagina in the offspring of treated women.

Other toxic effects of drugs can be associated with almost every organ system. The stiffness of the joints accompanied by optic nerve damage (SMON—subacute myelo-optic neuropathy) that was common in Japan in the 1960s was apparently a toxic side effect of chloroquinol (Enterovioform), an antidiarrhea drug. Teratogenesis can also be caused by drugs, with thalidomide being the most alarming example. Skin effects (dermatitis) are common side effects of drugs, for example, in the case of topically applied corticosteroids.

1. CNS Depressants

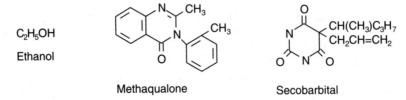

C₂H₅OH

Ethanol

Methaqualone   Secobarbital

2. CNS Stimulants

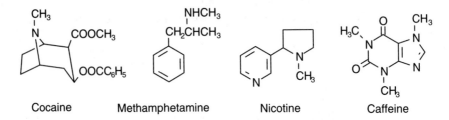

Cocaine   Methamphetamine   Nicotine   Caffeine

3. Opioids

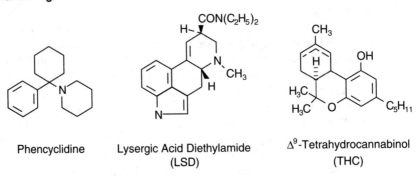

Meperidine   Morphine
(Heroine, OHs = OCOCH₃)

4. Hallucinogens

Phencyclidine   Lysergic Acid Diethylamide   Δ⁹-Tetrahydrocannabinol
(LSD)   (THC)

Figure 1.3. Some common drugs of abuse.

A number of toxic effects on the blood have been documented, including agranulocytosis caused by chlorpromazine, hemolytic anemia caused by methyldopa, and megaloblastic anemia caused by methotrexate. Toxic effects on the eye have also been noted, and range from the retinotoxicity caused by thioridazine to glaucoma caused by systemic corticosteroids.

It should be emphasized that, in general, toxic side effects are not common and may occur only in susceptible individuals or populations. At the same time, the wide variety of such effects and their frequent severity argue against indiscriminate or unnecessary use of therapeutic drugs.

1.3.1.6   Pesticides

Pesticides are used to control a wide variety of pests, to increase the production of food and fiber, and to facilitate modern agricultural production methods. By the very nature of their use in pest control, they are common contaminants of the environment, food and water, and domestic structures. Although selective toxicity toward target organisms is a desirable quality, it is not absolute, and most pesticides are toxic to a greater or lesser extent toward nontarget organisms, including humans. Thus, in an attempt to control unwanted toxic side effects and, at the same time, obtain the benefits to be derived from their use, a considerable body of law and regulation concerned with their registration and use has developed. The various classes of pesticides are shown in Table 1.2, and structures for some of the important pesticides are shown in Fig. 1.4.

1.3.1.7   Solvents

Although solvents are more a feature of the industrial environment, they are also found in the home. In addition to cutaneous effects of solvents, such as defatting and local irritation, many have systemic toxic effects, including effects on the nervous system or, as with benzene, on the blood-forming elements. Commercial solvents are frequently complex mixtures and may include nitrogen or sulfur-containing organics—gasoline and other oil-based products are excellent examples of this. The common solvents fall into the following classes:

1. *Aliphatic hydrocarbons*, such as hexane. These may be straight or branched chain compounds and are often present in mixtures.
2. *Halogenated aliphatic hydrocarbons.* The best known examples are methylene dichloride, chloroform, and carbon tetrachloride, although chlorinated ethylenes are also widely used.
3. *Aliphatic alcohols*, such as methanol and ethanol.
4. *Glycols and glycol ethers* such as ethylene and propylene glycols. Use in antifreeze gives rise to considerable exposure of the general public. The glycol ethers, such as methyl cellosolve, are also widely used.
5. *Aromatic hydrocarbons.* Benzene is probably the one of greatest concern, but others, such as toluene, are also used.

TABLE 1.2. CLASSIFICATION OF PESTICIDES, WITH EXAMPLES

Class	Principal Chemical Type	Example, Common Name
Algicide	Organotin	Brestar
Fungicide	Dicarboximide	Captan
	Chlorinated aromatic	Pentachlorophenol
	Dithiocarbamate	Maneb
	Mercurial	Phenylmercuric acetate
Herbicide	Amides, Acetamides	Propanil
	Bipyridyl	Paraquat
	Carbamates, Thiocarbamates	Barban
	Phenoxy	2,4-D
	Dinitrophenol	DNOC
	Dinitroaniline	Trifluralin
	Substituted urea	Monuron
	Triazine	Atrazine
Nematocide	Halogenated alkane	Ethylene dibromide (EDB)
Molluscide	Chlorinated hydrocarbon	Bayluscide
Insecticide	Chlorinated hydrocarbons	
	DDT analogs	DDT
	Chlorinated alicyclic	BHC
	Cyclodiene	Aldrin
	Chlorinated terpenes	Toxaphene
	Organophosphate	Parathion
	Carbamate	Carbaryl
	Thiocyanate	Lethane
	Dinitrophenols	DNOC
	Fluroacetates	Nissol
	Botanicals	
	Nicotinoids	Nicotine
	Rotenoids	Rotenone
	Pyrethroids	Pyrethrin
	Synthetic pyrethroids	Fenvalerate
	Juvenile hormone analogs	Methoprene
	Growth regulators	Dimilin
	Inorganics	
	Arsenicals	Lead arsenate
	Fluorides	Sodium fluoride
	Microbials	Thuricide, Avermectin
Insecticide synergists	Methylenedioxyphenyl	Piperonyl butoxide
	Dicarboximides	MGK-264
Acarides	Organosulfur compounds	Ovex
	Formamidine	Chlordimeform
	Dinitrophenols	Dinex
	DDT analogs	Chlorobenzilate
Rodenticides	Anticoagulants	Warfarin
	Botanicals	
	Alkaloids	Strychine sulfate
	Glycosides	Scillaren A and B
	Fluorides	Fluoroacetate
	Inorganics	Thallium sulfate
	Thioureas	ANTU

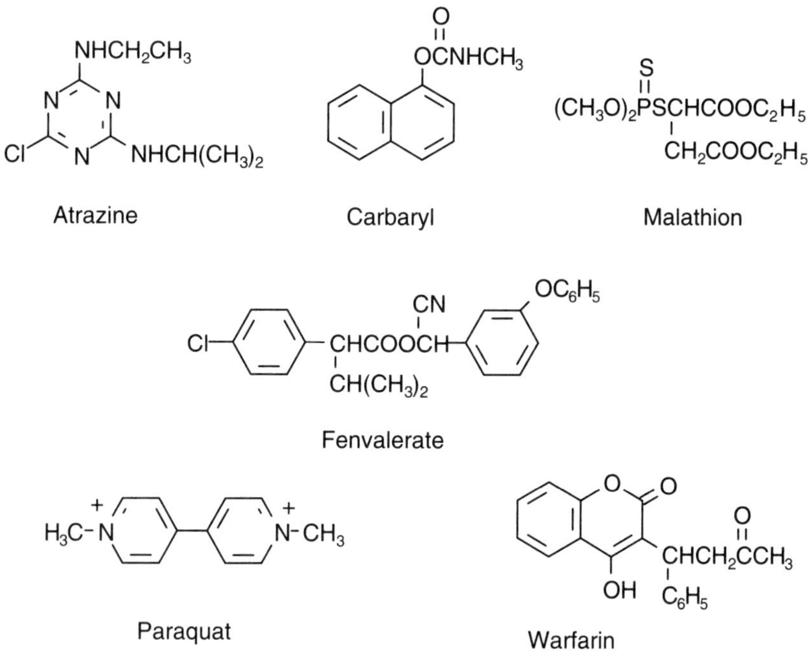

Figure 1.4. Chemical structures of some important pesticides.

1.3.1.8 Polycyclic Aromatic Hydrocarbons

Although some natural products such as coal and crude oil contain polycyclic aromatic hydrocarbons, they are generally associated with incomplete combustion of organic materials and are found in smoke from wood, coal, oil, tobacco, and so on, as well as in tar and broiled foods. Because some of them are carcinogens, they have been studied intensively from the point of view of metabolic activation, interaction with DNA, and chemical carcinogenesis. Some of these compounds are heterocyclic, containing nitrogen atoms in at least one of the rings. The chemical structures of a selection of the most studied polycyclic aromatic hydrocarbons are shown in Fig. 1.5.

1.3.1.9 Cosmetics

The most common deleterious effects of cosmetics are occasional allergic reactions and contact dermatitis. The highly toxic and/or carcinogenic azo or aromatic amine dyes are no longer in use; neither are the organometallics, which were used in even earlier times. Bromates, used in some cold-wave neutralizers, may be acutely toxic if ingested, as may the ethanol used as a solvent in hair dyes and perfumes.

Thioglycolates and thioglycerol used in cold-wave lotion and depilatories and sodium hydroxide used in hair straighteners are also toxic on ingestion. Used as di-

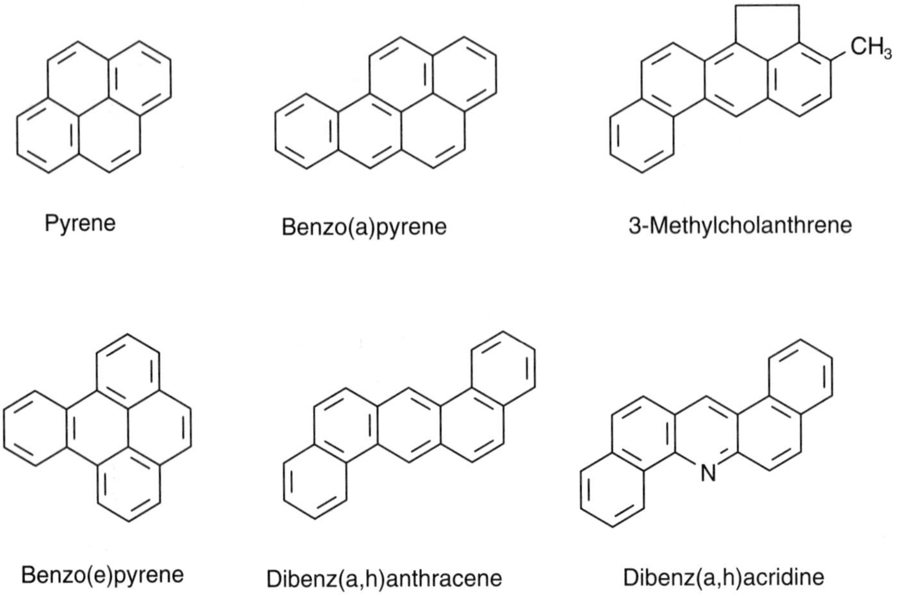

Pyrene   Benzo(a)pyrene   3-Methylcholanthrene

Benzo(e)pyrene   Dibenz(a,h)anthracene   Dibenz(a,h)acridine

Figure 1.5. Examples of carcinogenic polycyclic aromatic hydrocarbons.

rected, cosmetics appear to present little risk of systemic poisoning, due in part to the deletion of ingredients now known to be toxic and in part to the small quantities absorbed.

1.3.2   Naturally Occurring Toxins

1.3.2.1   Mycotoxins

The range of chemical structures and biologic activity among the broad class of fungal metabolites is large and cannot be summarized briefly. Mycotoxins do not constitute a separate chemical category, and they lack common molecular features.

Mycotoxins of most interest are those found in human food or in the feed of domestic animals. They include the ergot alkaloids produced by *Claviceps* sp., aflatoxins and related compounds produced by *Aspergillus* sp., and the tricothecenes produced by several genera of fungi imperfecti, primarily *Fusarium* sp.

The ergot alkaloids (Fig. 1.6) are known to affect the nervous system and to be vasoconstrictors. Historically, they have been implicated in epidemics of both gangrenous and convulsive ergotism (St. Anthony's fire), although such epidemics no longer occur in humans due to increased knowledge of the cause and to more varied modern diets. Outbreaks of ergotism in livestock do still occur frequently, however. These compounds have also been used as abortifacients. The ergot alkaloids are derivatives of ergotine, the most active being, more specifically, amides of lysergic acid.

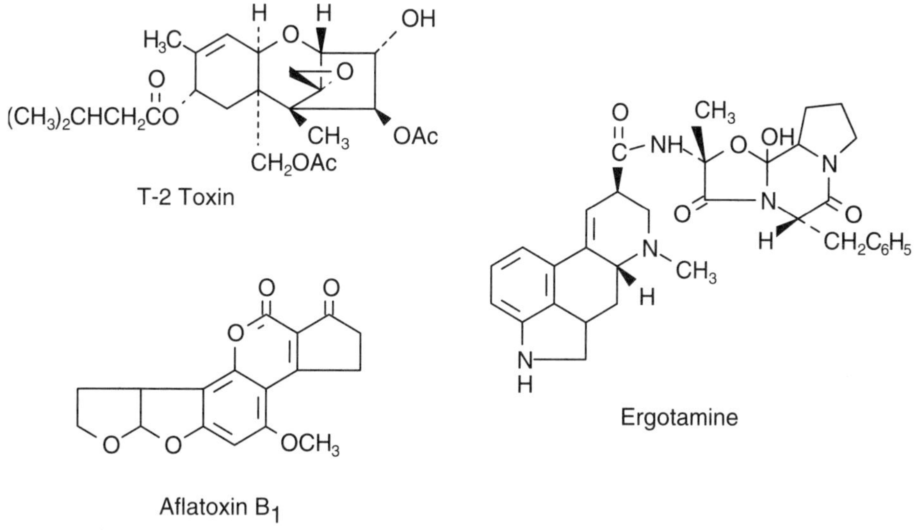

Figure 1.6. Selected mycotoxins.

Aflatoxins are products of species of the genus *Aspergillus,* particularly *A flavus,* a common fungus found as a contaminant of grain, maize, peanuts, and so on. First implicated in poultry diseases such as Turkey-X disease, they were subsequently shown to cause cancer in experimental animals and, from epidemiological studies, in humans. Aflatoxin B_1, the most toxic of the aflatoxins, must be activated enzymatically to exert its carcinogenic effect.

Tricothecenes are a large class of sesquiterpenoid fungal metabolites produced particularly by members of the genera *Fusarium* and *Tricoderma.* They are frequently acutely toxic, displaying bactericidal, fungicidal, and insecticidal activity, as well as causing various clinical symptoms in mammals, including diarrhea, anorexia, and ataxia. They have been implicated in natural intoxications in both humans and animals, such as Abakabi disease in Japan and Stachybotryotoxicosis in the former USSR, and are the center of a continuing controversy concerning their possible use as chemical warfare agents.

Mycotoxins may also be used for beneficial purposes. The mycotoxin avermectin is currently generating considerable interest both as an insecticide and for the control of nematode parasites of domestic animals.

1.3.2.2 Microbial Toxins

The term microbial toxin is usually reserved by microbiologists for toxic substances produced by microorganisms that are of high molecular weight and have antigenic properties; toxic compounds produced by bacteria that do not fit these criteria are referred to simply as poisons. Many of the former are proteins or mucoproteins and may

HCHO CH_3CHO

Formaldehyde   Acetaldehyde
Clostridium globosa

$CH_3CH_2CH_2CH_2OH$

n-Butanol
Clostridium acetobutylicum

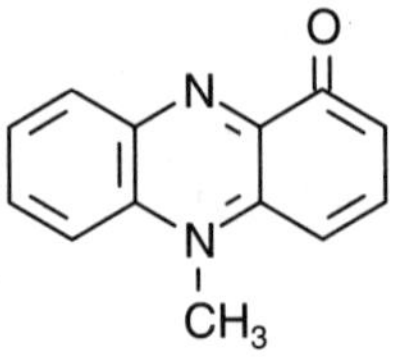

Pyocyanine
Pseudomonas aeruginosa

Figure 1.7. Some selected poisons from bacteria.

have a variety of enzymatic properties. They include some of the most toxic substances known, such as tetanus toxin, botulinus toxin, and diphtheria toxin. Bacterial toxins may be extremely toxic to mammals and may affect a variety of organ systems, including the nervous system and the cardiovascular system. A detailed account of their chemical nature and mode of action is beyond the scope of this volume.

The range of poisonous chemicals produced by bacteria is also large. Some examples are shown in Fig. 1.7. Again, such compounds may also be used for beneficial purposes, for example, the insecticidal properties of *Bacillus thuringiensis*, due to a toxin, have been utilized in agriculture for some time.

1.3.2.3   Plant Toxins

The large array of toxic chemicals produced by plants (phytotoxins), usually referred to as secondary plant compounds, are often held to have evolved as defense mechanisms against herbivorous animals, particularly insects and mammals. These compounds may be repellent, but not particularly toxic, or they may be acutely toxic to a wide range of organisms. They include sulfur compounds, lipids, phenols, alkaloids, glycosides, and many other types of chemicals. Many of the common drugs of abuse such as cocaine, caffeine, nicotine, morphine, and the cannabinoids are plant toxins. Some further examples are shown in Fig. 1.8. Many chemicals that have been shown to be toxic are constituents of plants that form part of the human diet. For example, the carcinogen safrole and related compounds are found in black pepper. Solanine and chaconine, which are cholinesterase inhibitors and possible teratogens, are found in potatoes, and quinones and phenols are widespread in food. Livestock poisoning by plants is still an important veterinary problem in some areas.

1.3.2.4   Animal Toxins

Some species from practically all phyla of animals produce toxins. Some are passively venomous, often following inadvertent ingestion, whereas others are actively venomous, injecting poisons through specially adapted stings or mouthparts. It may

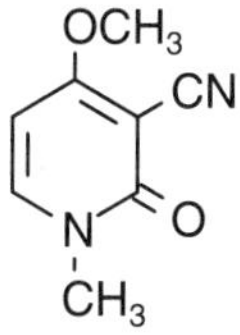

Ricinine

castor bean plant
Ricinus communis

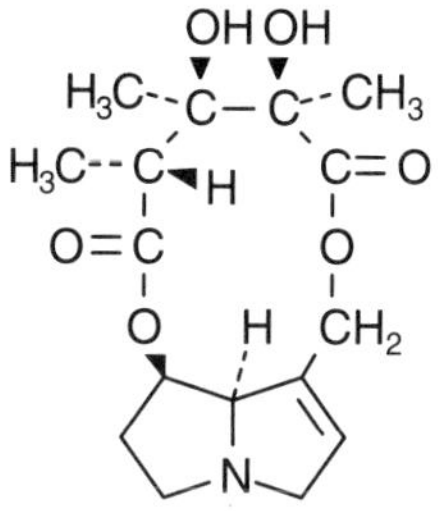

Monocrotaline

Senecio species

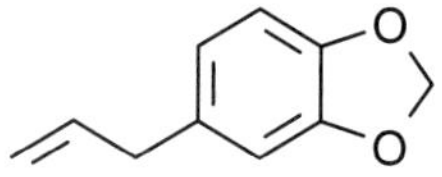

Safrole

black pepper,
oil of Sassafras, etc.

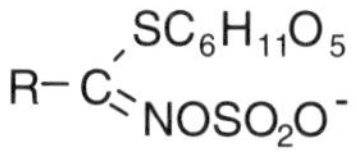

Glucosinolates

Cruciferous species
R = alkane or aromatic group

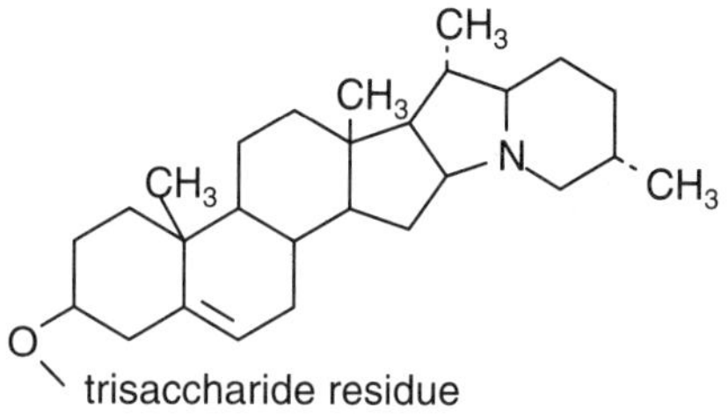

Solanine

Solanaceous species
particularly potato

Figure 1.8. Selected examples of plant toxins.

be more appropriate to refer to the latter group only as venomous and to refer to the former simply as poisonous. The chemistry of animal toxins extends from enzymes and neurotoxic and cardiotoxic peptides and proteins to many small molecules such as biogenic amines, alkaloids, glycosides, terpenes, and others (Fig. 1.9). In many cases, the venoms are complex mixtures that include both proteins and small molecules and depend on the interaction of the components for the full expression of their toxic effect. For example, bee venom contains a biogenic amine, histamine, three peptides, and two enzymes (Table 1.3). The venoms and defensive secretions of insects may also contain many relatively simple toxicants or irritants such as formic acid, benzoquinone, and other quinones, or terpenes such as citronellal.

Snake venoms have been studied extensively; their effects are due, in general, to toxins that are peptides with 60–70 amino acids. These toxins are cardiotoxic or neurotoxic and their effects are usually accentuated by the phospholipases, peptidases, proteases, and other enzymes present in venoms. These enzymes may affect the blood-clotting mechanisms and damage blood vessels.

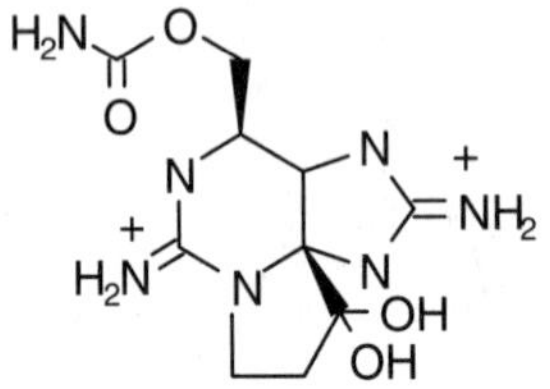

Saxitoxin

Produced by dinoflagelates
and taken up by mollusks

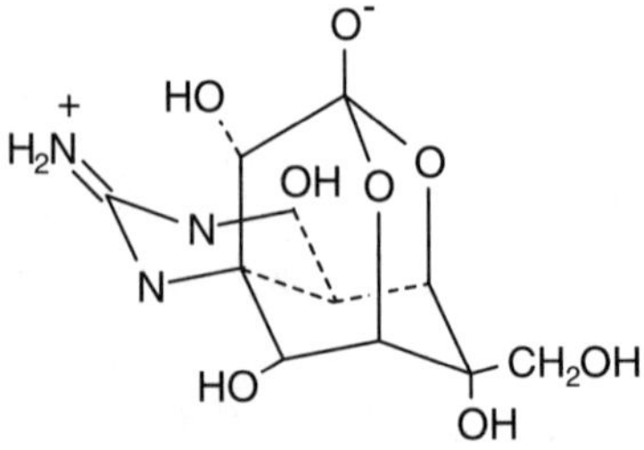

Tetrodotoxin

Produced by puffer and other fishes

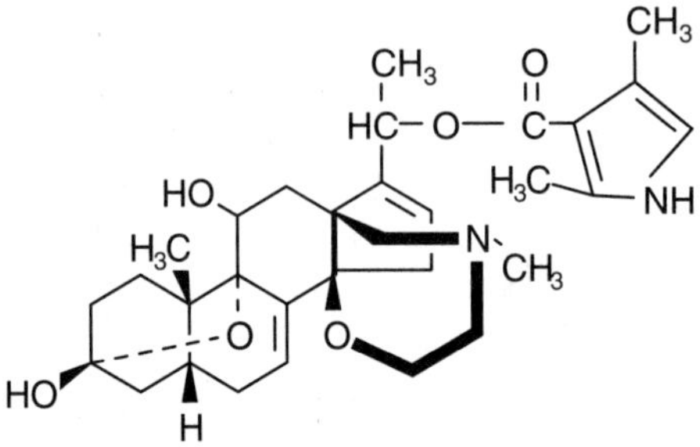

Batrachotoxin

Produced by poison-dart frogs

Figure 1.9. Selected animal toxicants.

TABLE 1.3. SOME COMPONENTS OF BEE VENOM

Compound	Effect
Biogenic amine	
Histamine	Pain, vasodilation, increased capillary permeability
Peptides	
Apamine	CNS effects
Melittin	Hemolytic, serotonin release, cardiotoxic
Mast cell degranulating peptide	Histamine release from mast cells
Enzymes	
Phospholipase A	Increased spreading and penetration of tissues
Hyaluronidase	

1.3.3 Inorganic Chemicals

In addition to the inorganic air pollutants such as nitrogen oxides and oxides of sulfur, probably the most important inorganic toxicants are metals. Some of the most important of these toxic metals are beryllium, used in the steel industry; cadmium, exposure to which occurs in welding and soldering and through tobacco smoking; and mercury, which is used in the electronics industry and in fungicides. Epidemics of mercury poisoning have resulted from the use of mercury compounds in the pulp and paper industries and in manufacturing plastic. Another metal of particular importance is lead, used in leaded gasoline and batteries and formerly in paint. Lead poisoning has been common in children, particularly in slum housing, and has been diagnosed frequently in livestock. Lead is still a widespread contaminant of water, air, and a common component of gasoline in many countries. Certain metals, such as mercury, can be converted into more toxic alkyl derivatives by bacteria in the environment. Organic lead compounds, such as tetraethyl lead, can be absorbed readily through the lungs and skin. In food and animal feeds, nitrite and nitrate are the toxic inorganic chemicals of most concern.

1.4

ENVIRONMENTAL MOVEMENT OF TOXICANTS

Chemicals released into the environment rarely remain in the form, or at the location, of release. Agricultural chemicals used as sprays may drift from the point of application as air contaminants or enter run-off water as water contaminants. Many of these chemicals are susceptible to bacterial and fungal degradation and are rapidly detoxified, frequently being broken down to compounds that can enter the carbon, nitrogen, and oxygen cycles. Others, particularly halogenated organics, are recalcitrant to a greater or lesser degree to metabolism by microorganisms and persist in the soil as contaminants; they may enter biologic food chains and move to higher trophic levels or persist in the processed crop as postharvest food contaminants. For example, DDT and its principal metabolite DDE were involved in all of these routes and can still be detected in many locations years after the use of DDT was discontinued. Soil fumigants, such as ethylene dibromide (EDB), have now been found in groundwater. Similarly, industrial chemicals released in wastewater may also become widely disseminated.

Although most transport between inanimate phases of the environment results in wider dissemination but, at the same time, dilution of the toxicant in question, transfer between living creatures may result in increased concentration or bioaccumulation. Lipid soluble toxicants are readily taken up by organisms following exposure in air, water, or soil. Unless rapidly metabolized, they persist in the tissues long enough to be transferred to the next trophic level. At each level, the lipophilic toxicant tends to be retained whereas the bulk of the food is digested, utilized, and excreted, thus increasing the toxicant concentration. At some point in the chain, the

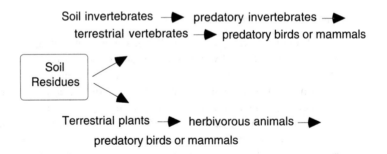

Figure 1.10. Food chain.

toxicant can become deleterious, particularly if the organism at that trophic level is more susceptible than those at the level proceeding it. Examples of such food chains are depicted in Fig. 1.10.

It seems fairly certain that the reproductive failure in certain raptorial birds such as the sparrow hawk, brought about by eggshell thinning, was due to the uptake of DDT through the food chain and their particular susceptibility to this type of toxicity.

It is clear that such transport can occur through both aquatic and terrestrial food chains, although in the former, higher members of the chains, such as fish, can accumulate large amounts of toxicants directly from the medium. This accumulation occurs because of the large area of the gill filaments, their intimate contact with the water, and the high flow rate of water over them. Given these characteristics and a toxicant with a high partition coefficient between water and lipid membranes, considerable uptake is inevitable.

Suggested Further Reading

Ames BW: Dietary carcinogens and anticarcinogens. *Science* **221**:1256–1264, 1983.

Bennett G, Vourakis C, Woolf DS (eds.): *Substance Abuse. Pharmacological, Developmental and Clinical Perspectives.* New York: Wiley, 1983, 453 pp.

Chivian E, McCally M, Hu H, Haines A (eds.): *Critical Condition, Human Health and the Environment.* Cambridge, MA: MIT Press, 1993, 244 pp.

Cockerham LG, Shane BS (eds): *Basic Environmental Toxicology.* Boca Raton, FL: CRC Press, 1994, 627 pp.

Esser HO, Moser P: An appraisal of problems related to the measurement and evolution of bioaccumulation. *Ecotoxicol Environ Safety* **6:**131–148, 1982.

Habermehl GG: *Venomous Animals and Their Toxins.* Berlin: Springer-Verlag, 1981, 195 pp.

Haley TJ, Berndt WO: *Toxicology.* Washington: Hemisphere, 1987, 697 pp.

Hardman JG, Limbird LE, Molinoff PB, Ruddon RW, Gilman AG (eds.): *Goodman and Gilman's The Pharmacological Basis of Therapeutics.* 9th ed. Columbus, OH: McGraw-Hill, 1996, 1936 pp.

Hayes AW (ed.): *Principles and Methods of Toxicology,* 2nd ed. New York: Raven Press, 1989, 929 pp.

Hodgson E, Levi PE (eds.): *Introduction to Biochemical Toxicology,* 2nd ed. Norwalk, CT: Appleton & Lange, 1994, 588 pp.

Hodgson E, Mailman RB, Chambers JE (eds.): *Dictionary of Toxicology,* 2nd ed. London: Macmillan, 1997, in press.

Klaassen CD, Amdur MO, Doull J (eds.): *Casarett and Doull's Toxicology. The Basic Science of Poisons,* 5th ed. New York: McGraw-Hill, 1996, 1111 pp.

Landis WG, Yu M-H: *Introduction to Environmental Toxicology.* Boca Raton, FL: Lewis Publishers, 1995, 328 pp.

Loomis TA, Hayes AW: *Essentials of Toxicology.* 4th ed. San Diego: Academic Press, 1996, 282 pp.

Lu FC: *Basic Toxicology,* 2nd ed. Washington: Hemisphere, 1991, 361 pp.

Matsumura F: *Toxicology of Insecticides.* New York: Plenum Press, 1985.

Ottoboni MA: *The Dose Makes the Poison,* 2nd ed. New York: Van Nostrand Reinhold, 1991, 244 pp.

Peterle TJ: *Wildlife Toxicology.* New York: Van Nostrand Reinhold, 1991, 322 pp.

Steyn PS (ed.): *The Biosynthesis of Mycotoxins: A Study in Secondary Metabolism.* New York: Academic Press, 1980.

Thomson WT: *Agricultural Chemicals Books I, II, III, and IV.* Fresno, CA: Thomson Publications, 1982.

Timbrell JA: *Principles of Biochemical Toxicology.* London: Taylor and Francis, 1991, 412 pp.

Wexler P: *Information Resources in Toxicology,* 2nd ed. New York: Elsevier, 1989, 510 pp.

ABSORPTION AND DISTRIBUTION OF TOXICANTS

2

ERNEST HODGSON • PATRICIA E. LEVI

2.1

INTRODUCTION

Until the middle of the twentieth century, the skin and other body barriers were believed to be relatively effective in preventing potential poisons from entering the body. Now, however, we know that almost every toxicant can pass through one or more portals of entry, although there may be considerable differences in rate. Thus at any given time, few, if any, chemicals will be excluded from entry. Toxicants, however, are usually metabolized between the time of entry and transport to the target tissue, and thus they may become either less harmful or activated to more toxic compounds. In addition, toxicants may be metabolized, either activated or detoxified, by the target tissue itself. It should be emphasized that toxicants do not pass through the body on a single linear pathway. Different routes of metabolism and modes of action are possible, and these routes are dependent on the organ to which that portion of the dose was distributed, the simultaneous presence of other toxicants, the dose level, and many other factors. Not only are these various pathways dynamically related to each other, but their relative contribution to the overall fate of the toxicant also can vary as a result of both extrinsic and intrinsic factors.

Each portal of entry permits a different rate of penetration and may also cause different metabolic patterns. The major routes of xenobiotic entry into the body are through the respiratory, gastrointestinal, and cutaneous systems. Depending on the chemical form and exposure of the organism to the chemical, the importance of a particular route may be either inconsequential or of key importance. In general, the respiratory system offers the most rapid route of entry and the dermal the least rapid, although overall entry depends on both the amount present and the saturability of the epithelium involved.

Many of the opportunities for entry into the body are related to the form of the toxicant and its location in the environment. For example, a chemical in the vapor phase may have very high probability for respiratory entry, but if the chemical is associated exclusively with water, then entry will be primarily through gastrointestinal (GI) absorption for terrestrial animals and through dermal and gill uptake for aquatic animals. If a chemical is strongly bound to an organic or inorganic component of the environment, there is little likelihood that it will be absorbed while in the bound form. Opportunities for transfer from one form (or substrate) to another make toxicity difficult to predict, however. For example, some very volatile compounds that could cause serious problems through lung entry have been found to be transported in water for considerable distances. They become GI problems during the transport phase and may again become respiratory hazards at termination of transport. For this reason, volatile toxic compounds do not always disappear as might be expected and may become chronic hazards at points far removed from their original entry into the environment. For instance, a volatile compound placed "safely" in a metal drum in a waste dump may enter groundwater following leakage from the resting drum. Eventually, this chemical could become a chronic problem in a house that, although built several miles from the disposal dump, receives small amounts of the contaminated water on a continuing basis.

As discussed in more detail later, the events occurring during toxic action are very dynamic. A chemical may enter the body and be metabolized and eliminated without toxic action. However, the toxicant may be absorbed, transported to the site of action, and quickly elicit an adverse action. Toxicokinetics refers to the rates of all metabolic processes related to the expression of toxic endpoints and includes the relationship between such rates and their integration into formal models that provide a mathematic description of any part or all of the overall process.

Often overlooked is the fact that the acute and chronic actions of a toxicant are often exerted on different systems. For example, many chlorinated hydrocarbons are central nervous system (CNS) depressants following relatively high acute doses. The same chemicals given in small chronic amounts for long periods have no important actions on the nervous system but, in time, may have a necrotic or carcinogenic action on such organs as the liver.

After a chemical enters the body, it is then transported through the body. The circulatory system offers an ideal transport system because it can easily move water-soluble as well as lipid-soluble compounds by virtue of either the aqueous medium or the proteins (including lipoproteins) it contains. These proteins may serve to bind the toxicants for release at some tissue distant from the site of entry. Such transport may carry a toxicant to a site of toxic action, to a site of metabolism, to a site of storage, or to organs of elimination. All these events occur simultaneously, and the resulting dynamic flux makes the study of toxicant movement quite complex.

2.2

MEMBRANES

Toxicants must pass through a number of barriers during entry into the body as well as when entering tissues, cells, and cellular compartments. Similar passages occur also when toxicants or metabolites are excreted from the body. These barriers include structures that vary from the relatively thick areas of the skin to the relatively thin lung membranes. Each step of this process involves translocation of the chemical across various membrane barriers, from the skin or mucosa through the capillary membranes, and through the cellular and organelle membranes (Fig. 2.1). In all cases, however, the membranes of tissue, cell, and cell organelle are similar.

The lipid constituents in the membrane permit considerable movement of macromolecules, and membrane constituents may move appreciably within membranes. All membranes appear to be bimolecular lipid leaflets containing proteins. Leaflets are oriented on opposing sides of the membrane so that they are approximately mirror images of each other. The average width of a membrane is 75 Å. The lipids are oriented so that the hydrophilic head is to the outside of the membrane and the lipophilic tail is to the inside of the membrane (Fig. 2.2).

Several types of lipids are found in membranes, with phospholipids and cholesterol predominating. Sphingolipids comprise the primary minor component. Phosphatidylcholine, phosphatidylserine, and phosphatidylethanolamine are the primary phosphatides, and their two fatty acid hydrocarbon chains (typically 16 to 18, but varying from 12 to 22) comprise the nonpolar region. Some of the fatty acids are unsaturated and contribute appreciably to the fluidity of the membrane.

Proteins, which have many physiological roles in normal cell function, are intimately associated with lipids and may be located variously throughout lipid bilayers. These proteins may be located on either surface or traverse the entire structure. Hydrophobic forces are responsible for maintaining the structural integrity of pro-

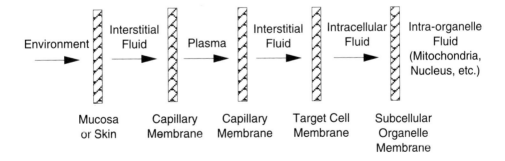

Figure 2.1. Schematic showing membranes that a chemical may need to cross during passage from the environment to the site of action. *(Source: Redrawn from Hodgson and Levi, eds.* Introduction to Biochemical Toxicology, *2nd ed. Norwalk CT: Appleton & Lange, 1994, p 12.)*

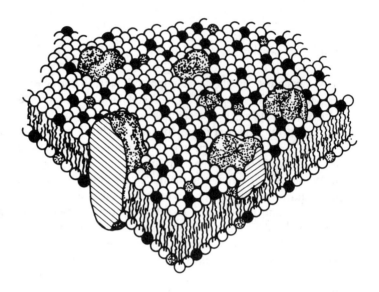

Figure 2.2. Schematic diagram of biological membrane. Head groups of lipids represented by spheres, tail ends by zigzag lines. Black, white, or stippled spheres indicate different kinds of lipids and illustrate asymmetry in certain cases. Large bodies are membrane-associated proteins. *(Source: Modified from Singer and Nicolson,* Science ***175:720,*** *1972.)*

teins and lipids within membranes, but movement within the membranes may occur.

The ratio of lipid to protein varies from 5:1 for the myelin membrane to 1:5 for the inner structure of the mitochondria. A more important feature with regard to the extent and rate of absorption may be the proportion of the membrane surface that is comprised of lipid bilayers. One hundred percent of the myelin membrane surface is lipid bilayer, whereas the inner membrane of the mitochondria may have only 40% lipid bilayer surface.

For ready movement of small molecules such as water through membranes, the presence of pores of approximately 4 Å has been postulated. Thus, certain molecules that ordinarily would be excluded can rapidly traverse the highly lipid membrane barrier. In specialized membranes such as those associated with the kidney, pore size may be as large as 45 Å, permitting the ready transfer of larger molecules with molecular weights approaching 50,000 daltons.

Many of the proteins that traverse the membrane are transport proteins that translocate their ligands, either by active or facilitated transport, across the membrane (see Section 2.5). The amphipathic nature of the membrane produces a barrier for ionized, highly polar compounds—although not an absolute barrier. The importance of nonionic, lipid-soluble characteristics of a xenobiotic is discussed in the following sections. It is worth noting that differences between membranes, such as the presence of different lipids, the amount of surface lipid, differences in size and shape of proteins, or physical features of bonding may cause differences in permeability between membranes.

2.3

IONIZATION

Because of their lipid nature, membranes are much less permeable to compounds that are in the ionized state than to those in the nonionized form. For example, alkaloids, such as strychnine, that are ionized as a result of introduction into the strongly acid stomach do not show toxic effects if the digestive tract is ligated between stomach and intestine. However, when such alkaloids are allowed to pass to the more alkaline intestine, where they became nonionized, toxicity becomes apparent because the toxic alkaloid is more easily absorbed. This is not an important criterion for most toxicants because they are incapable of being ionized and are thus unaffected by pH. A small number of toxicants, however, such as alkaloids and organic acids, are ionizable, and their absorption and thus their toxicity may be altered appreciably by pH.

The amount of the compound in the ionized or nonionized form depends on the pKa of the potential toxicant and the pH of the bathing medium. The pKa, the negative logarithm of the dissociation constant of a weak acid or base, is the pH at which the compound is 50% ionized, and is a physiochemical characteristic of that compound. Thus, when the pH of a solution is equal to the pKa of the dissolved compound, one half of the compound exists in the ionized form and one half exists in the nonionized form. The degree of ionization is given by the Henderson–Hasselbach equation:

$$\log \frac{\text{nonionized form}}{\text{ionized form}} = \text{pKa} - \text{pH (for weak acids)}$$

$$\log \frac{\text{ionized form}}{\text{nonionized form}} = \text{pKa} - \text{pH (for weak bases).}$$

For an organic acid ($RCOOH \longleftrightarrow RCOO^- + H^+$), acidic conditions (pH less than the pKa of the compound) will favor the formation of the nonionized RCOOH, whereas alkaline conditions (pH greater than pKa) will shift the equilibrium to the right. For an organic base ($RNH_2 + H^+ \rightleftharpoons RNH_3^+$) the reverse is true, and decreasing the pH (increasing the concentration of H^+) will favor formation of the ionized form, whereas increasing the pH (decreasing the concentration of H^+) will favor formation of the nonionized form.

Because the nonionized (more lipophilic) form of a weak electrolyte is the form most readily absorbed, weak organic acids are most readily absorbed from acid environments where they are nonionized, and weak organic bases from alkaline environments (Table 2.1). Thus some toxicants may be preferentially absorbed from the more acidic stomach whereas others are preferentially absorbed from the

TABLE 2.1. EFFECT OF PH ON ABSORPTION OF WEAK ORGANIC ACIDS AND BASES FROM RAT INTESTINE

Compound	pKa	Percent Absorbed at Various pH Values			
		3.6–4.3	4.7–5.0	7.0–7.2	7.8–8.0
Acids					
Nitrosalicyclic	2.3	40	27	< 02	< 02
Salicyclic	3.0	64	35	30	10
Benzoic	4.2	62	36	35	05
Bases					
Aniline	4.6	40	48	58	61
Aminopyrene	5.0	21	35	48	52
Quinine	8.4	09	11	41	54

Source: Adapted from Hogben et al: J Pharmacol Exp Ther *125:275, 1959.*

more alkaline intestine. In almost all cases, however, some degree of absorption occurs even when toxicants are not in the most lipid-soluble form, and even a small amount of absorption may produce serious effects with highly toxic compounds. There are the usual exceptions to the generalizations concerning ionization and some compounds, such as pralidoxime (2-PAM), paraquat, and diquat, are absorbed to an appreciable extent even in the ionized forms. The mechanisms allowing these exceptions are not understood.

2.4

PARTITION COEFFICIENT

A second parameter influencing penetration through membranes is the relative lipid solubility of the potential toxicant. The lipid solubility of a compound is measured by the partition coefficient, which is a measure of the compounds partitioning between aqueous and lipid phases (concentration in lipid phase/concentration in water phase). Thus, a high partition coefficient indicates greater lipophilicity. The lipid solvent used for measurement is usually octanol because it best mimics the carbon chain of phospholipids, but many other systems have been reported (chloroform/water, ether/water, olive oil/water). Obviously, each may give a different value, and there is often little consistency in correlation between penetration and partition coefficients derived from different solvent systems.

The correlation between high partition coefficient and rapid penetration has probably been more generally accepted than is warranted, although many studies show good correlation between high partition coefficients and rapid penetration, and this relationship has become generally accepted. Chemically related groups of compounds such as an analogous series of alcohols show the best correlation. Although lipid solubility is clearly necessary for initial uptake, once the toxicant has entered the membrane, other factors can complicate further penetration. For example, too high a lipid solubility may reduce penetration by restricting exit through the polar region of the membrane, and compounds that are extremely lipid soluble may tend to remain in membranes rather than pass through them. Thus a moderate degree of water solubility is often a facilitating factor in increased penetration; nevertheless, some very lipid soluble compounds such as DDT, polychlorinated biphenyls (PCBs), and synthetic pyrethroids are able to penetrate, in many cases without difficulty. If a large molecule has high water solubility, however, the penetration rate is invariably low. Chemical similarity of penetrants, size of molecule, and conformational similarities are other parameters that modify penetration similarities and differences among compounds, and measuring these characteristics is somewhat complex.

2.5

MECHANISMS OF ABSORPTION

The mechanisms of toxicant movement across membranes, particularly initial entry, has been a poorly researched area in general, although considerable work has been done in the specific case of drugs. There appear to be four primary mechanisms that allow toxicants to traverse membranes.

1. *Passive Transport.* For most toxicants, this mechanism appears to predominate. Passive transport involves movement of the compounds across the lipid membranes by simple diffusion with the water/lipid partition coefficients largely determining the rate of movement. Compounds in the ionized form do not move very readily by diffusion through membranes for several reasons. First, the ionized form tends to have low lipid solubility, a factor necessary for membrane diffusion. Second, there may be ionic interactions among xenobiotics, lipids, and proteins within the membrane.

2. *Filtration.* There are often pores in the membrane that allow compounds with molecular weights of less than 100 daltons to enter. Larger molecules, however, are excluded except in more highly porous tissues, such as the kidney and liver. Because many toxicants are relatively large molecules, this pathway is often of limited importance as a mechanism of absorption. Filtration is generally considered to be of more importance in the elimination of toxicants, especially by the kidney (see Chapter 5—Elimination of Toxicants).

3. *Special Transport.* A number of special transport systems, particularly in the GI tract, aid in transport of endogenous compounds across membranes. Such processes may require energy and permit passage against a concentration gradient (active transport) or may not require energy and be unable to move compounds against a gradient (facilitated transport). Although the results may differ, the mechanisms are somewhat similar and are discussed together. In both cases, a carrier protein that associates with the toxicant is

postulated. This protein assists the movement of the toxicant from one side of the membrane to the other and, on the other side, the chemical dissociates from the protein, which is then free to take up another toxicant molecule. Such penetration is more rapid than simple diffusion and, in the case of active transport, may proceed beyond the point at which concentrations are equal on both sides of the membrane.

These mechanisms may be important in those relatively rare instances in which toxicants have chemical or structural similarities to endogenous chemicals that rely on special transport mechanisms for normal physiological uptake and can thus utilize the same system. For example, 5-fluorouracil is transported by the thymidine transport system. Lead may be more quickly moved by a transport system that is normally involved in the uptake of calcium. As absorption mechanisms, such special transport systems are most manifest in GI absorption. These mechanisms become of much greater importance in the elimination of toxicants, however, in which special transport is important in the removal of xenobiotics and their metabolites. An important characteristic of the special transport systems, when operative, is that they allow movement of compounds with lesser lipid solubility, that is, compounds that would ordinarily be expected to move very slowly through highly lipid membranes. Many active transport systems are linked to energy producing enzymes (eg, ATPase), and both active and facilitated transport systems display saturation characteristics (ie, saturation of the available carrier proteins by toxicant molecules). Thus, the kinetics of special transport systems can best be described by using Michaelis–Menton enzyme kinetic models.

4. *Endocytosis*. Pinocytosis (for liquids) and phagocytosis (for solids) are specialized transport processes in which the membrane invaginates or flows around a toxicant allowing more ready transfer across membranes. Only in such isolated instances as absorption of carrageenens (mol wt ~40,000) in the gut have these mechanisms been found to be important in initial entry. Once inside the body, however, endocytosis is a rather common mechanism, and engulfment of compounds in the lung is common (lung phagocytosis).

2.6

RATES OF PENETRATION

The rate of penetration is determined by several factors: the concentration gradient across the membrane, the area and thickness of the membrane, and the diffusion constant of the toxicant. For a single vehicle and solvent system, the rate of penetration of nonpolar, nonionized toxicants by passive diffusion is believed to follow Fick's law of diffusion. One assumption of this pattern is that the concentration at the application site is much higher than the absorbed concentration, which can be considered negligible because it is removed quickly. Thus,

$$K = \frac{A(C)}{d}$$

where C = concentration, A = surface area directly related to transfer, d = thickness of membrane, and K = diffusion constant. This equation may be expanded to the more experimentally useful equation

$$J = \frac{K_m \, C_v \, D_m}{d}$$

where J = absorption rate per unit area at steady state (flux), K_m = vehicle partition coefficient, C_v = concentration of penetrant, D_m = diffusion constant of penetrant in the membrane, and d = the thickness of the membrane. The rate of absorption, then, depends on two easily controlled externally determined factors (partition coefficient and concentration of penetrant) and two innate factors (diffusion constant and membrane thickness). Permeability constants for human skin range from 1×10^{-6} to 5×10^{-2} cm/h.

The previous equation implies conditions of steady-state penetration, not attained until after a lag phase has occurred. A plot of the logarithm of the amount unpenetrated toxicant v time should be linear, indicating first-order kinetics.

This ideal situation may be an oversimplification except in the most rigid and nonphysiological terms, and deviations from first-order kinetics may be commonplace. When the absorption of a series of pesticides was compared in mice, no single equation seemed appropriate. Statistical tests of first-, second-, and third-order models generally showed significant departures from these kinetic models. Empirical models that used transformed responses (log P and arc sine P where P = percentage unpenetrated) and regressed on log (time) were much more effective in linearizing the response–time relationship, and the resulting $t_{0.5}$ estimates were then comparable because a single model fit was sufficient for all toxicants. Possible explanations for these variations from simple diffusion include differential shunts within the highly lipid membrane, contribution of appendagical shunts, for example, hair follicles, effects of the carrier necessary for application, injury to surface membranes, hydration of the stratum corneum, binding of the penetrant to the stratum corneum, and regional variations in skin permeability.

When first-order kinetics hold, a simple relationship exists between the penetration constant, K, and $t_{0.5}$ (time necessary for one-half of the applied dose to penetrate):

$$K = \frac{0.693}{t_{0.5}} \qquad \text{and the units of } K \text{ are percentage of change/time unit.}$$

When first-order kinetics do not apply, the only relevant number is $t_{0.5}$ itself, because the units of K change for any model other than first order.

TABLE 2.2. COMPARISON OF PHYSICAL PROPERTIES AND PENETRATION OF PESTICIDES IN MICE

Pesticide	Solubility Water (ppm)	Partition Coefficient Olive oil/water	$t_{0.5}$ (min) Dermal	$t_{0.5}$ (min) Oral
Carbaryl	40	46	12.8	17.0
Malathion	145	56	129.7	33.5
Chlorpyrifos	2	1044	20.6	78.1
DDT	0.001	1775	105.4	62.3
Nicotine	Miscible	0.02	18.2	23.1

Source: Adapted from Ahdaya SM, et al: Pestic Biochem Physiol **16**:38–46, 1981, and Shah PV, et al: Toxicol Appl Pharmacol **59**:414–423, 1981.

When oral and dermal administration were compared for in vivo experiments, the half-time penetration rates were found to vary considerably (Table 2.2). It is obvious that, in these experiments, no useful correlation between partition coefficients, animal species, or route of administration could be found. Although such comparisons may be interesting, it is perhaps not surprising to find large differences among higher animals. For example, one would have great difficulty in assuming that a skin area was similar in situations such as smooth versus hairy skin, or skin of a mammal versus that of a bird. Furthermore, comparisons of dermal application versus GI application have quite dissimilar patterns. A GI application will always be complicated by the much greater surface area of the gut as opposed to skin, immediate diffusion of the toxicant in the liquid of the GI tract, and the possibilities of binding of the administered dose to extraneous material in the gut contents. Thus, it is prudent to consider measurements of the penetration rates of toxicants derived from different animals or from different routes of application as estimates that may contain large errors.

2.7

ROUTES OF ABSORPTION IN MAMMALS

Because humans are the principal target of concern, this section is devoted primarily to animals that are usually chosen to assess toxicity to humans or to data derived from human tissue. Primary routes of entry are dermal, GI, and respiratory. Methods for studying these different routes are numerous, but they are perhaps best developed for the study of dermal penetration because this route is subject to more direct methodology, whereas methods for studying respiratory or GI absorption require more highly specialized instrumentation. Additional routes encountered in experimental studies include intraperitoneal, intramuscular, and subcutaneous routes. When direct entry into the circulatory system is desired, intravenous or intra-arterial injections can be used to bypass the absorption phase.

2.7.1   Dermal

The skin is a complex multilayered tissue with a large surface exposed to the environment. The skin is relatively impermeable to most ions as well as aqueous solutions, but is permeable to a large number of toxicants in the solid, liquid, or gaseous phases. Although most cases of poisoning occur after oral ingestion or respiratory entry, many toxicants can gain entry easily through the dermal route. Numerous examples of poisoning by the dermal route have been reported—organophosphorous pesticides in agricultural workers, chlorophenol in domestic and wild animals, and a large number of industrial solvents are a few examples.

A schematic representation of mammalian skin is shown in Fig. 2.3. Three distinct layers make up this important organ—epidermis, dermis, and subcutaneous tissue, but the epidermis is the only layer that is of significance in penetration of toxicants. In general, the vasculature is usually > 100 μm from the outer layer of skin. The outermost layer, the epidermis, is a multilayered tissue varying in thickness from about 0.1 to 0.8 mm, and it is this layer that presents the greatest deterrant to

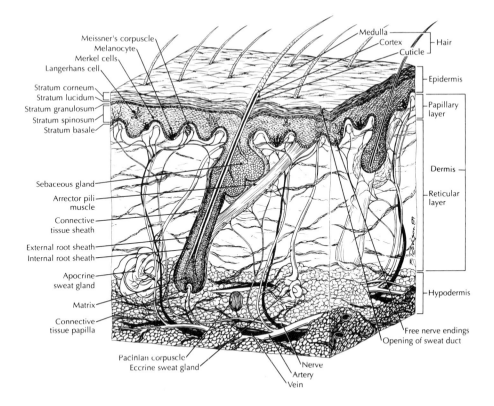

Figure 2.3. Schematic diagram of the microstructure of mammalian skin. *(Source: Monteiro-Riviere. In* Fundamentals and Methods of Dermal and Ocular Toxicology, *Hobson DW, (ed.). Boca Raton, FL: CRC Press, 1991, p 5).*

toxicant absorption. The thicker areas of the skin have a higher concentration of keratin than do the thinner areas. The basal cells of the epidermis proliferate and differentiate as they migrate outward toward the surface of the skin. The columnar basal cells become rounded and then flattened as they move through loosely defined layers and finally to the outer layer, the stratum corneum, which is the primary barrier to penetration. This layer consists of 8–16 layers of flattened, highly keratinized cells. It is approximately 25–40 μm wide, lies parallel to the skin surface, and forms a relatively impermeable, shingle-like layer approximately 10 μm thick. It requires about 26–28 days for cells to migrate from the basal layer to the stratum corneum, where they are eventually sloughed off. These dead, keratinized cells are, however, very water absorbant (hydrophilic), a property that keeps the skin soft and supple. Sebum, a natural oil covering the skin, functions in maintaining the water-holding ability of the epidermis.

A number of appendages are associated with the skin, including hair follicles, sebaceous glands, eccrine and apocrine sweat glands, and nails. Recently, it was found that removal of the stratum corneum does not allow complete absorption; thus, it is apparent that some role, although of lesser importance, is played by other parts of the skin.

The dermis and subcutaneous areas of the skin are less important in influencing penetration, and once a toxicant has penetrated the epidermis, the other layers are traversed rather easily. The dermis is highly vascular, a characteristic that provides maximal opportunity for further transport once molecules have gained entry through the epidermis or through skin appendages. The blood supply of the dermis is under neural and humoral influences whose temperature-regulating functions could thus affect penetration and distribution of toxicants. The subcutaneous layer of the skin is highly lipid in nature and serves as a shock absorber, an insulator, and a reserve depot of energy. The pH of the skin varies between 4 and 7 and is markedly affected by hydration.

The skin serves not only as a passive barrier to diffusion but may also have a function in the metabolism of topically applied substances before they enter the systemic circulation. The epidermal layer accounts for the major portion of biochemical transformations in skin, although the total skin activity is low (2–6% that of the liver). If activity is based on epidermis alone, however, that layer is as active as the liver or, in the case of certain toxicants, several times more active. Although skin metabolism usually deactivates toxicants, activation of some skin carcinogens is known to occur. For rapidly penetrating substances, metabolism by the skin is not presently considered to be of major significance; however, skin may have an important first-pass metabolic function, especially for compounds that are absorbed slowly.

Percutaneous absorption could occur through several routes, but it is generally believed that most lipid-soluble toxicants move directly through the stratum corneum rather than through hair follicles or sweat ducts. Arguments in favor of transepidermal absorption are that epidermal damage or partial removal increases penetration, epidermal penetration is markedly slower than dermal, and the epidermal surface area is much greater than the surface area of skin appendages. Initial penetration may be aided by appendages, but absorption through the general skin surface eventually becomes more important than appendicular absorption. Currently, there is no evidence for active transport in the skin, and it is thought that toxicants, whether gas, ion, or nonelectrolyte, move by simple diffusion.

Variations in areas of the body cause appreciable differences in penetration of toxicants, as has been shown for both pesticides and hydrocortisone in human skin (Table 2.3). Head, neck, and axilla (where environmental exposure is greatest) are areas of increased absorption. Also, hair follicle density may affect absorption of more polar compounds.

It is important to recognize that occlusion of the site of application by bandage, clothing, or ointment markedly increases absorption. Such action changes physical and physiological factors, affecting penetration as well as retarding mechanical abrasion of the applied compound.

Surfactants and soaps applied in conjunction with a toxicant may also affect penetration. Alterations of the stratum corneum appear to be the major factor. Organic solvents often decrease penetration and may be divided into damaging categories (acetone, methanol, ether, hexane) that alter lipids and increase permeability, or nondamaging categories (long-chain esters, olive oil, higher alcohols). Aqueous solutions of detergents also increase penetration markedly.

The choice of the most appropriate experimental animal to mimic penetration into human skin has always been controversial. Data in Fig. 2.4 show comparative results from one experiment. Although a suitable animal model has not been developed for all cases, primates and pigs seem to be better models, whereas mice and rabbits appear to absorb toxicants faster than humans. Whereas comparison of in vivo and in vitro data with human skin does not give consistent correlations, it has been possible to distinguish between compounds of low permeability using in vitro systems. Recent methodology has improved in vitro techniques, and it is hoped that these tools may become valuable in absorption studies because in vivo testing in humans is becoming much more impractical for ethical and legal reasons.

TABLE 2.3. PENETRATION OF HYDROCORTISONE IN HUMANS AT DIFFERENT ANATOMIC SITES

Anatomic Site	Penetration Ratio
Foot (plantar)	0.14
Ankle (lateral)	0.42
Palm	0.83
Forearm	1.0
Back	1.7
Scalp	3.5
Forehead	6.0
Scrotum	42.0

Source: Adapted from Feldman RJ, Maibach HI: J Invest Dermatol *48*:181–183, 1967.

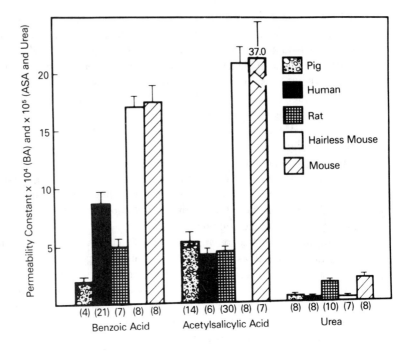

Figure 2.4. Permeability constants obtained with animal and human skin. *(Source: Modified from Bronough et al. Toxicol Appl Pharmacol **62**:481, 1982.)*

Other factors that have an effect on penetration include concentration of toxicant, age of animal, temperature, multiple dose application, skin condition, relative humidity, surface area of applied dose, and hyperemia.

2.7.2   Gastrointestinal

The oral route is especially important for accidental or deliberate ingestion of toxicants. Food additives, food toxins, licking or rubbing, and airborne particles excluded from passage to the alveoli and returned to the glottis are among potential avenues for accidental ingestion. Although the buccal cavity and the rectum are sometimes used to introduce drugs, with a few exceptions ingested toxicants enter the body through the stomach or intestine. Exceptions include nicotine, which enters readily through the buccal cavity, and cocaine, which enters through the nasal mucosa.

The digestive system (Fig. 2.5a) is lined by a layer of columnar cells protected by mucus, although the latter has little role in absorption. The distance from the outer membrane to the vasculature is about 40 μm, from which point further transport can easily occur. The route of venous blood flow from the stomach and intestine causes absorbed materials to have a first pass through the liver, a route that fa-

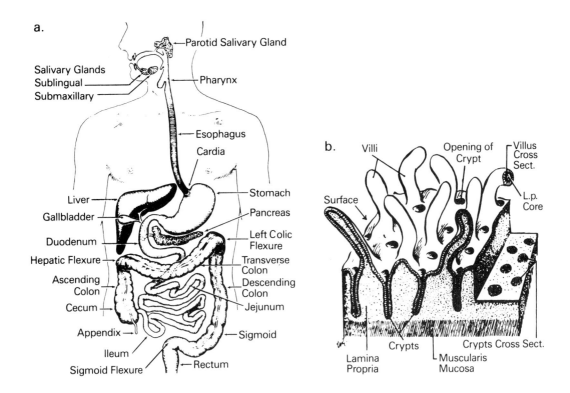

Figure 2.5. Schematic showing (a) alimentary canal and associated structures and (b) lining of the small intestine. *(Source: (a) Scholtelius and Scholtelius in* Textbook of Physiology, *St. Louis: Mosby, 1973, and (b) Ham and Cormack in* Histology, *8th ed, Philadelphia: Lippincott, 1979.)*

vors metabolism of the toxicant. However, absorption of toxicants through the skin or lungs follows more indirect routes to organs of detoxication, without a first pass directly through the liver. A major factor favoring absorption in the intestine is the presence of microvilli, which provide an extremely large surface area (Fig. 2.5b).

It is generally conceded that absorption is more rapid through the GI route than the dermal route, although meager data support this assumption. As stated earlier, it is difficult to make a direct comparison experimentally, but recent tests with mice indicate that differences in penetration between the dermal and oral routes are often either relatively small or even nonexistent (Table 2.2).

Although the greater surface area of the intestine favors absorption at that location rather than the stomach, compounds enter the stomach first and may be readily absorbed during residence in that organ.

Appreciable differences in pH exist within the GI tract, a factor that may change permeability characteristics of a toxicant. The stomach tends to be much more acidic than the intestine, and this pH difference can affect the rate and site of absorption of ionizable compounds. The measured pH of the GI contents may not be identical to the pH of the epithelium at the site of absorption, and this may explain the entrance of compounds whose pKa would normally suggest a much slower rate.

In contrast to the skin, active transport of toxicants is known to occur in the GI tract. For toxicants with structural similarities to compounds normally taken up by active transport mechanisms, entry is enhanced. For example, cobalt is absorbed by the same active transport mechanism that normally transports iron, and 5-bromouracil is absorbed by the pyrimidine transport system.

A feature of the GI tract that seems to contradict basic assumptions of absorption is the penetration of certain very large molecules. Compounds such as bacterial endotoxins, large particles of azo dyes, and carrageenans are apparently absorbed by endocytotic mechanisms.

Some factors contributing to GI absorption require brief mention. One important factor is that dissolution of a toxicant in the gut contents greatly increases absorption, because the compound must be in intimate contact with the epithelium for significant absorption to occur. Very lipid soluble compounds that are not miscible in the aqueous GI fluid are passed to the intestine, where they are brought into solution through the action of the detergent-like bile acids, such as cholic acid. Without the action of bile acids, the lipids would remain as an emulsion and be unavailable for absorption. Factors such as particle size, solvent effects, presence of emulsifiers, and rate of dissolution are also important. The presence of microorganisms and hydrolysis-promoting pH conditions, binding to gut contents, the rate of emptying of the stomach, the temperature of the contents, intestinal motility, dietary and health effects, and GI secretion are all related factors that may affect penetration.

Another important aspect of GI absorption is enterohepatic circulation. Following secretion of conjugated metabolites from the bile duct into the intestine, a water-soluble metabolite may be altered to a less polar compound, readsorbed through the intestine, and returned to the liver. Enterohepatic circulation is discussed in greater detail in Chapter 5.

2.7.3   Respiratory

The third major route for systemic absorption of toxicants is through the respiratory system. Although this organ is in direct contact with contaminated air, it is also equipped with a number of protective mechanisms to reduce the toxicity of airborne substances, especially particles. The respiratory system is especially vulnerable from two aspects, however. The rich capillary exchange at the deeper lung recesses, separated by only 1–2 μm from the circulation, is ideal not only for rapid exchange of O_2 and CO_2, but also enables exchange of gaseous toxicants in seconds or less. In addition, a thin film of aqueous fluid wets the alveolar walls, aiding in initial absorption of toxicants from alveolar air. In some cases, however, the phospholipid component of the surface monolayer may interact with very highly lipid toxicants to slow uptake. Moreover, the surface area of the lung is large—50–100 m², some 50 times the area of the skin.

The process of respiration involves the movement and exchange of air through several interrelated passages, including the nose, mouth, pharynx, trachea, bronchi, and successively smaller airways terminating in the alveoli, where gaseous exchange occurs (Fig. 2.6). The amount of air retained in the lung despite maximum expiratory effort is known as the residual volume. Thus toxicants in the respiratory air may not be cleared immediately because of slow release from the residual volume. The rate of entry of vapor-phase toxicants is controlled by the alveolar ventilation rate, with the toxicant being presented to the alveoli in an interrupted fashion approximately 20 times/min.

Although many definitions are used for airborne toxicants, these may be simplified to two general types. Compounds that are subject to gas laws include solvents, vapors, and gases. These are most easily carried to the alveolar areas. The second group is not subject to gas laws because they are in particulate form, and includes aerosols, clouds, particles, fumes, and so on.

Entry of aerosols and particulates is governed by a number of factors that may seem to facilitate or preclude their entry. The upper respiratory tract, beginning with

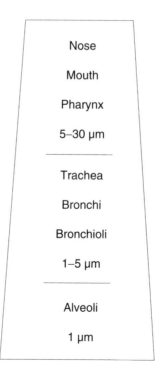

Figure 2.6. Schematic illustrating the regions where absorption may occur in the respiratory tract.

the nose and continuing down its tubular elements, is a very efficient filtration system for trapping particulates before they reach the alveoli. The efficiency of the system is illustrated by the fact than on average only 100 g of coal dust is found postmortem in the lungs of coal miners although they inhale approximately 6000 g during their lifetime. The parameters of air velocity and directional air change favor impaction of particles in the upper respiratory system. In addition to particle size, such factors as coagulation, sedimentation, electrical charge, and diffusion may be important. Particles of > 5 μm are usually deposited in the nasopharyngeal region (Fig. 2.6). Particles down to 2 μm are deposited in the tracheobronchiolar region, where they are cleared upward by the mucus blanket that covers the backward-beating cilia. The removal of particles may result in half-lives of < 5 hours (movement up to 1 mm/min), and 80% of lung clearance may occur in this way. Particles may be trapped temporarily in nasal passages or may move to the glottis, where they are swallowed. This could permit later absorption in the GI tract.

In addition to upper pathway clearance, lung phagocytosis is very active in both upper and lower pathways of the respiratory tract and may be coupled to the mucus cilia. Phagocytes may also direct engulfed toxicants into the lymph, where the toxicants may be stored for long periods. If not phagocytized, particles ≤ 1 μm may penetrate to the alveolar portion of the lung. Some particles do not desequamate but instead form a dust node in association with a developing network of reticular fibers. Overall, removal of alveolar particles is markedly slower than that achieved by the directed upper pulmonary mechanisms.

For very small particles and gaseous toxicants, absorption takes place in the alveolar region (Fig. 2.7). Gas in the alveoli equilibrates almost instantaneously with the blood passing through the pulmonary capillary bed. Release of gas into or out of the blood is dependent on its solubility in blood. If a substance has a low solubility, only a small amount of the gas in the lung is removed by the blood. In this case because of the low carrying capacity, the respiratory rate would not affect exchange. The rate of cardiac output would affect transfer into blood, however. The time for blood–gas to come in equilibrium with alveolar gas often exceeds 10 minutes for relatively insoluble gases.

The greater portion of highly blood-soluble gases is transferred to the blood with each breath, and little is left in the alveolus. The more soluble the toxicant, the more time it will take to reach equilibrium in the blood. Thus, the time required to equilibrate with blood will be longer than with low-solubility gases (~ 1 hour). For highly soluble gases, the principal factor limiting absorption is the rate of respiration. Increasing cardiac output does not appreciably increase rate of absorption.

There is little evidence for active transport in the respiratory system, although pinocytosis may be of importance. The lung is also an important excretory organ for metabolic end products (eg, CO_2), anesthetic gases, and certain gaseous toxicants, such as ethanol (see Chapter 5—Elimination of Toxicants).

Toxicants may produce irritation on exposure, may accumulate in the upper respiratory passages to cause irritation and damage, or may be absorbed into the circulatory system and result in systemic toxicity. In addition, the lung contains many

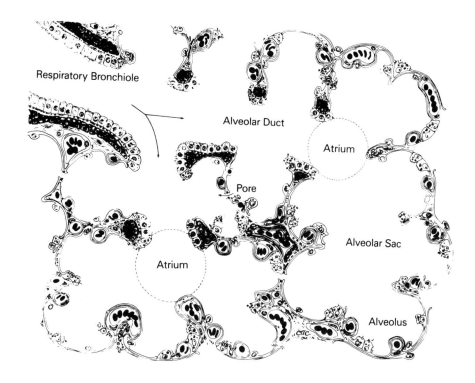

Figure 2.7. Schematic representation of the respiratory unit of the lung. (*Source: Bloom and Fawcett in* A Textbook of Histology, *Philadelphia: WB Saunders, 1975.)*

xenobiotic-metabolizing enzymes that play a role in the activation and detoxication of toxicants, either during the absorption phase or on exposure through the systemic route.

2.8

DISTRIBUTION

Body fluids are distributed between three primary components: plasma water, interstitial water, and intracellular water. Vascular fluid has the important role in the distribution of absorbed toxicants. Human plasma accounts for about 4% of body weight but 53% of total blood volume, whereas the interstitial tissue fluids account for 13% of body weight and intracellular fluids comprise 41%. The concentration a toxicant may achieve in the blood following exposure depends on the apparent volume of distribution. If the toxicant is distributed only in plasma, a high concentration is achieved in the vascular tissue. On the contrary, if the same quantity of toxicant is also distributed in the interstitial and intracellular water, concentrations will be much lower in the vascular system.

Following absorption, a toxicant may be distributed to the site of toxic action, transferred to a storage depot, transported to organs of detoxication or interaction, and eventually eliminated.

Although many compounds have sufficient solubility in the aqueous portion of the blood for simple solution to be the important route of distribution, toxicants are usually transported in association with plasma proteins. Cellular components, such as erythrocytes, may also be responsible for transport but usually to a minor degree. The transport of toxicants by lymph is quantitatively of little importance because blood flow is many times faster than that of lymph. It must be recognized, however, that both erythrocytes and lymph can have important roles on occasions. Highly water-soluble metabolites of toxicants are also bound to blood proteins, suggesting a role in transport to the kidney.

Studies on plasma proteins have shown the albumin fraction to be of particular importance in the binding of xenobiotics. Because many toxicants are very lipophilic, the plasma lipoproteins also play an important role in toxicant binding.

Toxicants are often distributed and stored in specific tissues, either at sites of storage, in the liver or kidney, or at the site of action (eg, binding to hemoglobin). Toxicants may be sequestered either physically, such as solubilization of lipophilic chemicals in fat or chemically by binding to tissue components, such as proteins. If a toxicant is stored in a depot removed from the site of action, such as PCBs in fat or lead in bone, no adverse effect may be manifested immediately. Although an equilibrium is established between tissue and blood, amounts escaping from the storage depot are usually very small at any given time. The large amount stored in the depot is a potential toxic hazard, however, because this is an opportunity for chronic action, or even acute action if the toxicant is suddenly mobilized.

If a compound is bound to a blood protein, it is immobilized away from the site of action. Other consequences of such binding are possible displacement of one toxicant by another, perhaps more toxic, chemical; facilitation of cellular absorption while bound to a lipoprotein; and dilution of the toxicant.

A ligand–protein interaction raises the apparent contradiction that, although many toxicants are chemically "unreactive" in the strict sense, they can be reversibly bound to a variety of biological constituents. In the case of ligand–protein interactions important to transport, mass action provides a remarkably efficient means whereby toxicants can be transported and then dissociate in various tissues.

$$T_f + \text{Free site} \underset{k_2}{\overset{k_1}{\rightleftharpoons}} T_b$$

T_f and T_b are free and bound toxicant molecules, and k_1 and k_2 are rate constants for association and dissociation. The rate constant, k_2, which governs the rate of binding to the protein, dictates the rate of toxicant release at a site of action, inaction, or storage. The ratio k_2/k_1 is identical with the dissociation constant, K_{diss}.

Among a group of binding sites on proteins, those with the smallest K_{diss} values for a given toxicant bind it most tightly. In contrast to reversible binding, some potentially carcinogenic metabolites (eg, epoxides) may be covalently bound to tissue proteins, in which case there is no true distribution mechanism operative in the sense used in this section, because k_2 is nonexistent and there is no opportunity for dissociation. In addition to cytotoxicity, such covalent binding may lead to allergies or other immune responses.

Once a molecule binds to a plasma protein, it moves throughout the circulation until it dissociates, perhaps for attachment to another large molecule or at a site where the concentration of unbound ligand is low. Dissociation occurs when the affinity of another molecule or tissue component is greater than that of the plasma protein to which the toxicant was originally bound. Concentration differential, innate affinity, pH change, ionic strength, and temperature change may all be involved. Forces of association must be strong enough to establish an initial interaction but weak enough to permit dissociation at another site. As long as binding is reversible, redistribution will occur whenever the concentration of one pool, blood or tissue, is diminished relative to the other. Redistribution must occur when a pool is diminished in order to maintain equilibrium.

Ligands complex with proteins in various ways. Covalent binding may have a pronounced effect on an organism due to the modification of an essential molecule, but such binding is usually a very minor portion of the total dose. Because covalently bound molecules dissociate very slowly, if at all, they are not considered further in this discussion.

Noncovalent binding is of primary importance to distribution because the ligand can dissociate more readily than it can in covalent binding. In rare cases, the noncovalent bond may be so stable that the toxicant remains bound for weeks or months, and for all practical purposes, the bond is equivalent to a covalent one. Types of interactions that lead to noncovalent binding under the proper physiological conditions include ionic binding, hydrogen bonding, van der Waals forces, and hydrophobic interactions.

Although drug studies have been numerous, other xenobiotic compounds have been studied less extensively. The major difference between drugs and most toxicants is the frequent ionizability and high water solubility of drugs as compared with the nonionizability and high lipid solubility of many toxicants. Thus, experience with drugs forms an important background, but one that may not always be relevant to other potentially toxic compounds.

Variation in chemical and physical features affect binding to plasma constituents. Table 2.4 shows the results of binding studies with a group of insecticides with greatly differing water and lipid solubilities. The affinity for albumin and lipoproteins is inversely related to water solubility, although the relation may be imperfect. Chlorinated hydrocarbons bind strongly to albumin but even more strongly to lipoproteins. Strongly lipophilic organophosphates bind to both protein groups, whereas more water-soluble compounds bind primarily to albumin. The most water-soluble compounds appear to be transported primarily in the aqueous phase.

TABLE 2.4. RELATIVE DISTRIBUTION OF INSECTICIDES INTO ALBUMIN AND LIPOPROTEINS

Insecticide	Percent Bound	Percent Distribution of Bound Insecticide		
		Albumin	LDL	HDL
DDT	99.9	35	35	30
Dieldrin	99.9	12	50	38
Lindane	98.0	37	38	25
Parathion	98.7	67	21	12
Diazinon	96.6	55	31	14
Carbaryl	97.4	99	< 1	< 1
Carbofuran	73.6	97	1	2
Aldicarb	30.0	94	2	4
Nicotine	25.0	94	2	4

LDL, low-density lipoprotein; HDL, high-density lipoprotein.
Source: Adapted from Maliwal BP, Guthrie FE: Chem Biol Interact *35:177–188, 1981.*

Movement of highly lipid soluble compounds is known to occur between different lipoproteins in the plasma, indicating the dynamic nature of binding phenomena. Such distribution may have important consequences in dictating which "pools" ultimately determine toxicity. For example, chlordecone (Kepone) has partitioning characteristics that cause it to bind in the liver whereas DDE, the metabolite of DDT, partitions into fatty depots. Thus, the toxicological implications for these two compounds may be quite different.

Many binding possibilities exist for attachment of a small molecule, such as a toxicant, to a large molecule, such as a blood protein. Although highly specific (high-affinity, low-capacity) binding is more common with drugs, examples of specific binding for toxicants seem less common. It seems probable that low-affinity, high-capacity binding describes most cases of toxicant binding. The number of binding sites can only be estimated, often with considerable error, because of the nonspecific nature of the interaction.

Several factors must be considered regarding the physiological and biological significance of protein binding. The number of ligand molecules bound per protein molecule, and the maximum number of binding sites, n, define the definitive capacity of the protein. Another consideration is the binding affinity $K_{binding}$ (or $1/K_{diss}$). If the protein has only one binding site for the toxicant, a single value, $K_{binding}$, describes the strength of the interaction. Usually more than one binding site is present, each site having its intrinsic binding constant, $k_1, k_2, \ldots, k_n$. Rarely does one find a case where $k_1 = k_2 = \ldots = k_n$, where a single value would describe the affinity constant at all sites. This is especially true when hydrophobic binding and van der Waals forces contribute to nonspecific, low-affinity binding. Obviously, the chemical nature of the binding site is of critical importance in determining binding. The three-dimensional molecular structure of the binding site, the environment of the protein, the general location in the overall protein molecule, and allosteric effects are all factors that influence binding. Studies with toxicants, and even more extensive studies with drugs, have not yet provided an adequate elucidation of these factors. Binding appears to be too complex a phenomenon to be accurately described by any one set of equations.

There are many methods for analyzing binding, but equilibrium dialysis is perhaps the most common. The examples presented here are greatly simplified to avoid the undue confusion engendered by a very complex subject.

Toxicant–protein complexes that utilize relatively weak bonds (energies of the order of hydrogen bonds or less) readily associate and dissociate at physiological temperatures, and the law of mass action applies to the thermodynamic equilibrium.

$$K_{binding} = \frac{[TP]}{[T][P]} = \frac{1}{K_{diss}}$$

where $K_{binding}$ is the equilibrium constant for association, $[TP]$ is the molar concentration of toxicant–protein complex, $[T]$ is the molar concentration of free toxicant, and $[P]$ is the molar concentration of free protein. This equation does not describe the binding site(s) or the binding affinity. To incorporate these parameters and estimate the extent of binding, double-reciprocal plots $1/[TP]$ *versus* $1/[T]$ may be used to test the specificity of binding. Regression lines passing through the origin imply infinite binding, and the validity of calculating an affinity constant under these circumstances is questionable. Figure 2.8a illustrates one such case with four pesticides, and the insert illustrates the low-affinity, "unsaturable" nature of binding in this example.

The two classes of toxicant–protein interactions encountered may be defined as (1) specific, high-affinity, low-capacity; and (2) nonspecific, low-affinity, high-capacity. The term high-affinity implies an affinity constant ($K_{binding}$) of the order of 10^8 M^{-1}, whereas low affinity implies concentrations of 10^4 M^{-1}. Nonspecific, low-affinity binding is probably most characteristic of nonpolar compounds, although most cases are not as extreme as that shown in Fig. 2.8a.

A well-accepted treatment for binding studies is the Scatchard equation:

$$v = \frac{nk[T]}{1 + k[T]}$$

which is simplified for graphic estimates to

$$\frac{v}{[T]} = k(n - v)$$

where v is the moles of ligand (toxicant) bound per mole of protein, $[T]$ is the concentration of free toxicant, k is the intrinsic affinity constant, and n is the number of sites exhibiting such affinity. When $v[T]$ is plotted against v, a straight line is obtained if only one class of binding sites is evident. The slope is $-k$ and the intercept on the v axis becomes n (number of binding sites). If more than one class of sites occurs (probably the most common situation for toxicants), a curve is obtained from which the constants may be obtained. This is illustrated in Fig. 2.8b, for which the data show not one but two species of binding sites: one with low capacity but high affinity and another with about three times the capacity but less affinity. Commonly used computer programs usually solve such data by determining one line for the

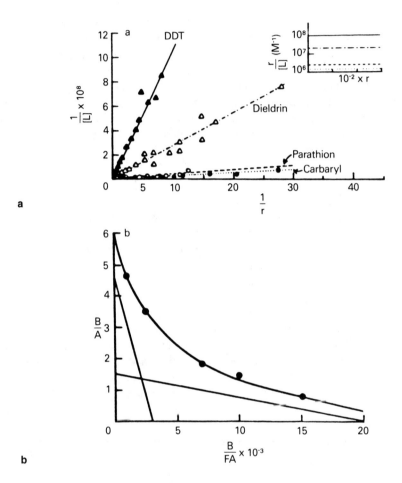

Figure 2.8. Binding of toxicants to blood proteins: (a) Double-reciprocal plot of binding of rat serum lipoprotein fraction with four insecticides. Insert illustrates magnitude of differences in slope with Scatchard plot. (b) Scatchard plot of binding of salicylate to human serum proteins. *(Source: (a) Skalsky and Guthrie, Pest Biochem Physiol 7:289, 1977. (b) Moran and Walker, Biochem Pharmacol 17:153, 1968.)*

specific binding and one line for nonspecific binding, the latter being an average of many possible solutions.

When hydrophobic binding of lipid toxicants occurs, as is the case for many environmental contaminants, binding is probably not limited to a single type of plasma protein. For example, the binding of the chlorinated hydrocarbon DDT is strongest for lipoproteins and albumin, but other proteins account for a significant part of overall transport. Similar results have been seen for several compounds with a range of physiochemical properties.

Protein-binding data are often expressed in terms of the percentage of ligand bound. A factor that must be noted, however, is that as ligand concentration is lowered, the percentage of bound ligand increases. Thus, if a compound has a high affinity for a ligand, as often occurs with albumin, the percentage bound falls sharply when the total ligand concentration (D_T) exceeds a critical value.

Competitive binding for the same sites on a protein can have an important toxicological significance. If a toxicant competes for sites already occupied by a previously applied compound, displacement may result. For example, the anticoagulant warfarin has an important therapeutic value in the treatment of heart disease, but many fatty acids and some drugs also bind to the same site. Concurrently applied phenylbutazone, an anti-inflammatory agent, displaces warfarin, and the resultant increase in free warfarin may appreciably increase anticoagulant effects. Many metals show competitive binding for the metal-binding protein metallothionein.

If a highly toxic compound has a very high affinity, the consequences of such interactions can be very important. For example, assume that compound A has low fractional binding (30%) and compound B displaces 10% of A from the protein. The net increase in free A is negligible (free A increases from 70% to 73%). If A were 98% bound and 10% were displaced, however, free A would increase from 2% to 12%, and a severe reaction might result.

2.9

TOXICODYNAMICS

The dynamic situation involving the constantly changing events following absorption and terminating with excretion is a relatively new field of research best described by appropriate mathematic equations. For this introduction to the subject, a very simplified discussion is presented.

Immediately on entering the body, a chemical begins changing location, concentration, or chemical identity. It may be transported independently by several components of the circulatory system, absorbed by various tissues, or stored; the chemical may effect an action, be detoxified, or be activated; the parent compound or its metabolite(s) may react with body constituents, be stored, or be eliminated—to name some of the more important actions (Fig. 2.9). Each of these processes may be described by rate constants. Thus, at no time is the situation stable but is constantly changing. For instance, how fast is the chemical absorbed? How long is it stored in the fat? How rapidly is it excreted from the body?

The explanation of the kinetics (pharmacokinetics or toxicokinetics) involved in these processes is a highly specialized branch of toxicology. In the physiological sense, one can divide the body into "compartments" that may represent discrete parts of the whole—blood, liver, urine, and so on—or the mathematical model describing the process may be a composite representing the pooling of parts of tissues involved in distribution and bioactivation. Usually pharmacokinetic compartments have no anatomical or physiological identity; they represent all locations within the body that have similar characteristics relative to the dynamics of the particular toxicant. Simple first-order kinetics are usually accepted to describe individual rate processes for the toxicant after entry. The resolution of the model necessitates mathematical estimates (as a function of time) concerning the absorption, distribution,

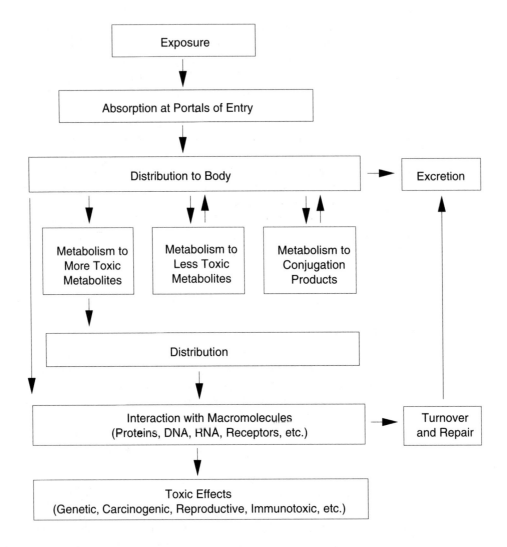

Figure 2.9. Sequence of events following exposure of an animal to exogenous chemicals.

biotransformation, and excretion of toxicant that ultimately provide information relative to innate toxicity. In addition to the chemical and biological processes involved in this complex transformation, physical processes such as diffusion, dissolution, and physical interaction with receptor sites must also be considered.

Thus, complexity is inherent in even the simplest one-compartment case. Measurements of blood and excretory products are usually taken as the simplest and most easily determined experimental parameters. Even here, the situation quickly becomes complex. If a radiolabeled compound is used, is the radioactivity the parent compound or metabolite(s)? Is the compound bound? If so, is it bound to one primary macromolecule or several? What proportion of the changes are occurring in which tissue? Many factors can perturb the dynamics of a toxicant. Some of these are rate of uptake, which can be affected by physical characteristics of the absorbing media; physiological factors, such as blood flow or peristalsis; GI functions, such as emptying and motility; and differences in membranes.

Each factor in the first phase of absorption may cause alteration of a first-order kinetic process, and as distribution and other factors come into play, the phases become the sum of a number of simultaneous and consecutive first-order reactions. A complete kinetic analysis for all routes of administration is a rarity, but the monitoring of blood and urine (and metabolites) is the most simple method of analysis and provides useful information concerning the onset and duration of toxic effects.

Several equations that measure the reaction(s) that occur have been described. One useful equation is

$$\ln \frac{a}{a-x} = kt$$

where a is the initial concentration, x is the amount reacted at time t, and k is a rate constant. A plot of the natural logarithm of the concentration measured at various time intervals against sampling time should yield a straight line of slope k and an intercept on the ordinate axis at 1n of the original concentration. Linearity of the line confirms first-order kinetics. When k has been determined in this way, $t_{0.5}$ can be determined from the relationship $t_{0.5} = 0.693/k$. Proceeding from the simple to the complex situation requires appropriate modifications of the model, but by similar procedures, equations for two-compartment and three-compartment models can be developed (Fig. 2.10). The rapid increase in complexity is illustrated by the observation that 13 different three-compound models are possible. Examination of the selected references is recommended for the interested reader.

The use of linear pharmacokinetics to assess potential bioaccumulation and toxic hazard of 2,3,7,8-tetrachlorodibenzo-p-dioxin (TCDD) is illustrative. TCDD is an unwanted contaminant in the manufacture of several commercial compounds involving reactions of chlorinated phenols. The high toxicity and physicochemical properties of the contaminant suggest that prolonged exposure to small amounts may lead to toxicity. A single dose of 1 µg/kg of TCDD in rats decreased at an apparent first-order rate ($t_{0.5}$ = 21–39 days) with elimination being through the feces. When rats were given 1.0 or 0.1 µg/kg/day, 5 days per week for 7 weeks, the amount of TCDD in the body increased but the rates of increase decreased with time. A plateau effect was noted despite continued exposure (Fig. 2.11). The rate constant for excretion was determined to be 0.0293 day^{-1} (half-life of 23.7 days), and the fraction of each dose absorbed was 0.861. From these values, it was calculated that if a given dose (D) were administered every day for an indefinite time, the steady-state body burden would be 29 times that dose (D × 29).

The calculations show that in the rat, small amounts of TCDD will not accumulate in the body, and this result has been tested experimentally. Whereas 1.0 or

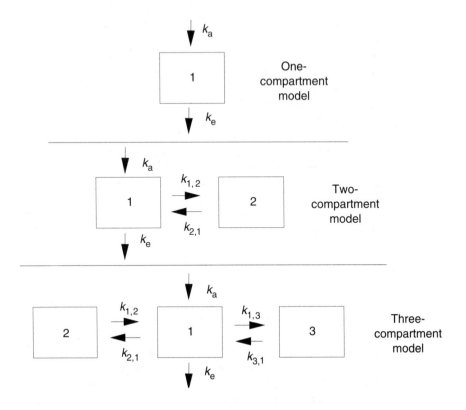

Figure 2.10. Open-compartment toxicokinetic models: k_a is the absorption rate constant and k_e is the excretion rate constant. The other rate constants are for transfers between compartments.

0.1 μg/kg/day caused toxic manifestations (hepatic pathology and functional changes), longer exposure at lower rates (0.01 μg/kg/day) did not cause accumulation. Because TCDD in the tissues reached a plateau within 90 days, more prolonged exposure of amounts < 0.1 μg/kg/day would not be expected to cause toxic levels of TCDD in body tissues.

Physiologically based pharmacokinetic (PBPK) models reflect the incorporation of basic physiology and anatomy. The compartments actually correspond to anatomic entities such as the liver, lung, and so on, and the blood flow conforms to the basic physiological pattern in mammals. The models may be as simple as two compartments or may rise in complexity to as many compartments as is needed. A PBPK model uses physiological and biochemical data to describe the distribution and disposition of chemicals in the body.

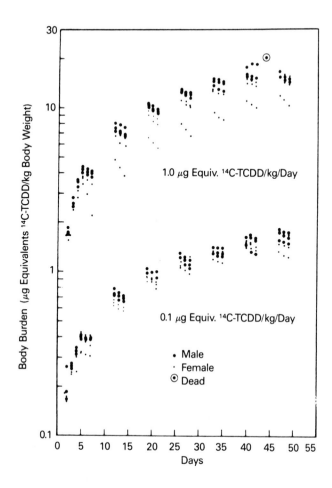

Figure 2.11. Concentration of microgram equivalents of 2,3,7,8-tetrachlorodibenzo-*p*-dioxin (TCDD) in rats given 0.1 or 1.0 μg/kg per day, 5 days per week for 7 weeks.*(Source: Gehring et al. Chapter 8 in Mehlman, Shapiro, Blumenthal, eds. New Concepts in Safety Evaluation, Pt. 1. Washington, DC: Halsted Press, 1976.)*

Suggested Further Reading

Bronough RL, Maibach HI (eds.): *Percutaneous Absorption,* 2nd ed. New York: Marcel Dekker, 1989.

Carrier G, Brunet RC, Brodeur J: Modeling of the toxicokinetics of polychlorinated dibenzo-*p* dioxins and dibenzofurans in mammalians, including humans. II. Kinetics of absorption and disposition of PCDDs/PCDFs. *Toxicol Appl Pharmacol* **131**:267–276, 1995.

Dallas CE, Gallo JM, Ramanathan R, Muralidhars S, Bruckner JV: Physiological pharmacokinetic modeling of inhaled trichloroethylene in rats. *Toxicol Appl Pharmacol* **110**: 303–314, 1991.

Dugard PH: Skin permeability theory in relation to measurements of percutaneous absorption in toxicology. In *Dermatotoxicology,* 2nd ed. Marzulli FN, Maibach HI, (eds.): Washington: Hemisphere, 1983, pp 91–116.

Gargas ML, Burgess RJ, Voisard DJ, Cason GH, Andersen ME: Partition coefficients of low molecular weight volatile compounds in various liquids and tissues. *Toxicol Appl Pharmacol.* **98:**87–99, 1989.

Kragh-Hansen U: Molecular aspects of ligand binding to serum albumin. *Pharmacol Rev* **33:**17–53, 1981.

Krishnan K, Andersen ME, Clewell III HJ, Yang RSH: Physiologically based pharmacokinetic modeling of chemical mixtures. In *Toxicology of Chemical Mixtures.* Yang RSH, (ed.). San Diego: Academic Press, 1994, pp 399–437.

Levy G: Effect of plasma protein binding on renal clearance of drugs. *J Pharmaceut Sci* **69:**482–483, 1980.

O'Flaherty EJ: Physiologically based models for bone-seeking elements. V. Lead absorption and disposition in childhood. *Toxicol Appl Pharmacol* **131:**297–308, 1995.

Riviere JE: Absorption and distribution. In *Introduction to Biochemical Toxicology,* 2nd ed. Hodgson E, Levi PE (eds.). Norwalk, CT: Appleton & Lange, 1994, pp 12–48.

Riviere JE, Bowman KF, Monteiro-Riviere NA, Carver MP, Dix LP: The isolated perfused porcine skin flap (IPPSF). I. A novel in vitro model for percutaneous absorption and cutaneous toxicology studies. *Fundam Appl Toxicol* **7:**444–453, 1986.

Riviere JE, Chang S-K: Transdermal penetration and metabolism of organophosphate insecticides. In *Organophosphates: Chemistry, Fate, and Effects.* Chambers JE, Levi PE (eds.). San Diego: Academic Press, 1992, pp 241–253.

Roxman KK, Klaassen CD: Absorption, distribution, and excretion of toxicants. In *Casarett & Doull's Toxicology, the Basic Science of Poisons,* 5th ed. Klaassen CD (ed.). New York: McGraw-Hill, 1996, pp 91–112.

Webster RC, Maibach HI: In vivo percutaneous absorption and decontamination of pesticides in humans. *J Toxicol Environ Health* **16:**25–37, 1985.

Yang RSH, Anderson ME: Pharmacokinetics. In *Introduction to Biochemical Toxicology,* 2nd ed. Hodgson E, Levi PE. (eds.). Norwalk, CT: Appleton & Lange, 1994, pp 49–73.

3

METABOLISM OF TOXICANTS*

ERNEST HODGSON

3.1

INTRODUCTION

Metabolism by a wide array of enzymes that are capable of using xenobiotics as substrates is the principle means by which the toxicity of endogenous chemicals is modified in vivo, either increased or decreased. This chapter is based on Chapters 4 and 5 in Hodgson and Levi (1994), the material being condensed and updated to reflect more recent findings.

Most xenobiotics that enter the body are lipophilic, a property that enables them to penetrate lipid membranes and to be transported by lipoproteins in the blood. Xenobiotic metabolism consists of two phases. In phase one, a polar reactive group is introduced into the molecule, rendering it a suitable substrate for phase-two enzymes. These latter enzymes bring about conjugations to various endogenous substrates such as sugars, amino acids, and so on, forming exceedingly water-soluble products that are readily excreted. Although this process is generally a detoxication sequence, reactive intermediates may be formed that are much more toxic than the parent compound. It is, however, usually a sequence that increases water solubility and hence decreases $t_{0.5}$ in vivo.

Formation of reactive intermediates is more frequently the case with phase-one monooxygenations because the products are often potent electrophiles capable of reacting with nucleophilic substituents on macromolecules, unless detoxified by some subsequent reaction. In the following discussion, examples of both detoxication and intoxication reactions are given.

---

*Throughout this chapter, cytochrome P450 is abbreviated to P450 and the flavin-containing monooxygenase to FMO.

3.2

PHASE-ONE REACTIONS

Phase-one reactions include microsomal monooxygenations, cytosolic and mito-chondrial oxidations, cooxidations in the prostaglandin synthetase reaction, reductions, hydrolyses, and epoxide hydration. All of these reactions introduce a polar group that, in most cases, can be conjugated during phase-two metabolism. The major phase-one reactions are summarized in Table 3.1.

3.2.1 The Endoplasmic Reticulum, Microsomes, and Monooxygenations

Monooxygenations of xenobiotics are catalyzed either by the cytochrome P450 (P450)–dependent monoxygenase system or by the flavin-containing monooxyge-nase (FMO). Both are located in the endoplasmic reticulum of the cell and have

TABLE 3.1. SUMMARY OF SOME IMPORTANT OXIDATIVE AND REDUCTIVE REACTIONS OF XENOBIOTICS

Enzymes and Reactions	Examples
Cytochrome P450	
Epoxidation/hydroxylation	Aldrin, benzo(a)pyrene, aflatoxin, bromobenzene
N-, O-, S-Dealkylation	Ethylmorphine, atrazine, p-nitroanisole, methylmercaptan
N-, S-, P-Oxidation	Thiobenzamide, chlorpromazine, 2-acetylaminofluorene
Desulfuration	Parathion, carbon disulfide
Dehalogenation	Carbon tetrachloride, chloroform
Nitro reduction	Nitrobenzene
Azo reduction	O-Aminoazotoluene
Flavin-containing monooxygenase	
N-, S-, P-Oxidation	Nicotine, imiprimine, thiourea, methimazole
Desulfuration	Fonofos
Prostaglandin synthetase cooxidation	
Dehydrogenation	Acetaminophen, benzidine, epinephrine
N-Dealkylation	Benzphetamine, dimethylaniline
Epoxidation/hydroxylation	Benzo(a)pyrene, 2-aminofluorene, phenylbutazone
Oxidation	FANFT, ANFT, bilirubin
Molybdenum hydroxylases	
Oxidations	Purines, pteridine, methotrexate, 6-deoxycyclovir
Reductions	Aromatic nitrocompounds, azo dyes, nitrosoamines
Alcohol dehydrogenase	
Oxidation	Methanol, ethanol, glycols, glycol ethers
Reduction	Aldehydes and ketones
Aldehyde dehydrogenase	
Oxidation	Aldehydes resulting from alcohol and glycol oxidations
Esterases and amidases	
Hydrolysis	Parathion, paraoxon, dimethoate
Epoxide hydrolase	
Hydrolysis	Benzo(a)pyrene epoxide, styrene oxide

been studied in many tissues and organisms. This is particularly true of P450, probably the most studied of all enzymes.

Microsomes are derived from the endoplasmic reticulum as a result of tissue homogenization and are isolated by ultracentrifugation of the postmitochondrial supernatant fraction. The endoplasmic reticulum is an anastomosing network of lipoprotein membranes extending from the plasma membrane to the nucleus and mitochondria, whereas the microsomal fraction derived from it consists of membranous vesicles contaminated with free ribosomes, glycogen granules, and fragments of other subcellular structures such as mitochondria and Golgi apparatus. The endoplasmic reticulum, and consequently the microsomes derived from it, consists of two types, rough and smooth, the former having the outer membrane studded with ribosomes, which the latter characteristically lack. Although both rough and smooth microsomes have all the components of the P450–dependent monooxygenase system, the specific activity of the smooth type is usually higher.

Monooxygenations, also previously known as mixed-function oxidations, are those oxidations in which one atom of a molecule of oxygen is incorporated into the substrate while the other is reduced to water. Because the electrons involved in the reduction of P450 or flavin enzymes are derived from NADPH, the overall reaction can be written as follows (where RH is the substrate):

$$RH + O_2 + NADPH + H^+ \longrightarrow NADP^+ + ROH + H_2O$$

3.2.2 The Cytochrome P450-Dependent Monooxygenase System

The cytochrome P450s, the carbon monoxide–binding pigments of microsomes, are hemoproteins of the b cytochrome type. Originally described as a single protein, there are now known to be more than 400 P450s, widely distributed throughout animals, plants, and microorganisms. A new system of nomenclature utilizing the prefix CYP has been devised for the genes and cDNAs corresponding to the different forms (see Section 3.2.2.3—Classification and Evolution of Cytochrome P450), although P450 is still appropriate as a prefix for the protein products. Unlike most cytochromes, the name cytochrome P450 is derived, not from the absorption maximum of the reduced form in the visible region but from the unique wavelength of the absorption maximum of the carbon monoxide derivative of the reduced form, namely 450 nm.

The role of P450 as the terminal oxidase in monooxygenase reactions is supported by considerable evidence. The initial proof was derived from the demonstration of the concomitant light reversibility of the CO complex of cytochrome P450 and the inhibition, by CO, of the C-21 hydroxylation of 17 α-hydroxy-progesterone by adrenal gland microsomes. This was followed by a number of indirect but nevertheless convincing proofs involving the effects on both P450 and monooxygenase activity of CO, inducing agents, spectra resulting from ligand binding, and the loss of activity on degradation of P450 to P420. Direct proof was subsequently provided by the demonstration that monooxygenase systems, reconstituted from apparently homogenous purified P450, NADPH-P450 reductase, and phosphatidyl-choline, can catalyze many monooxygenase reactions.

Cytochrome P450s, like other hemoproteins, have characteristic absorptions in the visible region. The addition of many organic, and some inorganic, ligands results in perturbations of this spectrum. Although the detection and measurement of these spectra requires a high-resolution spectrophotometer, these perturbations, measured as optical difference spectra, have been of tremendous use in the characterization of P450, particularly in the decades preceding the molecular cloning and expression of specific P450 isoforms.

The most important difference spectra of oxidized P450 are type I, with an absorption maximum at 385–390 nm and a minimum near 420 nm; and type II, with a peak at 420–435 nm and a trough at 390–410 nm. Type I ligands are found in many different chemical classes and include drugs, environmental contaminants, insecticides, and so on. They appear to be generally unsuitable, on chemical grounds, as ligands for the heme iron and are believed to bind to a hydrophobic site in the protein that is close enough to the heme to allow both spectral perturbation and interaction with the activated oxygen. Although most type I ligands are substrates, it has not been possible to demonstrate a quantitative relationship between K_s (concentration required for half-maximal spectral development) and K_m (Michaelis constant). Type II ligands, however, interact directly with the heme iron of P450 and are associated with organic compounds having nitrogen atoms with sp^2 or sp^3 nonbonded electrons that are sterically accessible. Such ligands are frequently inhibitors of P450 activity.

The two most important difference spectra of reduced P450 are the well-known CO spectrum, with its maximum at or about 450 nm, and the type III spectrum, with two pH-dependent peaks at approximately 430 nm and 455 nm. The CO spectrum forms the basis for the quantitative estimation of P450. The best known type III ligands for P450 are ethyl isocyanide and compounds such as the methylenedioxyphenyl synergists and SKF-525A, the last two forming stable type III complexes that appear to be related to the mechanism by which they inhibit monooxygenations.

In the catalytic cycle of P450, reducing equivalents are transferred from NADPH to P450 by a flavoprotein enzyme known as NADPH–P450 reductase. The evidence that this enzyme is involved in P450 monooxygenations was originally derived from the observation that cytochrome c, which can function as an artificial electron acceptor for the enzyme, is an inhibitor of such oxidations. This reductase is an essential component in P450 catalyzed enzyme systems reconstituted from purified components. Moreover, antibodies prepared from purified reductase are inhibitors of microsomal monooxygenase reactions. The reductase is a flavoprotein of approximately 80,000 daltons that contains 1 mole each of flavin mononucleotide (FMN) and flavinadevine dinucleotide (FAD) per mole of enzyme. The only other component necessary for activity in the reconstituted system is a phospholipid, phosphatidylcholine. This is not involved directly in electron transfer but appears to be involved in the coupling of the reductase to the cytochrome and in the binding of the substrate to the cytochrome.

The mechanism of P450 function has not been established unequivocally; however, the generally recognized steps are shown in Fig. 3.1. The initial step consists of the binding of substrate to oxidized P450 followed by a one-electron reduction catalyzed by NADPH–P450 reductase to form a reduced cytochrome substrate complex. This complex can interact with CO to form the CO-complex, which gives rise to the well-known difference spectrum with a peak at 450 nm and also inhibits monooxygenase activity. The next several steps are less well understood. They involve an initial interaction with molecular oxygen to form a ternary oxygenated complex. This ternary complex accepts a second electron, resulting in the further formation of one or more poorly understood complexes. One of these, however, is probably the equivalent of the peroxide anion derivative of the substrate-bound hemoprotein. Under some conditions, this complex may break down to yield hydrogen peroxide and the oxidized cytochrome substrate complex. Normally, however, one atom of molecular oxygen is transferred to the substrate and the other is reduced to water, followed by dismutation reactions leading to the formation of the oxygenated product, water, and the oxidized cytochrome.

The possibility that the second electron is derived from NADH through cytochrome b_5 has been the subject of argument for some time and has yet to be

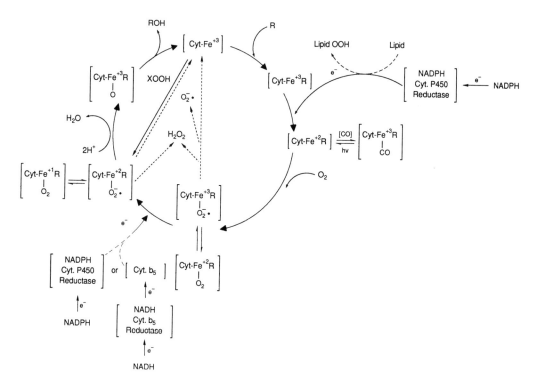

Figure 3.1. Generalized scheme showing the sequence of events for P450 monooxygenations.

completely resolved. Cytochrome b_5 is a widely distributed microsomal heme protein that is involved in metabolic reactions such as fatty acid desaturation that involve endogenous substrates. It is clear, however, that cytochrome b_5 is not essential for all P450–dependent monooxygenations because many occur in systems reconstituted from NADPH, O_2, phosphatidylcholine and highly purified P450 and NADPH–P450 reductase. Nevertheless, cytochrome b_5 is stimulatory in some cases and this stimulation is isoform and/or substrate specific. Thus, cytochrome b_5 may facilitate oxidative activity in the intact endoplasmic reticulum. The isolation of forms of P450 that bind avidly to cytochrome b_5 also tends to support this idea.

3.2.2.1   *Distribution of Cytochrome P450*

In vertebrates, the liver is the richest source of P450 and is most active in the monooxygenation of xenobiotics. P450 and other components of the P450–dependent monooxygenase system are found also in the skin, nasal mucosa, lung, and gastrointestinal tract (GI) tract, presumably reflecting the evolution of defense mechanisms at portals of entry. In addition to these organs, P450 has been demonstrated in the kidney, adrenal cortex and medulla, placenta, testes, ovaries, fetal and embryonic liver, corpus luteum, aorta, blood platelets, and the nervous system. In humans, P450 has been demonstrated in the fetal and adult liver, the placenta, kidney, testes, fetal and adult adrenal gland, skin, blood platelets, and lymphocytes.

Although P450s are found in many tissues, the function of the particular subset of isoforms in a particular organ, tissue, or cell type does not appear to be the same in all cases. In the liver, P450s oxidize a large number of xenobiotics as well as some endogenous steroids and bile pigments. The P450s of the lung also appear to be concerned primarily with xenobiotic oxidation, although the range of substrates is more limited than that of the liver. The skin and small intestine also carry out xenobiotic oxidations, but their activities have been less well characterized. In normal pregnant females, the placental microsomes display little or no ability to oxidize foreign compounds, appearing to function as a steroid hormone metabolizing system. On induction of the P450 enzymes, such as occurs in pregnant women who smoke, P450–catalyzed aryl hydrocarbon hydroxylase activity is readily apparent. The P450s of the kidney are active in the ω-oxidation of fatty acids, such as lauric acid, but are relatively inactive in xenobiotic oxidation. Mitochondrial P450s, such as those of the placenta and adrenal cortex, are active in the oxidation of steroid hormones rather than xenobiotics.

Distribution of P450s within the cell has been studied primarily in the mammalian liver, where it is present in greatest quantity in the smooth endoplasmic reticulum and in smaller but appreciable quantities in the rough endoplasmic reticulum. The nuclear membrane has also been reported to contain P450 and to have detectable aryl hydrocarbon hydroxylase activity, an observation that may be of considerable importance in studies of the metabolic activation of carcinogens.

3.2.2.2   *Multiplicity of Cytochrome P450, Purification, and Reconstitution of P450 Activity*

Even before appreciable purification of cytochrome P450 had been accomplished, it was already apparent from indirect evidence that mammalian liver cells contained more than one P450 enzyme. Subsequent direct evidence on the multiplicity of P450s included the separation and purification of P450 isozymes, distinguished from each other by chromatographic behavior, immunologic specificity, and/or substrate specificity after reconstitution and separation of distinct polypeptides by sodium dodecyl sulfate polyacrylamide gel electrophoresis (SDS-PAGE), which could then be related to distinct P450s present in the original microsomes. These different P450s probably have specific locations within the cell because microsomal fractions of different densities show qualitative differences in spectral characteristics related to P450.

Considerations of isoform multiplicity are of importance in several areas of toxicology, including developmental changes, sex differences, inhibition, induction, and comparative toxicology. Any of these effects on P450 or monooxygenase activity could involve specific expression of different P450s, specificity differences between the different cytochromes expressed or different proportions of the same cytochromes. Multiplicity of P450 in different organisms, organs, tissues, and cell types may be considered the usual state of affairs rather than the exception.

Purification of P450 and its constituent isoforms was, for many years, an elusive goal; one, however, that has been largely resolved. The problem of instability on solubilization was resolved by the use of glycerol and dithiothreitol as protectants, and the problem of reaggregation by maintaining a low concentration of a suitable detergent, such as Emulgen 911 (Kao-Atlas, Tokyo), throughout the procedure. Multiple forms, as discussed previously, may be separated from each other and purified as separate entities, although individual isoforms are now frequently cloned and expressed as single entities. It has been possible to purify P450 as well as NADPH–P450 reductase from mammalian liver, lung, and other tissues as well as from other organisms from several different taxonomic groups.

Systems reconstituted from purified P450, NADPH–P450 reductase and phosphatidylcholine will, in the presence of NADPH and O_2, oxidize xenobiotics such as benzphetamine, often at rates comparable to microsomes. Although systems reconstituted from this minimal number of components are enzymatically active, other microsomal components, such as cytochrome b_5, may facilitate activity either in vivo or in vitro or may even be essential for the oxidation of certain substrates.

One important finding from purification studies as well as cloning and expressing of individual isoforms is that the lack of substrate specificity of microsomes for monooxygenase activity is not an artifact caused by the presence of several specific cytochromes because it appears that many of the cytochromes isolated are relatively nonspecific. The relative activity toward different substrates does, however, vary greatly from one P450 isoform to another even when both are relatively nonspecific. This lack of specificity is illustrated in Table 3.2, using human isoforms as examples.

TABLE 3.2. SOME IMPORTANT HUMAN CYTOCHROME P450 ISOZYMES AND SELECTED SUBSTRATES

P450	Drugs	Carcinogens/Toxicants/ Endogenous Substrates	Diagnostic Substrates In Vivo [In Vitro]
1A1	Verlukast (very few drugs)	Benzo(a)pyrene, dimethylbenz(a)anthracene	[Ethoxyresorufin, benzo(a)pyrene]
1A2	Phenacetin, theophylline, acetamino-phen, warfarin, caffeine, cimetidine	Aromatic amines, arylhydrocarbons, NNK,[a] aflatoxin, estradiol	Caffeine, [acetanilide, methoxy-resorufin, ethoxyresorufin]
2A6	Coumarin, nicotine	Aflatoxin, diethylnitrosamine, NNK[a]	Coumarin
2B6	Cyclophosphamide, ifosphamide, nicotine	6 Aminochrysene, aflatoxin, NNK[a]	[7-ethoxy-4-trifluoro-methyl coumarin]
2C8	Taxol, tolbutamide, carbamazepine	—	[Chloromethyl fluorescein diethyl ether]
2C9	Tienilic acid, tolbutamide, warfarin, phenytoin, THC, hexobarbital, diclofenac	—	[Diclofenac (4'-OH)]
2C19	S-Mephenytoin, diazepam, phenytoin, omeprazole, indomethacin, impramine, propanolol, proguanil	—	[S-Mephentoin (4'-OH)]
2D6	Debrisosquine, sparteine, bufuralol, propanolol, thioridazine, quinidine, phenytoin, fluoxetine, numerous other drugs	NNK[a]	Dextromethorphan, [bufuralol (4'-OH)]
2E1	Chlorzoxazone, isoniazid, acetamino-phen, halothane, enflurane, meth-oxyflurane	Dimethylnitrosamine, benzene, halogenated alkanes (eg, CCl$_4$), acrylonitrile, alcohols, aniline, stryene, vinyl chloride	Chlorzoxazone (6-OH), [p-nitrophenol]
3A4	Nifedipine, ethylmorphine, warfarin, quinidine, taxol, ketoconazole, verapamil, erythromycin, diazepam, numerous other drugs	Aflatoxin, 1-nitropyrene, benzo(a)pyrene 7,8-diol, 6 aminochrysene, estradiol, progesterone, testosterone, other steroids, bile acids	Erythromycin, nifedipine, [testosterone (6-β)]
4A9/11	(Very few drugs)	fatty acids, prostaglandins, thromboxane, prostacyclin	[Lauric acid]

[a]NNK = 4-(methylnitrosamino)-1-(3-pyridyl)-1-butanone, a tobacco-smoke specific nitrosamine.

3.2.2.3 Classification and Evolution of Cytochrome P450

The techniques of molecular biology have been applied extensively to the study of P450. More than 400 genes have been characterized as of 1996, and the nucleotide and derived amino acid sequences compared. In some cases the location of the gene on a particular chromosome has been determined and the mechanism of gene expression investigated.

A system of nomenclature was proposed in 1987 and has been updated several times since, most recently in 1996. Under the most recent update of the system, P450 genes are designated *CYP* (or *cyp* in the case of mouse genes). This is followed by an arabic numeral designating the gene family, a letter designating the subfamily when more than one subfamily exists within the family, and finally, an arabic numeral designating the individual gene. If there are no subfamilies or if there is only a single gene within the family or subfamily, the letter and/or the sec-

TABLE 3.3. AN EXAMPLE OF NOMENCLATURE FOR CYTOCHROME P450 GENES AND GENE PRODUCTS

Gene symbol	Gene product	Trivial name	Species
CYP1A1	P4501A1 or CYP1A1	c, βNF-B	Rat
		P_1, c	Human
		form 6	Rabbit
		Dah1	Dog
Cyp1a-1	P4501A1 or CYP1A1	P_1	Mouse
CYP1A2	P4501A2 or CYP1A2	P-448, d, HCB	Rat
		P_3, d	Human
		LM_4	Rabbit
		Dah2	Dog
Cyp1a-2	P4501A2 or CYP1A2	P_2, P_3	Mouse

ond numeral may be omitted (eg, *CYP17*). The name of the gene is italicized, whereas the protein (enzyme) is not.

The protein sequence of any member of a gene family is equal to or less than 40% similar to that of any member of any other gene family. Protein sequences within subfamilies are greater than 55% similar in the case of mammalian genes, or 46% in the case of nonmammalian genes. So far, genes in the same subfamily have been found to lie on the same chromosome within the same gene cluster and are nonsegregating, suggesting a common origin through gene duplication events. Sequences showing less than 3% divergence are arbitrarly designated allelic variants unless other evidence exists to the contrary.

The genes' products, the P450 isoforms, may still be designated P450 followed by the same numbering system used for the genes, or the CYP designation may be used: for example, P4501A1 or CYP1A1. Common names may still be used, although this is not recommended, provided that no use is made of hyphens, subscripts, or superscripts. An example of this system of classification is shown in Table 3.3 and the rate and extent of P450 evolution is shown in Fig. 3.2.

3.2.2.4 *Cytochrome P450 Reactions*

Although microsomal monooxygenase reactions are basically similar in the role played by molecular oxygen and in the supply of electrons, the many P450 isoforms are nonspecific, with both substrates and products falling into many different chemical classes. In the following sections, therefore, these activities are classified on the basis of the overall chemical reaction catalyzed; one should bear in mind, however, that not only do these classes often overlap, but often a substrate may also undergo more than one reaction. See Table 3.1 for a listing of important oxidation and reduction reactions of P450.

EPOXIDATION AND AROMATIC HYDROXYLATION. Epoxidation is an extremely important microsomal reaction because not only can stable and environmentally persistent epoxides be formed (see aliphatic epoxidations, later in this chapter), but highly reactive intermediates of aromatic hydroxylations, such as arene oxides, can also be produced.

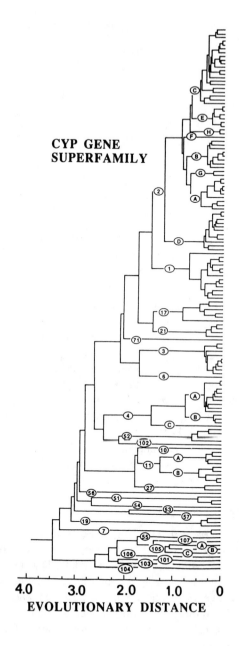

CYP GENE SUPERFAMILY

EVOLUTIONARY DISTANCE

Figure 3.2. Schematic of cytochrome P450 superfamily. *(Source: Nebert et al, DNA and Cell Biol **10:**1–14, 1991.)*

These highly reactive intermediates are known to be involved in chemical carcinogenesis as well as a chemically induced cellular and tissue necrosis.

The oxidation of naphthalene was one of the earliest examples of an epoxide as an intermediate in aromatic hydroxylations. As shown in Fig. 3.3, the epoxide can rearrange nonenzymatically to yield predominantly 1-naphthol, can interact with the enzyme epoxide hydrolase to yield the dihydrodiol, or can interact with glutathione *S*-transferase to yield the glutathione conjugate, which is ultimately metabolized to a mercapturic acid. These reactions are also of importance in the metabolism of other xenobiotics that contain an aromatic nucleus, such as the insecticide carbaryl and the carcinogen benzo(a)pyrene.

The ultimate carcinogens arising from the metabolic activation of benzo(a)pyrene are stereoisomers of benzo(a)pyrene 7,8-diol-9,10-epoxide (Fig. 3.3). These metabolites arise by prior formation of the 7,8-epoxide, which gives rise to the 7,8-dihydrodiol through the action of epoxide hydrolase. This is further me-

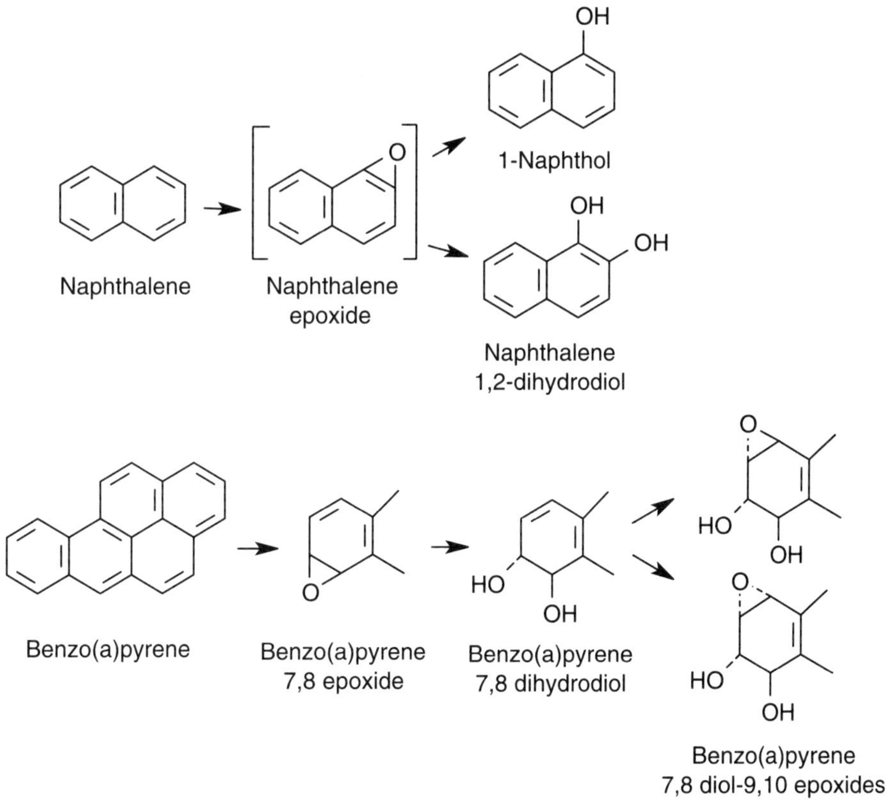

Figure 3.3. Examples of epoxidation and aromatic hydroxylation.

tabolized by the P450 to the 7,8-diol-9,10-epoxides, which are both potent muta-gens and unsuitable substrates for the further action of epoxide hydrolase. Stereo-chemistry is important in the toxicity of the final product. Of the four possible iso-mers of the diol epoxide, the (+)-benzo(a)pyrene diol epoxide-2 is the most active carcinogen.

ALIPHATIC HYDROXYLATION. Although simple aliphatic molecules such as *n*-butane, *n*-pentane, *n*-hexane, and so on, as well as alicyclic compounds such as cyclohexane, are known to be oxidized to alcohols, alkyl side chains of aromatic compounds are more readily oxidized, often at more than one position, and provide good examples of this type of oxidation. The *n*-propyl side chain of *n*-propyl benzene can be oxidized at any one of the three carbons to yield 3-phenylpropan-1-ol ($C_6H_5CH_2CH_2CH_2OH$) by ω-oxidation, benzylmethyl carbinol ($C_6H_5CH_2CHOHCH_3$) by ω-1 oxidation, and ethyl-phenylcarbinol ($C_6H_5CHOHCH_2CH_3$) by α-oxidation. Further oxidation of these alco-hols is also possible.

ALIPHATIC EPOXIDATION. Many aliphatic and alicyclic compounds containing unsaturated carbon atoms are thought to be metabolized to epoxide intermediates (Fig. 3.4). In the case of aldrin, the product, dieldrin, is an extremely stable epoxide and repre-sents the principal residue found in animals exposed to aldrin. Epoxide formation in the case of aflatoxin is believed to be the final step in formation of the ultimate car-cinogenic species and is, therefore, an activation reaction.

DEALKYLATION: *O-*, *N-*, AND *S-*DEALKYLATION. Probably the best known example of *O*-dealkyla-tion is the demethylation of *p*-nitroanisole. Due to the ease with which the product, *p*-nitrophenol, can be measured, it is a frequently used substrate for the demonstra-

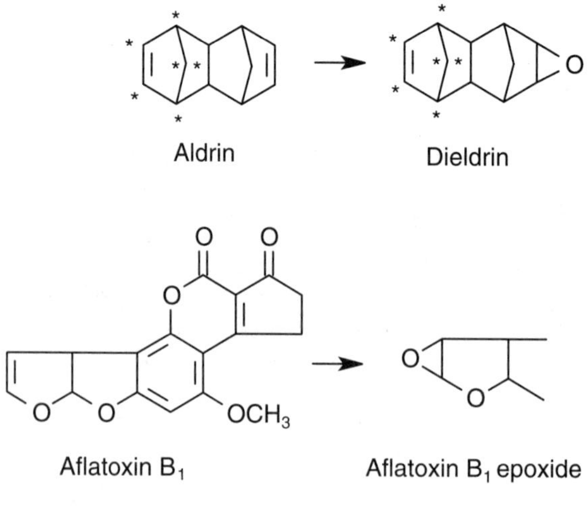

Aldrin   Dieldrin

Aflatoxin B$_1$ Aflatoxin B$_1$ epoxide

Figure 3.4. Examples of aliphatic epoxidation.

tion of P450 activity. The reaction is believed to proceed by an unstable methylol intermediate (Fig. 3.5).

The *O*-dealkylation of organophosphorus triesters differs from that of *p*-nitroanisole in that it involves the dealkylation of an ester rather than an ether. The reaction was first described for the insecticide chlorfenvinphos and is known to occur with a wide variety of vinyl, phenyl, phenylvinyl, and naphthyl phosphate and thionophosphate triesters (Fig. 3.5).

N-Dealkylation is a common reaction in the metabolism of drugs, insecticides, and other xenobiotics. The drug ethylmorphine is a useful model compound for this reaction. In this case, the methyl group is oxidized to formaldehyde, which can be readily detected by the Nash reaction.

S-Dealkylation is believed to occur with a number of thioethers, including methylmercaptan and 6-methylthiopurine, although with newer knowledge of the specificity of the flavin-containing monooxygenase (see Section 3.2.2.4), it is possible that the initial attack is through sulfoxidation mediated by FMO rather than P450.

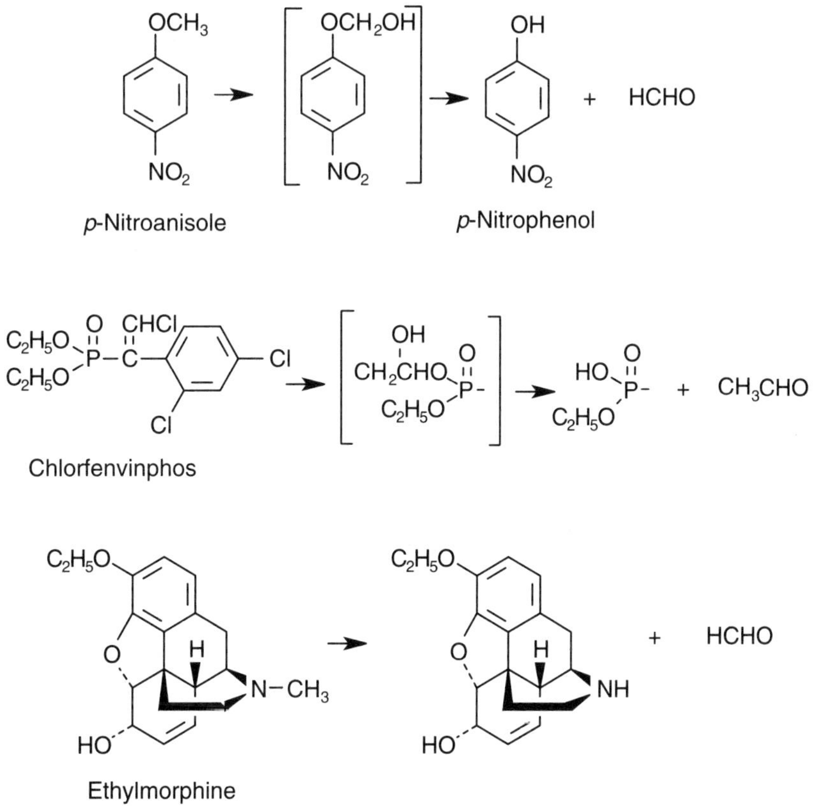

Figure 3.5. Examples of dealkylation.

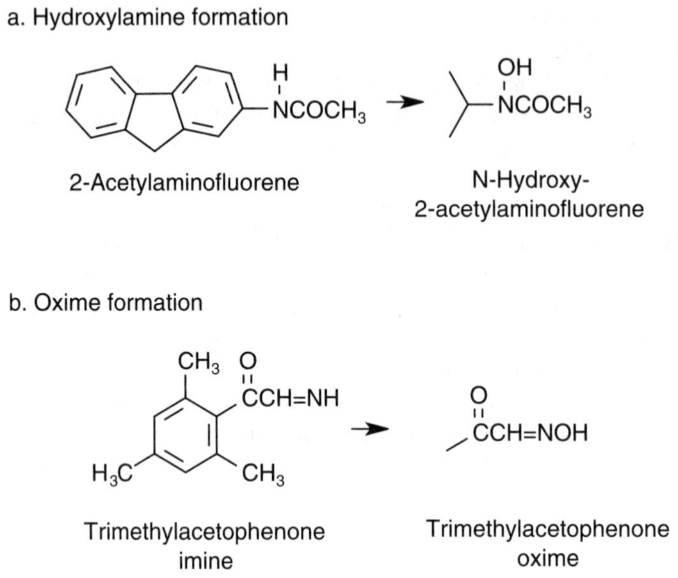

a. Hydroxylamine formation

2-Acetylaminofluorene

N-Hydroxy-
2-acetylaminofluorene

b. Oxime formation

Trimethylacetophenone
imine

Trimethylacetophenone
oxime

Figure 3.6. Examples of N-oxidation.

N-OXIDATION. N-Oxidation can occur in a number of ways, including hydroxylamine formation, oxime formation, and N-oxide formation, although the latter is primarily dependent on the FMO enzyme. Hydroxylamine formation occurs with a number of amines such as aniline and many of its substituted derivatives. In the case of 2-acetylaminofluorene, the product is a potent carcinogen and thus the reaction is an activation reaction (Fig. 3.6).

Oximes can be formed by the N-hydroxylation of imines and primary amines. Imines have been suggested as intermediates in the formation of oximes from primary amines (Fig. 3.6).

OXIDATIVE DEAMINATION. Oxidative deamination of amphetamine occurs in the rabbit liver but not to any extent in the liver of either the dog or the rat, which tend to hydroxylate the aromatic ring. A close examination of the reaction indicates that it is probably not an attack on the nitrogen but rather on the adjacent carbon atom, giving rise to a carbinol amine, which eliminates ammonia, producing a ketone.

$$R_2CHNH_2 \xrightarrow{O} R_2C(OH)NH_2 \xrightarrow{-NH_3} R_2C=O$$

The carbinol, by another reaction sequence, can also give rise to an oxime, which can be hydrolyzed to yield the ketone, which is thus formed by two different routes.

$$R_2C(OH)NH_2 \xrightarrow{-H_2O} R_2C=NH \xrightarrow{+O} R_2CNOH \xrightarrow{+H_2O} R_2C=O$$

S-OXIDATION. Thioethers in general are oxidized by microsomal monooxygenases to sulfoxides, some of which are further oxidized to sulfones. This reaction is very common among insecticides of several different chemical classes, including carbamates, organophosphates, and chlorinated hydrocarbons. The organophosphates include phorate, demeton, and others, whereas among the chlorinated hydrocarbons, endosulfan is oxidized to endosulfan sulfate and methiochlor to a series of sulfoxides and sulfones, eventually yielding the *bis*-sulfone. Among carbamates, methiocarb yields the sulfoxide and sulfone, and drugs such as chloropromazine and solvents such as dimethyl sulfoxide are also subject to *S*-oxidation. The current knowledge that the FMO is also a versatile sulfur oxidase carrying out many of the previously mentioned reactions raises important questions as to the relative role of this enzyme versus that of P450. Thus, a reexamination of earlier work in which many of these reactions were ascribed to P450 is required.

P-OXIDATION. *P*-Oxidation, a little-known reaction, involves the conversion of trisubstituted phosphines to phosphine oxides, for example, diphenylmethylphosphine to diphenylmethylphosphine oxide. Although described as a typical P450–dependent monooxygenation, it too is now known to be catalyzed by the FMO also.

DESULFURATION AND ESTER CLEAVAGE. The phosphorothionate $[(R^1O)_2P(S)OR^2]$ and phosphorodithioate $[(R^1O)_2P(S)SR^2]$ owe their insecticidal activity and their mammalian toxicity to an oxidative reaction in which the P=S group is converted to P=O, thereby converting the compounds from chemicals relatively inactive toward cholinesterases into potent cholinesterase inhibitors (see Chapter 7 for a discussion of the mechanism of cholinesterase inhibition). This reaction is known for many organophosphorus compounds but has been studied most intensively in the case of parathion. Much of the splitting of the phosphorus ester bonds in organophosphorus insecticides, formerly believed to be due to hydrolysis, is now known to be due to oxidative dearylation. This is a typical P450–dependent monooxygenation, requiring NADPH and O_2 and being inhibited by CO. Current evidence supports the hypothesis that this reaction and oxidative desulfuration involve a common intermediate of the "phosphooxithirane" type (Fig. 3.7). Some organophosphorus insecticides, all phosphonates, are activated by the FMO as well as by P450.

METHYLENEDIOXY (BENZODIOXOLE) RING CLEAVAGE. Methylenedioxyphenyl compounds, such as safrole or the insecticide synergist, piperonyl butoxide, many of which are effective inhibitors of P450 monooxygenations, are themselves metabolized to catechols. The most probable mechanism appears to be an attack on the methylene carbon, followed by elimination of water to yield a carbene. The highly reactive carbene either reacts with the heme iron to form a P450–inhibitory complex or breaks down to yield the catechol (Fig. 3.8).

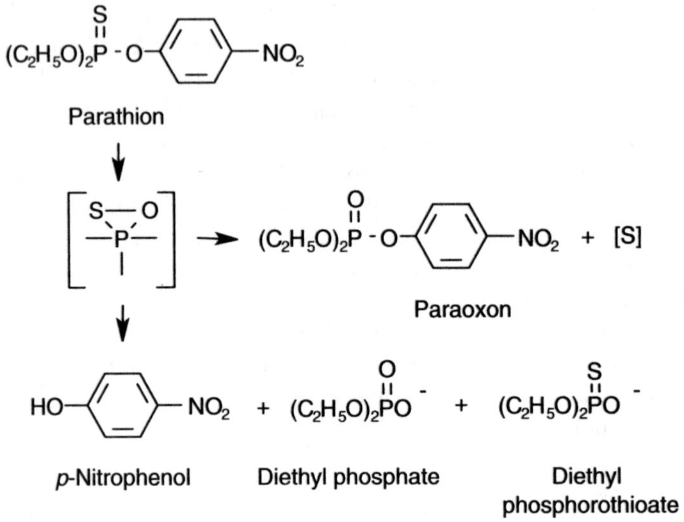

Figure 3.7. Desulfuration and oxidative dearylation.

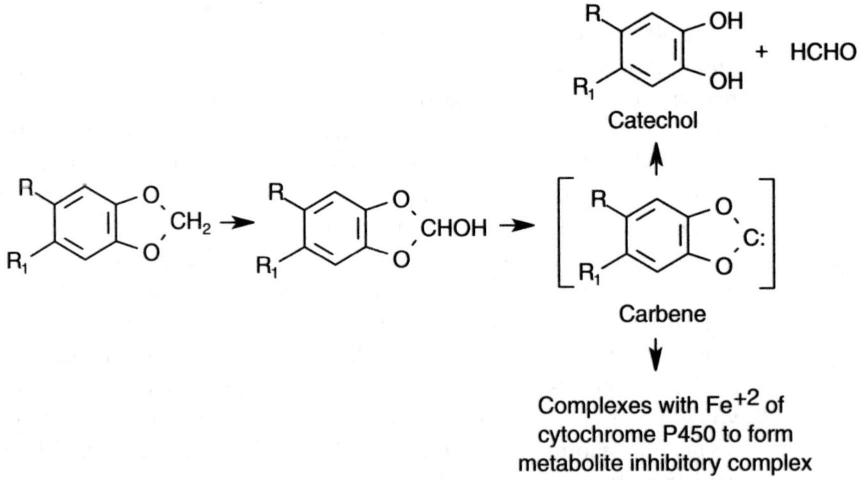

Figure 3.8. Monooxygenation of methylenedioxyphenyl compounds.

3.2.3 The Flavin-containing Monooxygenase

Tertiary amines such as trimethylamine and dimethylaniline had long been known to be metabolized to N-oxides by a microsomal amine oxidase that was not dependent on P450. This enzyme, now known as the microsomal flavin-containing monooxygenase, is also dependent on NADPH and O_2, and has been purified to homogeneity from a number of species. It has a monomeric molecular mass of about 56,000/mol of FAD.

The FMO is now known to have a much wider substrate specificity than formerly supposed. It includes tertiary and secondary amines as well as a number of different types of sulfur compounds such as sulfides, thioethers, thiols, and thiocarbamates. More recently still, this enzyme has been shown to attack organophosphorus compounds in the case of phosphines and in the activation of phosphonates to their oxons (Fig. 3.9).

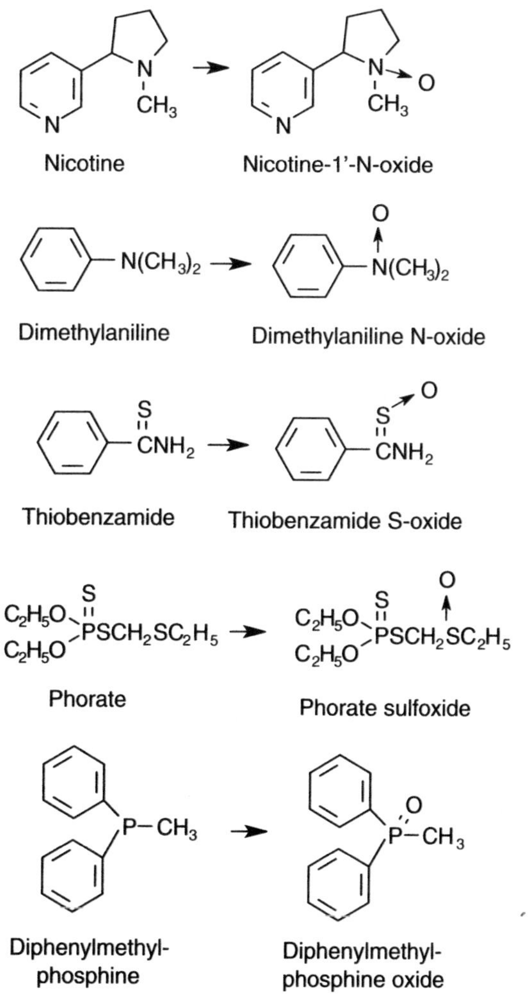

Figure 3.9. Examples of oxidations catalyzed by the flavin-containing monooxygenase (FMO).

Many of these compounds are also known to be substrates for P450, and current research is being directed toward an assessment of the relative importance of P450 and the FMO in both detoxication and activation reactions.

Toxicologically, it is of interest that this enzyme is responsible for the oxidation of nicotine to nicotine-1'-N-oxide, whereas the oxidation of nicotine to cotinine is catalyzed by two enzymes acting in sequence: P450 and a soluble aldehyde dehydrogenase. Thus, nicotine is metabolized by two different routes, the relative contributions of which may vary with both the extrinsic and intrinsic factors outlined in Chapter 6.

3.2.4 Nonmicrosomal Oxidations

In addition to the microsomal monooxygenases, other enzymes are involved in the oxidation of xenobiotics. These enzymes are located in the mitochondria or in the soluble cytoplasm of the cell.

3.2.4.1 Alcohol Dehydrogenases

Alcohol dehydrogenases catalyze the conversion of alcohols to aldehydes or ketones:

$$RCH_2OH + NAD^+ \longrightarrow RCHO + NADH + H^+$$

This reaction should not be confused with the monooxygenation of ethanol by P450 that occurs in the microsomes. The alcohol dehydrogenase reaction is reversible, with the carbonyl compounds being reduced to alcohols.

This enzyme is found in the soluble fraction of the liver, kidney, and lung and is probably the most important enzyme involved in the metabolism of foreign alcohols. Alcohol dehydrogenase is a dimer, the subunits of which can occur in several forms that are under genetic control, thus giving rise to a large number of variants of the enzyme. It can use either NAD or NADP as a coenzyme, but the reaction proceeds at a much slower rate with NADP. In the intact organism, the reaction proceeds in the direction of alcohol consumption, because aldehydes are further oxidized to acids. Because aldehydes are toxic and are not readily excreted because of their lipophilicity, alcohol oxidation may be considered an activation reaction, the further oxidation of the aldehyde to an acid being a detoxication step.

Primary alcohols are oxidized to aldehydes, n-butanol being the substrate oxidized at the highest rate. Although secondary alcohols are oxidized to ketones, the rate is less than that for primary alcohols, and tertiary alcohols are not readily oxidized. Alcohol dehydrogenase is inhibited by a number of heterocyclic compounds such as pyrazole, imidazole, and their derivatives.

3.2.4.2 Aldehyde Dehydrogenases

This enzyme catalyzes the formation of acids from aliphatic and aromatic aldehydes; the acids are then available as substrates for conjugating enzymes:

$$RCHO + NAD^+ \longrightarrow RCOOH + NADH + H^+$$

The enzyme from mammalian liver has been isolated, and many aldehydes can serve as substrates. Other enzymes in the soluble fraction of liver that oxidize aldehydes are aldehyde oxidase and xanthine oxidase, both flavoproteins that contain molybdenum; however, their primary role seems to be the oxidation of endogenous aldehydes formed as a result of deamination reactions.

3.2.4.3   *Amine Oxidases*

The most important function of amine oxidases appears to be the oxidation of amines formed during normal processes. Two types of amine oxidases are concerned with the oxidative deamination of both endogenous and exogenous amines. Typical substrates are shown in Fig. 3.10.

MONOAMINE OXIDASES. The monoamine oxidases are a family of flavoproteins found in the mitochondria of a wide variety of tissues: liver, kidney, brain, intestine, and blood platelets. They are a group of similar enzymes with overlapping substrate specificities and inhibition. Although the enzyme in the central nervous system is concerned primarily with neurotransmitter turnover, that in the liver will deaminate primary, secondary, and tertiary aliphatic amines, reaction rates with the primary amines being faster. Electron-withdrawing substitutions on an aromatic ring increase the reaction rate, whereas compounds with a methyl group on the α-carbon such as amphetamine and ephedrine are not metabolized.

a. Monoamine oxidase

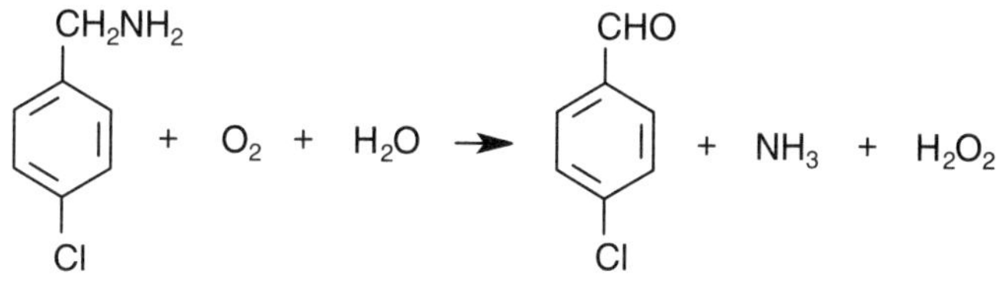

p-Chlorobenzylamine   *p*-Chlorobenzaldehyde

b. Diamine oxidase

$$H_2N(CH_2)_5NH_2 + O_2 + H_2O \rightarrow H_2N(CH_2)_4CHO + NH_3 + H_2O_2$$

Cadaverine

Figure 3.10. Examples of oxidations catalyzed by amine oxidases.

DIAMINE OXIDASES. Diamine oxidases are enzymes that also oxidize amines to aldehydes. The preferred substrates are aliphatic diamines in which the chain length is four (putrescine) or five (cadaverine) carbon atoms. Diamines with carbon chains longer than nine will not serve as substrates but can be oxidized by monoamine oxidases. Secondary and tertiary amines are not metabolized. Diamine oxidases are typically soluble pyridoxal phosphate-containing proteins that also contain copper. They have been found in a number of tissues, including liver, intestine, kidney, and placenta.

3.2.5 Cooxidation During Prostaglandin Biosynthesis

During the biosynthesis of prostaglandins, a polyunsaturated fatty acid, such as arachidonic acid, is first oxygenated to yield a hydroperoxy endoperoxide, prostaglandin G. This is then further metabolized to prostaglandin H_2, both reactions being catalyzed by the same enzyme, prostaglandin synthase (Fig. 3.11). This enzyme is located in the microsomal membrane and is found in high levels in such tissues as seminal vesicle. It is a glycoprotein with a subunit molecular mass of about 70,000 daltons, containing one heme per subunit. During the second step of the previous sequence (peroxidase), many xenobiotics can be cooxidized, and investigations of the mechanism have shown that the reactions are hydroperoxide-dependent reactions catalyzed by a peroxidase that uses prostaglandin G as a substrate. In at least some of these cases, the identity of this peroxidase has been established as prostaglandin synthase. Many of the reactions are similar or identical to those catalyzed by other peroxidases and also by microsomal monooxygenases; they include both detoxication and activation reactions. This mechanism is important in xenobiotic metabolism, particularly in tissues that are low in P450 and/or the FMO but high in prostaglandin synthase.

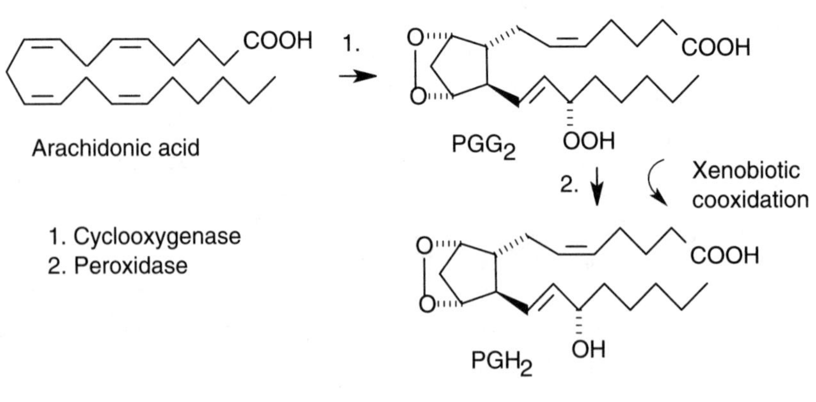

Figure 3.11. Cooxidation during prostaglandin biosynthesis.

3.2.6 Reduction Reactions

A number of functional groups, such as nitro, diazo, carbonyl, disulfide sulfoxide, alkene, pentavalent arsenic, and so on, are susceptible to reduction, although in many cases it is difficult to tell whether the reaction proceeds enzymatically or nonenzymatically by the action of such biologic reducing agents as reduced flavins or reduced pyridine nucleotides. In some cases, such as the reduction of the double bond in cinnamic acid ($C_6H_5CH=CHCOOH$), the reaction has been attributed to the intestinal microflora. Examples of reduction reactions are shown in Fig. 3.12.

NITRO REDUCTION. Aromatic amines are susceptible to reduction by both bacterial and mammalian nitroreductase systems. Convincing evidence has been presented that this reaction sequence is catalyzed by P450. It is inhibited by oxygen, although NADPH is still consumed. Earlier workers had suggested a flavoprotein reductase was involved, and it is not clear if this is incorrect or if both mechanisms occur. It is true, however, that high concentrations of FAD or FMN will catalyze the nonenzymatic reduction of nitro groups.

AZO REDUCTION. Requirements for azoreduction are similar to those for nitroreduction, namely, anaerobic conditions and NADPH. They are also inhibited by CO, and presumably they involve P450. The ability of mammalian cells to reduce azo bonds is rather poor, and intestinal microflora may play a role.

DISULFIDE REDUCTION. Some disulfides, such as the drug disulfiram (Antabuse), are reduced to their sulfhydryl constituents. Many of these reactions are three-step sequences, the last reaction of which is catalyzed by glutathione reductase, using glutathione (GSH) as a cofactor.

$$RSSR + GSH \longrightarrow RSSG + RSH$$
$$RSSG + GSH \longrightarrow GSSG + RSH$$
$$GSSG + NADPH + H^+ \longrightarrow 2GSH + NADP^+$$

KETONE AND ALDEHYDE REDUCTION. In addition to the reduction of aldehyde and ketones through the reverse reaction of alcohol dehydrogenase (Section 3.2.4.1), a family of aldehyde reductases also reduces these compounds. These reductases are NADPH-dependent, cytoplasmic enzymes of low molecular weight and have been found in liver, brain, kidney, and other tissues.

SULFOXIDE REDUCTION. The reduction of sulfoxides has been reported to occur in mammalian tissues. Soluble thioredoxin-dependent enzymes in the liver are known to be responsible in some cases. It has been suggested that oxidation in the endoplasmic reticulum followed by reduction in the cytoplasm may be a form of recyling that could extend the in vivo half-life of certain toxicants.

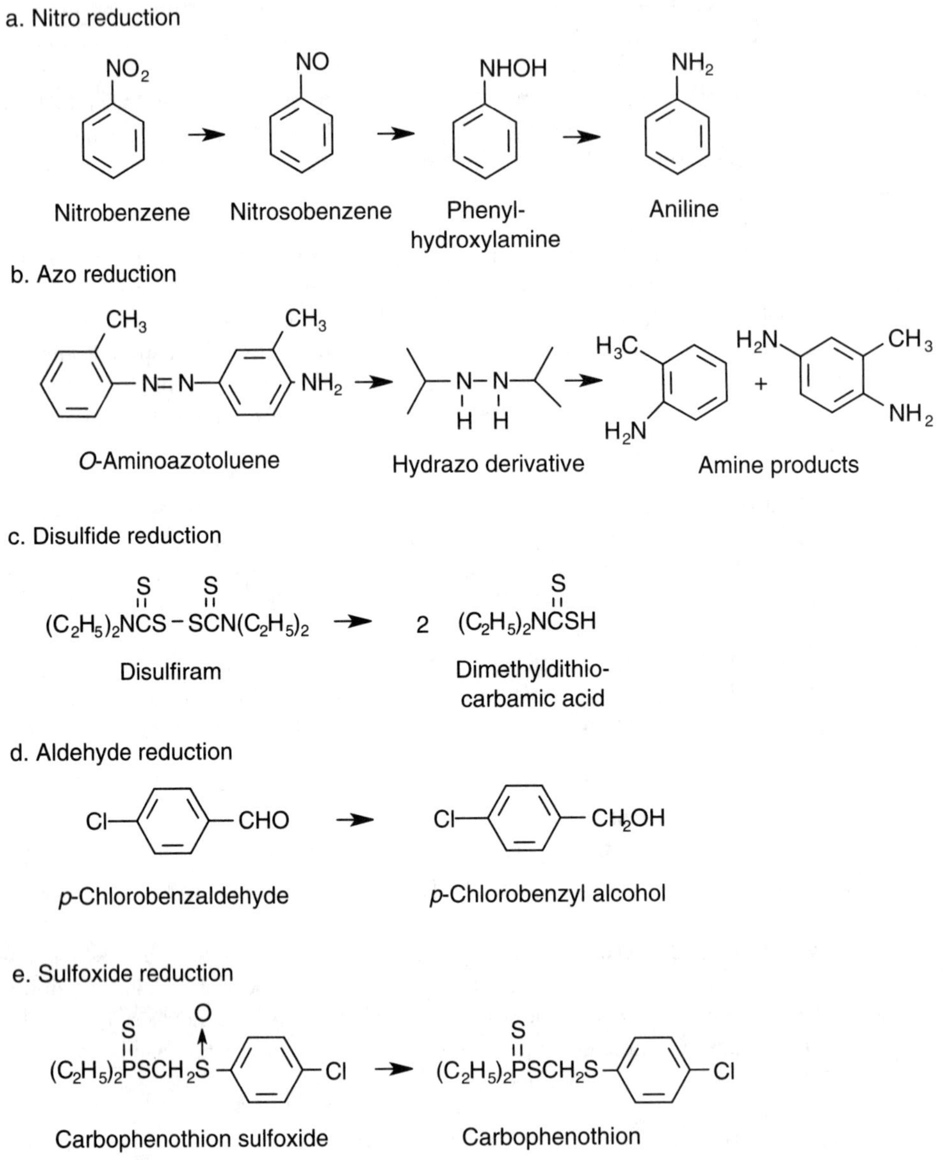
a. Nitro reduction
NO2
NO
NHOH
NH2
Nitrobenzene
Nitrosobenzene
Phenyl-hydroxylamine
Aniline
b. Azo reduction
CH3
CH3
N=N
NH2
N-N
H H
H3C
H2N
H2N
CH3
NH2
+
O-Aminoazotoluene
Hydrazo derivative
Amine products
c. Disulfide reduction
S S
(C2H5)2NCS-SCN(C2H5)2
2 (C2H5)2NCSH
S
Disulfiram
Dimethyldithio-carbamic acid
d. Aldehyde reduction
Cl
CHO
Cl
CH2OH
p-Chlorobenzaldehyde
p-Chlorobenzyl alcohol
e. Sulfoxide reduction
O
S
(C2H5)2PSCH2S
Cl
S
(C2H5)2PSCH2S
Cl
Carbophenothion sulfoxide
Carbophenothion

Figure 3.12. Examples of metabolic reduction reactions.

3.2.7 Hydrolysis

Enzymes with carboxylesterase and amidase activity are widely distributed in the body, occurring in many tissues and in both microsomal and soluble fractions. They catalyze the following general reactions:

$$RC(O)OR' + H_2O \longrightarrow RCOOH + HOR' \quad \text{Carboxylester hydrolysis}$$
$$RC(O)NR'R'' + H_2O \longrightarrow RCOOH + HNR'R'' \quad \text{Carboxyamide hydrolysis}$$
$$RC(O)SR' + H_2O \longrightarrow RCOOH + HSR' \quad \text{Carboxythioester hydrolysis}$$

Although carboxylesterases and amidases were thought to be different, no purified carboxylesterase has been found that does not have amidase activity toward the corresponding amide. Similarly, enzymes purified on the basis of their amidase activity have been found to have esterase activity. Thus, these two activities are now regarded as different manifestations of the same activity, specificity depending on the nature of R, R', and R'' groups and, to a lesser extent, on the atom (O, S, or N) adjacent to the carboxyl group.

In view of the large number of esterases in many tissues and subcellular fractions, as well as the large number of substrates hydrolyzed by them, it is difficult to derive a meaningful classification scheme. The division into A-, B-, and C-esterases on the basis of their behavior toward such phosphate triesters as paraoxon, first devised by Aldridge, is still of some value, although not entirely satisfactory.

B-Esterases, the most important group, are all inhibited by paraoxon, and all have a serine residue in their active site that is phosphorylated by this inhibitor. This group includes a number of different enzymes and their isozymes, many of which have quite different substrate specificities. For example, the group contains carboxylesterase/amidases, cholinesterases, monoacylglycerol lipases, and arylamidases. Many of these enzymes hydrolyze physiological (endogenous) substrates as well as xenobiotics. Several examples of their activity toward xenobiotic substrates are shown in Fig. 3.13.

A-Esterases, often referred to as arylesterases, are not inhibited by phosphotriesters such as paraoxon, but hydrolyze them instead.

C-Esterases, or acetylesterases, are defined as those esterases that prefer acetyl esters as substrates, and for which paraoxon serves as neither substrate nor inhibitor.

3.2.8 Epoxide Hydration

Epoxide rings of alkene and arene compounds are hydrated by enzymes known as epoxide hydrolases, the animal enzyme forming the corresponding *trans*-diols, although bacterial hydrolases are known that form *cis*-diols. In some cases, such as benzo(a)pyrene, the hydration of an epoxide is the first step in an activation sequence that ultimately yields highly toxic *trans*-dihydrodiol intermediates. In

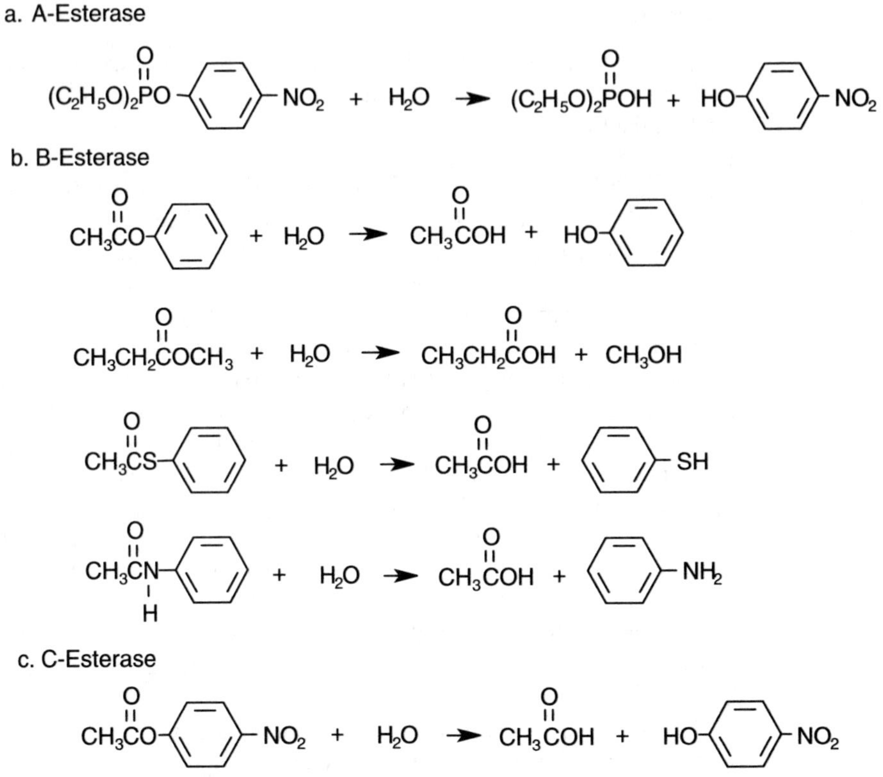

a. A-Esterase

$$(C_2H_5O)_2PO{-}\underset{}{\bigcirc}{-}NO_2 \;+\; H_2O \;\longrightarrow\; (C_2H_5O)_2POH \;+\; HO{-}\underset{}{\bigcirc}{-}NO_2$$

b. B-Esterase

$$CH_3CO{-}\underset{}{\bigcirc} \;+\; H_2O \;\longrightarrow\; CH_3COH \;+\; HO{-}\underset{}{\bigcirc}$$

$$CH_3CH_2COCH_3 \;+\; H_2O \;\longrightarrow\; CH_3CH_2COH \;+\; CH_3OH$$

$$CH_3CS{-}\underset{}{\bigcirc} \;+\; H_2O \;\longrightarrow\; CH_3COH \;+\; \underset{}{\bigcirc}{-}SH$$

$$CH_3CN{-}\underset{H}{\bigcirc} \;+\; H_2O \;\longrightarrow\; CH_3COH \;+\; \underset{}{\bigcirc}{-}NH_2$$

c. C-Esterase

$$CH_3CO{-}\underset{}{\bigcirc}{-}NO_2 \;+\; H_2O \;\longrightarrow\; CH_3COH \;+\; HO{-}\underset{}{\bigcirc}{-}NO_2$$

Figure 3.13. Example of esterase/amidase reactions involving xenobiotics.

others, reactive epoxides are detoxified by both glutathione transferase and epoxide hydrolase. The reaction probably involves a nucleophilic attack by –OH on the oxirane carbon. The most studied epoxide hydrolase is microsomal, and the enzyme has been purified from hepatic microsomes of several species. Although less well known, soluble epoxide hydrolases with different substrate specificities have also been described. Examples of epoxide hydrolase reactions are shown in Fig. 3.14.

3.2.9   DDT-Dehydrochlorinase

DDT-Dehydrochlorinase is an enzyme that occurs in both mammals and insects and has been studied most intensively in DDT-resistant houseflies. It catalyzes the dehydrochlorination of DDT to DDE and occurs in the soluble fraction of tissue homogenates. Although the reaction requires glutathione, it apparently serves in a cat-

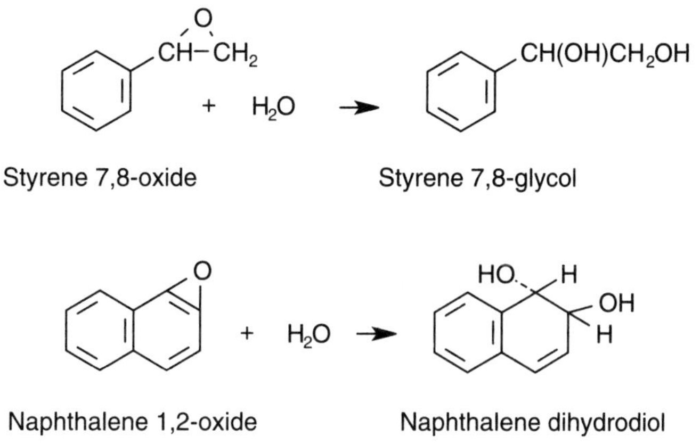

Styrene 7,8-oxide   Styrene 7,8-glycol

Naphthalene 1,2-oxide   Naphthalene dihydrodiol

Figure 3.14. Examples of epoxide hydrolyase reactions.

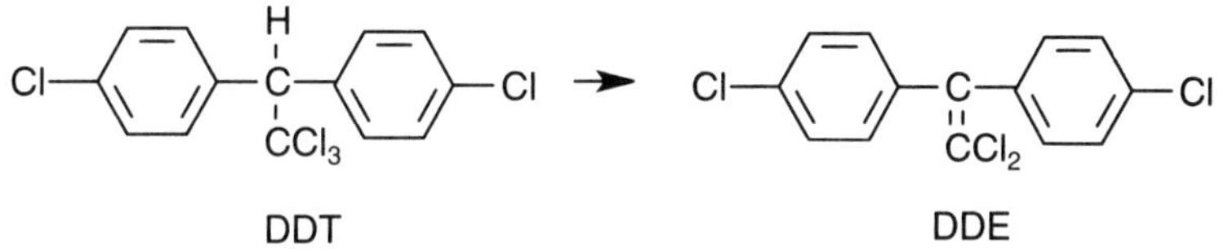

DDT   DDE

Figure 3.15. DDT-dehydrochlorinase.

alytic role because it does not appear to be consumed during the reaction. The K_m for DDT is 5×10^{-7} mol/L with optimum activity at pH 7.4. The monomeric form of the enzyme has a molecular mass of about 36,000 daltons, but the enzyme normally exists as a tetramer. In addition to catalyzing the dehydrochlorination of DDT to DDE and DDD (2,2-*bis*(*p*-chlorophenyl)-1,1-dichloroethane) to TDE (2,2-*bis*(*p*-chlorophenyl)-1-chlorothylene), DDT dehydrochlorinase also catalyzes the dehydrohalogenation of a number of other DDT analogs. In all cases, the *p,p* configuration is required, *o,p* and other analogs are not utilized as substrates. The reaction is illustrated in Fig. 3.15.

3.3

PHASE-TWO REACTIONS

Metabolism of phase-one products and other xenobiotics containing functional groups such as hydroxyl, amino, carboxyl, epoxide, or halogen can undergo conjugation reactions with endogenous metabolites, these conjugations being collectively termed phase-two reactions. The endogenous metabolites in question include sugars, amino acids, glutathione, sulfate, and so on. Conjugation products, with only rare exceptions, are more polar, less toxic, and more readily excreted than are their parent compounds.

Conjugation reactions usually involve activation by some high energy intermediate and have been classified into two general types: type I, in which an activated conjugating agent combines with the substrate to yield the conjugated product, and type II, in which the substrate is activated and then combines with an amino acid to yield a conjugated product. The formation of sulfates and glycosides are examples of type I, whereas type II consists primarily of amino acid conjugations.

3.3.1   Glucuronide Conjugation

The final step of glucuronide formation involves the reaction of uridine diphosphate glucuronic acid (UDPGA) with the aglycone, the latter being, in many cases, a xenobiotic. The reaction involves a nucleophilic displacement (SN_2 reaction) of the functional group of the substrate with Walden inversion. UDPGA is in the α-configuration whereas, due to the inversion, the glucuronide formed is in the ß-configuration. The enzyme involved, glucuronosyl transferase, is found in the microsomal fraction of liver, kidney, and other tissues. Examples of various types of glucuronides are shown in Fig. 3.16.

Whether this is one enzyme or a family of closely related enzymes is not entirely clear, although the latter is indicated from both purification and induction studies. Homogeneous glucuronosyl transferase has been isolated as a single polypeptide chain of about 59,000 daltons, apparently containing carbohydrate, the activity of which appears to be dependent on reconstitution with microsomal lipid. There appears to be an absolute requirement for UDPGA; related UDP-sugars will not suffice. This enzyme, as it exists in the microsomal membrane, does not exhibit its maximal capacity for conjugation; activation by some means (detergents, for example) is required.

A wide variety of reactions are mediated by glucuronosyltransferases. O-Glucuronides, N-glucuronides, and S-glucuronides have all been identified.

3.3.2   Glucoside Conjugation

Although rare in vertebrates, glucosides formed from xenobiotics are common in insects and plants. Formed from UDP-glucose, they appear to fall into the same classes as the glucuronides. An example is shown in Fig. 3.16.

3.3.3   Sulfate Conjugation

Sulfate esters, which are water soluble and readily eliminated from the organism, are formed with xenobiotics such as alcohols, arylamines, and phenols. This process requires the prior activation of sulfate ions to 3'-phospho-adenosine-5'-phosphosul-

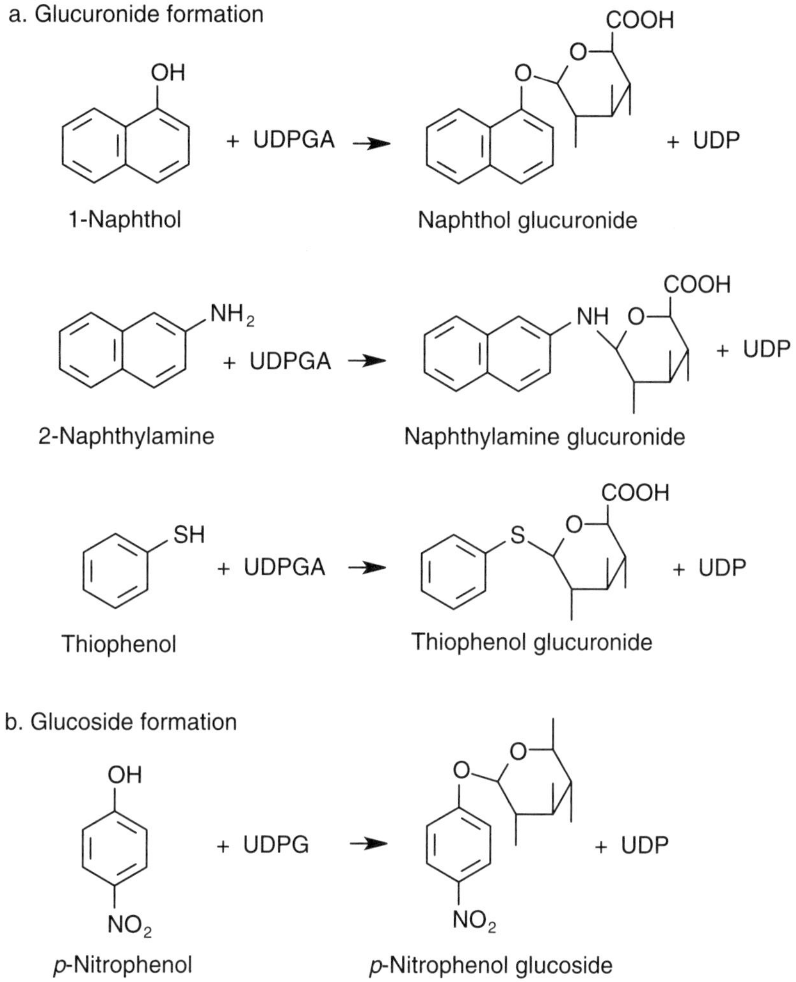

a. Glucuronide formation

1-Naphthol + UDPGA → Naphthol glucuronide + UDP

2-Naphthylamine + UDPGA → Naphthylamine glucuronide + UDP

Thiophenol + UDPGA → Thiophenol glucuronide + UDP

b. Glucoside formation

p-Nitrophenol + UDPG → p-Nitrophenol glucoside + UDP

Figure 3.16. Glycoside formation.

fate (PAPS), a reaction sequence (Fig. 3.17) requiring the consumption of ATP and hence using a considerable amount of energy.

In addition to inorganic sulfate and adenosine triphosphate (ATP), the formation of PAPS requires the sequential action of ATP sulfurylase and adenosine 5′-phosphosulfate kinase. ATP sulfurylase from rat liver is a large molecule of about 500,000 daltons. Several group VI anions other than sulfate can also serve as substrates, although the resultant anhydrides are unstable. Because this instability would lead to the overall consumption of ATP, these other anions can exert a toxic effect by depleting the cell of ATP. The second enzyme, the kinase, is not well

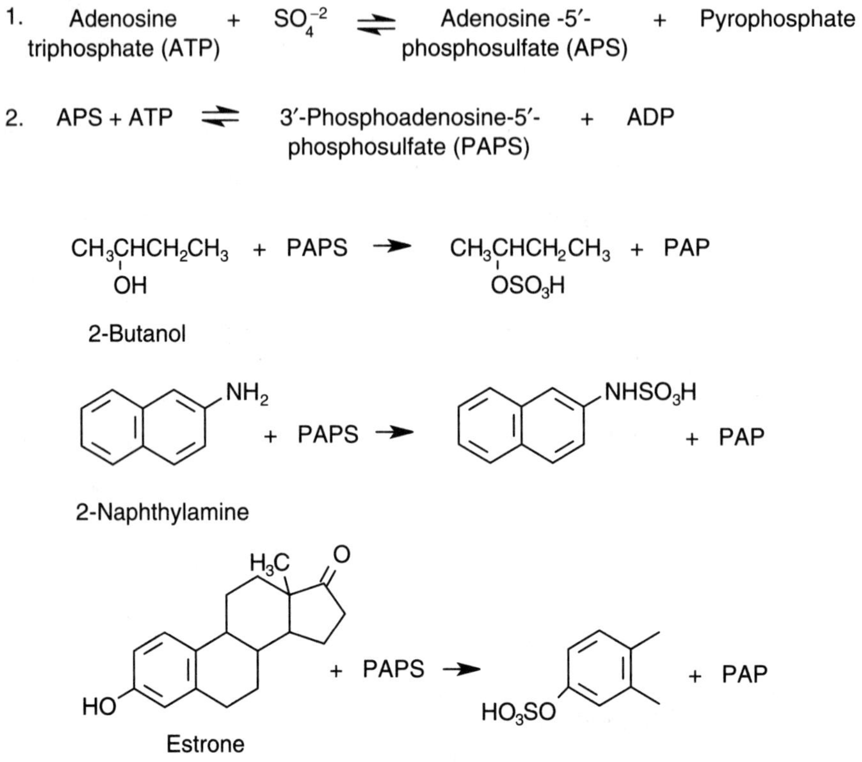

1. Adenosine   + SO_4^{-2} ⇌   Adenosine -5'-   +   Pyrophosphate
   triphosphate (ATP)   phosphosulfate (APS)

2. APS + ATP ⇌   3'-Phosphoadenosine-5'-   +   ADP
                   phosphosulfate (PAPS)

$CH_3CHCH_2CH_3$ + PAPS → $CH_3CHCH_2CH_3$ + PAP
     | |
     OH OSO_3H

2-Butanol

[structure] NH$_2$ + PAPS → [structure] NHSO$_3$H + PAP

2-Naphthylamine

[structure of Estrone] + PAPS → [structure] + PAP

Estrone

Figure 3.17. Sulfate ester formation.

known from mammalian tissues, but that from yeast shows a high affinity for adenosine-5'-phosphosulfate (APS) and the reaction is essentially irreversible.

The final step is catalyzed by a family of related sulfotransferases that have been classified as follows: aryl sulfotransferase; hydroxysteroid sulfotransferase; estrone sulfotransferase; and bile salt sulfotransferase. Aryl sulfotransferases from rat liver have been separated into four distinct forms, each of which catalyzes the sulfation of various phenols and catecholamines. They differ, however, in pH optimum, relative substrate specificity, and immunologic properties. The molecules of all of them are in the range of 61,000–64,000 daltons.

Hydroxysteroid sulfotransferase also appears to exist in several forms. This reaction is now known to be important, not only as a detoxication mechanism, but also in the synthesis and possibly the transport of steroids. Hydroxysteroid sulfotransferase will react with hydroxysterols and primary and secondary alcohols but not with hydroxy groups on the aromatic rings of steroids.

The third sulfotransferase, estrone sulfotransferase, has been purified from bovine adrenal gland. This enzyme will conjugate hydroxyl groups on the A ring of sterols.

Bile salt sulfotransferase appears to have the function of detoxifying bile salts, the toxic properties of which are well documented. This enzyme has been purified from both the liver and the kidney, the two forms appearing to be distinct entities.

3.3.4   Methyltransferases

A large number of both endogenous and exogenous compounds can be methylated by several N-, O-, and S-methyl transferases. The most common methyl donor is S-adenosyl methionine (SAM), formed from methionine and ATP. Even though these reactions may involve a decrease in water solubility, they are generally detoxication reactions. Examples of biologic methylation reactions are seen in Fig. 3.18.

N-METHYLATION. Several enzymes are known that catalyze N-methylation reactions. They include histamine N-methyltransferase, a highly specific enzyme that occurs

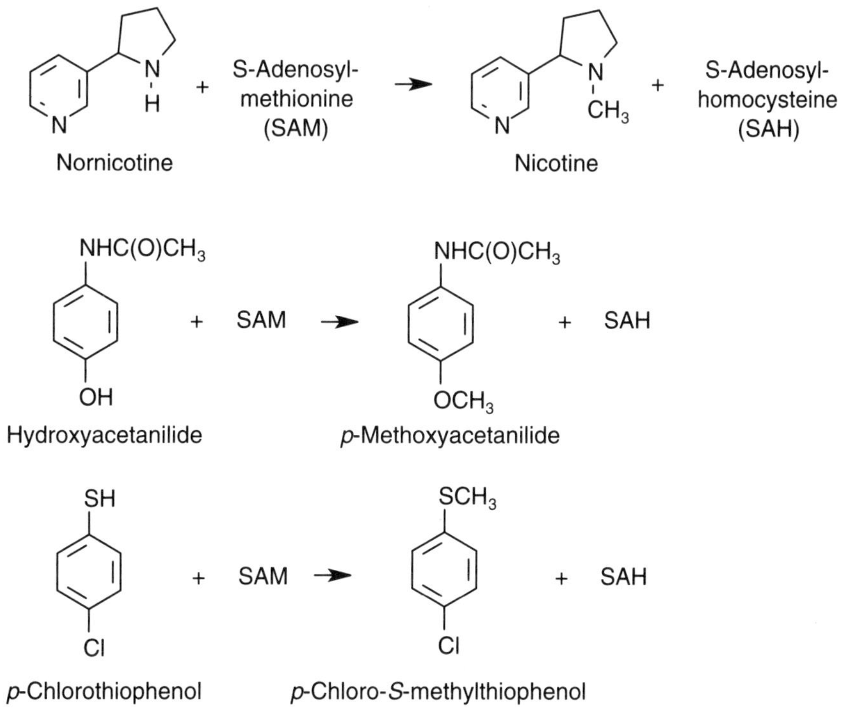

Figure 3.18. Examples of methyl transferase reactions.

in the soluble fraction of the cell, phenylethanolamine *N*-methyltransferase, which catalyzes the methylation of noradrenaline to adrenaline as well as the methylation of other phenylethanolamine derivatives. A third *N*-methyltransferase is the indoethylamine *N*-methyltransferase, or nonspecific *N*-methyltransferase. This enzyme is known to occur in various tissues. It methylates endogenous compounds such as serotonin and tryptamine and exogenous compounds such as nornicotine and norcodeine. The relationship between this enzyme and phenylethanolamine *N*-methyltransferase is not yet entirely clear.

O-METHYLATION. Catechol *O*-methyltransferase occurs in the soluble fraction of several tissues and has been purified from rat liver. The purified form has a molecular weight of 23,000 daltons, requires *S*-adenosylmethionine and Mg^+, and catalyzes the methylation of epinephrine, norepinephrine, and other catechol derivatives. There is evidence that this enzyme exists in multiple forms.

A microsomal *O*-methyltransferase that methylates a number of alkyl-, methoxy-, and halophenols has been described from rabbit liver and lungs. These methylations are inhibited by SKF-525A, *N*-ethyl-maleimide and *p*-chloromer-curibenzoate.

A hydroxyindole *O*-methyltransferase, which methylates *N*-acetyl-serotonin to melatonin and, to a lesser extent, other 5-hydroxyindoles and 5,6-dihydroxyindoles, has been described from the pineal gland of mammals, birds, reptiles, amphibians, and fish.

S-METHYLATION. Thiol groups of some foreign compounds are also methylated, the reaction being catalyzed by the enzyme, thiol *S*-methyltransferase. This enzyme is microsomal and, as with most methyl transferases, utilizes *S*-adenosylmethionine. It has been purified from rat liver and is a monomer of about 28,000 daltons. A wide variety of substrates are methylated, including thioacetanilide, mercaptoethanol, and phenylsulfide. This enzyme may also be important in the detoxication of hydrogen sulfide, which is methylated in two steps, first to the highly toxic methanethiol and then to dimethylsulfide.

Methylthiolation, or the transfer of a methylthio (CH_3S-) group to a foreign compound may occur through the action of another recently discovered enzyme, cysteine conjugate ß-lyase. This enzyme acts on cytsteine conjugates of foreign compounds as follows:

$$RSCH_2CH(NH_2)COOH \longrightarrow RSH + NH_3 + CH_3C(O)COOH$$

The thiol group can then be methylated to yield the methylthio derivative of the original xenobiotic.

BIOMETHYLATION OF ELEMENTS. The biomethylation of elements is carried out primarily by microorganisms and is important in environmental toxicology, particularly in the case of heavy metals, because the methylated compounds are absorbed through the membranes of the gut, the blood–brain barrier, and the placenta more readily than are the inorganic forms. For example, inorganic mercury can be methylated first to monomethylmercury and subsequently to dimethylmercury:

$$Hg^{2+} \longrightarrow CH_3\,Hg^+ \longrightarrow (CH_3)_2Hg$$

The enzymes involved are reported to use either S-adenosylmethionine or vitamin B_{12} derivatives as methyl donors and, in addition to mercury, the metals, lead, tin, and thallium, as well as the metalloids, arsenic, selenium, tellurium, and sulfur, are methylated. Even the unreactive metals, gold and platinum, are reported as substrates for these reactions.

3.3.5   Glutathione Transferases and Mercapturic Acid Formation

Although mercapturic acids, the N-acetylcysteine conjugates of xenobiotics, have been known since the early part of the twentieth century, only since the early 1960s has the source of the cysteine moiety (glutathione) and the enzymes required for the formation of these acids been identified and characterized. The overall pathway is shown in Fig. 3.19.

The initial reaction is the conjugation of xenobiotics having electrophilic substituents with glutathione, a reaction catalyzed by one of the various forms of

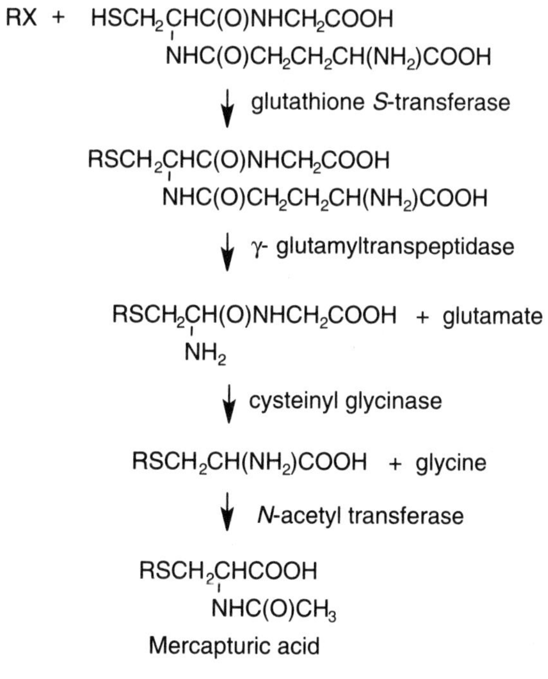

RX +   HSCH$_2$CHC(O)NHCH$_2$COOH
                 NHC(O)CH$_2$CH$_2$CH(NH$_2$)COOH

        ↓ glutathione S-transferase

RSCH$_2$CHC(O)NHCH$_2$COOH
            NHC(O)CH$_2$CH$_2$CH(NH$_2$)COOH

        ↓ γ- glutamyltranspeptidase

RSCH$_2$CH(O)NHCH$_2$COOH + glutamate
    NH$_2$

        ↓ cysteinyl glycinase

RSCH$_2$CH(NH$_2$)COOH + glycine

        ↓ N-acetyl transferase

RSCH$_2$CHCOOH
      NHC(O)CH$_3$
Mercapturic acid

Figure 3.19. Glutathione transferase reaction and formation of mercapturic acids.

glutathione transferase. This is followed by transfer of the glutamate by γ-glutamyltranspeptidase, by loss of glycine through cysteinyl glycinase, and finally by acetylation of the cysteine amino group. The overall sequence, particularly the initial reaction, is extremely important in toxicology because, by removing reactive electrophiles, vital nucleophilic groups in macromolecules such as proteins and nucleic acids are protected. The mercapturic acids formed can be excreted either in the bile or in the urine.

The glutathione transferases, the family of enzymes that catalyzes the initial step, are widely distributed, being found in essentially all groups of living organisms. Although the best known examples have been described from the soluble fraction of mammalian liver, these enzymes have also been demonstrated in microsomes. All forms appear to be highly specific with respect to glutathione but nonspecific with respect to xenobiotic substrates, although the relative rates for different substrates can vary widely from one form to another.

The types of reactions catalyzed include the following: alkyltransferase, aryltransferase, aralkyltransferase, alkenetransferase, and epoxidetransferase. Examples are shown in Fig. 3.20.

Multiple forms of glutathione transferase have been demonstrated in the liver of many mammalian species; multiple forms occur also in insects. Seven forms have been purified from rat liver and five forms from human liver. These enzymes have molecular weights in the range of 45,000–50,000 daltons and consist of two subunits. All forms appear to be nonspecific with respect to the reaction types described, although the kinetic constants for particular substrates vary from one form to another. They are usually identified and named from their chromatographic behavior. One of them, form B, appears to be identical to the binding protein ligandin.

γ-Glutamyltranspeptidase is a membrane-bound glycoprotein that has been purified from both the kidney and the liver of several species. Molecular weights for the kidney enzyme are in the range of 68,000-90,000 daltons, and the enzyme appears to consist of two unequal subunits; the different forms appear to differ in the degree of sialalylation. This enzyme, which exhibits wide specificity toward γ-glutamyl peptides and has a number of acceptor amino acids, catalyzes two types of reactions:

$$\text{Hydrolysis} \quad \gamma\text{-Glu-R} + H_2O \longrightarrow \text{Glu} + \text{HR}$$
$$\text{Transpeptidation} \quad \gamma\text{-Glu-R} + \text{Acceptor} \longrightarrow \gamma\text{-Glu-Acceptor} + \text{HR}$$
$$\gamma\text{-Glu-R} + \gamma\text{-Glu-R} \longrightarrow \gamma\text{-Glu } \gamma\text{-Glu-R} + \text{HR}$$

Aminopeptidases that catalyze the hydrolysis of cysteinyl peptides are known. The membrane-bound aminopeptidases are glycoproteins, usually with molecular weights of about 100,000 daltons. They appear to be metalloproteins, one of the better known being a zinc-containing enzyme. Other enzymes, such as the leucine aminopeptidase, are cytosolic, but, at least in this case, are also zinc-

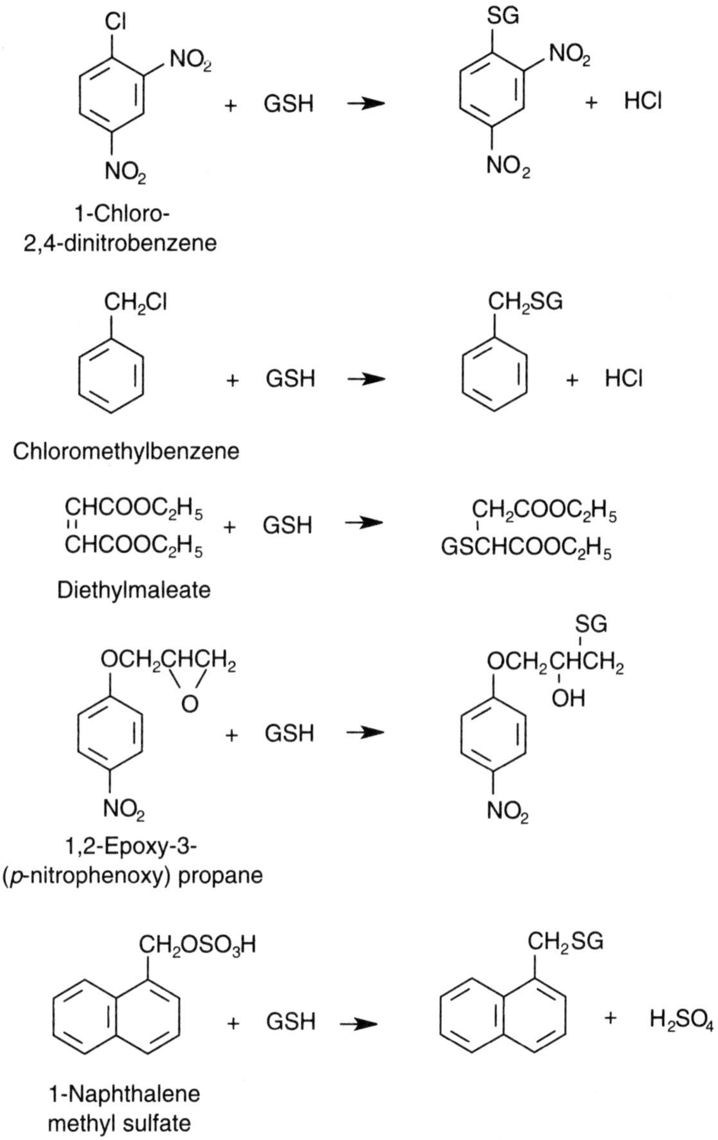

Figure 3.20. Examples of glutathione transferase reactions.

containing. The substrate specificity of these enzymes varies, but most are relatively nonspecific.

Little is known of the *N*-acetyltransferase(s) responsible for the acetylation of *S*-substituted cysteine. It is found in the microsomes of the kidney and liver, however, and is specific for acetyl CoA as the acetyl donor. It is distinguished from other *N*-acetyltransferases by its substrate specificity and subcellular location.

3.3.6   Cysteine Conjugate ß-Lyase

This enzyme uses cysteine conjugates as substrates, releasing the thiol of the xenobiotic, pyruvic acid, and ammonia, with subsequent methylation giving rise to the methylthio derivative. The enzyme from the cytosolic fraction of rat liver is a pyridoxal phosphate requiring protein of about 175,000 daltons. Cysteine conjugates of aromatic compounds are the best substrates and it is necessary for the cysteine amino and carboxyl groups to be unsubstituted for enzyme activity.

3.3.7   Acylation

Acylation reactions are of two general types, the first involving an activated conjugation agent, CoA, and the second involving activation of the foreign compounds and subsequent acylation of an amino acid. This type of conjugation is commonly undergone by exogenous carboxylic acids and amides and, although the products are often less water soluble than the parent compound, they are usually less toxic. Examples of acylation reactions are shown in Fig. 3.21.

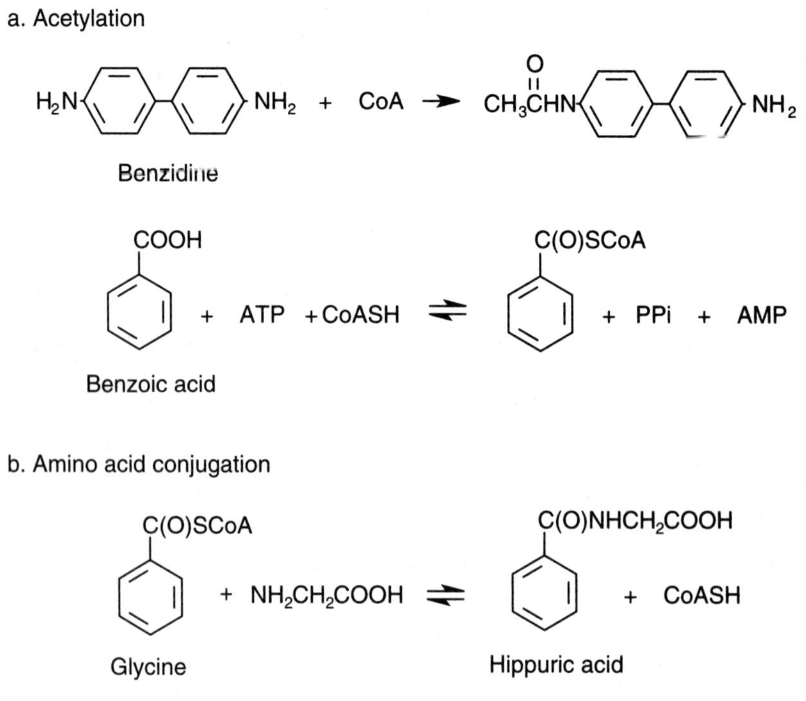

a. Acetylation

Benzidine

Benzoic acid

b. Amino acid conjugation

Glycine   Hippuric acid

Figure 3.21. Examples of acylation reactions.

ACETYLATION. Acetylated derivatives of foreign exogenous amines are acetylated by *N*-acetyl transferase, the acetyl donor being CoA. This enzyme is cytosolic, has been purified from rat liver, and is known to occur in several other organs. Evidence exists for the existence of multiple forms of the enzyme. Although endogenous amino, hydroxy, and thiol compounds are acetylated in vivo, the acetylation of exogenous hydroxy and thiol groups is presently unknown.

Acetylation of foreign compounds is influenced by both development and genetics. Newborn mammals generally have a low level of the transferase whereas, due to the different genes involved, fast and slow acetylators can be identified in both rabbit and human populations. Slow acetylators are more susceptible to the effects of compounds detoxified by acetylation.

N,O-ACYLTRANSFERASE. This enzyme is believed to be involved in the carcinogenicity of arylamines These compounds are first *N*-oxidized, and then, in species capable of their *N*-acetylation, acetylated to arylhydroxamic acids. The effect of *N,O*-transacetylation is shown in Fig. 3.22. The *N*-acyl group of the hydroxamic acid is first removed and is then transferred, either to an amine to yield a stable amide, or to the oxygen of the hydroxylamine to yield a reactive *N*-acyloxyarylamine. These compounds are highly reactive in the formation of adducts with both proteins and nucleic acids, and *N,O*-acyltransferase, added to the medium in the Ames test, increases the mutagenicity of compounds such as *N*-hydroxy-2-acetylaminofluorene. In spite of its great instability, this enzyme has been purified from the cytosolic fraction of rat liver.

AMINO ACID CONJUGATION. In the second type of acylation reaction, exogenous carboxylic acids are activated to form *S*-CoA derivatives in a reaction involving ATP and CoA. These CoA derivatives then acylate the amino group of a variety of amino acids. Glycine and glutamate appear to be the most common acceptor of amino acids in mammals; in other organisms, other amino acids are involved. These include ornithine in reptiles and birds and taurine in fish.

The activating enzyme occurs in the mitochondria and belongs to a class of enzymes known as the ATP-dependent acid:CoA ligases (AMP), but has also been

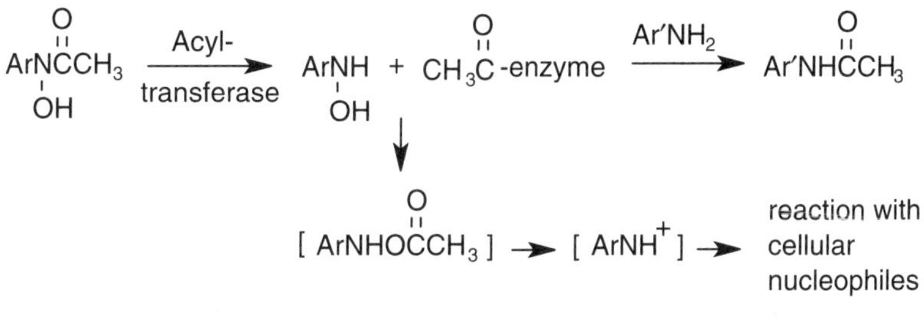

Figure 3.22. *N-, O*-Acyltransferase reactions of arylhydroxamic acid. Ar, aryl group.

known as acyl CoA synthetase and acid-activating enzyme. It appears to be identical to the intermediate chain length fatty acyl-CoA synthetase.

Two acyl-CoA:amino acid N-acyltransferases have been purified from liver mitochondria of cattle, Rhesus monkeys, and humans. One is a benzoyltransferase that utilizes benzoyl-CoA, isovaleryl-CoA, and tiglyl-CoA, but not phenylacetyl-CoA, malonyl-CoA, or indoleacetyl-CoA. The other is a phenylacetyl transferase that utilizes phenylacetyl-CoA and indoleacetyl-CoA but is inactive toward benzoyl-CoA. Neither is specific for glycine, as had been supposed from studies using less defined systems; both also utilize asparagine and glutamine, although at lower rates than glycine.

Bile acids are also conjugated by a similar sequence of reactions involving a microsomal bile acid:CoA ligase and a soluble bile acid-CoA amino acid N-acyltransferase. The latter has been extensively purified, and differences in acceptor amino acids, of which taurine is the most common, have been related to the evolutionary history of the species.

DEACETYLATION. Deacetylation occurs in a number of species, but there is a large difference between species, strains, and individuals in the extent to which the reaction occurs. Because acetylation and deacetylation are catalyzed by different enzymes, the levels of which vary independently in different species, the importance of acetylation as a xenobiotic metabolizing mechanism also varies between species. This can be seen in a comparison of the rabbit and the dog. The rabbit, which has high acetyltransferase activity and low deacetylase, excretes significant amounts of acetylated amines. The dog, in which the opposite situation obtains, does not.

A typical substrate for the aromatic deacetylase of the liver and kidney is acetanilide, which is deacetylated to yield aniline.

3.3.8   Phosphate Conjugation

Phosphorylation of xenobiotics is not a widely distributed conjugation reaction, insects being the only major group of animals in which it is found. The enzyme from the gut of cockroaches utilizes ATP, requires Mg^+, and is active in the phosphorylation of 1-naphthol and p-nitrophenol.

Suggested Further Reading

Armstrong RN: Glutathione S-transferases: reaction mechanism, structure, and function. In *Frontiers in Molecular Toxicology.* Marnett LJ, (ed.). Washington, DC: American Chemical Society, 1992, pp 115–124.

Beckett GJ, Hayes JD: Glutathione S-transferases: biomedical applications. *Adv Clin Chem* **30:**281–380, 1993.

Bertilsson L: Geographical/interracial differences in polymorphic drug oxidation: current state of knowledge of cytochromes P450 (CYP) 2D6 and 2C19. *Clin Pharmacokinet* **29:**192–209, 1995.

Brittebo EB: Metabolism of xenobiotics in the nasal olfactory mucosa: implications for local toxicity. *Pharmacol Toxicol* **72**(suppl III):50–52, 1993.

Cashman JR: Structural and catalytic properties of the mammalian flavin-containing monooxygenase. *Chem Res Toxicol* **8:**165–181, 1995.

Foth H: Role of the lung in accumulation and metabolism of xenobitotic compounds–implications for chemically induced toxicity. *Crit Rev Toxicol* **25:**165–205, 1995.

Daniel V: Glutathione *S*-transferases: gene structure and regulation of expression. *Crit Rev Biochem Mol Biol* **28:**173–207, 1993.

Eling T, Thompson DC, Foureman GL, et al: Prostaglandin H synthase and xenobiotic oxidation. *Ann Rev Pharmacol Toxicol* **30:**1–45, 1990.

Gillette JR: Keynote address: man, mice, microsomes, metabolites, and mathematics 40 years after the revolution. *Drug Metabol Rev* **27:**1–44, 1995.

Goeptar AR, Scheerens H, Vermeulen NPE: Oxygen and xenobiotic reductase activities of cytochrome P450. *Crit Rev Toxicol.* **25:**25–65, 1995.

Gonzalez FJ, Gelboin HV: Role of human cytochromes P450 in the metabolic activation of chemical carcinogens and toxins. *Drug Metabol Rev* **26:**165–183, 1994.

Guengerich FP: Bioactivation and detoxication of toxic and carcinogenic chemicals. *Drug Metabol Disp* **21:**1–6, 1993.

Guengerich FP: Cytochrome P450 enzymes. *American Scientist* **81:**440–447, 1993.

Guengerich FP: Metabolic activation of carcinogens. *Pharmac Ther* **54:**17–61, 1992.

Hodgson E, Levi PE (eds.): *Introduction to Biochemical Toxicology.* Norwalk, CT: Appleton & Lange, 1994.

Kitada M, Kamataki T: Cytochrome P450 in human fetal liver: significance and fetal-specific expression. *Drug Metabol Rev* **26:**305–323, 1994.

Krisna DR, Klotz U: Extrahepatic metabolism of drugs in humans. *Clin Pharmacokinet* **26:**144–160, 1994.

Lawton MP, Cashman JR, Cresteil T, Dolphin CT, Elfarra AA, Hines RN, Hodgson E, Kimura T, Ozols J, Phillips IR, Philpot RM, Poulsen LL, Rettie AE, Shephard EA, Williams DE, Zeigler DM: A nomenclature for the mammalian flavin-containing monooxygenase gene family based on amino acid sequence identities. *Arch Biochem Biophys* **308:**254–257, 1994.

Nelson DR, Koymans L, Kamatake T, Stegman JJ, Freyereisen R, Wasman DJ, Waterman MR, Gotoh L, Coon MJ, Estabrook RW, Gunsalus IC, Nebert DW: P450 Superfamily: update on new sequences, gene mapping, accession numbers and nomenclature. *Pharmacogenetics* **6:**1–42, 1996.

Parkinson A: Biotransformation of xenobiotics. In *Casarett & Doull's Toxicology, The Basic Science of Poisons,* 56th ed. Klaassen CD (ed.). New York: McGraw-Hill, 1996, pp 113–186.

Smith CAD, Smith G, Wolf CR: Genetic polymorphisms in xenobiotic metabolism. *Eur J Cancer* **30A:**1935–1941, 1994.

Tephly TR: Isolation and purification of UDP-glucuronosyltransferases. In *Frontiers in Molecular Toxicology.* Marnett LJ (ed.). Washington, DC: American Chemical Society, 1992, pp 125–132.

REACTIVE METABOLITES

PATRICIA E. LEVI

4.1

INTRODUCTION

Between uptake from the environment and excretion from the body, many exogenous compounds (xenobiotics) undergo metabolism to highly reactive intermediates. These metabolites may interact with cellular constituents in numerous ways, such as binding covalently to macromolecules and/or stimulating lipid peroxidation. This biotransformation of relatively inert chemicals to highly reactive intermediary metabolites is commonly referred to as *metabolic activation* or *bioactivation* and is known to be the initial event in many chemically induced toxicities. Some toxicants are direct acting and require no activation, whereas other chemicals may be activated nonenzymatically. The focus of this chapter, however, relates to toxicants requiring metabolic activation and to those processes involved in activation.

In the 1940s and 1950s the pioneering studies of James and Elizabeth Miller provided early evidence for in vivo conversion of chemical carcinogens to reactive metabolites. They found that reactive metabolites of the aminoazo dye *N,N*-dimethyl-4-aminoazobenzene (DAB), a hepatocarcinogen in rats, would bind covalently to proteins and nucleic acids. The Millers coined the term metabolic activation to describe this process. Moreover, they demonstrated that covalent binding of these chemicals was an essential part of the carcinogenic process.

The overall scheme of metabolism for potentially toxic xenobiotics is outlined in Fig. 4.1. As can be seen from this diagram, metabolism of a chemical can produce not only nontoxic metabolites, which are more polar and readily excreted (detoxication), but also highly reactive metabolites, which can interact with vital intracellular macromolecules, resulting in toxicity. In addition, reactive metabolites can be detoxified—for example, by reaction with glutathione. In general, reactive metabolites, are *electrophiles* (molecules containing positive centers). These elec-

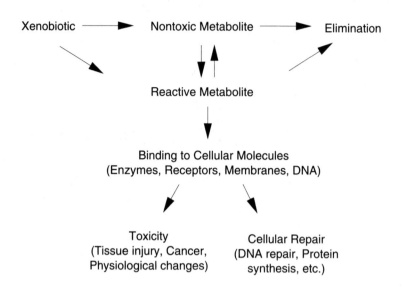

Figure 4.1. The relationship between metabolism, activation, detoxication, and toxicity of a chemical.

trophiles in turn can react with cellular *nucleophiles* (molecules containing negative centers), such as glutathione, proteins, and nucleic acids. Other reactive metabolites may be *free radicals* or act as radical generators that interact with oxygen to produce *reactive oxygen* species that are capable of causing damage to membranes, DNA, and other macromolecules.

Although a chemical can be metabolized by several routes, the activation pathway is often a minor route with the remainder of the pathways resulting in detoxication. Activation, however, may become a more dominant pathway in certain situations, thus leading to toxicity. Several examples illustrating these situations are discussed later in this chapter. Some important terms that are often used when discussing activation include: *parent compound*, sometimes referred to as *procarcinogen* in the case of a carcinogen or *prodrug* for pharmacological compounds; *proximate toxic metabolite* or *proximate carcinogen* for one or more of the intermediates; and *ultimate toxic metabolite* or *ultimate carcinogen* for the reactive species that binds to macromolecules and DNA.

4.2

ACTIVATION ENZYMES

Whereas most, if not all, of the enzymes involved in xenobiotic metabolism can form reactive metabolites (Table 4.1), the enzyme systems most frequently involved in the activation of xenobiotics are those which catalyze oxidation reactions (see

TABLE 4.1. ENZYMES IMPORTANT IN CATALYZING METABOLIC ACTIVATION REACTIONS

Type of Reaction	Enzyme
Oxidation	Cytochrome P450s
	Prostaglandin synthetase (PGS)
	Flavin-containing monooxygenases (FMO)
	Alcohol and aldehyde dehydrogenases
Conjugation	Glutathione transferases
	Sulfotransferases
	Glucuronidases
Deconjugation	Cysteine S-conjugate β-lyase
Hydrolysis and reduction	Gut microflora: hydrolases, reductases

Chapter 3). The cytochrome P450 monooxygenases (P450) are by far the most important enzymes involved in the oxidation of xenobiotics. This is because of the abundance of P450 (especially in the liver), the numerous isozymes of P450, and the ability of P450 to be induced by xenobiotic compounds.

Although the P450 enzymes are most abundant in the liver, they are also present in other tissues, including the skin, kidney, intestine, lung, placenta, and nasal mucosa. Because P450 exists as multiple isozymes with different substrate specificities, the presence or absence of a particular P450 isozyme may contribute to tissue-specific toxicities. Many drugs and other foreign compounds are known to induce one or more of the cytochrome P450 isozymes, resulting in an increase, decrease, or an alteration in the metabolic pathway of chemicals metabolized by the P450 isozymes involved. Specific examples of these types of interactions are given later in this section.

In addition to activations catalyzed by cytochrome P450, phase two conjugations, cooxidation during prostaglandin biosynthesis, oxidation by the flavin-containing monooxygenase (FMO), and metabolism by intestinal microflora may also lead to the formation of reactive toxic products. With some chemicals, only one enzymatic reaction is involved, whereas with other compounds, several reactions, often involving multiple pathways, are necessary for the production of the ultimate reactive metabolite.

4.3

NATURE AND STABILITY OF REACTIVE METABOLITES

Reactive metabolites include such diverse groups as epoxides, quinones, free radicals, reactive oxygen species, and unstable conjugates. Figure 4.2 gives some examples of activation reactions, the reactive metabolites formed, and the enzymes catalyzing their bioactivation.

As a result of their high reactivity, reactive metabolites are often considered to be short-lived. This is not always true, however, because reactive intermediates can

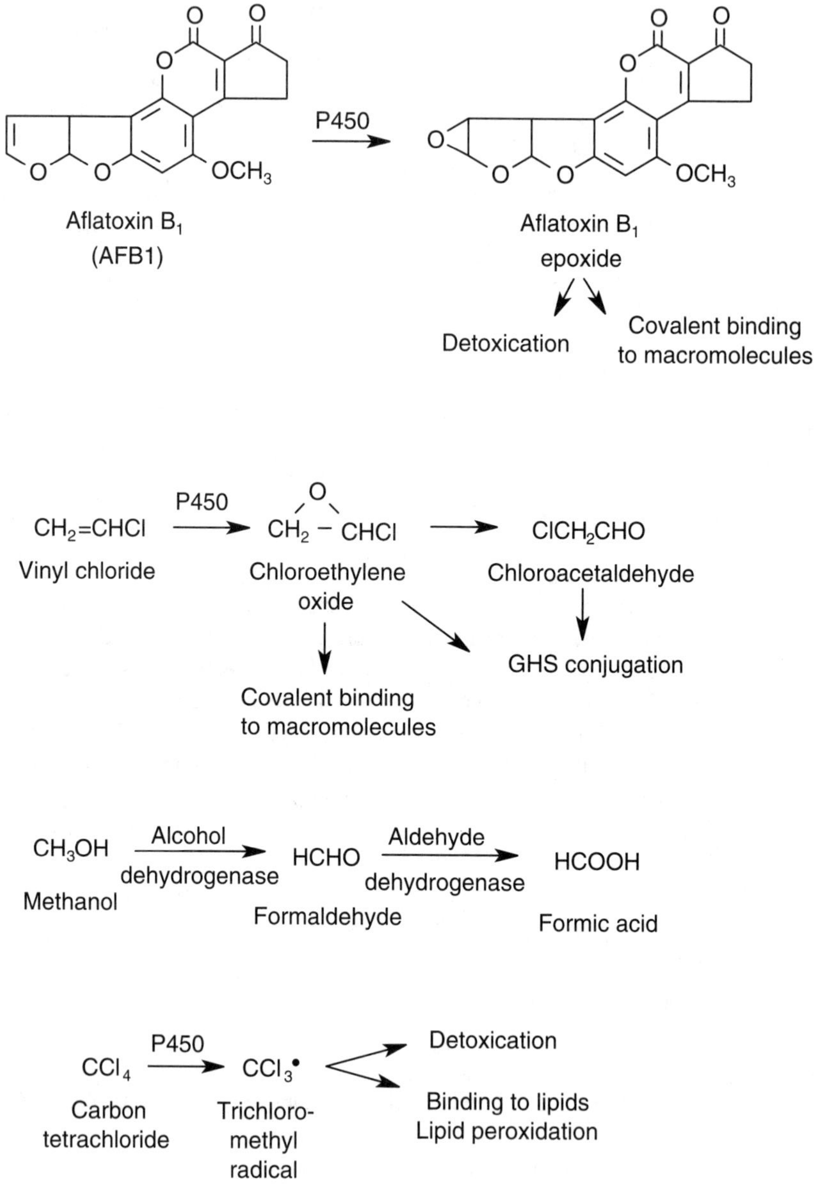

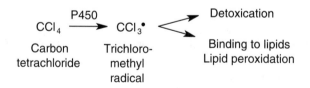

Figure 4.2. Examples of some activation reactions.

be transported from one tissue to another, where they may exert their deleterious effects. Thus, reactive intermediates can be divided into several categories depending on how far they are transported from the site of activation.

ULTRASHORT-LIVED METABOLITES. These are metabolites that bind primarily to the parent enzyme. This category includes substrates that form enzyme-bound intermediates that react with the active site of the enzyme. Such chemicals are known as "suicide substrates." A number of compounds are known to react in this manner with P450, and such compounds are often used experimentally as P450 inhibitors (see discussion of piperonyl butoxide in Chapter 3). Other compounds, although not true suicide substrates, produce reactive metabolites that bind primarily to the activating enzyme or adjacent proteins altering the function of the protein.

SHORT-LIVED METABOLITES. These metabolites remain in the cell or travel only to nearby cells. In this case, covalent binding is restricted to the cell of origin and to adjacent cells. Many metabolites fall into this group and give rise to localized tissue damage occurring at the site of activation. For example, in the lung, the Clara cells contain high concentrations of P450 and several lung toxicants that require activation often result in damage primarily to the Clara cells.

LONGER LIVED METABOLITES. These metabolites may be transported to other cells and tissues so that although the site of activation may be the liver, the target site may be in a distal organ. Reactive intermediates may also be transported to other tissues, not in their original form but as conjugates, which then release the reactive intermediate under the specific conditions in the target tissue. For example, carcinogenic aromatic amines are metabolized in the liver to the *N*-hydroxylated derivatives that, following glucuronide conjugation, are transported to the bladder, where the *N*-hydroxy derivative is released under the acidic conditions of urine.

4.4

FATE OF REACTIVE METABOLITES

If production of reactive metabolites is the initial process in the role of reactive metabolites in toxicity, then the fate of these metabolites is the next step to understand in the process. Within the tissue, a variety of reactions may occur depending on the nature of the reactive species and the physiology of the organism.

BINDING TO CELLULAR MACROMOLECULES. As mentioned previously, most reactive metabolites are electrophiles that can bind covalently to nucleophilic sites on cellular macromolecules such as proteins, polypeptides, RNA, and DNA. This covalent binding is considered to be the initiating event for many toxic processes such as mutagenesis, carcinogenesis, and cellular necrosis, and is discussed in greater detail in Chapters 7–9.

LIPID PEROXIDATION. Radicals such as $CCl_3\cdot$, produced during the oxidation of carbon tetrachloride, may induce lipid peroxidation and subsequent destruction of lipid membranes. Because of the critical nature of various cellular membranes (nuclear, mitochondrial, lysosomal, etc.), lipid peroxidation can be a pivotal event in cellular necrosis. (This mechanism is discussed more fully in Chapter 9, Section 9.1.5.)

TRAPPING AND REMOVAL: ROLE OF GLUTATHIONE. Once reactive metabolites are formed, mechanisms within the cell may bring about their rapid removal or inactivation. Toxicity then depends primarily on the balance between the rate of metabolite formation and the rate of removal. With some compounds, reduced glutathione plays an important protective role by trapping electrophilic metabolites and preventing their binding to hepatic proteins and enzymes. Although conjugation reactions occasionally result in bioactivation of a compound, the acetyl-, glutathione-, glucuronyl-, or sulfotransferases usually result in the formation of a nontoxic, water-soluble metabolite that is easily excreted. Thus, availability of the conjugating chemical is an important factor in determining the fate of the reactive intermediates.

4.5

EXAMPLES OF ACTIVATION REACTIONS

The following examples have been selected to illustrate the various concepts of activation and detoxication discussed in the preceeding sections.

4.5.1   Aflatoxin B₁

Aflatoxin B_1 (AFB1) is one of the mycotins produced by *Aspergillus flavus* and *A parasiticus* and is a well-known hepatotoxicant and hepatocarcinogen. It is generally accepted that the activated form of AFB1 that binds covalently to DNA is the 2,3-epoxide (Fig. 4.2). AFB1-induced hepatotoxicity and carcinogenicity is known to vary among species of livestock and laboratory animals. The selective toxicity of AFB1 appears to be dependent on quantitative differences in formation of the 2,3-epoxide, which is related to the particular enzyme complement of the organism. Table 4.2 shows the relative rates of AFB1 metabolism by liver microsomes from different species. Because the epoxides of foreign compounds are frequently further metabolized by epoxide hydrolases or are nonenzymatically converted to the corresponding dihydrodiols, existance of the dihydrodiol is considered as evidence for prior formation of the epoxide. Because epoxide formation is catalyzed by P450 enzymes, the amount of AFB1-dihydrodiol produced by microsomes is reflective of the P450 isozyme complement involved in AFB1 metabolism. In Table 4.2, for example, it can been seen that in rat microsomes in which specific P450 isozymes have been induced by phenobarbital (PB), dihydrodiol formation is considerably higher than that in control microsomes.

TABLE 4.2. FORMATION OF AFLATOXIN B₁ DIHYDRODIOL BY LIVER MICROSOMES

Source of Microsomes	Dihydrodiol Formation[a]
Rat	0.7
C57 mouse	1.3
Guinea pig	2.0
PB-induced rat	3.3
Chicken	4.8

[a] Micrograms dihydrodiol formed per milligram microsomal protein/30 min.
Source: Adapted from Neal et al, Toxicol Appl Pharmacol **58**:431–437, 1981.

4.5.2 Acetylaminofluorene

In the case of the hepatocarcinogen 2-acetylaminofluorene (2-AAF), two activation steps are necessary to form the reactive metabolites (Fig. 4.3). The initial reaction, N-hydroxylation, is a P450-dependent phase one reaction, whereas the second reaction, formation of the unstable sulfate ester, is a phase two conjugation reaction that results in the formation of the reactive intermediate. Another phase two reaction, glucuronide conjugation, is a detoxication step, with its conjugation product being readily excreted.

In some animal species 2-AAF is known to be carcinogenic, whereas in other species it is noncarcinogenic. The carcinogenic potential of 2-AAF can be correlated with the animal's ability to form N-hydroxy-2-AAF or the sulfate ester of the N-hydroxy-2-AAF. For example, hepatocarcinogenicity is considerably higher in male rats who possess high sulfotransferase activity than in female rats who have much lower levels of this enzyme.

In addition to N-hydroxylation, 2-AAF can also undergo various ring hydroxylations that are detoxication pathways. Because both N-hydroxylation and ring hydroxylation are catalyzed by cytochrome P450, the difference in the levels of the

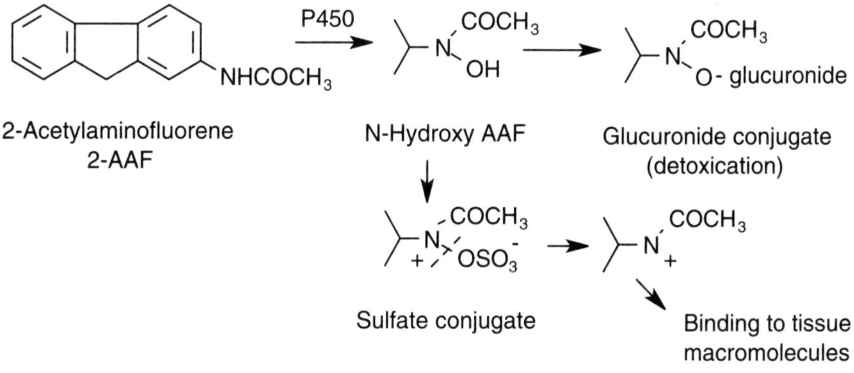

Figure 4.3. Bioactivation of 2-acetylaminofluorene.

various cytochrome P450 isozymes will affect the balance between activation and detoxication and thus the carcinogenicity of the compound. For example, 2-AAF is not carcinogenic to the guinea pig, an animal that does not form the *N*-hydroxylated metabolite.

4.5.3   Acetaminophen

A good example of the importance of tissue availability of the conjugating chemical is found with acetaminophen. At normal therapeutic doses, acetaminophen is safe, but can be hepatotoxic at high doses. The major portion of acetaminophen is conjugated with either sulfate or glucuronic acid to form water-soluble, readily excreted metabolites and only small amounts of the reactive intermediate, believed to be a quinoneimine, are formed by the P450 enzymes (Fig. 4.4).

When therapeutic doses of acetaminophen are ingested, the small amount of reactive intermediate formed is efficiently deactivated by conjugation with glutathione. When large doses are ingested, however, the sulfate and glucuronide cofactors (PAPS and UDPGA) become depleted, resulting in more of the acetaminophen being metabolized to the reactive intermediate.

As long as glutathione (GSH) is available most of the reactive intermediate can be detoxified. When the concentration of glutathione in the liver also becomes depleted, however, covalent binding to sulfhydryl (–SH) groups of various cellular proteins increases, resulting in hepatic necrosis. If sufficiently large amounts of acetaminophen are ingested, as in drug overdoses and suicide attempts, extensive liver damage and death may result.

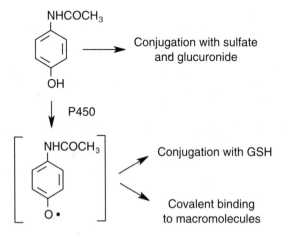

Figure 4.4. Formation of reactive metabolite from acetaminophen.

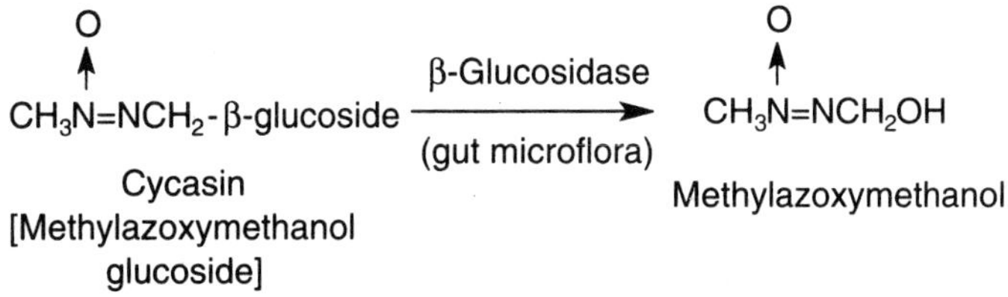

$$
\begin{array}{ccc}
& O & \\
& \uparrow & \\
CH_3N{=}NCH_2{\text{-}}\beta\text{-glucoside} & \xrightarrow[\text{(gut microflora)}]{\beta\text{-Glucosidase}} & CH_3N{=}NCH_2OH \\
\text{Cycasin} & & \text{Methylazoxymethanol} \\
\text{[Methylazoxymethanol} & & \\
\text{glucoside]} & &
\end{array}
$$

Figure 4.5. Bioactivation of cycasin by intestinal microflora to the carcinogen methylazoxymethanol.

4.5.4   Cycasin

When flour from the cycad nut, which is used extensively among residents of South Pacific islands, is fed to rats, it leads to cancers of the liver, kidney, and digestive tract. The active compound is cycasin, the ß-glucoside of methylazoxymethanol (Fig. 4.5). If this compound is injected intraperitoneally (IP) rather than given orally, or if the compound is fed to germ-free rats, no tumors occur. Intestinal microflora possess the necessary enzyme, ß-glucosidase, to form the active compound methylazoxymethanol, which is then absorbed into the body. The parent compound cycasin is carcinogenic only if administered orally because ß-glucosidases are not present in mammalian tissues but are present in the gut. However, it can be demonstrated that the metabolite, methylazoxymethanol, will lead to tumors in both normal and germ-free animals regardless of the route of administration.

4.6

FACTORS AFFECTING TOXICITY OF REACTIVE METABOLITES

A number of factors can influence the balance between the rate of formation of reactive metabolites and the rate of removal, thereby affecting toxicity. The major factors discussed in this chapter are summarized in the following subsections. A more in-depth discussion of factors affecting metabolism and toxicity are presented in Chapter 6.

LEVELS OF ACTIVATING ENZYMES. Specific isozymes of cytochrome P450 are often important in determining metabolic activation of a foreign compound. As mentioned previously, many xenobiotics induce specific forms of cytochrome P450. Frequently, the P450 forms induced are those involved in the metabolism of the inducing agent. Thus, a carcinogen or other toxicant has the potential of inducing its own activation. In addition, there are species and gender differences in enzyme levels as well as specific differences in the expression of particular isozymes.

LEVELS OF CONJUGATING ENZYMES. Levels of conjugating enzymes, such as glutathione transferases, are also known to be influenced by gender and species differences as well as by drugs and other environmental factors. All of these factors will, in turn, affect the detoxication process.

LEVEL OF COFACTORS OR CONJUGATING CHEMICALS. Treatment of animals with N-acetylcysteine, a precursor of glutathione, protects animals against acetaminophen-induced hepatic necrosis, possibly by reducing covalent binding to tissue macromolecules. However, depletion of glutathione potentiates covalent binding and hepatotoxicity.

4.7

FUTURE DEVELOPMENTS

The current procedures for assessing safety and carcinogenic potential of chemicals using whole animal studies are expensive and time-consuming as well as becoming less socially acceptable. Moreover, the scientific validity of such tests for human risk assessment is also being questioned. Currently, a battery of short-term mutagenicity tests are used extensively as early predictors of mutagenicity and possible carcinogenicity.

Most of these systems use test organisms—for example, bacteria, that lack suitable enzyme systems to bioactivate chemicals, and therefore an exogenous activating system is used. Usually the postmitochondrial fraction from rat liver, containing both phase one and phase two enzymes, is used as the activating system. The critical question is to what extent does this rat system represent the true in vivo situation, especially in humans. If not this system, then what is a better alternative? As some of the examples in this chapter illustrate, a chemical that is toxic or carcinogenic to one species or gender may be inactive in another, and this phenomenom is often related to the complement of enzymes, either activation or detoxication, expressed in the exposed organism.

Another factor to consider is the ability of many foreign chemicals to selectively induce the P450 enzymes involved in their metabolism, especially if this induction results in activation of the compound. With molecular techniques now available, considerable progress is being made in defining the enzyme and isozyme complements of humans and laboratory species and understanding their mechanisms of control. Another area of active research is the use of in vitro expression systems to study the oxidation of foreign chemicals (eg, bacteria containing genes for specific human P450 isozymes).

In summary, in studies of chemical toxicity, pathways and rates of metabolism as well as effects resulting from toxicokinetic factors and receptor affinities are critical in the choice of animal species and experimental design. Therefore, it is important that the animal species chosen as a model for humans in safety evaluations metabolize the test chemical by the same routes as humans and, furthermore, that quantitative differences be considered in the interpretation of animal toxicity data.

Risk assessment methods involving the extrapolation of toxic or carcinogenic potential of a chemical from one species to another must consider the metabolic and toxicokinetic characteristics of both species.

Suggested Further Reading

Anders MW, Dekant W, Vamvakas S: Glutathione-dependent toxicity. *Xenobiotics* **22:** 1135–1145, 1992.

Gonzalez FJ, Gelboin HV: Role of human cytochromes P450 in the metabolic activation of chemical carcinogens and toxins. *Drug Metabol Rev* **26:**165–183, 1994.

Guengerich FP: Bioactivation and detoxication of toxic and carcinogenic chemicals. *Drug Metabol Disp* **21:**1–6, 1993.

Guengerich FP: Catalytic selectivity of human cytochrome P450 enzymes—relevance to drug metabolism and toxicity. *Toxicol Letters* **70:**133–138, 1994.

Guengerich FP: Metabolic activation of carcinogens. *Pharmac Ther* **54:**17–61, 1992.

Levi PE: Reactive metabolites and toxicity. In *Introduction to Biochemical Toxicology,* 2nd edition. Hodgson E, Levi PE (eds.). Norwalk, CT: Appleton & Lange, 1994, pp 219–239.

Miller EC, Miller JA: Some historical perspectives on the metabolism of xenobiotic chemicals to reactive electrophiles. In *Bioactivation of Foreign Compounds*, Anders MW (ed.). New York: Academic Press, 1985, pp 3–28.

Monks TJ, Lau SS: Reactive intermediates and their toxicological significance. *Toxicology* **52:**1–53, 1988.

Osawa Y, Davila JC, Nakatsuka M, et al: Inhibition of P450 cytochromes by reactive intermediates. *Drug Metabol Rev* **27:**61–72, 1995.

Parkinson A: Biotransformation of xenobiotics. In *Casarett and Doull's Toxicology, the Basic Science of Poisons,* 5th ed. Klaassen CD (ed.). New York: McGraw-Hill, 1996, pp 113–186.

Smith CAD, Smith G, Wolf CR: Genetic polymorphisms in xenobiotic metabolism. *Eur J Cancer* **30A:**1935–1941, 1994.

ELIMINATION OF TOXICANTS

5

PATRICIA E. LEVI • ERNEST HODGSON • GERALD A. LEBLANC

5.1

INTRODUCTION

Simple forms of life eliminate toxicants ingested with food or otherwise passively absorbed by diffusion into the surrounding medium, which is usually water. As organisms evolved to freshwater, where water and CO_2 balance needed to be regulated, and to land, where, in addition, water needed to be conserved, elimination became a complex regulatory function. Thus, elimination of toxicants became part of a broader specialized system of elimination that maintained the delicate balance of nutrients, minerals, and other substances necessary to life in terrestrial and other environments. Therefore, evolution of mechanisms for the elimination of endogenous and exogenous substances was a prerequisite for the evolution of more complex forms of life, greater size, movement to freshwater and, ultimately, to land.

Although it might seem peculiar that a wide variety of synthetic chemicals that are very recent, relative to the evolutionary time scale, can be eliminated without special physiological systems, it has become apparent that such xenobiotics are not readily eliminated until they are in a form similar to that utilized for the elimination of endogenous substances. Thus, absorbed xenobiotics must first be metabolized by one or more reactions to progressively more polar forms, a process that eventually permits excretion, primarily by renal and hepatic routes. Other routes of excretion may serve to eliminate the parent compounds intact (eg, polychlorinated biphenyls [PCBs] in milk, ethanol in expired air). Such routes of elimination as milk, lungs, alimentary excretion, sweat, hair, and so on, are generally of minor importance as compared with urine and bile.

5.2

RENAL EXCRETION

The kidneys are primarily excretory organs. Elimination by this route accounts for most byproducts of normal body metabolism; in addition, the kidneys are also the primary organ for excretion of polar xenobiotics and the hydrophilic metabolites of lipophilic xenobiotics. The nephron, the functional unit of the kidney, is depicted in Fig. 5.1. Transport of a toxicant or its metabolite to the kidney may occur by dissolution in blood or by binding to blood proteins as discussed in Chapter 2.

GLOMERULAR FILTRATION. The initial step in urine formation is glomerular filtration. The blood plasma is passively filtered as it passes through the numerous large glomerular pores of approximately 70–100 Å in diameter. This filtration system is under pressure generated by the heart. The rate of glomerular filtration is about 180 L/day in an average adult human. No specificity is shown except for molecular size; any solute in the plasma that is small enough to pass through the pores will appear in the ultrafiltrate. Molecules that are too large to pass through the pores or those bound to proteins will not appear in the filtrate and must be either further altered or eliminated by other avenues. Any factor that affects the hydrostatic pressure of the glomerulus may affect the rate of filtration and perhaps result in elevated concentrations of excretory products in the plasma.

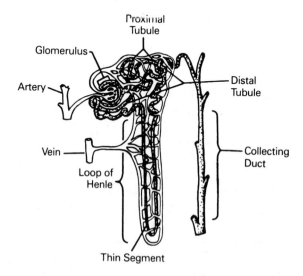

Figure 5.1. Diagrammatic illustration of major components of a typical nephron in the mammalian kidney. *(Source: Hodgson E, Guthrie FE (eds.). Introduction to Biochemical Toxicology. New York: Elsevier, 1980.)*

TUBULAR REABSORPTION. The second major process occurring in the kidney is tubular re-absorption. The glomerular filtrate contains water and a large number of solutes necessary for normal body function—amino acids, glucose, salts, and so on. These solutes must be recovered from the filtrate during the elimination process. Many of the reabsorption mechanisms take place in the cells of the proximal segment of the tubule; in fact, this portion of the tubule accounts for about 75% of reabsorption from the glomerular filtrate. For this reason, the proximal tubule is often the site of toxic action of many reabsorbed toxicants. Both active and passive mechanisms occur, thus permitting varying degrees of selective action. Amino acids, some cations, glucose, peptides, and organic acids are actively reabsorbed, whereas water, chloride, and other ions are passively reabsorbed as a result of the osmotic and electrochemical gradients generated by the active transport of sodium and potassium. Henle's loop functions to establish regulation of osmolarity of fluid in the collecting duct. The remainder of the water and ion reabsorption occurs in the distal tubule and collecting duct.

Reabsorption of xenobiotics is usually passive and is regulated by the same principle that controls passage of endogenous molecules across membranes—that is, lipophilic compounds traverse cell membranes more readily than do polar compounds. Thus, passive reabsorption of lipophilic toxicants is greater than reabsorption of more polar ones, and renal excretion of lipophilic xenobiotics is less than that of excretion of polar, water-soluble compounds.

TUBULAR SECRETION. Another major mechanism for the excretion of solutes by the kidney is tubular secretion. This mechanism permits transport of solutes from the peritubular fluid to the lumen of the tubule, and the process may be either active or passive. One active mechanism permits secretion of a number of organic acids, including glucuronide and sulfate conjugates, whereas a second active process secretes strong organic bases. Passive secretion of some weak basic and acidic organic compounds occurs as a result of pH differences. The nonionized and therefore more lipophilic form of the toxicant is readily diffusible through the tubule membranes. In the tubular lumen, however, the pH is such that the compound becomes ionized and unable to diffuse back across the cell membrane. This mechanism, known as diffusion trapping, is very sensitive to fluctuations of pH in the urine, and in some cases the modification of the urine pH by the oral administration of bicarbonate can be used to help eliminate unwanted compounds. For example, alkalinization of the urine results in an increase in the excretion of phenobarbital and salicylate.

FACTORS AFFECTING RENAL EXCRETION. As previously mentioned, toxicants are excreted by the same mechanisms that govern elimination of endogenous substances. Polar xenobiotics of a size permitting glomerular passage are removed from the plasma and concentrated in the tubules. Minimal tubular reabsorption of such polar compounds occurs, and thus they are readily excreted.

Xenobiotics bound to plasma proteins, however, are unable to pass the glomerulus but are subject to tubular secretion as long as protein binding is readily reversible. As the free fraction of a toxicant is removed from the plasma and secreted by the tubular cells, more toxicant dissociates from the bound form to maintain the equilibrium of free and bound toxicant in the plasma. This equilibrium is governed by both the solubility of the toxicant in the plasma and its binding affinity to plasma proteins. (See Chapter 2 for a discussion of pKa, pH, ionization, and solubility of toxicants.) The newly freed fraction is now available for tubular secretory processes. This process will eventually allow significant excretion of previously bound toxicants. Highly lipophilic toxicants, however, would not be expected to be excreted by this mechanism because they easily diffuse back across the membrane.

5.3

HEPATIC EXCRETION

The second most significant route of elimination is biliary, or hepatic excretion. Although bile was first recognized as a route of excretion for xenobiotics late in the nineteenth century, only in recent years has it been recognized as a major mechanism for toxicant excretion, second only to urine. More than 200 foreign compounds have been detected in bile, and an appreciable fraction of many xenobiotics can be found in bile.

A major problem in investigating hepatic excretion in humans is the difficulty of obtaining bile under physiological conditions. Surgery appreciably depresses bile flow, and studies are also greatly limited because relatively few drugs have warranted careful investigation. Within these constraints, evidence continues to mount for a significant role of the bile in the elimination of foreign comounds. Studies with laboratory animals are also confounded by the effects of anesthesia and surgery, and some investigators have implanted chronic cannulae in the bile duct to measure biliary excretion in unrestrained animals. This technique has the disadvantage of continued loss of bile salts and other biliary constituents, but recent experimental techniques, including using a cannula that redirects bile flow to the duodenum, promise to overcome these objections.

LIVER MORPHOLOGY. The liver is interposed between the intestinal tract and the general blood circulation and thus is ideally located to effect metabolism of both endogenous and exogenous compounds. The products of liver metabolism may be released into either the circulating blood or the bile. The bulk of the liver is comprised of hepatic cells arranged in plates two cells thick (Fig. 5.2). These plates are arranged around the terminal branches of the hepatic veins and exposed to venous and arterial blood flowing through interconnecting spaces (hepatic sinusoids). The sinusoid walls are very permeable to relatively large molecules. In addition, solutes may be transferred from the hepatic cells to the bile or blood by active or passive processes. There is, however, little transfer of lipophilic compounds prior to metabolism to more water-soluble forms.

BILE FORMATION AND SECRETION. Bile secretion is relatively independent of hydrostatic pressure, and bile flow may be either bile salt–dependent, the most important mechanism, or bile salt–independent. The compounds actively secreted by bile are usually amphipathic molecules, having both polar and nonpolar moieties. Bile salts are classic examples of endogenous amphipathic molecules of exogenous origin. As the pKa of most conjugates is 3–4, they are 99% nonionized at physiological pH, thus facilitating active transport.

Foreign compounds can be classified according to their bile/plasma concentration ratios. Class A compounds have a ratio of approximately 1 and are largely excreted by diffusion. They appear in blood or bile in approximately equal ratios. Class B compounds have a ratio greater than unity and tend to be concentrated in bile. These include conjugates of many xenobiotics, and active transport is involved. Class C compounds have a ratio less than 1 and tend to be excluded from bile. These compounds are usually macromolecules such as insulin, phospholipids, and protein.

Bile is secreted by the liver cells into the bile canaliculi, where it flows into the terminal branches of the bile duct and then into the hepatic duct and gallbladder. The gallbladder acts as a reservoir where bile is held until a meal is ingested. Hormonal secretions then cause the gallbladder to release its contents into the duodenum where the bile acids, such as cholic acid, emulsify lipids and facilitate their absorption from the small intestines. Some species (eg, rat, whale, deer) have no gallbladder, and bile flows continuously into the duodenum as it is formed.

Compounds representing nearly every class of pharmacologic agents appear in bile to some extent. Most toxicants found in the bile occur as metabolites. Molecular weight is a major factor that determines the pathway of elimination. A threshold exists, below which compounds are excreted primarily in the urine and above which they are excreted primarily in the bile. Such threshold figures are only approxima-

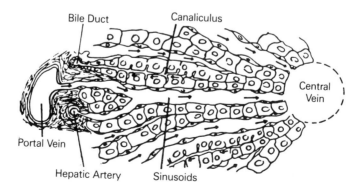

Figure 5.2. Flow of blood from the portal vein and hepatic artery into the sinusoids that empty into the central vein. Bile flows in the opposite direction through canaliculi to empty into the bile ducts. *(Source: Hodgson E, Guthrie FE (eds.).* Introduction to Biochemical Toxicology. *New York: Elsevier, 1980.)*

TABLE 5.1. EFFECT OF MOLECULAR WEIGHT ON ROUTE OF EXCRETION IN THE RAT

Xenobiotic	Mol. Wt.	Urine (%)	Feces (%)
Biphenyl	154	80	20
4-Monochlorobiphenyl	188	50	50
4,4'-Dichlorobiphenyl	223	34	66
2,4,5,2',5'-Pentachlorobiphenyl	326	11	89
2,3,6,2',3',6'-Hexachlorobiphenyl	361	01	99

Source: Matthews HB. In Introduction to Biochemical Toxicology. Hodgson E, Guthrie FE (eds.). New York: Elsevier, 1980, p 171.

tions and vary widely between species. The approximate molecular-weight threshold is 325 in rats, 400 in guinea pigs, 475 in rabbits, and 500–700 in humans. This implies that a range of molecular weights may be excreted in both urine and bile to appreciable extents. Table 5.1 shows urinary versus biliary elimination for a series of compounds of increasing molecular weights. The molecular weight concept does not appear to be operative for all chemical classes, and some water-soluble compounds, such as certain highly water-soluble polymers, with molecular weights of more than 1000, are readily eliminated in urine.

ENTEROHEPATIC CIRCULATION. An important aspect of biliary elimination concerns enterohepatic circulation. Following absorption and transfer to the liver, a nonpolar toxicant is usually oxidized and then conjugated. Depending on the molecular weight it is either eliminated in the urine or secreted in the bile. When conjugates enter the intestine, they may be hydrolyzed by microflora or other intestinal conditions. The compound is again in a less polar form and can be absorbed by the intestine and returned to the liver through the portal circulation. This process may be repeated a number of times, significantly increasing the biologic half-life and possible adverse effects to the liver (Fig. 5.3). Some of the compound may be excreted while in the intestinal lumen, and some of the reabsorbed compound may enter the general circulation. In many cases, however, most of the compound goes into enterohepatic circulation, and thus a much longer biologic half-life is permitted. It may be possible to introduce compounds into the alimentary canal to bind to the newly hydrolyzed compound and thus hasten removal. For example, in methyl mercury therapy a polythiol resin is introduced into the intestine, and for treatment of chlordecone (Kepone) toxicity, cholestyramine is used.

5.4

RESPIRATORY EXCRETION

Although the renal and biliary systems are the most important routes of elimination, many volatile compounds are eliminated through the respiratory system. Other compounds, temporarily taken into the respiratory system but not absorbed, are eliminated.

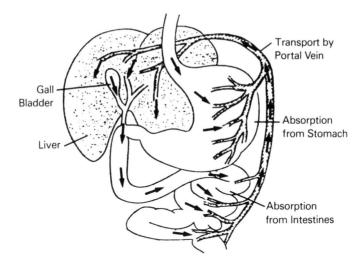

Figure 5.3. Enterohepatic circulation.

The functional structure of the lungs consists of myriad, thin, highly vascularized alveoli. This highly specialized part of the lung with its great surface area and thin membranes has the primary function of exchanging O_2 from air to blood and CO_2 from blood to air (see Chapter 2, Fig. 2.7). The exchange is primarily passive, and any toxicant in the blood with adequate volatility may pass from blood to air for elimination. Ethanol is a well-recognized example, a fact that forms the basis for the forensic determination of alcohol use.

The rate of elimination of volatile toxicants depends on solubility in blood, rate of respiration, and blood flow to the lungs. If a compound has considerable blood solubility, as does ether, hyperventilation will cause it to be eliminated more rapidly. If a compound has low blood solubility, as does ethylene, hyperventilation has little additional effect.

The best-known examples of respiratory elimination are among the anesthetic gases, but pesticide fumigants, many volatile organic solvents, and volatile metabolites of nonvolatile toxicants are eliminated to a significant extent by the lungs. In metabolic studies, carbon from compounds that are appropriately labeled with ^{14}C are often found in expired air, usually as $^{14}CO_2$. Disposition studies reveal that as much as 50% of some radiolabeled compounds can be eliminated in expired air.

Another mechanism for pulmonary elimination of xenobiotics is by way of the alveolobronchiolar transport mechanisms. These mechanisms include fluids secreted by the bronchi and trachea, the lipoprotein surfactant layer secreted by cells in the alveolar structures, and material ingested by macrophages. These secretions may contain dissolved xenobiotics, and macrophages often contain particulates. As discussed in Chapter 2, most of the inhaled particulate matter is deposited in the upper respiratory tract and is moved up and out by the mucociliary bronchotracheal escalator. The mucociliary bronchotracheal escalator is a term used to describe the ciliated surfaces of the upper respiratory tract that are in constant movement to carry the mucus generated by the lung cells and any associated xenobiotics, including particulate material, into the pharynx. More than 90% of inhaled particulate matter is delivered to the pharynx by the mucociliary bronchotracheal escalator within 1 hour after it is inhaled. Once in the pharynx, this material is usually swallowed and passed out through the gastrointestinal tract.

5.5

SEX-LINKED ROUTES

Certain routes of xenobiotic elimination, such as through milk, eggs, and fetus, are restricted to the female of the species. In most instances these routes of elimination offer minimal benefit to the mother, but may have serious effects on the health or survival of the offspring.

MILK. Because milk is an emulsion of lipid in an aqueous solution of protein, a wide variety of xenobiotics have the potential to be found in the milk. Compounds eliminated in milk range from polar compounds such as alcohol and caffeine to less polar compounds, including many drugs, vitamins, and hormones, to very lipophilic compounds such as halogenated insecticides and industrial chemicals. When the mother has accumulated considerable quantities of highly lipid-soluble toxicants (such as DDT or PCBs in fatty depots), a ready route of elimination is in milk. An exchange of toxicants occurs between fatty depots and blood and those toxicants that readily cross the mammary cell membrane.

Elimination of toxicants in milk is highly dependent on the half-life of the xenobiotic. Whereas the short half-lives of more polar compounds dictate a minor role for elimination in milk, for some compounds with long half-lives, milk may become an important mechanism of elimination. For example, in experimental studies with chlorinated insecticides, elimination in cow's milk of 25% of the administered dose may occur. In some South American countries, the DDT content of mother's milk is close to the Acceptable Daily Intake (ADI) recommended by the World Health Organization. Although adverse effects to infants have not been reported in these cases, documented instances of adverse effects have resulted when nursing mothers were accidentally exposed to high concentrations of hexachlorobenzene or PCBs. Large numbers of people were exposed to hexachlorobenzene in Turkey and to PCBs in Japan. In each case a number of infants showed signs of intoxication.

EGGS. Another sex-linked route can be observed with the eggs of birds. Polar toxicants and metabolites may be eliminated primarily in the egg white. Adverse effects are usually quite transient or not noted in these cases. With lipophilic compounds, elimination occurs in the egg yolk, and such compounds are metabolized with difficulty. The effect of such elimination on the survival of the young bird makes the use of these compounds as agricultural chemicals highly controversial. Thus, although elimination of toxic xenobiotics in eggs may have some limited beneficial effects for the mother, xenobiotic elimination in eggs may endanger the survival of the young and possibly the survival of the species if environmental contamination is widespread.

FETUS. A final sex-linked route of elimination is in the fetus. The placental barrier may be important in preventing entry of a number of polar toxicants and their metabolites, but it is no longer considered an important barrier to entry of lipophilic compounds that can cross the placenta by passive diffusion. Although the fetus contains relatively small amounts of toxicants in most cases, the tragic examples of teratologic effects of thalidomide, toxic effects of mercury, and carcinogenic effects of diethylstilbesterol (DES) are well documented.

5.6
ALIMENTARY ELIMINATION

When toxicants equilibrate with body fluids and have the necessary lipophilicity to traverse membranes, they may move through the alimentary canal into the lumen. There is some evidence for active transport of penicillin through the salivary glands and of compounds of ammonia in the intestine, but usually the process is passive. Passive elimination in the alimentary canal usually results in the excretion of quantitatively unimportant amounts of toxicants; in some cases, however, this may be an important route of elimination. The contaminant chlordecone (Kepone) appears to be eliminated primarily in the intestine (although the rate is slow). The therapy for chlordecone poisoning is the administration of cholestyramine, which binds chlordecone and prevents its reabsorption (enterohepatic circulation); thus, in time, appreciable amounts of chlordecone may be eliminated.

5.7
OBSCURE ROUTES

Finally, elimination of toxicants may also involve some very obscure and poorly understood routes. Because diffusion of toxicants can occur across any of the cell membranes of the body, hair, feathers, oil, sweat, and so on may be expected to be involved in the elimination of trace quantities of lipophilic compounds. Such elimination may also be possible when compounds of the body are continuously removed—for example, in sloughing of the skin when toxicants adhere to the tissue.

Cells that have a secretory function or much growth may be of some importance as routes of elimination. In secretory cells a favorable gradient for the passive elimination of xenobiotics is maintained by the constant renewal of the cell contents. The sweat glands have been shown to eliminate a large number of metal ions and a smaller number of polar xenobiotics. Sebaceous glands secrete oils that keep skin and hair soft and pliable. These oily secretions are probably responsible for the lipophilic xenobiotics, such as insecticides and PCBs that have been detected on human hair samples.

In cells responsible for growth of hair, feathers, and nails, a favorable gradient for xenobiotic elimination is maintained by new growth. Such compounds as mercury, selenium, and arsenic are well-known examples of toxicants associated with hair and such compounds have been detected at concentrations that are proportional to the dose received.

Although the benefit to the individual from elimination by these minor routes is thought to be negligible, one or more of these routes may be used to provide a nonintrusive method of estimating total body burden of certain toxicants. For example, bird feathers are ideal for assessment of heavy metals as they accumulate certain heavy metals in proportion to blood levels at the time of feather formation and the procedure is noninvasive. The measurement of cotinine, a major metabolite of nicotine, in saliva can be used as as indicator of nicotine uptake and is of importance in epidemiology. Several references concerning such biomonitoring procedures are listed under further reading.

5.8

CELLULAR ELIMINATION

The cellular elimination of xenobiotics must be sufficiently efficient to ensure that toxicants do not accumulate at target sites and that they can be readily effluxed from excretory cells such as hepatocytes. Active elimination processes have a prominent role in providing for the efficient cellular elimination of xenobiotics. Considering that the canalicular membrane of the hepatocyte constitutes only 13% of the total cell surface membrane, active transport processes at this site are necessary for the selective transport of xenobiotics across this membrane into the bile canaliculus. Furthermore, biotransformation processes within the hepatocyte render xenobiotics more polar. Although these changes facilitate the mobilization of the xenobiotic within intracellular and extracellular aqueous compartments, they reduce the ability of the xenobiotic to diffuse passively across membranes. Active transport of the biotransformation products surmounts this obstacle to elimination.

Hepatocytes and other cell types express a family of active transport proteins that are responsible for the elimination of many xenobiotics. Two members of this family that contribute to xenobiotic elimination are the *multidrug resistance–associated protein* (MRP), also called the multispecific organic anion transporter, and *p-glycoprotein* (P-gp). Both of these proteins were identified initially because of their overexpression in cells that were resistant to the toxic effects of anticancer drugs. Subsequently it was demonstrated that these proteins contributed to drug resistance by actively transporting drugs out of the cells. These active transporters are embedded in the cell membrane, across which the xenobiotic requires transport. The protein conforms to a pore traversing the membrane, and the xenobiotic binds to the transport site at the intracellular component of the protein. Adenosine triphosphate (ATP) hydrolysis provides the energy required to pump the xenobiotic, perhaps by changing the confirmation of the protein, through the pore and into the extracellular space.

MRP is capable of transporting ligands that are conjugated to glutathione, glucuronic acid, or sulfate. Thus, phase-two conjugation processes not only increase the water solubility of a xenobiotic, but also target the compound for active elimination. P-gp transports a diverse array of structurally diverse xenobiotics. Characteristics common to most P-gp transport ligands include a molecular mass of 300–500 daltons, aromatic components, lipophilicity, and amphipathic properties often associated with cationic amine groups on one side of the molecule.

Active transporters are very important in protecting organisms against chemical toxicity. In an effort to establish the physiological role of P-gp, transgenic mice were produced that lacked a functional isoform of the protein. Although these mice appeared normal, when the mouse colony was treated with the acaricide ivermectin to control a mite infestation, the transgenic mice died. Further study revealed that ivermectin accumulated in the brain of the transgenic animals, presumably because of the absence of P-gp at the blood–brain barrier. Studies using inhibitors of P-gp have shown that inhibition of the transporter results in the increased accumulation and half-life of P-gp substrates. Accordingly, active elimination is now often referred to as phase-three detoxication following the biotransformation processes incurred during phase-one and phase-two detoxication.

Suggested Further Reading

Burger J: Metals in avian feathers: bioindicators of environmental pollution. *Rev Environ Toxicol* **5:**197–306, 1994.

Burger J, Gochfeld M: Biomonitoring of heavy metals in the Pacific Basin using avian feathers. *Environ Toxicol Chem* **14:**1233–1239, 1995.

Klaassen CD: Biliary excretion of metals. *Drug Metab Rev* **5:**165–196, 1976.

LeBlanc GA: Hepatic vectorial transport of xenobiotics. *Chemical-Biol Interact* **90:**101–120, 1994.

Matthews HB: Excretion and elimination of toxicants and their metabolites. In *Introduction to Biochemical Toxicology,* 2nd ed. Hodgson E, Levi PE (eds.). Norwalk, CT: Appleton & Lange, 1994, pp 177–192.

Pritchard JB, Miller DS: Mechanisms mediating renal secretion of organic anions and cations. *Physiol Rev* **73:**765–796, 1993.

Rozman K. Fecal excretion of toxic substances. In *Gastrointestinal Toxicology.* Rozman K, Hanninen O (eds.). Amsterdam/New York: Elsevier, 1986, pp 119–145.

Rozman KK, Klaassen CD: Absorption, distribution, and excretion of toxicants. In *Casarett & Doull's Toxicology, the Basic Science of Poisons,* 5th ed. Klaassen CD (ed.). New York: McGraw-Hill, 1996, pp 91–112.

Wilson JT: Determinants and consequences of drug excretion in breast milk. *Drug Metab Rev* **14:**619–652, 1983.

MODIFICATION OF XENOBIOTIC METABOLISM

6

ERNEST HODGSON

6.1

INTRODUCTION

The metabolism of toxicants and their overall toxicity can be modified by many factors both extrinsic and intrinsic to the normal functioning of the organism. It is entirely possible that many changes in toxicity are due to changes in metabolism, because most sequences of events that lead to overt toxicity involve activation and/or detoxication of the parent compound. In many cases, the chain of cause and effect is not entirely clear, due to the difficulty of relating single events, measured in vitro, to the complex and interrelated effects that occur in vivo. This relationship between in vitro and in vivo studies is important and is discussed in connection with enzymatic inhibition and induction (see Section 6.5). It is important to note that the chemical, nutritional, physiological, and other effects noted herein have been described primarily from experiments carried out on experimental animals. These studies indicate that similar effects may occur in humans or other animals, but not that they must occur, or that they occur at the same magnitude in all species, if they occur at all.

6.2

NUTRITIONAL EFFECTS

Many nutritional effects on xenobiotic metabolism have been noted, but the information is scattered and often appears contradictory. This is one of the most important of several neglected areas of toxicology. This section is concerned only with the effects of nutritional constituents of the diet; the effects of other xenobiotics in the diet are discussed under chemical effects (see Section 6.5).

6.2.1 Protein

Low protein diets generally decrease monooxygenase activity in rat liver micro-somes, and gender and substrate differences may be seen in the effect. For example, aminopyrine N-demethylation, hexobarbital hydroxylation, and aniline hydroxyla-tion are all decreased, but the effect on the first two is greater in males than in fe-males. In the third case, aniline hydroxylation, the reduction in males is equal to that in females. Tissue differences may also be seen. These changes are presumably related to the reductions in the levels of cytochrome P450 and NADPH–cytochrome P450 reductase that are also noted. One might speculate that the gender and other variations are due to differential effects on P450 isozymes. Even though enzyme levels are reduced by low protein diets, they can still be induced to some extent by compounds such as phenobarbital. Such changes may also be reflected in changes in toxicity. Changes in the level of azoreductase activity in rat liver brought about by a low protein diet are reflected in an increased severity in the carcinogenic effect of dimethylaminoazobenzene. The liver carcinogen, dimethylnitrosamine, which must be activated metabolically, is almost without effect in protein-deficient rats. Strychnine, which is detoxified by microsomal monooxygenase action, is more toxic to animals on low protein diets, whereas octamethylpyrophosphoramide, car-bon tetrachloride, and heptachlor, which are activated by monooxygenases, are less toxic. Phase-two reactions may also be affected by dietary protein levels. Chloram-phenicol glucuronidation is reduced in protein-deficient guinea pigs, although no effect is seen on sulfotransferase activity in protein-deficient rats.

6.2.2 Carbohydrates

High dietary carbohydrate levels in the rat tend to have much the same effect as low dietary protein, decreasing such activities as aminopyrine N-demethylase, pentobar-bital hydroxylation, and p-nitrobenzoic acid reduction along with a concomitant de-crease in the enzymes of the cytochrome P450 monooxygenase system. Because rats tend to regulate total caloric intake, this may actually reflect low protein intake.

6.2.3 Lipids

Dietary deficiencies in linoleic or in other unsaturated fats generally bring about a reduction in P450 and related monooxygenase activities in the rat. The increase in effectiveness of breast and colon carcinogens brought about in animals on high fat diets, however, appears to be related to events during the promotion phase rather than the activation of the causative chemical. Lipids also appear to be necessary for the effect of inducers, such as phenobarbital, to be fully expressed.

6.2.4 Micronutrients

Vitamin deficiencies in general bring about a reduction in monooxygenase activity, although exceptions can be noted. Riboflavin deficiency causes an increase in P450 and aniline hydroxylation, although at the same time it causes a decrease in P450 reductase and benzo(a)pyrene hydroxylation. Ascorbic acid deficiency in the guinea pig not only causes a decrease in P450 and monooxygenase activity but also causes a reduction in microsomal hydrolysis of procaine. Deficiencies in vitamins A and E cause a decrease in monooxygenase activity, whereas thiamine deficiency causes an increase. The effect of these vitamins on different P450 isozymes has not been investigated. Changes in mineral nutrition have also been observed to affect monooxygenase activity. In the immature rat, calcium or magnesium deficiency causes a decrease, whereas, quite unexpectedly, iron deficiency causes an increase. This increase is not accompanied by a concomitant increase in P450, however. An excess of dietary cobalt, cadmium, manganese, and lead all cause an increase in hepatic glutathione levels and a decrease in P450 content.

6.2.5   Starvation and Dehydration

Although in some animals starvation appears to have effects similar to those of protein deficiency, this is not necessarily the case. For example, in the mouse, monooxygenation is decreased but reduction of p-nitrobenzoic acid is unaffected. In male rats, hexobarbital and pentabarbital hydroxylation as well as aminopyrine N-demethylation are decreased, but aniline hydroxylation is increased. All of these activities are stimulated in the female. Water deprivation in gerbils causes an increase in P450 and a concomitant increase in hexobarbital metabolism, which is reflected in a shorter sleeping time.

6.2.6   Nutritional Requirements in Xenobiotic Metabolism

Because xenobiotic metabolism involves many enzymes with different cofactor requirements, prosthetic groups, or endogenous cosubstrates, it is apparent that many different nutrients are involved in their function and maintainence. Determination of the effect of deficiencies, however, is more complex because reductions in activity of any particular enzyme will be effective only if it affects a change in a rate limiting step in a process. In the case of multiple deficiencies, the nature of the rate limiting step may change with time.

PHASE-ONE REACTIONS. Nutrients involved in the maintainence of the cytochrome P450 monooxygenase system are shown in Fig. 6.1. The B complex vitamins niacin and riboflavin are both involved, the former in the formation of NADPH, the latter in the formation of FAD and FMN. Essential amino acids are, of course, required for the synthesis of all of the proteins involved. The heme of the cytochrome requires iron, an essential inorganic nutrient. Other nutrients required in heme synthesis include pantothenic acid, needed for the synthesis of the coenzyme A used in the formation of acetyl Co-A, pyridoxine, a cofactor in heme synthesis and copper, required in the ferroxidase system that converts ferrous to ferric iron prior to its incorporation into heme. Although it is clear that dietary deficiencies could reduce the ability of the P450 system to metabolize xenobiotics, it is not clear how this effect will be manifested in vivo unless there is an understanding of the rate-limiting

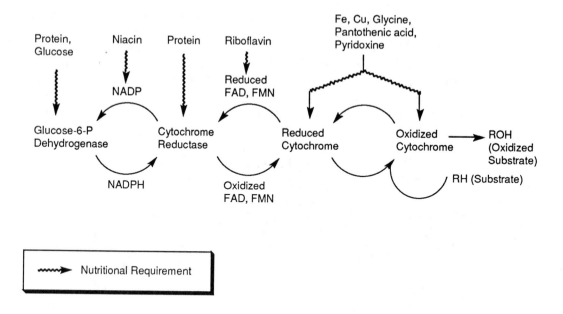

Figure 6.1. Nutritional requirements with potential effects on the cytochrome P450 monooxygenase system. *(Source: Donaldson WE: Nutritional factors. In Hodgson E, Levi PE [eds]. Introduction to Biochemical Toxicology, 2nd ed. Norwalk CT: Appleton & Lange, 1994, p. 306.)*

factors involved, a considerable task in such a complex of interrelated reactions. Similar considerations could be made for other phase-one reaction systems such as arachidonic acid cooxidations, the glutathione peroxidase system, and so on.

PHASE-TWO REACTIONS. As with phase-one reactions, phase-two reactions usually depend on several enzymes with different cofactors and different prosthetic groups and, frequently, different endogenous cosubstrates. All of these many components can depend on nutritional requirements, including vitamins, minerals, amino acids, and others. Mercapturic acid formation can be cited to illustrate the principles involved. The formation of mercapturic acids starts with the formation of glutathione conjugates, reactions catalyzed by the glutathione S-transferases. This is followed by removal of the glutamic acid and the glycine residues followed by acetylation of the remaining cysteine. Essential amino acids are required for the synthesis of the proteins involved, pantothenic acid for coenzyme A synthesis and phosphorus for synthesis of the ATP needed for glutathione synthesis. Similar scenarios can be developed for glucuronide and sulfate formation, acetylation and other phase-two reaction systems.

6.3

PHYSIOLOGICAL EFFECTS

6.3.1   Development

Birth, in mammals, initiates an increase in the activity of many hepatic enzymes, including those involved in xenobiotic metabolism. The ability of the liver to carry out monooxygenation reactions appears to be very low during gestation and to increase after birth, with no obvious differences being seen between immature males and females. This general trend has been observed in many species, although the developmental pattern may vary according to gender and genetic strain. The component enzymes of the P450 monooxygenase system both follow the same general trend although there may be differences in the rate of increase. In the rabbit, the postnatal increase in P450 and its reductase is parallel; in the rat, the increase in the reductase is slower than that of the cytochrome.

Phase-two reactions may also be age dependent. Glucuronidation of many substrates is low or undetectable in fetal tissues but increases with age. The inability of newborn mammals of many species to form glucuronides is associated with deficiencies in both glucuronosyltransferase and its cofactor, uridine diphosphate glucuronic acid (UDPGA). A combination of this deficiency, as well as slow excretion of the bilirubin conjugate formed, and the presence in the blood of pregnanediol, an inhibitor of glucuronidation, may lead to neonatal jaundice. Glycine conjugations are also low in the newborn, resulting from a lack of available glycine, an amino acid that reaches normal levels at about 30 days of age in the rat and 8 weeks in the human. Glutathione conjugation may also be impaired, as in fetal and neonatal guinea pigs, because of a deficiency of available glutathione. In the serum and liver of perinatal rats, glutathione transferase is barely detectable, increasing rapidly until adult levels are reached at about 140 days (Fig. 6.2). This pattern is not followed in all cases, because sulfate conjugation and acetylation appear to be fully functional and at adult levels in the guinea pig fetus. Thus, some compounds that are glucuronidated in the adult can be acetylated or conjugated as sulfates in the young.

An understanding of how these effects may be related to the expression of individual isoforms is now beginning to emerge. It is known that in immature rats of either gender, P450s 2A1, 2D6, and 3A2 predominate, whereas in mature rats the males show a predominance of P450s 2C11, 2C6, and 3A2 and the females P450s 2A1, 2C6, and 2C12.

The effect of senescence on the metabolism of xenobiotics has not been studied extensively. In rats monooxygenase activity, which reaches a maximum at about 30 days of age, begins to decline some 250 days later, a decrease that may be associated with reduced levels of sex hormones. Glucuronidation also decreases in old animals, whereas monoamine oxidase activity increases. These changes in the ability to metabolize xenobiotics are often reflected in changes in overall toxicity. The sleeping time for hexobarbital, which is detoxified by monooxygenase action, may be greatly extended in the newborn, whereas the hepatotoxicity of paracetamol,

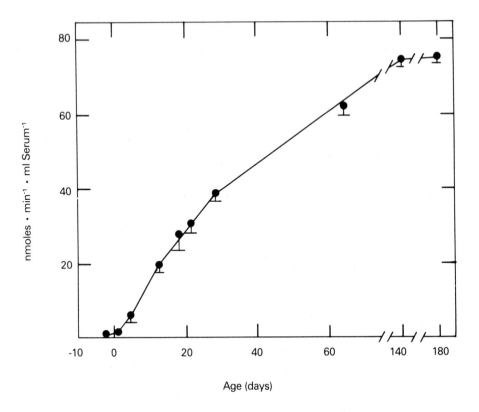

Figure 6.2. Developmental pattern of serum glutathione *S*-transferase activity in female rats. *(Source: Redrawn from Mukhtar and Bend. Life Sci **21**:1277, 1977.)*

which is activated by the same enzymes, is much lower in the newborn than in adults. Again, we are now beginning to understand how these changes may be reflected in changes in specific isoforms. For example, in old male rats, P450s 2C11 and 3A2 decrease while 2C12 increases, effects that may be related to decreases in circulating sex hormones.

6.3.2   Gender Differences

Metabolism of xenobiotics may vary with the gender of the organism. Gender differences become apparent at puberty and are usually maintained throughout adult life. Adult male rats metabolize many compounds at rates higher than females, for example, hexobarbital hydroxylation, aminopyrine *N*-demethylation, glucuronidation of *o*-aminophenol and glutathione conjugation of aryl substrates; however, with other substrates, such as aniline and zoxazolamine, no gender differences are seen. In other species, including humans, the gender difference in xenobiotic metabolism is less pronounced. The differences in microsomal monooxygenase activity between males and females have been shown to be under the control of sex hormones, at least in some species. Some enzyme activities are decreased by castration in the male, and administration of androgens to castrated males increases the activity of these sex-dependent enzyme activities without affecting the independent ones. Procaine hydrolysis is faster in male than female rats, and this compound is less toxic to the male. Gender differences in enzyme activity may also vary from tissue to tissue. Hepatic microsomes from adult male guinea pigs are less active in the conjugation of p-nitrophenol than are those from females, but no such gender difference is seen in the microsomes from lung, kidney, and small intestines.

Many differences in overall toxicity between males and females of various species are known (Table 6.1). Although it is not always known whether metabolism is the only or even the most important factor, such differences may be related to gender-related differences in metabolism. Hexobarbital is metabolized faster by male rats; thus, female rats have longer sleeping times. Parathion is activated to the cholinesterase inhibitor paraoxon more rapidly in female than in male rats, and thus is more toxic to females. Presumably many of the gender-related differences, as with developmental differences, are related to quantitative or qualitative differences in the isozymes of the xenobiotic-metabolizing enzymes that exist in multiple forms, but this aspect has not been investigated extensively.

In the rat, sexually dimorphic P450s appear to arise by programming, or imprinting, that occurs in neonatal development. This imprinting is brought about by a surge of testosterone that occurs in the male, but not the female, neonate and appears to imprint the developing hypothalamus so that in later development growth hormone is secreted in a gender-specific manner. Growth hormone production is pulsatile in adult males with peaks of production at aproximately 3-hour intervals and more continuous in females, with smaller peaks. This pattern of growth hormone production and the higher level of circulating testosterone in the male maintain the expression of male-specific isoforms such as P450 2C11. The more continuous pattern of growth hormone secretion and the lack of circulating testosterone appears to be responsible for the expression of female specific isoforms such as P450 2C12. The high level of sulfotransferases in the female appears to be under similar control, raising the possibility that this is a general mechanism for the expression of gender-specific xenobiotic-metabolizing enzymes or their isoforms. A schematic version of this proposed mechanism is seen in Fig. 6.3.

TABLE 6.1. GENDER-RELATED DIFFERENCES IN TOXICITY

Species	Toxicant	Susceptibility
Rat	EPN, warfarin, strychnine, hexobarbital, parathion	F > M
	Aldrin, lead, epinephrine, ergot alkaloids	M > F
Cat	Dinitrophenol	F > M
Rabbit	Benzene	F > M
Mouse	Folic acid	F > M
Nicotine	M > F	
Dog	Digitoxin	M > F

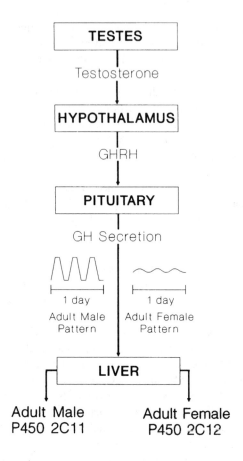

Figure 6.3. Hypothetical scheme for neonatal imprinting of the hypothalamus-pituitary-liver axis resulting in sexually dimorphic expression of hepatic enzymes in the adult rat. Neonatal surges of testosterone appear to play a role in imprinting. *(Source: Ronis MJJ, Cunny HC: Physiological (endogenous) factors affecting the metabolism of xenobiotics. In Hodgson E, Levi PE [eds],* Introduction to Biochemical Toxicology, 2nd ed. *Norwalk CT: Appleton & Lange, 1994, p 136.)*

Gender-specific expression is also seen in the flavin-containing monooxygenases. In the mouse liver FMO1 is higher in the female than in the male, and FMO3, present at high levels in female liver, is not expressed in male liver. FMO5, however, is expressed equally in the livers of both male and female mice. The mechanism for this unusual gender-specific pattern is not yet known.

6.3.3   Hormones

Hormones other than sex hormones are also known to affect the levels of xenobiotic metabolizing enzymes, but these effects are much less studied or understood.

THYROID HORMONE. Treatment of rats with thyroxin increases hepatic microsomal NADPH oxidation in both male and female rats, with the increase being greater in females. Cytochrome P450 content decreases in the male but not in the female. Hyperthyroidism causes a decrease in gender-dependent monooxygenase reactions and appears to interfere with the ability of androgens to increase the activity of the enzymes responsible. Gender differences are not seen in the response of mice and rabbits to thyroxine. In mice, aminopyrine N-demethylase, aniline hydroxylase, and hexobarbital hydroxylase are decreased, whereas p-nitrobenzoic acid reduction is unchanged. In rabbits, hexobarbital hydroxylation is unchanged, whereas aniline hydroxylation and p-nitrobenzoic acid reduction increase. Thyroid hormone can also affect enzymes other than microsomal monooxygenases. For example, liver monoamine oxidase activity is decreased whereas the activity of the same enzymes in the kidney is increased.

ADRENAL HORMONES. Removal of adrenal glands from male rats results in a decrease in the activity of hepatic microsomal enzymes, impairing the metabolism of aminopyrine and hexobarbital, but the same operation in females has no effect on their metabolism. Cortisone or prednisolone restores activity to normal levels.

INSULIN. The effect of diabetes on xenobiotic metabolism is quite varied and, in this regard, alloxan-induced diabetes may not be a good model for the natural disease. The in vitro metabolism of hexobarbital and aminopyrine is decreased in alloxan-diabetic male rats, but is increased in similarly treated females. Aniline hydroxylase is increased in both males and females with alloxan diabetes. The induction of P450 2E1 in diabetes (and in fasting) is believed to be due to the high circulating levels of endogenously generated ketones. Studies of activity of the enzymes mentioned show no gender differences in the mouse; both sexes show an increase. Some phase-two reactions, such as glucuronidation, are decreased in diabetic animals. This appears to be due to a lack of UDPGA caused by a decrease in UDPG dehydrogenase, rather than a decrease in transferase activity, and the effect can be reversed by insulin.

OTHER HORMONES. Pituitary hormones regulate the function of many other endocrine glands and hypophysectomy in male rats results in a decrease in the activity of xenobiotic metabolizing enzymes. Administration of adrenocorticotropic hormone (ACTH) also results in a decrease of those oxidative enzyme activities that are gender dependent. In contrast, ACTH treatment of female rats causes an increase in aminopyrine N-demethylase but no change in other activities.

6.3.4   Pregnancy

Many xenobiotic metabolizing enzyme activities decrease during pregnancy. Catechol O-methyltransferase and monoamine oxidase decrease, as does glucuronide conjugation. The latter may be related to the increasing levels of progesterone and pregnanediol, both known to be inhibitors of glucuronosyltransferase in vitro. A similar effect on sulfate conjugation has been seen in pregnant rats and guinea pigs. In some species, liver microsomal monooxygenase activity may also decrease during pregnancy, this decrease being accompanied by a concomitant decrease in P450 levels. An increased level of FMO2 is seen in the lung of pregnant rabbits.

6.3.5 Disease

Quantitatively, the most important site for xenobiotic metabolism is the liver; thus, effects on the liver are likely to have a pronounced effect on the organism's overall capacity in this regard. At the same time, effects on other organs can have consequences no less serious for the organism. Patients with acute hepatitis frequently have an impaired ability to oxidize drugs, with a concomitant increase in plasma half-life. Impaired oxidative metabolism has also been shown in patients with chronic hepatitis or cirrhosis. The decrease in drug metabolism that occurs in obstructive jaundice may be a consequence of the accumulation of bile salts, which are known inhibitors of some of the enzymes involved. Phase-two reactions may also be affected, decreases in acetylation, glucuronidation, and a variety of esterase activities having been seen in various liver diseases. Hepatic tumors, in general, have a lower ability to metabolize foreign compounds than does normal liver tissue, although in some cases the overall activity of tumor-bearing livers may be no lower than that of controls. Kidney diseases may also affect the overall ability to handle xenobiotics, because this organ is one of the main routes for elimination of xenobiotics and their metabolites. The half-lives of tolbutamide, thiopental, hexobarbital, and chloramphenicol are all prolonged in patients with renal impairment.

6.3.6 Diurnal Rhythms

Diurnal rhythms, both in P450 levels and in the susceptibility to toxicants, have been described, especially in rodents. Although such changes appear to be related to the light cycle, they may, in fact, be activity dependent because feeding and other activities in rodents are themselves markedly diurnal.

6.4

COMPARATIVE AND GENETIC EFFECTS

Comparative toxicology is the study of the variation in toxicity of exogenous chemicals toward different organisms, either of different genetic strains or of different taxonomic groups. Thus, the comparative approach can be used in the study of any aspect of toxicology, such as absorption, metabolism, mode of action, and acute or chronic effects. Most comparative data for toxic compounds exist in two areas—acute toxicity and metabolism. The value of the comparative approach can be summarized under four headings:

1. *Selective Toxicity.* If toxic compounds are to be used for controlling diseases, pests, and parasites, it is important to develop selective biocides, toxic to the target organism but less toxic to other organisms, particularly humans.
2. *Experimental Models.* Comparative studies of toxic phenomena are necessary to select the most appropriate model for extrapolation to humans and for testing and development of drugs and biocides. Taxonomic proximity does not necessarily indicate which will be the best experimental animal

because in some cases primates are less valuable for study than are other mammals.

3. *Environmental Xenobiotic Cycles.* Much concern over toxic compounds springs from their occurrence in the environment. Different organisms in the complex ecological foodwebs metabolize compounds at different rates and to different products; the metabolic end-products are released back to the environment, either to be further metabolized by other organisms or to exert toxic effects of their own. Clearly, it is desirable to know the range of metabolic processes possible. Laboratory microecosystems have been developed, and with the aid of ^{14}C-labeled compounds, chemicals and their metabolites can be followed through the plants and terrestrial and aquatic animals involved.

4. *Comparative Biochemistry.* Some researchers believe that the proper role of comparative biochemistry is to put evolution on a molecular basis, and that detoxication enzymes, like other enzymes, are suitable subjects for study. Xenobiotic-metabolizing enzymes were probably essential in the early stages of animal evolution because secondary plant products, even those of low toxicity, are frequently lipophilic and as a consequence would, in the absence of such enzymes, accumulate in lipid membranes and lipid depots. The evolution of cytochrome P450 isoforms, with more than 400 isoform cDNA sequences known, is proving a useful tool for the study of biochemical evolution.

6.4.1 Variations Among Taxonomic Groups

There are few differences in xenobiotic metabolism that are specific for large taxonomic groups. The formation of glucosides by insects and plants rather than the glucuronides of other animal groups is one of the most distinct. Although differences between species are common and of toxicologic significance, they are usually quantitative rather than qualitative in nature and tend to occur within as well as between taxonomic groups. Although the ultimate explanation of such differences must be at the level of biochemical genetics, they are manifested at many other levels, the most important of which are summarized in the following sections.

6.4.1.1 In Vivo Toxicity

Toxicity is a term used to describe the adverse effects of chemicals on living organisms. Depending on the degree of toxicity, an animal may die, suffer injury to certain organs, or have a specific functional derangement in a subcellular organelle. Sublethal effects of toxicants may be reversible. Available data on the toxicity of selected pesticides to rats suggest that herbicide use, in general, provides the greatest human safety factor by selectively killing plants. As the evolutionary position of the target species approaches that of humans, however, the human safety factor is narrowed considerably. Thus, as far as direct toxicity to humans and other mammals is concerned, biocide toxicity seems to be in the following progression: herbicides = fungicides < molluscicides < acaricides < nematocides < insecticides < rodenticides. This relationship is obviously oversimplified because marked differences in lethality are observed when different members of each group of biocides is tested against laboratory test animals and target species. One should also bear in mind that any chemical can be environmentally dangerous if misused because many possible targets are interrelated in complex ecological systems.

Interspecific differences are also known for some naturally occurring poisons. Nicotine, for instance, is used as an insecticide and kills many insect pests at low doses, yet tobacco leaves constitute a normal diet for several species. As indicated earlier, most strains of rabbit eat *Belladonna* leaves without ill effects, whereas other mammals are easily poisoned. Natural tolerance to cyanide poisoning in millipedes and the high resistance to the powerful axonal blocking agent tetrodotoxin in puffer fish are examples of the tolerance of animals to the toxins they produce.

The specific organ toxicity of chemicals also exhibits wide species differences. Carbon tetrachloride, a highly potent hepatotoxicant, induces liver damage in many species, but chickens are almost unaffected by it. Dinitrophenol causes cataracts in humans, ducks, and chickens, but not in other experimental animals. The eggshell thinning associated with DDT poisoning in birds is observed in falcons and mallard ducks, whereas this reproductive toxicity is not observed in gallinaceous species. Delayed neurotoxicity caused by organophosphates such as leptophos and tri-*o*-cresyl phosphate occurs in humans and can be easily demonstrated in chickens, but can be produced only with difficulty in most common laboratory mammals.

6.4.1.2   In Vivo Metabolism

Many ecological and physiological factors affect the rates of penetration, distribution, biotransformation, and excretion of chemicals, and thus govern their biological fate in the body. In general, the absorption of xenobiotics, their tissue distribution, and penetration across the blood–brain barrier and other barriers are dictated by their physicochemical nature and, therefore, tend to be similar in various animal species. The biologic effect of a chemical depends on the concentration of its active form and its duration inside the body; this is governed in turn by the rates of its biotransformation and excretion and the magnitude and nature of its binding to tissue macromolecules. Thus, substantial differences in these variables should confer species specificity in the biologic response to any metabolically active xenobiotic. The biologic half-life is governed by the rates of metabolism and excretion and thus reflects the most important variables explaining interspecies differences in toxic response. Striking differences between species can be seen in the biologic half-lives of various drugs. Humans, in general, metabolize xenobiotics more slowly than do various experimental animals. For example, phenylbutazone is metabolized slowly in humans, with a half-life averaging 3 days. In the monkey, rat, guinea pig, rabbit, dog, and horse, however, this drug is metabolized readily, with half-lives ranging between 3 and 6 hours. The interdependence of metabolic rate, half-life, and pharmacologic action is well illustrated in the case of hexobarbital. The duration of sleeping time is directly related to the biologic half-life and is inversely proportional to the in vitro degradation capacity of liver enzymes from the respective species. Thus, mice inactivate hexobarbital readily, as reflected in a brief biologic half-life in vivo and short sleeping time, whereas the reverse is true in dogs.

Xenobiotics, once inside the body, undergo a series of biotransformations. Those reactions that introduce a new functional group into the molecule, either by oxidation, reduction, or hydrolysis, are designated phase-one reactions, whereas the conjugation reactions by which phase-one metabolites are combined with endogenous substrates in the body are referred to as phase-two reactions. Chemicals may undergo any one of these reactions or any combination of them, either simultaneously or consecutively. Because biotransformations are catalyzed by a large number of enzymes, it is to be expected that they will vary between species. Qualitative differences imply the occurrence of different enzymes, whereas quantitative differences imply variations in the rate of biotransformation along a common metabolic pathway, the variations resulting from differences in enzyme levels, in the extent of competing reactions, or in the efficiency of enzymes capable of reversing the reaction.

Even in the case of a xenobiotic undergoing oxidation primarily by a single reaction, there may be remarkable species differences in relative rates. Thus, in humans, rats, and guinea pigs, the major route of papaverine metabolism is *O*-demethylation to yield phenolic products, but very little of these products is formed in dogs. Aromatic hydroxylation of aniline is another example. In this case, both *ortho* and *para* positions are susceptible to oxidative attack yielding the respective aminophenols. The biological fate of aniline has been studied in many species and striking selectivity in hydroxylation position has been noted (Table 6.2). These data show a trend, in that carnivores generally display a high aniline *ortho*-hydroxylase ability with a *para/ortho* ratio of ≤1, whereas rodents exhibit a striking preference for the *para* position, with a *para/ortho* ratio of from 2.5 to 15. Along with extensive *p*-aminophenol, substantial quantities of *o*-aminophenol are also produced from

TABLE 6.2. IN VIVO HYDROXYLATION OF ANILINE IN FEMALES OF VARIOUS SPECIES

Species	Percent Dose Excreted as Aminophenol		P/O Ratio
	Ortho	*Para*	
Dog	18.0	9.0	0.5
Cat	32.0	14.0	0.4
Ferret	26.0	28.0	1.0
Rat	19.0	48.0	2.5
Mouse	4.0	12.0	3.0
Hamster	5.5	53.0	10.0
Guinea pig	4.2	46.0	11.0
Rabbit	8.8	50.0	6.0
Hen	10.5	44.0	4.0

*Source: Adapted from Parke DV, Biochem J **77**:493, 1960.*

aniline administered to rabbits and hens. The major pathway is not always the same in any two animal species. 2-Acetylaminofluorene may be metabolized in mammals by two alternative routes: N-hydroxylation, yielding the carcinogenic N-hydroxy derivative; and aromatic hydroxylation, yielding the noncarcinogenic 7-hydroxy metabolite. The former is the metabolic route in the rat, rabbit, hamster, dog, and in humans in which the parent compound is known to be carcinogenic. In contrast, the monkey carries out aromatic hydroxylation and the guinea pig appears to deacetylate the N-hydroxy derivative; thus, both escape the carcinogenic effects of this compound.

The hydrolysis of esters by esterases and of amides by amidases constitutes one of the most common enzymatic reactions of xenobiotics in humans and other animal species. Because both the number of enzymes involved in hydrolytic attack and the number of substrates for them is large, it is not surprising to observe interspecific differences in the disposition of xenobiotics due to variations in these enzymes. In mammals, the presence of a carboxylesterase that hydrolyzes malathion but is generally absent in insects explains the remarkable selectivity of this insecticide. As with esters, wide differences exist between species in the rates of hydrolysis of various amides in vivo. Fluoracetamide is less toxic to mice than to the American cockroach. This is explained by the faster release of the toxic fluoroacetate in insects as compared with mice. The insecticide dimethoate is susceptible to the attack of both esterases and amidases, yielding nontoxic products. In the rat and mouse, both reactions occur, whereas sheep liver contains only the amidase and that of guinea pig only the esterase. The relative rates of these degradative enzymes in insects are very low as compared with those of mammals, however, and this correlates well with the high selectivity of dimethoate.

The various phase-two reactions are concerned with the conjugation of primary metabolites of xenobiotics produced by phase-one reactions. Factors that alter or govern the rates of phase-two reactions may play a role in interspecific differences in xenobiotic metabolism. Xenobiotics, frequently in the form of conjugates, can be eliminated through urine, feces, lungs, sweat, saliva, milk, hair, nails, or placenta, although comparative data are generally available only for the first two routes. Interspecific variation in the pattern of biliary excretion may determine species differences in the relative extent to which compounds are eliminated in the urine or feces. Fecal excretion of a chemical or its metabolites tends to be higher in species that are good biliary excretors, such as the rat and dog, than in species that are poor biliary excretors, such as the rabbit, guinea pig, and monkey. For example, the fecal excretion of stilbestrol in the rat accounts for 75% of the dose, whereas in the rabbit about 70% can be found in the urine. Dogs, like humans, metabolize indomethacin to a glucuronide but, unlike humans that excrete it in the urine, dogs excrete it primarily in the feces—apparently due to inefficient renal and hepatic blood clearance of the glucuronide. These differences may involve species variation in enterohepatic circulation, plasma levels, and biologic half-life.

Interspecific differences in the magnitude of biliary excretion of a xenobiotic excretion product largely depend on molecular weight, the presence of polar groups in the molecule, and the extent of conjugation. Conjugates with molecular weights of less than 300 are poorly excreted in bile and tend to be excreted with urine, whereas the reverse is true for those with molecular weights higher than 300. The critical molecular weight appears to vary between species, and marked species differences are noted for biliary excretion of chemicals with molecular weights of about 300. Thus, the biliary excretion of succinylsulfathioazole is 20- to 30-fold greater in the rat and the dog than in the rabbit and the guinea pig, and more than 100-fold greater than in the pig and the rhesus monkey. The cat and sheep are intermediate and excrete about 7% of the dose in the bile.

The evidence reported in a few studies suggests some relationship between the evolutionary position of a species and its conjugation mechanisms (Table 6.3). In humans and most mammals, the principal mechanisms involve conjugations with glucuronic acid, glycine, glutamine, and sulfate, mercapturic acid synthesis, acetylation, methylation, and thiocyanate synthesis. In some species of birds and reptiles, ornithine conjugation replaces glycine conjugation; in plants, bacteria, and insects, conjugation with glucose instead of glucuronic acid results in the formation of glucosides. In addition to these predominant reactions, certain other conjugative processes are found involving specific compounds in only a few species. These reactions include conjugation with phosphate, taurine, N-acetyl-glucosamine, ribose, glycyltaurine, serine, arginine, formic acid, and succinate. Certain species of spiders use glutamic acid and arginine for the conjugation of aromatic acids.

From the standpoint of evolution, similarity might be expected between humans and other primate species as opposed to the nonprimates. This phylogenic relationship is obvious from the relative importance of glycine and glutamine in the conjugation of arylacetic acids. The conjugating agent in humans is exclusively glutamine, and the same is essentially true with Old World monkeys. New World monkeys, however, use both the glycine and glutamine pathways. Most nonprimates and lower primates carry

TABLE 6.3. OCCURRENCE OF COMMON AND UNUSUAL CONJUGATION REACTIONS

Conjugating Group	Common	Unusual
Carbohydrate	Glucuronic acid (animals) Glucose (insects, plants)	N-Acetylglucosamine (rabbits) Ribose (rats, mice)
Amino acids	Glycine Glutathione Methionine	Glutamine (insects, humans) Ornithine (birds) Arginine (ticks, spiders) Glycyltaurine (cats) Glycylglycine (cats) Serine (rabbits)
Acetyl	Acetyl group from acetyl-CoA	
Formyl		Formylation (dogs, rats)
Sulfate	Sulfate group from PAPS	
Phosphate		Phosphate monoester formation (dogs, insects)

Source: Modified from Kulkarni AP, Hodgson E: Comparative Toxicology. In Introduction to Biochemical Toxicology. *Hodgson E, Guthrie FE (eds.). New York: Elsevier, 1980, p 115.*

out glycine conjugation selectively. A similar evolutionary trend is also observed in the *N*-glucuronidation of sulfadimethoxine and in the aromatization of quinic acid; both reactions occur extensively in humans, and their importance decreases with increasing evolutionary divergence from humans. When the relative importance of metabolic pathways is considered, one of the simplest cases of an enzyme-related species difference in the disposition of a substrate undergoing only one conjugative reaction is the acetylation of 4-aminohippuric acid. In the rat, guinea pig, and rabbit, the major biliary metabolite is 4-acetamidohippuric acid; the cat excretes nearly equal amounts of free acid and its acetyl derivative; and the hen excretes mainly the unchanged compound. In the dog, 4-aminohippuric acid is also passed into the bile unchanged because this species is unable to acetylate aromatic amino groups.

Defective operation of phase-two reactions usually causes a striking species difference in the disposition pattern of a xenobiotic. The origin of such species variations is usually either the absence or a low level of the enzyme(s) in question and/or its cofactors. Glucuronide synthesis is one of the most common detoxication mechanisms in most mammalian species. The cat and closely related species have a defective glucuronide-forming system, however. Although cats form little or no glucuronide from *o*-aminophenol, phenol, *p*-nitrophenol, 2-amino-4-nitrophenol, 1- or 2-naphthol, and morphine, they readily form glucuronides from phenolphthalein, bilirubin, thyroxine, and certain steroids. Recently, polymorphism of UDP glucuronyl-transferase has been demonstrated in rat and guinea pig liver preparations; thus, defective glucuronidation in the cat is probably related to the absence of the appropriate transferase rather than that of the active intermediate, UDPGA, which is known to occur in cat liver in normal concentrations. Insects are incapable of synthesizing glucuronide conjugates. This may be due to the lack of UDP glucuronyl-transferase, UDPGA, or UDP glucose dehydrogenase, which converts UDP glucose into UDPGA.

Studies on the metabolic fate of phenol in several species have indicated that four urinary products are excreted (Fig. 6.4). Although extensive phenol metabolism takes place in most species, the relative proportions of each metabolite produced varies from species to species. In contrast to the cat, which selectively forms sulfate conjugates, the pig excretes phenol exclusively as the glucuronide. This defect in sulfate conjugation in the pig is restricted to only a few substrates, however, and may be due to the lack of a specific phenyl sulfotransferase because the formation of substantial amounts of the sulfate conjugate of 1-naphthol clearly indicates the occurrence of other forms of sulfotransferase.

Certain unusual conjugation mechanisms have been uncovered during comparative investigations, but this may be a reflection of inadequate data on other species. Future investigations may demonstrate a wider distribution. A few species of birds and reptiles use ornithine for the conjugation of aromatic acids rather than glycine, as do mammals. For example, the turkey, goose, duck, and hen excrete ornithuric acid as the major metabolite of benzoic acid, whereas pigeons and doves excrete it exclusively as hippuric acid.

Taurine conjugation with bile acids, phenylacetic acid, and indolylacetic acid seems to be a minor process in most species, but in the pigeon and ferret it occurs

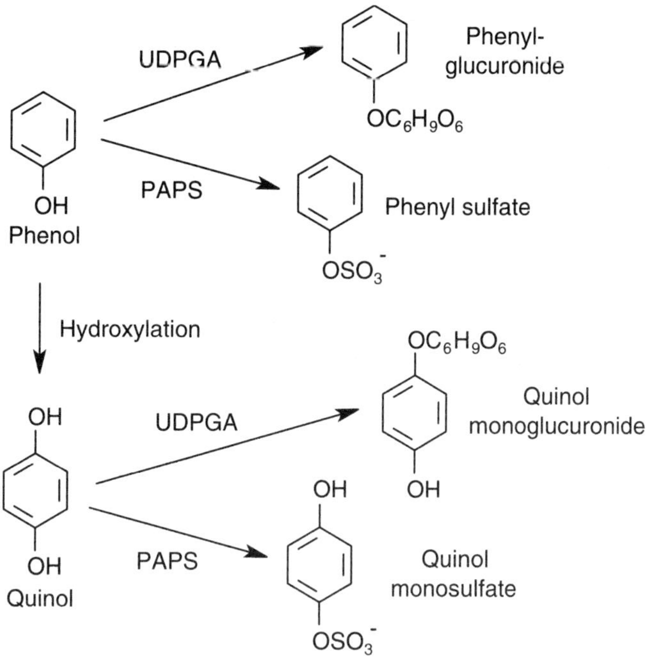

Species	Percent of 24-hr Excretion as Glucuronide		Percent of 24-hr Excretion as Sulfate	
	Phenol	*Quinol*	*Phenol*	*Quinol*
Pig	100	0	0	0
Indian fruit bat	90	0	10	0
Rhesus monkey	35	0	65	0
Cat	0	0	87	13
Human	23	7	71	0
Squirrel monkey	70	19	10	0
Rat-tail monkey	65	21	14	0
Guinea pig	78	5	17	0
Hamster	50	25	25	0
Rat	25	7	68	0
Ferret	41	0	32	28
Rabbit	46	0	45	9
Gerbil	15	0	69	15

Figure 6.4. Species variation in the metabolic conversion of phenol in vivo.

extensively. Other infrequently reported conjugations include serine conjugation of xanthurenic acid in rats; excretion of quinaldic acid as quinaldylglycyltaurine and quinaldylglycylglycine in the urine of the cat, but not of the rat or rabbit; phosphate conjugation of 2-naphthylamine in the dog, but not in the rat or rabbit; and conversion of furfural to furylacrylic acid in the dog and rabbit, but not in the rat, hen, or human. The dog and human but not the guinea pig, hamster, rabbit, or rat excrete the carcinogen 2-naphthyl hydroxylamine as a metabolite of 2-naphthylamine, which, as a result, has carcinogenic activity in the bladder of humans and dogs.

6.4.1.3   In Vitro Metabolism

Numerous variables simultaneously modulate the in vivo metabolism of xenobiotics; therefore, their relative importance cannot be studied easily. This problem is alleviated to some extent by in vitro studies of the underlying enzymatic mechanisms responsible for qualitative and quantitative species differences. Quantitative differences may be related directly to the absolute amount of active enzyme present and the affinity and specificity of the enzyme toward the substrate in question. Because many other factors alter enzymatic rates in vitro, caution must be exercised in interpreting data in terms of species variation. In particular, enzymes are often sensitive to the experimental conditions used in their preparation. Because this sensitivity varies from one enzyme to another, their relative effectiveness for a particular reaction can be sometimes miscalculated.

Species variation in the oxidation of xenobiotics, in general, is quantitative (Table 6.4), whereas qualitative differences, such as the apparent total lack of parathion oxidation by lobster hepatopancreas microsomes, are seldom observed. Although the amount of P450 or the activity of NADPH–cytochrome P450 reductase seems to be related to the oxidation of certain substrates, this explanation is not

TABLE 6.4. SPECIES VARIATION IN HEPATIC MICROSOMAL OXIDATION OF XENOBIOTICS IN VITRO

Substrate Oxidation	Rabbit	Rat	Mouse	Guinea Pig	Hamster	Chicken	Trout	Frog
Coumarin 7-hydroxylase[a]	0.86	0.00	0.00	0.45	—	—	—	—
Biphenyl 4-hydroxylase[b]	3.00	1.50	5.70	1.40	3.80	1.70	0.22	1.15
Biphenyl 2-hydroxylase[b]	0.00	0.00	2.20	0.00	1.80	0.00	0.00	0.15
2-Methoxybiphenyl demethylase[a]	5.20	1.80	3.40	2.20	2.30	2.00	0.60	0.40
4-Methoxybiphenyl demethylase[a]	8.00	3.00	3.20	2.30	2.30	1.70	0.40	0.90
p-Nitroanisole O-demethylase[b]	2.13	0.32	1.35	—	—	0.76	—	—
2-Ethoxybiphenyl deethylase[a]	5.30	1.60	1.40	2.10	2.50	1.70	0.60	0.40
4-Ethoxybiphenyl deethylase[a]	7.80	2.80	1.80	2.30	1.80	1.50	0.40	0.90
Ethylmorphine N-demethylase[b]	4.00	11.60	13.20	5.40	—	—	—	—
Aldrin epoxidase[b]	0.34	0.45	3.35	—	—	0.46	0.006	—
Parathion desulfurase[b]	2.11	4.19	5.23	8.92	7.75	—	—	—

[a] nmol/mg/hr.
[b] nmol/mg/min.
Source: Modified from Kulkarni AP, Hodgson E: Comparative Toxicology. In Introduction to Biochemical Toxicology. Hodgson E, Guthrie FE (eds.). New York: Elsevier, 1980, p 120.

always satisfactory because the absolute amount of cytochrome P450 is not necessarily the rate-limiting characteristic. It is clear that there are multiple forms of P450 isozymes in each species, and that these forms differ from one species to another. Presumably, both quantitative and qualitative variation in xenobiotic metabolism depend in variations on the particular isoforms expressed and the extent of this expression.

Reductive reactions, like oxidations, are carried out at different rates by enzyme preparations from different species. Microsomes from mammalian liver are 18 times or more higher in azoreductase activity and more than 20 times higher in nitroreductase activity than those from fish liver. Although relatively inactive in nitroreductase, fish can reduce the nitro group of parathion, suggesting multiple forms of reductase enzymes.

Hydration of epoxides catalyzed by epoxide hydrolase is involved in both detoxication and intoxication reaction. With high concentrations of styrene oxide as a substrate, the relative activity of hepatic microsomal epoxide hydrolase in several animal species is rhesus monkey > human = guinea pig > rabbit > rat > mouse. With some substrates, such as epoxidized lipids, the cytosolic hydrolase may be much more important than the microsomal enzyme.

Blood and various organs of humans and other animals contain esterases capable of acetylsalicylic acid hydrolysis. A comparative study has shown that the liver is the most active tissue in all animal species studied except for the guinea pig, in which the kidney is more than twice as active as the liver. Human liver is least active; the enzyme in guinea pig liver is the most active. The relatively low toxicity of some of the new synthetic pyrethroid insecticides appears to be related to the ability of mammals to hydrolyze their carboxyester linkages. Thus, mouse liver microsomes catalyzing (+)-*trans*-resmethrin hydrolysis are more than 30-fold more active than insect microsomal preparations. The relative rates of hydrolysis of this substrate in enzyme preparations from various species are mouse >> milkweed bug >> cockroach >> cabbage looper > housefly.

The toxicity of the organophosphorus insecticide dimethoate depends on the rate at which it is hydrolyzed in vivo. This toxicant undergoes two main metabolic detoxication reactions, one catalyzed by an esterase and the other by an amidase. Although rat and mouse liver carry out both reactions, only the amidase occurs in sheep liver, and the esterase in guinea pig liver. The ability of liver preparations from different animal species to degrade dimethoate is as follows: rabbit > sheep > dog > rat > cattle > hen > guinea pig > mouse > pig, these rates being roughly inversely proportioned to the toxicity of dimethoate to the same species. Insects degrade this compound much more slowly than do mammals and hence are highly susceptible to dimethoate.

Hepatic microsomes of several animal species possess UDP glucuronyltransferase activity and, with *p*-nitrophenol as a substrate, a 12-fold difference in activity due to species variation is evident. Phospholipase-A activates the enzyme and results of activation experiments indicate that the amount of constraint on the activity of this enzyme is variable in different animal species.

Glutathione S-transferase in liver cytosol from different animal species also shows a wide variation in activity. Activity is low in humans, whereas the mouse and guinea pig appear to be more efficient than other species. The ability of the guinea pig to form the initial glutathione conjugate contrasts with its inability to readily N-acetylate cysteine conjugates; consequently, mercapturic acid excretion is low in guinea pigs.

6.4.2   Selectivity

Selective toxic agents have been developed to protect crops, animals of economic importance, and humans from the vagaries of pests, parasites, and pathogens. Such selectivity is conferred primarily through distribution and comparative biochemistry.

Selectivity through differences in uptake permits the use of an agent toxic to both target and nontarget cells, provided that lethal concentrations accumulate only in target cells, leaving nontarget cells unharmed. An example is the accumulation of tetracycline by bacteria, but not by mammalian cells, the result being drastic inhibition of protein synthesis in the bacteria, leading to death.

Certain schistosome worms are parasitic in humans and their selective destruction by antimony is accounted for by the differential sensitivity of phosphofructokinase in the two species, the enzyme from schistosomes being more susceptible to inhibition by antimony than is the mammalian enzyme.

Sometimes both target and nontarget species metabolize a xenobiotic by the same pathways but differences in rate determine selectivity. Malathion (see Fig. 1.4), a selective insecticide, is metabolically activated by P450 enzymes to the cholinesterase inhibitor malaoxon. In addition to this activation reaction, several detoxication reactions also occur. Carboxylesterase hydrolyzes malathion to form the monoacid, phosphatases hydrolyze the P-O-C linkages to yield nontoxic products, and glutathione S-alkyltransferase converts malathion to desmethylmalathion. Although all of these reactions occur in both insects and mammals, activation is rapid in both insects and mammals, whereas hydrolysis to the monoacid is rapid in mammals but slow in insects. As a result, malaoxon accumulates in insects but not in mammals, resulting in selective toxicity.

A few examples are also available in which the lack of a specific enzyme in some cells in the human body has enabled the development of a therapeutic agent. For example, guanine deaminase is absent from the cells of certain cancers but is abundant in healthy tissue; as a result, 8-azaguanine can be used therapeutically.

Distinct differences in cells with regard to the presence or absence of target structures or metabolic processes also offer opportunities for selectivity. Herbicides such as phenylureas, simazine, and so on, block the Hill reaction in chloroplasts, thereby killing plants without harm to animals. This is not always the case, because paraquat, which blocks photosynthetic reactions in plants, is a pulmonary toxicant in mammals, due apparently to analogous free-radical reactions (see Fig. 9.6) involving enzymes different from those involved in photosynthesis.

6.4.3   Genetic Differences

Just as the xenobiotic-metabolizing ability in different animal species seems to be related to evolutionary development and therefore to different genetic constitutions, different strains within a species may differ from one another in their ability to metabolize xenobiotics.

6.4.3.1   In Vivo Toxicity

The toxicity of organic compounds has been found to vary between different strains of laboratory animals. For example, mouse strain C_3H is resistant to histamine, the LD50 being 1523 mg/kg in C_3H/Jax mice as compared with 230 in Swiss/ICR mice; that is, the animals of the former strain are 6.6 times less susceptible to the effects of histamine. Striking differences in the toxicity of thiourea, a compound used in the treatment of hyperthyroidism, are seen in different strains of the Norway rat. Harvard rats were 11 times more resistant and wild Norway rats were 335 times more resistant than were rats of the Hopkins strain.

Genetic polymorphism is well known in the metabolism of drugs such as isoniazid. Such differences are related to the rate of acetylation of isoniazid and have a genetic basis. "Slow acetylators" are homozygous for a recessive gene; this is believed to lead to the lack of the hepatic enzyme acetyltransferase, which in normal homozygotes or heterozygotes (rapid acetylators) acetylates isoniazid as a step in the metabolism of this drug (see Fig. 10.14). This effect is seen also in humans, the gene for slow acetylation showing marked differences in distribution between different human populations. It is very low in Eskimos and Japanese, with 80% to 90% of these populations being rapid acetylators, whereas 40% to 60% of Blacks and some European populations are rapid acetylators. Rapid acetylators often develop symptoms of hepatotoxicity and polyneuritis at the dosage necessary to maintain therapeutic blood levels of isoniazid.

The development of strains resistant to insecticides is an extremely widespread phenomenon that is known to have occurred in more than 200 species of insects and mites, and resistance of up to several hundred–fold has been noted. The different biochemical and genetic factors involved have been studied extensively and well characterized. Relatively few vertebrate species are known to have developed pesticide resistance and the level of resistance in vertebrates is low compared to that often found in insects. Susceptible and resistant strains of pine voles exhibit a 7.4-fold difference in endrin toxicity. Similarly, pine mice of a strain resistant to endrin were reported to be 12-fold more tolerant than a susceptible strain. Other examples include the occurrence of organochlorine insecticide-resistant and -susceptible strains of mosquito fish, and resistance to *Belladonna* in certain rabbit strains.

6.4.3.2   Metabolite Production

Strain variation in response to hexobarbital also depends on its degradation rate. For example, male mice of the AL/N strain are long sleepers, and this trait is correlated with slow inactivation of the drug. The reverse is true in CFW/N mice, which have a short sleeping time due to rapid hexobarbital oxidation. This close relationship is further evidenced by the fact that the level of brain hexobarbital at awakening is essentially the same in all strains. Similar strain differences have been reported for zoxazolamine paralysis in mice.

Studies on the induction of aryl hydrocarbon hydroxylase by 3-methylcholanthrene have revealed several responsive and nonresponsive mouse strains, and it is now well established that the induction of this enzyme is controlled by a single gene. In the accepted nomenclature, Ah[b] represents the allele for responsiveness, whereas Ah[d] denotes the allele for nonresponsiveness.

In rats, both age and gender seem to influence strain variation in xenobiotic metabolism. Male rats exhibit about twofold variation between strains in hexobarbital metabolism, whereas female rats may display up to sixfold variation. In either gender the extent of variations depending on age. The ability to metabolize hexobarbital is related to the metabolism of other substrates and the interstrain differences are maintained.

A well-known interstrain difference in phase-two reactions is that of glucuronidation in Gunn rats. This is a mutant strain of Wistar rats that is characterized by a severe, genetically determined defect of bilirubin glucuronidation. Their ability to glucuronidate o-aminophenol, o-aminobenzoic acid, and a number of other substrates is also partially defective. This deficiency does not seem to be related to an inability to form UDPGA but rather to the lack of a specific UDP glucuronyltransferase. It has been demonstrated that Gunn rats can conjugate aniline by N-glucuronidation and can form the O-glucuronide of p-nitrophenol.

Rabbit strains may exhibit up to 20-fold variation, particularly in the case of hexobarbital, amphetamine, and aminopyrine metabolism. Relatively smaller differences between strains occur with chlorpromazine metabolism. Wild rabbits and California rabbits display the greatest differences from other rabbit strains in hepatic drug metabolism.

6.4.3.3   Enzyme Differences

Variation in the nature and amount of constitutively expressed microsomal P450s have not been studied extensively in different strains of the same vertebrate. The only thorough investigations, those of the Ah locus, which controls aryl hydrocarbon hydroxylase induction, have shown that, in addition to quantitative differences in the amount of P450 after induction in different strains of mice, there may also be a qualitative difference in the P450 isozymes induced. (See Section 6.5.2, Induction.)

6.5

CHEMICAL EFFECTS

With regard to both logistics and scientific philosophy, the study of the metabolism and toxicity of xenobiotics must be initiated by considering single compounds. Unfortunately, humans and other living organisms are not exposed in this way; rather,

TABLE 6.5. SOME ESTIMATES OF THE NUMBER OF CHEMICALS IN USE IN THE UNITED STATES

Number	Type	Source of Estimate[a]
1500	Active ingredients of pesticides	EPA
4000	Active ingredients of drugs	FDA
2000	Drug additives (preservatives, stabilizers, etc.)	FDA
2500	Food additives (nutritional value)	FDA
3000	Food additives (preservatives, stabilizers, etc.)	FDA
50,000	Additional chemicals in common use	EPA

[a] EPA, Environmental Protection Agency; FDA, Food and Drug Administration.

they are exposed to many xenobiotics simultaneously, involving different portals of entry, modes of action, and metabolic pathways. Some estimation of the number of chemicals in use in the United States are given in Table 6.5. Because it bears directly on the problem of toxicity-related interactions between different xenobiotics, the effect of chemicals on the metabolism of other exogenous compounds is one of the more important areas of biochemical toxicology.

Xenobiotics, in addition to serving as substrates for a number of enzymes, may also serve as inhibitors or inducers of these or other enzymes. Many examples are known of compounds that first inhibit and subsequently induce enzymes such as the microsomal monooxygenases. The situation is even further complicated by the fact that although some substances have an inherent toxicity and are detoxified in the body, others without inherent toxicity can be metabolically activated to potent toxicants. The following examples are illustrative of the situations that might occur involving two compounds:

- Compound A, without inherent toxicity, is metabolized to a potent toxicant. In the presence of an inhibitor of its metabolism, there would be a reduction in toxic effect.
- Compound A, given after exposure to an inducer of the activating enzymes, would appear more toxic.
- Compound B, a toxicant, is metabolically detoxified. In the presence of an inhibitor of the detoxifying enzymes, there would be an increase in the toxic effect.
- Compound B, given after exposure to an inducer of the detoxifying enzymes, would appear less toxic.

In addition to the previously mentioned cases, the toxicity of the inhibitor or inducer, as well as the time dependence of the effect, must also be considered because, as mentioned, many xenobiotics that are initially enzyme inhibitors ultimately become inducers.

6.5.1 Inhibition

As previously indicated, inhibition of xenobiotic-metabolizing enzymes can cause either an increase or a decrease in toxicity. Several well-known inhibitors of such

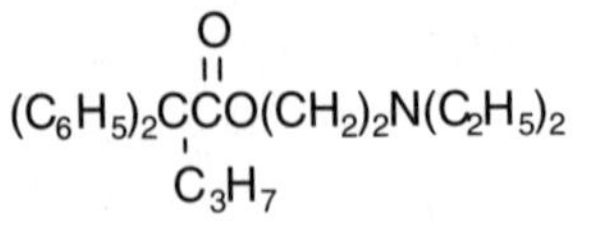

$$(C_6H_5)_2\overset{\overset{\displaystyle O}{\|}}{\underset{\underset{\displaystyle C_3H_7}{|}}{C}}CO(CH_2)_2N(C_2H_5)_2$$

SKF-525A [P450]
2-(Diethylamino)ethyl-
2,2-diphenylpentanoate

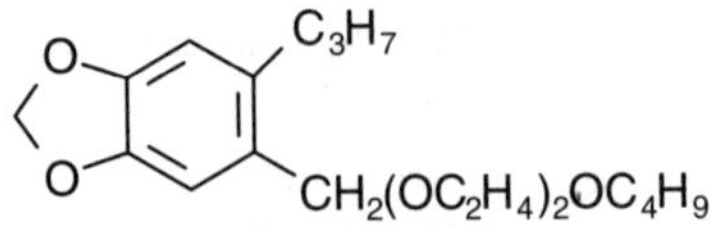

Piperonyl Butoxide [P450]
3,4-Methylenedioxy-6-proplybenzyl
n-butyl diethyleneglycol ether

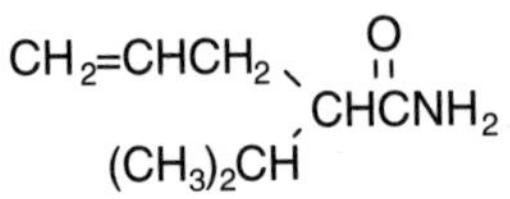

$$CH_2=CHCH_2 \diagdown \overset{\overset{\displaystyle O}{\|}}{\underset{(CH_3)_2CH \diagup}{CHCNH_2}}$$

Allylisopropylacetamide
[P450]

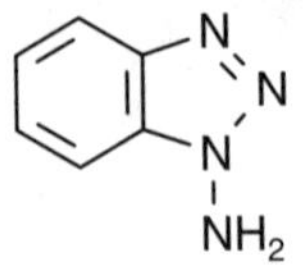

1-Aminobenzotriazole (1-ABT)
[P450]

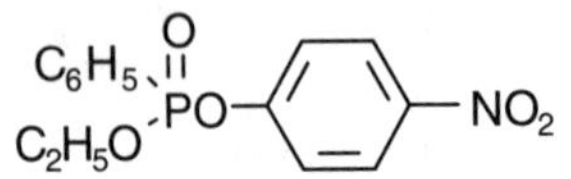

$$\overset{C_6H_5 \diagdown}{\underset{C_2H_5O \diagup}{\overset{\overset{\displaystyle O}{\|}}{P}O}} \!\!-\!\!\langle \underline{\quad} \rangle\!\!-\!\! NO_2$$

EPN [esterases]
O-Ethyl-O-p-nitrophenyl
phenylphosphonothioate

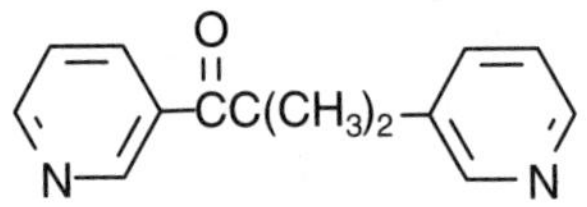

Metyrapone
[P450]

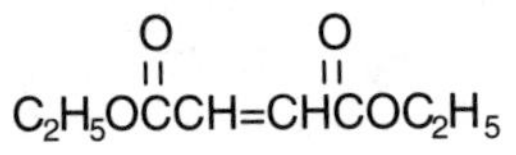

$$\overset{\overset{\displaystyle O}{\|}}{C_2H_5OC}CH=CH\overset{\overset{\displaystyle O}{\|}}{COC_2H_5}$$

Diethyl maleate
[glutathione S-transferase]

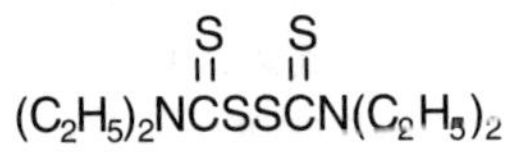

$$(C_2H_5)_2N\overset{\overset{\displaystyle S}{\|}}{C}SS\overset{\overset{\displaystyle S}{\|}}{C}N(C_2H_5)_2$$

Disulfiram (Antabuse)
[aldehyde dehydrogenase]

Figure 6.5. Some common inhibitors of xenobiotic-metabolizing enzymes.

enzymes are shown in Fig. 6.5 and are discussed in this section. Inhibitory effects can be demonstrated in a number of ways at different organizational levels.

6.5.1.1 Types of Inhibition: Experimental Demonstration

IN VIVO SYMPTOMS. The measurement of the effect of an inhibitor on the duration of action of a drug in vivo is the most common method of demonstrating its action. These methods are open to criticism, however, because effects on duration of action can be mediated by systems other than those involved in the metabolism of the drug. Furthermore, they cannot be used for inhibitors that have pharmacological activity similar or opposite to the compound being used.

Previously, the most used and most reliable of these tests involved the measurement of effects on the hexobarbital sleeping time and the zoxazolamine paralysis time. Both of these drugs are fairly rapidly deactivated by the hepatic microsomal monooxygenase system; thus, inhibitors of this system prolong their action. For example, treatment of mice with chloramphenicol (Fig. 6.5) 0.5 to1.0 hr before pentobarbital treatment prolongs the duration of the pentobarbital sleeping time in a dose-related manner; it is effective at low doses (<5 mg/kg) and has a greater than tenfold effect at high doses (100–200 mg/kg). The well-known inhibitor of drug metabolism, SKF-525A, causes an increase in both hexobarbital sleeping time and zoxazolamine paralysis time in rats and mice, as do the insecticide synergists piperonyl butoxide and tropital, the optimum pretreatment time being about 0.5 hr before the narcotic is given. As a consequence of the availability of single expressed isoforms for direct studies of inhibitory mechanisms, these methods are now used much less often.

In the case of activation reactions, such as the activation of the insecticide azinphosmethyl to its potent anticholinesterase oxon derivative, a decrease in toxicity is apparent when rats are pretreated with the P450 inhibitor SKF-525A.

Cocarcinogenicity may also be an expression of inhibition of a detoxication reaction, as in the case of the cocarcinogenicity of piperonyl butoxide, a P450 inhibitor, and the carcinogens, freons 112 and 113.

DISTRIBUTION AND BLOOD LEVELS. Treatment of an animal with an inhibitor of foreign compound metabolism may cause changes in the blood levels of an unmetabolized toxicant and/or its metabolites. This procedure may be used in the investigation of the inhibition of detoxication pathways; it has the advantage over in vitro methods of yielding results of direct physiological or toxicological interest because it is carried out in the intact animal. For example, if animals are first treated with either SKF-525A, glutethimide, or chlorcyclizine, followed in 1 hr or less by pentobarbital, it can be shown that the serum level of pentobarbital is considerably higher in treated animals than in controls within 1 hr of its injection. Moreover, the time sequence of the effects can be followed in individual animals, a factor of importance when inhibition is followed by induction—a not uncommon event.

EFFECTS ON METABOLISM IN VIVO. A further refinement of the previous technique is to determine the effect of an inhibitor on the overall metabolism of a xenobiotic in vivo, usually by following the appearance of metabolites in the urine and/or feces. In some cases, the appearance of metabolites in the blood or tissue may also be followed. Again, the use of the intact animal has practical advantages over in vitro methods, although little is revealed about the mechanisms involved.

Studies of antipyrine metabolism may be used to illustrate the effect of inhibition on metabolism in vivo; in addition, these studies have demonstrated variation between species in the inhibition of the metabolism of xenobiotics. In the rat, a dose of piperonyl butoxide of at least 100 mg/kg was necessary to inhibit antipyrine metabolism, whereas in the mouse a single intraperitoneal (IP) or oral dose of 1 mg/kg produced a significant inhibition. In humans an oral dose of 0.71 mg/kg had no discernible effect on the metabolism of antipyrine.

Disulfiram (Antabuse) inhibits aldehyde dehydrogenase irreversibly, causing an increase in the level of acetaldehyde, formed from ethanol by the enzyme alcohol dehydrogenase. This results in nausea, vomiting, and other symptoms in the human—hence its use as a deterrent in alcoholism. Inhibition by disulfiram appears to be irreversible, the level returning to normal only as a result of protein synthesis.

EFFECTS ON IN VITRO METABOLISM FOLLOWING IN VIVO TREATMENT. This method of demonstrating inhibition is of variable utility. The preparation of enzymes from animal tissues usually involves considerable dilution with the preparative medium during homogenization, centrifugation, and resuspension. As a result, inhibitors not tightly bound to the enzyme in question are lost, either in whole or in part, during the preparative processes. Therefore, negative results can have little utility because failure to inhibit and loss of the inhibitor give identical results. Positive results, however, not only indicate that the compound administered is an inhibitor but also provide a clear indication of excellent binding to the enzyme, most probably due to the formation of a covalent or slowly reversible inhibitory complex. The inhibition of esterases following treatment of the animal with organophosphorus compounds, such as paraoxon, is a good example, because the phosphorylated enzyme is stable and is still inhibited after the preparative procedures. Inhibition by carbamates, however, is greatly reduced by the same procedures, because the carbamylated enzyme is unstable and, in addition, the residual carbamate is highly diluted.

Microsomal monooxygenase inhibitors that form stable inhibitory complexes with P450, such as SKF-525A, piperonyl butoxide and other methylenedioxyphenyl compounds (see Fig. 3.8), and amphetamine and its derivatives, can be readily investigated in this way because the microsomes isolated from pretreated animals have a reduced capacity to oxidize many xenobiotics.

Another form of chemical interaction, resulting from inhibition in vivo, that can then be demonstrated in vitro, involves those xenobiotics that function by causing destruction of the enzyme in question, so-called suicide substrates. Exposure of rats to vinyl chloride results in a loss of cytochrome P450 and a corresponding reduction in the capacity of microsomes subsequently isolated to metabolize foreign compounds. Allyl isopropylacetamide and other allyl compounds have long been known to have a similar effect.

IN VITRO EFFECTS. In vitro measurement of the effect of one xenobiotic on the metabolism of another is by far the most common type of investigation of interactions involving inhibition. Although it is the most useful method for the study of inhibitory mechanisms, particularly when purified enzymes are used, it is of more limited utility in assessing the toxicological implications for the intact animal. The principal reason for this is that in vitro measurement does not assess the effects of factors that affect absorption, distribution, and prior metabolism, all of which occur before the inhibitory event under consideration.

Although the kinetics of inhibition of xenobiotic-metabolizing enzymes can be investigated in the same ways as any other enzyme mechanism, a number of problems arise that may decrease the value of this type of investigation. They include the following:

- The P450 system, a particulate enzyme system, has been investigated many times, but using methods developed for single soluble enzymes. As a result, Lineweaver–Burke or other reciprocal plots are frequently curvilinear, and the same reaction may appear to have quite different characteristics from laboratory to laboratory, species to species, and organ to organ.
- The nonspecific binding of substrate and/or inhibitor to membrane components is a further complicating factor affecting inhibition kinetics.
- Both substrates and inhibitors are frequently lipophilic, with low solubility in aqueous media.
- Xenobiotic-metabolizing enzymes commonly exist in multiple forms (eg, glutathione S-transferases and P450s). These isozymes are all relatively nonspecific but differ from one another in the relative affinities of the different substrates.

The primary considerations in studies of inhibition mechanisms are reversibility and selectivity. The inhibition kinetics of reversible inhibition give considerable insight into the reaction mechanisms of enzymes and, for that reason, have been well studied. In general, reversible inhibition involves no covalent binding, occurs rapidly, and can be reversed by dialysis or, more rapidly, by dilution. Reversible inhibition is usually divided into competitive inhibition, uncompetitive inhibition, and noncompetitive inhibition. Because these types are not rigidly separated, many intermediate classes have been described.

Competitive inhibition is usually caused by two substrates competing for the same active site. Following classic enzyme kinetics, there should be a change in the apparent K_m but not in V_{max}. In microsomal monooxygenase reactions, type I ligands, which often appear to bind as substrates but do not bind to the heme iron, might be expected to be competitive inhibitors, and this frequently appears to be the case. Examples are the inhibition of the O-demethylation of p-nitroanisole by aminopyrene, aldrin epoxidation by dihydroaldrin, and N-demethylation of aminopyrene by nicotinamide. More recently, some of the polychlorinated biphenyls (PCBs), notably dichlorobiphenyl, but also, less effectively, tetrachlorobiphenyl and hexachlorobiphenyl have been shown to have a high affinity as type I ligands for rabbit liver P450 and to be competitive inhibitors of the O-demethylation of p-nitroanisole.

Uncompetitive inhibition has seldom been reported in studies of xenobiotic metabolism. It occurs when an inhibitor interacts with an enzyme-substrate complex but cannot interact with free enzyme. Both K_m and V_{max} change by the same ratio, giving rise to a family of parallel lines in a Lineweaver–Burke plot.

Noncompetitive inhibitors can bind to both the enzyme and enzyme-substrate complex to form either an enzyme-inhibitor complex or an enzyme-inhibitor-substrate complex. The net result is a decrease in V_{max} but no change in K_m. Metyrapone (Fig. 6.5), a well-known inhibitor of monooxygenase reactions, can also, under some circumstances, stimulate metabolism in vitro. In either case, the effect is noncompetitive, in that the K_m does not change, whereas V_{max} does, decreasing in the case of inhibition and increasing in the case of stimulation.

Irreversible inhibition, which is much more important toxicologically, can arise from various causes. In most cases, the formation of covalent or other stable bonds or the disruption of the enzyme structure is involved. In these cases, the effect cannot be readily reversed in vitro by either dialysis or dilution.The formation of stable inhibitory complexes may involve the prior formation of a reactive intermediate that then interacts with the enzyme. An excellent example of this type of inhibition is the effect of the insecticide synergist piperonyl butoxide (Fig. 6.3) on hepatic microsomal monooxygenase activity. This methylenedioxyphenyl compound can form a stable inhibitory complex that blocks CO binding to P450 and also prevents substrate oxidation. This complex results from the formation of a reactive intermediate, which is shown by the fact that the type of inhibition changes from competitive to irreversible as metabolism, in the presence of NADPH and oxygen, proceeds. It appears probable that the metabolite in question is a carbene formed spontaneously by elimination of water following hydroxylation of the methylene carbon by the cytochrome (see Fig. 3.8 for metabolism of methylenedioxyphenyl compounds). Piperonyl butoxide inhibits the in vitro metabolism of many substrates of the monooxygenase system, including aldrin, ethylmorphine, aniline, and aminopyrene, as well as carbaryl, biphenyl, hexobarbital, *p*-nitroanisole, and many others. Although most of the studies carried out on piperonyl butoxide have involved rat or mouse liver microsomes, they have also been carried out on pig, rabbit, and carp liver microsomes, and in various preparations from houseflies, cockroaches, and other insects. Certain classes of monooxygenase inhibitors, in addition to methylenedioxyphenyl compounds, are now known to form "metabolite inhibitory complexes," including amphetamine and its derivatives and SKF-525A and its derivatives.

The inhibition of the carboxylesterase that hydrolyzes malathion by organophosphorus compounds such as EPN is a further example of xenobiotic interaction resulting from irreversible inhibition, because in this case the enzyme is phosphorylated by the inhibitor.

Another class of irreversible inhibitors of toxicological significance consists of those compounds that bring about the destruction of the xenobiotic-metabolizing enzymes, hence the designation "suicide substrates." The drug allylisopropylacetamide (Fig. 6.5), as well as other allyl compounds, has long been known to cause the breakdown of P450 and the resultant release of heme. More recently, the hepatocarcinogen vinyl chloride has also been shown to have a similar effect, probably also mediated through the generation of a highly reactive intermediate (see Fig. 10.10). Much information has accumulated since the mid 1970s on the mode of action of the hepatotoxicant carbon tetrachloride, which effects a number of irreversible changes in both liver proteins and lipids, such changes being generated by reactive intermediates formed during its metabolism (Figs. 9.1 and 9.3).

The less specific disruptors of protein structure, such as urea, detergents, strong acids, and so on, are probably of significance only in in vitro experiments.

6.5.1.2 Synergism and Potentiation

The terms synergism and potentiation have been used and defined in various ways but, in any case, they involve a toxicity that is greater when two compounds are given simultaneously or sequentially than would be expected from a consideration of the toxicities of the compounds given alone. Some toxicologists have used the term synergism for cases that fit this definition, but only when one compound is toxic alone whereas the other has little or no intrinsic toxicity. This is the case with the toxicity of insecticides to insects and mammals and the effects on this toxicity of methylenedioxyphenyl synergists such as piperonyl butoxide, sesamex, and tropital. The term potentiation is then reserved for those cases in which both compounds have appreciable intrinsic toxicity, such as in the case of malathion and EPN. Unfortunately, other toxicologists have used the terms in precisely the opposite manner.

Historically, pharmacologists have used the term synergism to refer to simple additive toxicity and potentiation either as a synonym or for examples of greater than additive toxicity or efficacy. In an attempt to make uniform the use of these terms, it is suggested that insofar as toxic effects are concerned, the terms be used according to the following: *Both synergism and potentiation involve toxicity greater than would be expected from the toxicities of the compounds administered separately, but in the case of synergism one compound has little or no intrinsic toxicity when administered alone, whereas in the case of potentiation both compounds have appreciable toxicity when administered alone. It is further suggested that no special term is needed for simple additive toxicity of two or more compounds.*

An example of synergism has already been mentioned. Piperonyl butoxide, sesamex, and related compounds increase the toxicity of insecticides to insects by inhibiting insect P450. Other insecticide synergists that interact with P450 include aryloxyalkylamines such as SKF-525A, Lilly 18947, and their derivatives; compounds containing acetylenic bonds such as aryl-2-propynyl phosphate esters containing propynyl functions; phosphorothionates; benzothiadiazoles; and some imidazole derivatives.

The best known example of potentiation involving insecticides and an enzyme other than the monooxygenase system is the increase in the toxicity of malathion to mammals that is brought about by certain other organophosphates. Malathion has a low mammalian toxicity due primarily to its rapid hydrolysis by a carboxylesterase. EPN (Fig. 6.5), another organophosphate insecticide, causes a dramatic increase in malathion toxicity to mammals at dose levels, which, given alone, cause essentially no inhibition of cholinesterase. In vitro studies have shown that the oxygen analog of EPN, as well as oxons of many other organophosphate compounds, increase the toxicity of malathion by inhibiting the carboxylesterase responsible for its degradation.

6.5.1.3 Antagonism

In toxicology, antagonism may be defined as that situation in which the toxicity of two or more compounds administered together or sequentially is less than would be expected from a consideration of their toxicities when administered individually. Strictly speaking, this definition includes those cases in which the lowered toxicity results from induction of detoxifying enzymes (this situation is considered separately in Section 6.5.2). Apart from the convenience of treating such antagonistic phenomena together with the other aspects of induction, they are frequently considered separately because of the significant time that must elapse between treatment with the inducer and subsequent treatment with the toxicant. The reduction of hexobarbital sleeping time and the reduction of zoxazolamine paralysis time by prior treatment with phenobarbital to induce drug-metabolizing enzymes are obvious examples of such induction effects at the acute level of drug action, whereas protection from the carcinogenic action of benzo(a)pyrene, aflatoxin B_1, and diethylnitrosamine by phenobarbital treatment are examples of inductive effects at the level of chronic toxicity. In the latter case, the P450 isozymes induced by phenobarbital metabolize the chemical to less toxic metabolites.

Antagonism not involving induction is a phenomenon often seen at a marginal level of detection and is consequently both difficult to explain and of marginal significance. In addition, several different types of antagonism of importance to toxicology that do not involve xenobiotic metabolism are known but are not appropriate for discussion in this chapter. They include competition for receptor sites, such as the competition between CO and O_2 in CO poisoning, or situations in which one toxicant combines nonenzymatically with another to reduce its toxic effects, such as in the chelation of metal ions. Physiological antagonism, in which two agonists act on the same physiological system but produce opposite effects, is also of importance.

6.5.2 · Induction

In the early 1960s, during investigations on the *N*-demethylation of aminoazo dyes, it was observed that pretreatment of mammals with the substrate or, more remarkably, with other xenobiotics, caused an increase in the ability of the animal to metabolize these dyes. It was subsequently shown that this effect was due to an increase in the microsomal enzymes involved. A symposium in 1965 and a landmark review by Conney in 1967 established the importance of induction in xenobiotic interactions. Since then, it has become clear that this phenomenon is widespread and nonspecific. Several hundred compounds of diverse chemical structure have been shown to induce monooxygenases and other enzymes. These compounds include drugs, insecticides, polycyclic hydrocarbons, and many others; the only obvious common denominator is that they are organic and lipophilic. It has also become apparent that, even though all inducers do not have the same effects, the effects tend to be nonspecific to the extent that any single inducer induces more than one enzymatic activity. Other enzymes can also be induced, such as glutathione *S*-transferase, epoxide hydrolase, and so on, and induction can extend even to cellular organelles, such as smooth endoplasmic reticulum, peroxisomes, and mitochondria.

6.5.2.1   Specificity of Monooxygenase Induction

Many inducers of monooxygenase activity fall into two principal classes, one exemplified by phenobarbital and containing many types of chemicals, especially drugs and insecticides, and the other exemplified by TCDD, 3-methylcholanthrene, and benzo(a)pyrene and containing primarily polycyclic hydrocarbons. However, other inducers with different isoform specificities are known. Many inducers require either fairly high dose levels or repeated dosing to be effective, frequently >10 mg/kg and some as high as 100 to 200 mg/kg. Some insecticides, however, such as mirex, can induce at dose levels as low as 1 mg/kg, and the most potent inducer known, 2,3,7,8-tetrachlorodibenzo-p-dioxin (TCDD), is effective at 1 μg/kg in some species.

In the liver, phenobarbital-type inducers cause a marked proliferation of the smooth endoplasmic reticulum as well as an increase in the amount of P450. A wide range of oxidative activities are induced, including O-demethylation of p-nitroanisole, N-demethylation of benzphetamine, pentobarbital hydroxylation, and aldrin epoxidation. The primary isoforms induced are P450 2B1 and 2B2 in the rat and 2B10 in the mouse. Some phenobarbital-type inducers also induce P450 3A isozymes, although in the latter case the mechanism may be different.

Induction by TCDD and polycyclic hydrocarbons, however, causes no increase in smooth endoplasmic reticulum although the P450 content is increased. The main isozymes induced are P450 1A1 and 1A2 along with other non-P450 proteins, including uridine diphosphoglucuronyl transferase. A relatively narrow range of oxidative activities, primarily aryl hydrocarbon hydroxylase, is induced by polycyclic hydrocarbons, with the best known reaction being the hydroxylation of benzo(a)pyrene.

All inducers do not fall readily into one or the other of these two classes. Some oxidative processes can be induced by either type of inducer, such as the hydroxylation of aniline and the N-demethylation of chlorcyclizine. Some inducers, such as the mixture of PCBs designated Arochlor 1254, can induce a broad spectrum of P450 isoforms. Many variations also exist in the relative stimulation of different oxidative activities within the same class of inducer, particularly of the phenobarbital type.

Pregnenolone-16α-carbonitrile (PCN) induces P450 3A1 and represents a third type of inducer, in that the substrate specificity of the microsomes from treated animals differs from that of the microsomes from either phenobarbital-treated or 3-methylcholanthrene-treated animals.

Ethanol and a number of other chemicals, including acetone and certain imidazoles, induce P450 2E1. Piperonyl butoxide, isosafrole, and other methylenedioxyphenyl compounds are known to induce P450 1A2 by a non–Ah receptor-dependent mechanism. Peroxisome proliferators, including the drug, clofibrate, and the herbicide synergist tridiphane induce a P450 4A isozyme that catalyzes the ω-oxidation of lauric acid.

It appears reasonable that because several types of P450 are associated with the hepatic endoplasmic reticulum, various inducers may induce one or more of them. Because each of these types has a relatively broad substrate specificity, differences may be caused by variations in the extent of induction of different cytochromes. Now that methods are available for gel electrophoresis of microsomes and identification of specific isoforms by immunoblotting blotting and isoform-specific antibodies, the complex array of inductive phenomena is being more logically explained in terms of specific isozymes.

Although the bulk of published investigations of the induction of monooxygenase enzymes has dealt with the mammalian liver, induction has been observed in other mammalian tissues and in nonmammalian species, both vertebrate and invertebrate. Cytochromes characteristic of all of these types of inducers have now been purified from rabbit and rat livers and, in some cases, from other organisms. It is also clear that many of these induced P450s represent only a small percentage of the total P450 in the uninduced animal. For this reason, the "constitutive" isozymes, those already expressed in the uninduced animal, must be fully characterized because they represent the available xenobiotic-metabolizing capacity of the normal animal.

6.5.2.2   Mechanism and Genetics of Induction in Mammals

It has been known for some time that in most, but not necessarily all, cases of increase in monooxygenase activity there is a true induction involving synthesis of new enzyme, and not the activation of enzyme already synthesized, since induction is prevented by inhibitors of protein synthesis. For example, aryl hydrocarbon hy-

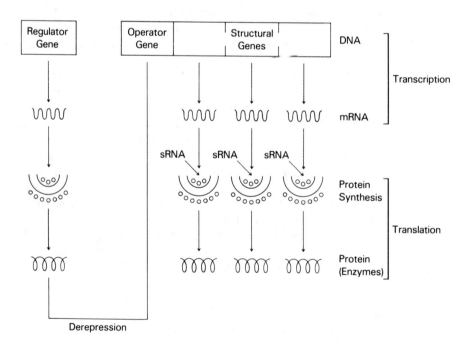

Figure 6.6. Simplified scheme for gene expression in animals.

droxylase induction is inhibited by puromycin, ethionine, and cycloheximide. A simplified scheme for gene expression and protein synthesis is shown in Fig. 6.6.

The use of suitable inhibitors of RNA and DNA metabolism has shown that inhibitors of RNA synthesis such as actinomycin D and mercapto(pyridethyl)benzimidazole block aryl hydrocarbon hydroxylase induction, whereas hydroxyurea, at levels that completely block the incorporation of thymidine into DNA, has no effect. Thus, it appears that the inductive effect is at the level of transcription and that DNA synthesis is not required.

These findings imply that compounds that induce xenobiotic-metabolizing enzymes play a role as derepressors of regulator or other genes in a manner analogous to steroid hormones—namely, combining with a cytosolic receptor followed by movement into the nucleus and then derepression of the appropriate gene. In the case of TCDD, the cytosolic receptor protein has been identified. The involvement of regulator and operator genes is more speculative; in view of the extremely variable results obtained with regard to the ratio of different enzymes induced by different inducers, it should be regarded with caution, particularly with inducers of the phenobarbital type.

The case is better argued with polycyclic hydrocarbon inducers, at least in the case of the mouse, because much genetic work has been done using "aromatic hydrocarbon-responsive" strains and "nonresponsive" strains. Thus, it has been demonstrated that facile inducibility of aryl hydrocarbon hydroxylase activity is due to a single dominant gene locus, Ah, even though it can be induced in so-called nonresponsive strains by more potent inducers such as TCDD.

Although phenobarbital induction has been known for a long time and is known to require de novo protein synthesis, little is known either of how the cell recognizes the inducer or of how the inducer affects transcription. Phenobarbital-like inducers are of low potency, requiring concentrations several orders of magnitude higher than a potent inducer such as TCDD. Although to date there is no evidence that a phenobarbital receptor exists, genomic DNA sequences have been described that are associated with phenobarbital-type induction.

Ah receptor-mediated induction, to date, is the only receptor-based mechanism for the induction of xenobiotic-metabolizing enzymes that has been defined clearly. This is due in large part to the observation that TCDD is more than 20,000 times more potent as an aryl hydrocarbon hydroxylase inducer than the compound previously regarded as the prototypical inducer in this class, namely 3-methylcholanthrene. Thus TCDD provided a high affinity ligand for investigations of the Ah receptor.

The general hypothesis for Ah receptor-dependent induction is as follows:

1. TCDD, or other lipophilic ligand of appropriate structure, enters the cell through the plasma membrane and binds to the cytosolic Ah receptor protein.
2. The receptor-ligand complex is transformed into a form that can associate with specific DNA sequences and migrates into the nucleus.
3. The transformed receptor-inducer complex combines with one or more regulatory sites on the P450 1A1 or other genes, bringing about increased transcription, followed by increased protein synthesis (Fig. 6.7).

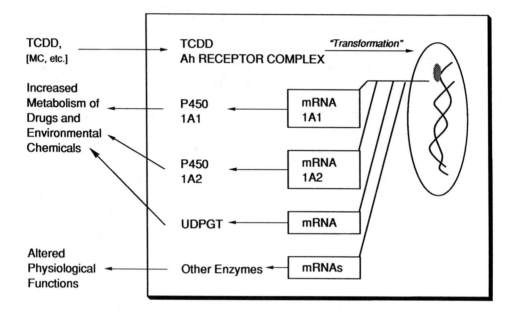

Figure 6.7. General model for Ah receptor regulation by TCDD and 3MC type chemicals. Ah-receptor ligands enter the cell by diffusion through the plasma membrane. After the ligand binds to the soluble Ah-receptor protein, the ligand receptor complex is transformed into a form that associates with specific DNA sequences. In the nucleus, the Ah-receptor–ligand complex appears to enhance the transcription of P450 1A and other genes. *(Source: Adapted from Okey AB: Enzyme induction in the cytochrome P450 system.* Pharmacol Ther *45:241–298, 1990.)*

Several independent lines of evidence support the role of the Ah receptor in the induction of P450 1A1 and other proteins. They include:

1. Structure-activity relationships that correlate relative ability to induce with relative affinity for the receptor, particularly in chemically related series of ligands.
2. Genetic variation.

Strains of mice are known that are Ah-responsive (eg, C57) or Ah-unresponsive (eg, DBA). The nonresponsive strains require some 15-fold more ligand to bring about a similar level of induction, a finding correlated with the presence of a low-affinity Ah receptor; molecular biology studies have shown good correlation between levels of TCDD-receptor complex and P450 1A1 mRNA, a finding subsequently confirmed using mutant mouse hepatoma cell lines that were either TCDD-inducible or TCDD nonindicible; antagonist studies using 6-methyl-1,3,8-trichlorobenzodifuran (MCDF), a weak inducer but a potent antagonist for induction by TCDD, an effect paralleled by inhibition of TCDD binding to the Ah receptor.

The Ah receptor–ligand complex appears to function by interaction with specific DNA sequences found c. 1000 base pairs upstream from the P450 1A1 transcription site. Two of these are transcription enhancer sites whereas the third is probably an inhibitor or suppressor site (Fig. 6.8).

In pregnenolone 16α-carbonitrile (PCN)-type induction of P450 3A1, it appears that not only transcriptional but also posttranscriptional events are important. Dexamethasone, for example, appears to increase P450 3A1 by message stabilization and erythromycin by protein stabilization. This is a complex class of inducers including synthetic and endogenous glucocorticoids, glucocorticoid and mineralocorticoid antagonists, phenobarbital-type inducers, macrolide antibiotics, and imidazoles.

Although P450 2E1 induction was discovered largely as a result of interest in ethanol metabolism, induction can be brought about by other chemicals such as acetone and imidazole, some of which are more potent than ethanol. It might also be noted that 2E1 is in the same family as 2B1 and 2B2; it is not induced by phenobarbital-type inducers. Its induction by either fasting or diabetes is believed

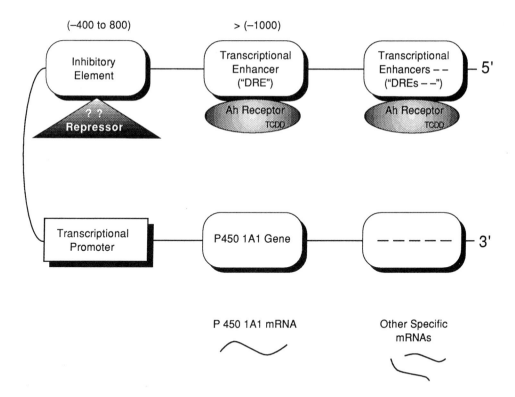

Figure 6.8. Interaction of the Ah-receptor–ligand complex with the 5' flanking region of the P450 1A1 gene. Two dioxin-responsive elements (DREs) appear to lie approximately 1000 or more base pairs upstream from the 1A1 transcriptional start site. These elements apear to be transcriptional enhancers, whereas less direct evidence indicates an inhibitory element ("negative control element") between 400 and 800 bases upstream. The negative control element may inhibit the 1A1 promoted although the conditions for this inhibition are, as yet, undefined. *(Source: Adapted from Okey AB: Enzyme induction in the cytochrome P450 system. Pharmacol Ther **45**:241–298, 1990.)*

to be due to the high levels of ketones likely to be present in either of these conditions. Although the mechanism of 2E1 induction is not well understood, transcriptional events appear to play little, if any, part; induction appearing to be dependent almost entirely on protein and/or mRNA stabilization.

Peroxisome proliferators, including hypolipidemic drugs such as clofibrate, phthalate plasticizers, and herbicides bring about the induction of a P450 4A isoform that catalyze the ω-oxidation of lauric acid. This is part of a pleiotropic response in the rodent liver, other components of which include increase in the number of peroxisomes and in peroxisomal enzymes such as catalase and an increase in liver weight. Peroxisome proliferators are often epigenetic carcinogens in rodents but, since the effect is primarily seen in rodents, its significance for other species such as humans is unclear. Evidence is accumulating that a peroxisome proliferator receptor exists and is involved in the inductive phenomenon.

6.5.2.3   Effects of Induction

The effects of inducers are usually the opposite of those of inhibitors; thus, their effects can be demonstrated by much the same methods, that is, by their effects on pharmacological or toxicological properties in vivo or by the effects on enzymes in vitro following prior treatment of the animal with the inducer. In vivo effects are frequently reported; the most common ones are the reduction of the hexobarbital sleeping time or zoxazolamine paralysis time. These effects have been reported for numerous inducers and can be quite dramatic. For example, in the rat, the paralysis time resulting from a high dose of zoxazolamine can be reduced from 11 hr to 17 min by treatment of the animal with benzo(a)pyrene 24 hr before the administration of zoxazolamine.

The induction of monooxygenase activity may also protect an animal from the effect of carcinogens by increasing the rate of detoxication. This has been demonstrated in the rat with a number of carcinogens including benzo(a)pyrene, N-2-fluorenylacetamide, and aflatoxin B_1. Effects on carcinogenesis may be expected to be complex because some carcinogens are both activated and detoxified by monooxygenase enzymes, while epoxide hydrolase, which can also be involved in both activation and detoxication, may also be induced. For example, the toxicity of the carcinogen 2-naphthylamine, the hepatotoxic alkaloid monocrotaline, and the cytotoxin cyclophosphamide are all increased by phenobarbital induction—an effect mediated by the increased population of reactive intermediates.

Organochlorine insecticides are also well-known inducers. Treatment of rats with either DDT or chlordane, for example, will decrease hexobarbital sleeping time and offer protection from the toxic effect of warfarin.

Effects on xenobiotic metabolism in vivo are also widely known in both humans and animals. Cigarette smoke, as well as several of its constituent polycyclic hydrocarbons, is a potent inducer of aryl hydrocarbon hydroxylase in the rat placenta, liver, and other organs. Examination of the term placentas of smoking human mothers revealed a marked stimulation of aryl hydrocarbon hydroxylase and related activities—remarkable in an organ that, in the uninduced state, is almost inactive toward foreign chemicals. Similarly, cigarette smoking lowers the plasma levels of phenacetin by induction of the enzymes responsible for its oxidation to N-acetyl-p-aminophenol. Persons exposed to DDT and lindane metabolized antipyrine twice as fast as a group not exposed, whereas those exposed to DDT alone had a reduced half-life for phenylbutazone and increased excretion of 6-hydroxycortisol.

The effects of inducers on the metabolic activity of hepatic microsomes subsequently isolated from treated animals have often been reported. Whereas the polycyclic hydrocarbons primarily induce aryl hydrocarbon hyroxylase activity and a few related activities, inducers such as phenobarbital, DDT, and so on, have been shown to induce many oxidative reactions, including benzphetamine N-demethylation, p-nitroanisole O-demethylation, N-demethylation of ethylmorphine, aldrin epoxidation, and many others. Some enzyme activities, such as zoxazolamine hydroxylase, chlorpromazine N-demethylation, and aniline hydroxylation, are induced by both types of inducers.

6.5.2.4 Induction of Xenobiotic-Metabolizing Enzymes Other than Monooxygenases

Although less well studied, xenobiotic-metabolizing enzymes other than those of the P450 system are also known to be induced, frequently by the same inducers that induce the oxidases. These include glutathione S-transferases, epoxide hydrolase, and UDP glucuronyltransferase. The selective induction of one pathway over another can greatly affect the metabolism of a xenobiotic.

6.5.3 Biphasic Effects: Inhibition and Induction

Many inhibitors of mammalian monooxygenase activity can also act as inducers. Inhibition of microsomal monooxygenase activity is fairly rapid and involves a direct interaction with the cytochrome, whereas induction is a slower process. Therefore, following a single injection of a suitable compound, an initial decrease due to inhibition would be followed by an inductive phase. As the compound and its metabolites are eliminated, the levels would be expected to return to control values. Some of the best examples of such compounds are the methylenedioxyphenyl synergists, such as piperonyl butoxide. Because P450 combined with methylenedioxyphenyl compounds in an inhibitory complex cannot interact with CO, the cytochrome P450 titer, as determined by the method of Omura and Sato (dependent upon CO-binding to reduced cytochrome), would appear to follow the same curve.

It is apparent from extensive reviews of the induction of monooxygenase activity by xenobiotics that many compounds other than methylenedioxyphenyl compounds have the same effect. It may be that any synergist that functions by inhibiting microsomal monooxygenase activity could also induce this activity on longer exposure, resulting in a biphasic curve as described previously for methylenedioxyphenyl compounds. This curve has been demonstrated for NIA 16824 (2-methylpropyl-2-propynyl phenylphosphonate) and WL 19255 (5,6-dichloro-1,2,3-benzothiadiazole), although the results were less marked with R05-8019

[2,(2,4,5-trichlorophenyl)-propynyl ether] and MGK 264 [*N*-(2-ethylhexyl)-5-nor-bornene-2,3-dicarboximide].

6.6

ENVIRONMENTAL EFFECTS

Because the in vitro effects of light, temperature, and so on, on xenobiotic-metabolizing enzymes are not different from their effects on other enzymes or enzyme systems, we are not concerned with them at present. This section deals with the effects of environmental factors on the intact animal as they relate to in vivo metabolism of foreign compounds.

6.6.1 Temperature

Although it might be expected that variations in ambient temperature would not affect the metabolism of xenobiotics in animals with homeothermic control, this is not the case. Temperature variations can be a form of stress and thereby produce changes mediated by hormonal interactions. Such effects of stress require an intact pituitary–adrenal axis and are eliminated by either hypothysectomy or adrenalectomy. There appear to be two basic types of temperature effect on toxicity: either with increase in toxicity at both high and low temperature, or an increase in toxicity with an increase in temperature. For example, both warming and cooling increases the toxicity of caffeine to mice, whereas the toxicity of *D*-amphetamine is lower at reduced temperatures and shows a regular increase with increases in temperature.

In many studies, it is unclear whether the effects of temperature are mediated through metabolism of the toxicant or via some other physiological mechanism. In other cases, however, temperature clearly affects metabolism. For example, in cold-stressed rats, there is an increase in the metabolism of 2-naphthylamine to 2-amino-1-naphthol.

6.6.2 Ionizing Radiation

In general, ionizing radiation reduces the rate of metabolism of xenobiotics both in vivo and in enzyme preparations subsequently isolated. This has occurred in hydroxylation of steroids, in the development of desulfuration activity toward azinphosmethyl in young rats, and in glucuronide formation in mice. Pseudocholinesterase activity is reduced by ionizing radiation in the ileum of both rats and mice.

6.6.3 Light

Because many enzymes, including some of those involved with xenobiotic metabolism, show a diurnal pattern that can be keyed to the light cycle, light cycles rather than light intensity would be expected to affect these enzymes. In the case of hydroxyindole-*O*-methyltransferase in the pineal gland, there is a diurnal rhythm with greatest activity at night; continuous darkness causes maintenance of the high level. Cytochrome P450 and the microsomal monooxygenase system show a diurnal rhythm in both the rat and the mouse, with greatest activity occurring at the beginning of the dark phase.

6.6.4   Moisture

No moisture effect has been shown in vertebrates, but in insects it was noted that housefly larvae reared on diets containing 40% moisture had four times more activity for the epoxidation of heptachlor than did larvae reared in a similar medium saturated with water.

6.6.5   Altitude

Altitude can either increase or decrease toxicity. It has been suggested that these effects are related to the metabolism of toxicants rather than to physiological mechanisms involving the receptor system, but in most examples this has not been demonstrated clearly. Examples of altitude effects include the observations that at altitudes of ≥ 5000 ft, the lethality of digitalis or strychnine to mice is decreased, whereas that of *D*-amphetamine is increased.

6.6.6   Other Stress Factors

Noise has been shown to affect the rate of metabolism of 2-napthylamine, causing a slight increase in the rat. This increase is additive with that caused by cold stress.

6.7

GENERAL SUMMARY AND CONCLUSIONS

It is apparent from the material presented in this chapter and the previous chapters related to metabolism that the metabolism of xenobiotics is complex, involving many enzymes; that it is susceptible to a large number of modifying factors, both physiological and exogenous; and that the toxicological implications of metabolism are important. In spite of the complexity, summary statements of considerable importance can be abstracted:

1. Phase-one metabolism generally introduces a functional group into a xenobiotic, which enables conjugation to an endogenous metabolite to occur during phase-two metabolism.
2. The conjugates produced by phase-two metabolism are considerably more water-soluble than either the parent compound or the phase-one metabolite(s) and hence are more excretable.

3. During the course of metabolism, and particularly during phase-one reactions, reactive intermediates that are much more toxic than the parent compound may be produced. Thus, xenobiotic metabolism may be either a detoxication or an activation process.

4. Because the number of enzymes involved in phase-one and phase-two reactions is large and many different sites on organic molecules are susceptible to metabolic attack, the number of potential metabolites and intermediates that can be derived from a single substrate is frequently very large.

5. Because both qualitative and quantitative differences exist between species, strains, individual organs, and cell types, a particular toxicant may have different effects in different circumstances.

6. Because exogenous chemicals can be inducers and/or inhibitors of the xenobiotic-metabolizing enzymes of which they are substrates; such chemicals may interact to bring about toxic sequelae different from those that might be expected from any of them administered alone.

7. Because endogenous factors also affect the enzymes of xenobiotic metabolism, the toxic sequelae to be expected from a particular toxicant will vary with developmental stage, nutritional status, health or physiological status, stress, or environment.

8. It has become increasingly clear that most enzymes involved in xenobiotic metabolism occur as several isozymes, which coexist within the same individual and, frequently, within the same subcellular organelle. An understanding of the biochemistry and molecular genetics of these isozymes may lead to an understanding of the variation between species, individuals, organs, sexes, developmental stages, and so on.

Suggested Further Reading

Anderson KE, Kappas A: Dietary regulation of cytochrome P450. *Ann Rev Nutr* **11**:141–167, 1991.

Batt AM, Siest G, Magdalou J, Galteau M-M: Enzyme induction by drugs and toxins. *Clin Chem Acta* **209**:109–121, 1992.

Conney AH: Pharmacological implications of microsomal enzyme induction. *Pharmacol Rev* **19**:317, 1967.

Denison MS, Whitlock JP Jr: Minireview: xenobiotic-inducible transcription of cytochrome P450 genes. *J Biol Chem* **270(31)**: 18175–18178, 1995.

Donaldson WE: Nutritional factors. In *Introduction to Biochemical Toxicology*, 2nd ed. Hodgson E, Levi PE (eds.), Norwalk, CT: Appleton & Lange, 1994, pp 297–317.

Goldstein A, Aronow L, Kalman SM: *Principles of Drug Action: The Basis of Pharmacology.* 3d ed. New York: Wiley, 1985.

Halpert JR, Guengerich FP, Bend JR, Correia MA: Contemporary issues in toxicology: selective inhibitors of cytochromes P450. *Toxicol Appl Pharmacol* **125**:163–175, 1994.

Hodgson E: Comparative toxicology: cytochrome P450 and mixed-function oxidase activity in target and non-target organisms. *Essays Toxicol* **7**:73, 1976.

Hodgson E: Chemical and environmental factors affecting metabolism of xenobiotics. In *Introduction to Biochemical Toxicology,* 2nd ed. Hodgson E, Levi PE, (eds). Norwalk, CT: Appleton & Lange, 1994, pp 153–175.

Hodgson E, Philpot RM: Interaction of methylenedioxyphenyl (1,3-benzodioxole) compounds with enzymes and their effects on mammals. *Drug Metab Rev* **3:**231, 1974.

Loomis TA. Hayes AW: *Loomis's Essentials of Toxicology,* 4th ed. San Diego: Academic Press, 1996. Chapters of interest: Biologic factors that influence toxicity; Chemical factors that influence toxicity; Influence of route of administration on systemic toxicity; Genetic factors that influence toxicity; The basis of selective toxicity.

Meyer, UA: The molecular basis of genetic polymorphisms of drug metabolism. *J Pharm Pharmacol* **46**(suppl 1)**:** 409–415, 1994.

Newton DJ, Wang RW, Lu AYH: Cytochrome P450 inhibitors: evaluation of specificities in the in vitro metabolism of therapeutic agents by human liver microsomes. *Drug Metab Disp* **23:**154–158, 1995.

Okey AB: Enzyme induction in the cytochrome P450 system. *Pharmacol Ther* **45:**141, 1990.

Ronis MJJ, Cunny HC: Physiological (endogenous) factors affecting the metabolism of xenobiotics. In *Introduction to Biochemical Toxicology,* 2nd ed. Hodgson E, Levi PE, (eds.). Norwalk, CT: Appleton and Lange, 1994, pp 133–151.

Smith CAD, Smith G, Wolf CR: Genetic polymorphisms in xenobiotic metabolism. *Eur J Cancer* **30A:**1935–1941, 1994.

Timbrell JA: *Principles of Biochemical Toxicology,* 2nd ed. London: Taylor & Francis, 1991.

Walker C: Comparative toxicology. In *Introduction to Biochemical Toxicology,* 2nd ed. Hodgson E, Levi PE (eds). Norwalk, CT: Appleton & Lange, 1994, pp 193–217.

7

ACUTE TOXICITY

PATRICIA E. LEVI

7.1

INTRODUCTION

The toxic effects of chemicals can be classified in a variety of ways. Frequently, toxicity is classified by effects to target organs (liver, lung, kidney, etc.), by types of responses (carcinogenic, developmental, etc.), and by toxic agents (pesticides, metals, etc.). For the most part, this approach is followed in this text. However, because this text is designed for the beginning toxicology student, the authors believe that it is important also to include a brief chapter focusing attention on some of the well-known chemicals and mechanisms associated with acute toxicity. Obviously there is overlap with other chapters—for example, acute effects of pesticides are discussed in some detail in this section and only briefly discussed in the section on toxic effects of pesticides. Furthermore, because certain classes of pesticides are nervous system toxicants, pesticide toxicity is also discussed under nervous system toxicity. For these reasons, students are encouraged to make use of the index to research a particular topic.

Acute effects are those that occur soon after a brief exposure to a chemical agent. Acute exposure can be the result of either a single exposure or multiple exposures occurring within a short time (generally less than 24 hours). The acute effect is an effect that is generally observed within hours to days of exposure but, in any case, within the first 2 weeks. Acute exposure to an agent that is absorbed rapidly is likely to produce an immediate toxic effect, but acute exposure can also produce a delayed effect. Chronic effects, however, are those effects that appear only after repetitive exposure to a substance, and many compounds require months of continuous exposure.

7.2

NERVOUS SYSTEM TOXICANTS

7.2.1   Pesticides

The reader is referred to Chapter 10, Section 10.5 for a discussion of pesticides, classification, and chemical structures.

ORGANOPHOSPHORUS AND CARBAMATE COMPOUNDS impair the function of the nervous system, their acute toxic effects resulting from binding to and inhibition of the enzyme acetylcholinesterase (AChE), which is found at synapses within the central and autonomic nervous systems and at the nerve endings in striated muscles.

Normally, acetylcholine (ACh), a neurotransmitter, is released from the presynapse and then binds to a protein receptor at the postsynapse. This binding leads

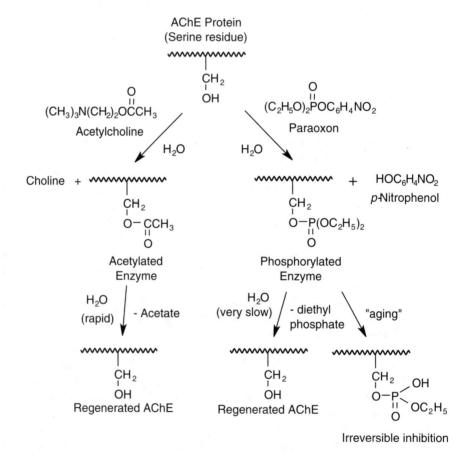

Figure 7.1. Schematic illustrating hydrolysis of ACh and parathion by the enzyme AChE.

to opening of ionic channels and a depolarization of the postsynaptic membrane. When ACh is released by the receptor, it is hydrolyzed by AChE to choline and acetate (Fig. 7.1) and its stimulatory activity is terminated. If AChE is inhibited, however, hydrolysis is prevented, ACh accumulates, and excessive nerve excitation occurs.

Exposure to organophosphorus compounds produces a broad spectrum of clinical effects that are indicative of overstimulation of the cholinergic system. These effects fall into three categories: (1) Inhibition of AChE at the neuromuscular junctions leads to muscular twitching from excessive contraction of muscles, extreme weakness, and often paralysis (nicotinic effects). The main muscles of concern in this type of acute poisoning are the respiratory muscles because paralysis of the diaphragm and chest muscles can result in respiratory failure and death. (2) Inhibition in the autonomic nervous system (muscarinic receptors) results in abdominal pain; diarrhea; involuntary urination; increased secretions in the respiratory system, filling the bronchioles with fluids; spasms of the smooth muscles in the respiratory tract, causing constriction of the airways; and a marked constriction of the pupils (miosis). (3) Central nervous system (CNS) effects include tremors, confusion, slurred speech, lack of coordination, and convulsions at very high exposures.

AChE inhibition results from blockage by the pesticide of the active site normally occupied by ACh. The organophosphorus compounds, if they are used as the P=S compound, such as parathion or malathion, first require metabolic activation to the P=O analog, termed the oxon, in order to possess anticholinesterase (anti-AChe) activity. This activation reaction is usually catalyzed by the cytochrome P450 system and is discussed in detail in Chapter 3. The oxon then becomes bound at the active site and undergoes cleavage to release the corresponding alcohol or thiol, leaving behind the phosphorylated enzyme (Fig. 7.1). The inactivation of the enzyme will persist until hydrolysis of the phosphorylated enzymes occurs. The time required for reactivation of free enzyme varies with different organophosphorates from a few hours to several days. With some compounds such as paraoxon, an additional reaction, known as "aging," occurs. This reaction stabilizes the phosphorylated enzyme so that the enzyme is irreversibly inhibited. In such cases, synthesis of new AChE is necessary for enzyme activity to be restored.

Carbamate pesticides are similar to organophosphorus pesticides in that they also act by binding to the active site of AChE, forming a carbamylated enzyme. The carbamylated enzyme, unlike the phosphorylated enzyme, is rapidly hydrolyzed and reactivated. The signs and symptoms of carbamate poisoning are typical of cholinesterase inhibition: lightheadedness, nausea and vomiting, increased sweating, blurred vision, increased salivation, weakness, chest pains, miosis, and in severe cases, convulsions. For a discussion of the treatment of anti-AChE poisoning, the reader is referred to Chapter 14.

PYRETHRINS AND PYRETHROIDS. Powders from pyrethrum flowers (*Chrysanthemum*) have been used commercially as insecticides since the late nineteenth century. In addition to their insect-killing activity, these natural compounds have two other attractive features—lack of environmental persistence and a rapid "knock-down" activity rendering flying insects unable to fly. Problems associated with the natural pyrethrins, such as poor light stability and high cost, have been largely overcome with the development of synthetic pyrethroids.

On the basis of the signs of acute toxicity in animals, the synthetic pyrethroids can be separated into two classes: type I and type II. Type I pyrethroids produce tremor in mice and rats that is noticed first in the limbs and then gradually spreads to involve the entire body. Body temperature increases dramatically during tremor. These effects are similar to those produced by DDT. Type II pyrethroids produce intense salivation followed by the development of a whole-body tremor. Convulsions are common before death.

All of the pyrethroids affect sodium channels in nerve membranes and bind with very high affinity. This binding results in changes in the gating kinetics of the sodium channel, including the prolongation of open time and a shifting of activation voltage toward hyperpolizarization. These effects lead to a hyperactivity of the nervous system. Type II pyrethroids produce longer delays in sodium channel inactivation than do type I compounds. Although interaction with the sodium channels represents a primary site of action of pyrethroids, this is not their only effect. In addition, some pyrethroids bind to the γ-amino butyric acid (GABA) receptor–chloride channel complex in the CNS, with type II pyrethroids being much more potent. Others inhibit Ca^{2+}, Mg^{2+}-ATPase, resulting in increased intracellular calcium levels, increased neurotransmitter release, and postsynaptic depolarization.

Of all the insecticides in use, pyrethrum and its derivatives are probably the least toxic to mammals. Injury to humans from pyrethrins has resulted most frequently from the allergenic properties of the material rather than its direct toxicity. Contact dermatitis is by far the most common. So far there has been little indication that acute or chronic use exposures to pyrethrins and pyrethroids are likely to produce significant neurologic concerns in humans.

DDT. Although exposure to DDT or its derivatives can result in an acute toxic response, very few deaths have been reported. After ingestion, the earliest effects involve paresthesia of the tongue, lips, and face and altered motor function leading to ataxia and abnormal stepping. These symptoms are typically followed by dizziness, confusion, vomiting, headache, and fatigue. Tremor, particularly of the hands, is a common symptom of DDT poisoning. Onset of symptoms may be as early as 30 minutes after ingesting large doses or may be delayed as much as 6 hours after ingesting smaller amounts. Dermal and inhalation exposures have rarely been reported to result in measurable neurotoxic effects.

The mechanism by which DDT produces its acute effects results from its action on the nervous system, probably by slowing down the closure of the gates in the sodium channels. The result of this is a repetitive firing in sensory and motor nerves. In addition, DDT affects the permeability of the neuronal membrane to potassium ions and inhibits neuronal ATPases that play vital roles in neuronal repolarization.

7.2.2   Natural Toxicants

Many exogenous chemicals can affect the presynaptic and postsynaptic binding sites of the neuromuscular junction, and some highly poisonous compounds owe their toxic action to their ability to alter nerve impulse transmission at this junction. A number of naturally occurring toxicants fall into this category.

TUBOCURARINE from the plant *Chondrodendron tomentosuni* is a deadly poison that owes its toxic action to its ability to block irreversibly the Ach receptor site of certain motor neurons. Curare and similar drugs act as competitive antagonists of Ach at the postjunctional membrane of muscle fibers, reducing or blocking Ach's transmitter action. These compounds are used pharmacologically as "muscle relaxants."

BOTULINUM TOXINS are heat-labile neurotoxins produced by the microorganism *Clostridium botulinum*. Botulinum toxin binds irreversibly to the axon terminal, thus preventing release of Ach. Botulism, one of the most dreaded of the bacterial foodborne diseases because it is so frequently fatal, results primarily from eating improperly preserved canned food in which the bacterium has grown and produced the toxin. Boiling food prior to eating, however, will destroy the toxin.

TETRODOTOXIN (see Fig. 1.9) has been responsible for deaths in humans as a result of consumption of improperly prepared puffer fish (Tetraodontidae). In Japan, puffer fish, known as *fugu*, are considered a great delicacy and are sold widely in restaurants. The toxins are found in the roe, liver, and skin of puffer fish, and food handlers must be specially trained in the preparation of this fish for human consumption. It is thought that tetrodotoxin selectively blocks sodium channels along the nerve axon, preventing the inward sodium current of the action potential while leaving unaffected the outward potassium current. Approximately 60% of all cases of poisoning due to puffer fish result in death.

BATRACHOTOXIN (see Fig. 1.9) has been used as an arrow poison and is found in the skin of the South American frog *Phyllobates aurotaenia*. The action of batrachotoxin is opposite to the effects of tetradotoxin on the sodium channels in that batrachotoxin increases the permeability of the resting membranes to sodium ions.

7.3

ELECTRON TRANSPORT INHIBITORS

The electron transport system consists of a series of linked, or coupled, oxidations and reductions, or redux reactions, with the final step being the reduction of O_2 to water. In the process energy in the form of ATP is generated. The enzymes involved in cellular respiration are located in the mitochondria. Because of the critical role of cellular respiration and ATP production, chemicals that inhibit or "uncouple" respiration can be extremely acute and potent toxicants.

7.3.1   Cyanide

Cyanide is one of the most rapidly acting of all poisons. It is readily absorbed through all routes, including the skin and mucous membranes, and by inhalation. Ingestion of very small amounts of cyanide can cause death within minutes or hours, depending on the route of exposure. Inhalation of hydrogen cyanide gas leads to death in a few minutes. The chemist Karl Wilhelm Scheele, discoverer of hydrocyanic acid (prussic acid), was killed by its vapors. Cyanide is a common component in some rat and pest poisons, silver and metal polishes, ore refining processes, photographic solutions, and fumigating products. Cyanide is also present in the seeds of apples, peaches, plums, apricots, cherries, and almonds in the form of amygdalin, a cyanogenic glycoside. Laetrile, a once popular, alleged anticancer drug, contains amygdalin. Cyanide can be released from the amygdalin glucoside by the action of ß-glucosidase, present in the pulp from crushed seeds and in mammalian intestinal microflora. Laetrile was known to be responsible for cases of human cyanide poisoning, as were apricot kernels, the latter being widely available in health food stores.

Another potential source of cyanide poisoning is the drug sodium nitroprusside, which is used in the treatment of hypertension. Overdoses of this drug have led to cyanide toxicity. Cyanide exerts its toxic effect by interrupting electron transport in the mitochondrial cytochrome chain. This system consists of three enzymes: cytochrome c and cytochromes a and a_3. Cytochromes a and a_3 form part of a large multiprotein complex known as cytochrome oxidase (Fig. 7.2). Cyanide

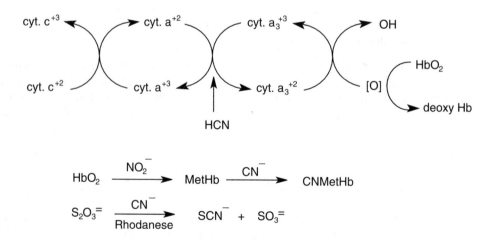

Figure 7.2. Cyanide poisoning and treatment.

complexes with the heme of the terminal cytochrome, thus preventing the heme's binding with oxygen. As a result of cyanide inhibition, electron transfer to molecular oxygen is blocked and cell death occurs. Death from cyanide poisoning is due to respiratory arrest. The symptoms, which occur in quick succession, are salivation, giddiness, headache, palpitation, difficulty in breathing, and unconsciousness.

Typically, cyanide has a bitter, burning taste; in addition, there is a faint odor of almonds. It has been estimated, however, that 20% to 40% of the population are genetically unable to detect the cyanide odor and thus are insensitive to this property. The accepted treatment for cyanide poisonings (Fig. 7.2) is a three-step procedure. First, amyl nitrite is given to the patient by inhalation. The second step is intravenous (IV) administration of sodium nitrite. These chemicals oxidize the heme iron of hemoglobin from the ferrous (+2) to the ferric (+3) state; the resulting greenish-brown to black pigment is known as methemoglobin. The ferric iron of the methemoglobin combines with cyanide from the plasma, causing dissociation of the cyanide bound to cytochrome oxidase. The third step is injection of sodium thiosulfate. This chemical provides a substrate for the enzyme rhodanese (thiosulfate sulfur transferase) that catalyzes the conversion of cyanide to thiocyanate, a form that is nontoxic and readily excreted.

7.2.2   Other Inhibitors

Azide, like cyanide, inhibits cytochrome oxidase and produces similar biochemical lesions. **Hydrogen sulfide** is also an inhibitor of cytochrome oxidase in vitro and is thought to have the same mode of action as hydrogen cyanide. **Carbon monoxide**, however, combines directly with hemoglobin, forming a stable carboxyhemoglobin complex, thus preventing the association of molecular oxygen with hemoglobin.

7.4
UNCOUPLERS OF OXIDATIVE PHOSPHORYLATION

Uncoupling agents allow electron transport to continue but prevent the phosphorylation of ADP to adenosine triphosphate (ATP). In vitro uncouplers can be shown to stimulate the rate of oxygen uptake by mitochondria, even in the absence of ADP or inorganic phosphate ions, and to induce ATPase activity, which is normally low in mitochondria. The first uncoupling agent described was the herbicide 2,4-dinitrophenol. Most uncoupling compounds arc lipophilic, weak acids, usually containing an aromatic ring. Many different uncoupling agents are known, including halogenated and nitrophenols, dicoumarin, carbonylcyanide phenylhydrazone, salicylanilides, atebrin (an antimalarial drug), and arsenate (Fig. 7.3).

Uncoupling agents are thought to function by breaking down or discharging a high energy state or intermediate generated by electron transport. They can "short-

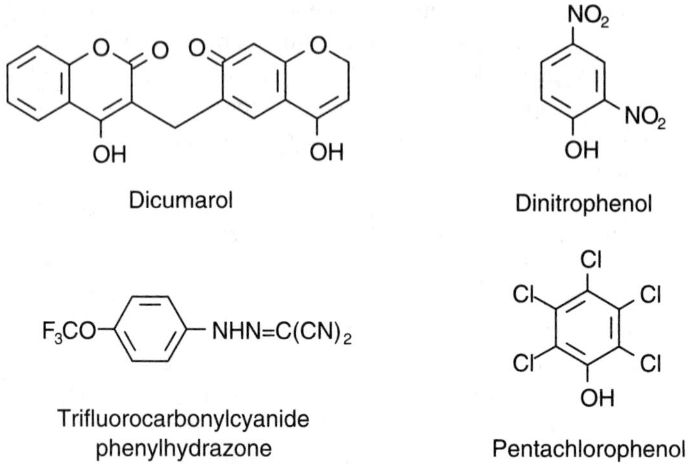

Figure 7.3. Examples of some compounds that uncouple oxidative phosphorylation.

circuit" the proton current by transporting protons directly through the mitochondrial membrane, which normally is impermeable. This "uncoupling" increases oxygen consumption and heat production. In humans, the result is hyperthermia, and the symptoms include fast respiratory and heart rates, flushed skin, sweating, nausea, and coma. The illness runs a rapid course, with either death from hyperthermia or recovery generally occurring within 24 to 48 hours.

In some natural situations the uncoupling of respiration from phosphorylation may be desirable. Many mammals, for example those that hibernate and those that are adapted to cold, have a special need to maintain body temperature. Such animals have a special tissue, called brown fat, in the neck and upper back. Mitochondria in this tissue are specialized to generate heat from fat oxidation, uncoupled from phosphorylation. These mitochondria are especially rich in cytochromes, which give this tissue its brown color.

7.5

SUICIDE SUBSTRATES

Suicide substrates are compounds that are not by themselves toxic to cells but resemble normal metabolites closely enough to undergo metabolic transformation to a product that can inhibit crucial enzymes. Thus the cell "commits suicide" by transforming the analog to a toxic product. This mechanism of toxicity was established by Sir Rudolph Peters, who used the term "lethal synthesis" to describe this type of biochemical lesion.

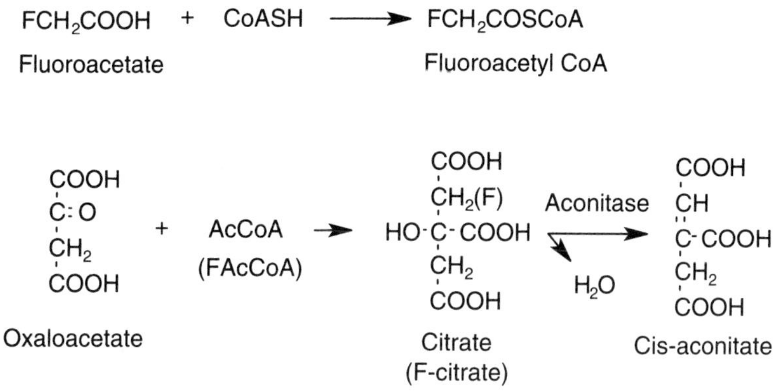
FCH2COOH + CoASH → FCH2COSCoA
Fluoroacetate
Fluoroacetyl CoA
COOH
C:O
CH2
COOH
Oxaloacetate
+ AcCoA
(FAcCoA)
COOH
CH2(F)
HO-C-COOH
CH2
COOH
Citrate
(F-citrate)
Aconitase
H2O
COOH
CH
C-COOH
CH2
COOH
Cis-aconitate

Figure 7.4. Inhibition of citric acid cycle by fluoroacetate. The enzyme aconitase is inhibited by the intermediate fluorocitrate.

FLUOROACETATE is a compound found naturally in certain plants in South Africa, where it has been known to cause livestock poisoning. Products of these plants are used as rodenticides (Compound 1080, sodium fluoroacetate and Compound 1081, fluoroacetamide). Because of their extreme toxicity to most animals, these chemicals are not available for household or general use. Fluoroacetate produces its toxic action by inhibiting the citric acid cycle (Fig. 7.4). The fluorine-substituted acetate becomes incorporated, by the mechanism for endogenous acetate, into fluoroacetyl coenzyme A, which combines with oxaloacetate to form fluorocitrate. The next enzyme in the cycle, aconitase, is inhibited by fluorocitrate, resulting in a large accumulation of citrate and disruption of the mitochondrial energy supply. The heart and nervous system are the most critical of the tissues involved when there is general inhibition of oxidative energy metabolism. The symptoms of fluoroacetate poisoning include nausea, convulsions, and defects in cardiac rhythm. Death may result from ventricular fibrillation or respiratory failure.

SUGGESTED FURTHER READING

Abou-Donia MB: Gases and vapors; Pesticides; Drugs of abuse; and Naturally occurring toxins. In *Neurotoxicology*, Abou-Donia MB (ed.). Boca Raton: CRC Press, 1992, pp 423–505.

Baumann H, Gauldie J: The acute phase response. *Immunol Today.* **15:**74–80, 1994.

Ellenhorn MJ, Barcelous DG: *Medical Toxicology, Diagnosis and Treatment of Human Poisoning.* New York: Elsevier, 1988.

Gregus Z, Klaassen CD: Mechanisms of toxicity. In *Casarett & Doull's Toxicology, the Basic Science of Poisons,* 5th ed. Klaassen CD (ed.). New York: McGraw-Hill, 1996, pp 35–74.

Leaning J: War and the environment: human health consequences of the environmental damage of war. In *Critical Condition. Human Health and the Environment.* Chivian E, McCally M, Hu H, Haines A, (eds.). Cambridge, MA: MIT Press, 1993, pp 123–137.

Loomis TA, Hayes AW: Classification of harmful effects of chemicals; Normal toxic effects of chemicals; Abnormal response to chemicals; The basis of selective toxicity; and The basis of antidotal therapy. In *Essentials of Toxicology,* 4th ed. San Diego: Academic Press, 1996, pp 101–168.

Margos L: The clinical and experimental aspects of carbon disulfide intoxication. In *Rev Environ Health* **2(1):**65–68, 1975.

Morgan DP: *Recognition and Management of Pesticide Poisoning,* EPA pub. No 540/9-88-001. Washington, DC: US Government Printing Office, 1989.

Moses M: Pesticide-related health problems and farmworkers. *Am Assoc Occup Health Nurses J* **37:**115–130, 1989.

Narahashi T: Nerve membrane Na^+ channels as targets of insecticides. *Trends Pharmacol Sci* **13:**236–241, 1992.

Nelson SD, Pearson PG: Covalent and noncovalent interactions in acute lethal cell injury caused by chemicals. *Ann Rev Pharmacol Toxicol* **30:**169–195, 1990.

US Congress, Office of Technology Assessment: *Neurotoxicity: Identifying and Controlling Poisons of the Nervous System,* OTA-BA-436. Washington, DC: US Government Printing Office, 1990.

CHRONIC TOXICITY: CARCINOGENESIS, MUTAGENESIS, TERATOGENESIS

PATRICIA E. LEVI

8.1

CARCINOGENESIS

8.1.1   Historic Perspective

The fact that certain agents in the environment may lead to various forms of cancer has been since the late eighteenth century. The evidence that environmental chemicals had the potential to cause cancer usually came first from observations of a high cancer incidence among certain occupational groups, but it was not until much later that direct experimental evidence confirmed these suggestions (Table 8.1). Two early recorded observations were those of John Hill in 1761 and Sir Percival Pott in 1775. Hill observed an increased incidence of nasal cancer among snuff users whereas Pott observed that many of his patients with cancer of the scrotum were chimney sweeps. Pott related this cancer to their exposure to soot and coal tar. These observations were not confirmed until around 1916, when it was shown that skin cancer could be produced on rabbit ears by the application of coal tar. In the 1920s and 1930s, coal tar was fractionated, and the active components were shown to be polycyclic aromatic hydrocarbons such as dimethylbenz(a)anthracene and benzo(a)pyrene (Fig. 8.1).

In the 1860s, Germany became the center for the manufacture of synthetic dyes that were based on aromatic amines or their products. About 30 years later came the first warning that exposure to the dyes or their intermediates was hazardous. In 1895, Ludwig Rehn, a surgeon in Frankfurt, reported a cluster of bladder carcinomas in workmen from nearby dye factories. Epidemiologic evidence suggested that 2-naphthylamine (Fig. 8.1) was the probable carcinogen, but this was not directly confirmed until 1938, when Hueper and coworkers demonstrated bladder tumors in dogs fed 2-naphthylamine. The structure of some synthetic chemical

TABLE 8.1. HISTORY OF DISCOVERY OF ENVIRONMENTAL AGENTS CAUSING CANCER IN HUMANS

Carcinogen	Organ	Discoverer	Year
Snuff	Nose	Hill	1761
Soot	Scrotum	Pott	1775
Pipe smoking	Lips	Sommering	1795
Coal tar	Skin	Volkman	1875
Dye intermediates	Bladder	Rehn	1895
X-rays	Skin	Van Trieben	1902
Tobacco juice	Oral cavity	Abbe	1915
Radioactive watch dial dyes	Bone	Martland	1929
Sunlight	Skin	Molesworth	1937
Cigarette smoke	Lung	Muller	1939
Asbestos	Pleura	Wagner	1960
Cadmium	Prostate	Kipling; Waterhouse	1967

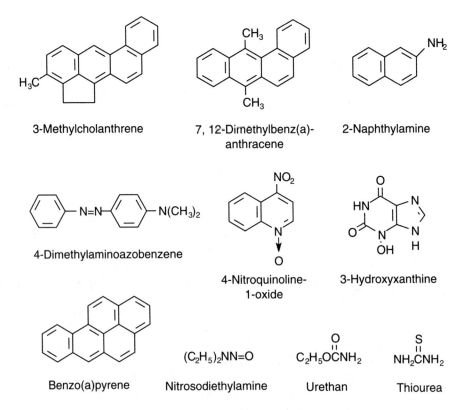

3-Methylcholanthrene

7, 12-Dimethylbenz(a)-anthracene

2-Naphthylamine

4-Dimethylaminoazobenzene

4-Nitroquinoline-1-oxide

3-Hydroxyxanthine

Benzo(a)pyrene

Nitrosodiethylamine

Urethan

Thiourea

Figure 8.1. Structures of some synthetic chemical carcinogens.

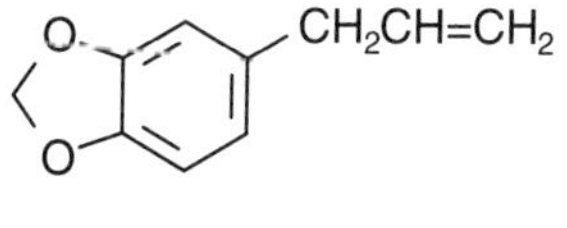

Safrole
(sassafras)

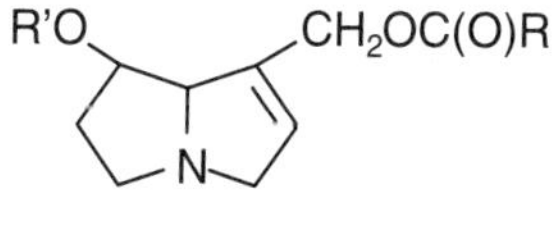

Pyrrolizidine alkaloids
(Senecio, Crotolaria, Heliotropium)

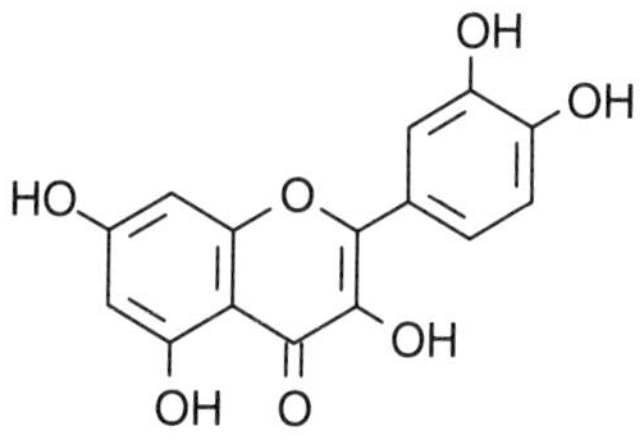

Quercetin
(bracken fern)

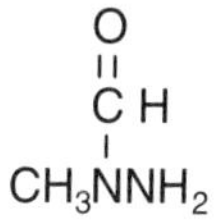

N-Methyl-*N*-formylhydrazine
(edible false morel mushroom)

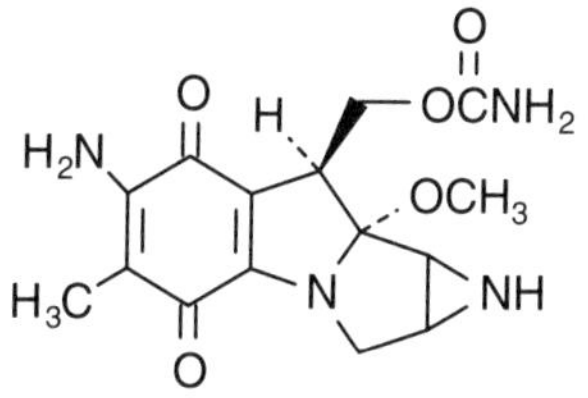

Mitomycin C
(*Streptomyces caespitosus*)

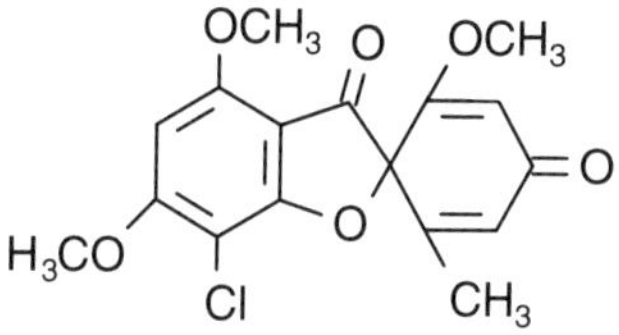

Griseofulvin
(*Penicillium griseofulvum*)

Figure 8.2. Structures of some naturally occurring chemical carcinogens.

carcinogens are shown in Fig. 8.1, and structures of some naturally occurring carcinogens are shown are shown in Fig. 8.2.

8.1.2 Initiation, Promotion, and Progression

The induction of cancer by chemicals is a complex multistep process involving interactions between environmental and endogenous factors. Carcinogenesis usually proceeds through several sequential stages before the formation of a malignant neoplasm (Fig. 8.3). In experimental models, carcinogenesis can be divided into at least three stages termed *initiation*, *promotion*, and *progression*.

INITIATION. The initiation stage is considered to be a rapid, essentially irreversible alteration in the cell's genetic material that "primes" the cell for subsequent neoplastic development. This cell, often referred to as an "initiated cell," requires a round of replication to "fix" the genetic change. The initiating chemical is either an elec-

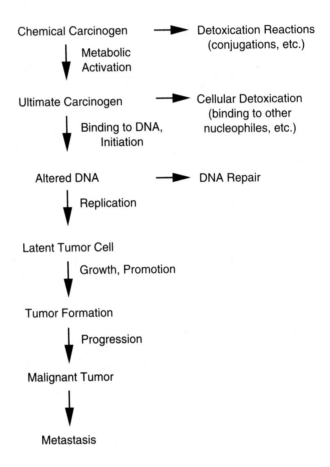

Figure 8.3. Schematic of main events in chemical carcinogenesis.

trophile or is metabolically activated to an electrophile. This reactive chemical then binds to DNA to form a permanent and heritable, but not yet expressed, change in the cell genome. According to this model, the initiated cell may remain dormant until exposed to a tumor promoting agent that then allows the growth of clones from initiated cells to eventually produce a tumor.

PROMOTION. Promoting agents are chemicals that are not in themselves carcinogens, but which, when given repetitively after a low dose of an initiating agent, increase cancer incidence. Promoters may either increase the number of tumors or decrease the latency period. Promoters are not usually electrophiles and do not bind to DNA.

PROGRESSION. The development of a malignant tumor from a benign tumor encompasses a third step termed progression, and is thought to involve further genetic changes.

8.1.3   Initiation–Promotion Model

The initiation–promotion model of multistage carcinogenesis was first shown in mouse skin, and this model has now been well characterized. In a typical experiment, an initiating chemical such as dimethylbenz(a)anthracene is applied to mouse skin at a low dose so that very few, if any, tumors are produced in the animal's lifetime. After an interval of 1 week to 1 year, the treated skin is exposed to multiple applications of a promoter such as the phorbol esters found in croton oil. Tumors begin to appear as early as 5 to 6 weeks after application of the promoter, and most mice yield tumors by 10 to 12 weeks after application.

Experimentally, the initiation–promotion process has now been demonstrated in several tissues including liver, lung, colon, mammary gland, prostate, and bladder. Tumor promoters are usually organ specific—for example, 12-O-tetradecanoylphorbol-13-acetate (TPA), a phorbol ester isolated from croton oil, is active almost exclusively on skin. Phenobarbital, DDT, chlordane, and TCDD are hepatic tumor promoters, bile acids are colon and liver tumor promoters, and mirex is active in skin and liver. Although tumor promoters have different mechanisms of action and many are organ specific, all have certain common operational features in the initiation–promotion protocol.

- The initiator must be given first; no tumors or very few tumors result if the promoter is given first.
- The initiator, if given once at a subcarcinogenic dose, does not produce tumors during the life of the animal; however, repeated doses of the initiator may elicit tumors even in the absence of the promoter.
- The action of the initiator is irreversible; tumors result in nearly the same yield if the interval between initiation and promotion is extended from 1 week to 1 year.
- The initiator is an electrophile, or is metabolically activated to an electrophile, which binds covalently to DNA to bring about a mutagenic change.
- The essential function of the tumor promoter is to complete the carcinogenic process started by the initiator.
- Promoters have not been found to be electrophilic, and there is no evidence of covalent binding to macromolecules.
- The action of the promoter is reversible at an early stage and usually requires repeated exposure; thus, there is probably a threshold level of exposure.

8.1.4   Examples of Promoters

In addition to promotion of skin carcinogenesis by the phorbol esters, there are known or suspected promoters for tumors in other organs. Bile acids are known to be promoters of colon carcinogenesis in experimental animals. In humans, there is a strong association between high intake of dietary fat and cancer of the colon; because ingestion of fat increases the amount of bile acids in the colon, the increased colon cancer may be due to the promotion effect of the bile acids.

In the rat bladder, saccharin and cyclamate are promoters for tumors after an initiating dose of methylnitrosourea; tryptophan is a promoter for urinary bladder tumors in dogs treated with an initiating dose of 4-aminobiphenyl or 2-naphthylamine.

Hormones are also known to be modifiers of chemical carcinogenesis. An oral or IV injection of dimethylbenzanthracene (DMBA) produces mammary tumors in susceptible female mice. Prolactin will increase tumor development, whereas in animals that have had the ovaries removed there will be very few tumors.

8.1.5   Cocarcinogenesis

A cocarcinogen is an agent that is applied either just before or together with a carcinogen and results in significantly higher tumor yields than with the carcinogen alone. Note the contrast to the experimental promotion model, which defines a promoter as a chemical administered after initiation. Some chemicals, however, can act as both promoters and cocarcinogens. Cocarcinogenesis can result from such factors as hormones, viruses, immunologic factors, nutritional factors, physical trauma, and skin abrasion. Several possible mechanisms by which cocarcinogens may affect the initiating process are summarized in Table 8.2.

Several cocarcinogens have been investigated in connection with tumors of the respiratory tract. Silicon dioxide dust in combination with benzo(a)pyrene is cocarcinogenic for carcinoma of the larynx, trachea, and lungs in experimental animals. Among uranium miners, uranium dust exposure has a synergistic effect on the formation of lung tumors among cigarette smokers.

A similar effect has been observed in connection with lung carcinoma among asbestos workers. Compared with controls who neither smoke nor work with asbestos, asbestos workers had a death rate from lung cancer that was five times higher. For smokers who were not asbestos workers, the rate was 11 times higher, but for asbestos workers who also smoked, the rate of lung cancer was approximately 50 times higher than in the control population.

Hormones may also play an important role as modulators of carcinogenesis. For example, male rats are generally more susceptible to tumor induction by 2-AAF than are female rats. This is due in part to higher sulfotransferase activity in male

TABLE 8.2. SOME PROPOSED MECHANISMS OF COCARCINOGENESIS

Increased uptake of carcinogen by cells
Increased bioactivation of procarcinogen
Depletion of detoxifying nucleophiles
Inhibition of DNA repair mechanisms
Increased conversion of DNA lesions to permanent changes

Source: Modified from Williams, G: Fund Appl Toxicol 4:325–344, 1984.

rats (Chapter 4, Section 4.5.2). This activity can be depressed in castrated males by the administration of estradiol. This treatment results in a lower susceptibility of male rats to 2-AAF carcinogenesis.

Although tobacco smoke contains only relatively small amounts of genotoxic carcinogens such as polycyclic aromatic hydrocarbons and nitrosamines, it does contain a number of cocarcinogens and promoters in the form of catechol and other phenolic compounds. The cocarcinogenic and promotional factors in tobacco smoke are thought to play an important role in the overall induction of cancer in cigarette smokers.

These concepts of initiation, promotion, and cocarcinogenesis are extremely important because many chemicals that are structurally unrelated to known carcinogens and appear not to be carcinogenic may turn out to be promoters or cocarcinogens. For this reason it is important that hazard assessment include testing for promotional activity.

8.1.6   Genotoxic and Epigenetic Carcinogens

In the study of chemical carcinogenesis, two important ideas have evolved. First, many carcinogenic chemicals alter cellular DNA irreversibly, resulting in a heritable change. Second, cancer formation is a multistep process, with the simplest model being that of initiation and promotion. In this multistep process, at least one step must involve a change in the DNA; the additional steps affect the growth and development of tumor cells. Thus, a carcinogen may be defined as any agent that induces neoplasms not usually observed, that causes the earlier appearance of neoplasms, or that increases the number of tumors. Using this operational definition, carcinogens can be divided into two main categories: *genotoxic* and *epigenetic* (Table 8.3).

Genotoxic chemicals are chemicals that are capable of damaging or modifying DNA, whereas epigenetic carcinogens exert their oncogenic effect by means other than genotoxic action. This includes such indirect mechanisms as alteration in gene expression, immunosuppression, hormonal imbalances, cytotoxicity, cocarcinogenic action, and promoting effects. The differences in chemical actions and mechanisms between the two types of carcinogens suggest that chemical reactivity and short-term tests for genetic effects could be used to distinguish genotoxic from epigenetic chemicals.

TABLE 8.3. EXAMPLES OF GENOTOXIC AND EPIGENETIC CARCINOGENS

Genotoxic Carcinogens	Epigenetic Carcinogens
Alkylating agents	Plastics, asbestos
Benzo(a)pyrene	Estrogen, androgen
Vinyl chloride	Phorbol ester
Dimethylnitrosoamine	Bile acid
Arsenic, nickel, chromium	Organochlorines
Radiation	Saccharin

8.1.7   Activation of Carcinogens and Binding to Macromolecules

An important advance in understanding chemical carcinogenesis came from the investigations of Drs. Elizabeth and James Miller, who demonstrated that many carcinogens are not intrinsically carcinogenic but require metabolic activation in order to express their carcinogenic potential. The Millers introduced the terms *procarcinogen*, *proximate carcinogen*, and *ultimate carcinogen* to describe this metabolic process. Chemical carcinogens that require metabolism to exert their carcinogenic effect are called procarcinogens; metabolites between procarcinogens and ultimate carcinogens are proximate carcinogens; and the products that interact with cellular components and are responsible for carcinogenic activity are ultimate carcinogens.

Not all carcinogens, however, require metabolic activation, and those compounds that do not are referred to as direct acting or primary carcinogens (Fig. 8.4). Generally, these chemicals are extremely reactive or are converted nonenzymatically to reactive electrophiles. Frequently, direct-acting carcinogens cause tumors at the site of exposure. Such compounds are usually too reactive to pose an environmental problem.

Most chemical carcinogens, however, require metabolic activation in vivo to exert their carcinogenic action (see Chapter 4, Metabolic Activation, for examples). The reactive metabolites, or ultimate carcinogens, are strong electrophiles, such as carbonium and nitrenium ions. These chemicals can form covalent adducts nonenzymatically with a wide variety of nucleophilic sites in cellular macromolecules such as peptides, proteins, RNA, and DNA. Binding to proteins, because of their relative abundance in cells, is usually the major macromolecular interaction of carcinogens.

Electrophilic carcinogens also bind to nucleic acids, and this covalent binding to DNA is considered the critical reaction of genotoxic carcinogens in the initiation of tumors. Such electrophiles attack nucleophilic oxygen as well as nitrogen atoms of the DNA bases. The exact mechanisms by which the mutation of DNA brings about carcinogenesis are unknown, but it is clear that these changes involve activa-

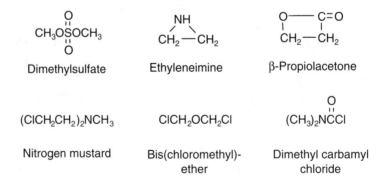

Figure 8.4. Structures of some primary carcinogens.

tion or inactivation of numerous cellular genes, such as oncogenes and tumor suppressor genes.

8.1.8   DNA Repair

Experimental and clinical evidence indicates that the development of cancer following exposure to chemical carcinogens is a relatively rare event. In part, this can be explained by the cell's numerous defense mechanisms, including its ability to recognize and repair damaged DNA.

Numerous repair mechanisms exist to repair the various types of DNA damage, and it has been estimated that more than 100 genes are related to DNA repair. In one mechanism, excision repair, the DNA region containing the adduct is removed, and a new area of DNA is synthesized using the opposite intact strand as a template. The new segment is then ligated into the DNA molecule in place of the defective one. To be effective in restoring the cell to normal, DNA repair must occur prior to cell division. If repair is not complete before DNA replication, the presence of the adducts can give rise to mispairing of bases and probably other genetic effects, such as rearrangements and translocations of segments of DNA. Thus, an agent that alters the repair process or the rate of cell division can itself affect the frequency of neoplastic transformation.

Clinical studies have shown that persons with an impaired ability to repair damaged DNA frequently develop cancers at an early age. In one syndrome, xeroderma pigmentosum, the person is unable to excise thymine dimers induced by ultraviolet (UV) light from the sun. These people are extremely sensitive to sunlight, and their incidence of skin cancer is nearly 100% by early adulthood.

8.1.9   Radiation Carcinogenesis

The effects of ionizing radiation on cells are initiated by the absorption of energy sufficient to expel electrons from molecules, resulting in the formation of positively charged ions. The expelled electrons react with nearby molecules, forming negatively charged ions. Because water is the principle component of the cell, it absorbs most of the ionizing radiation, forming free radicals that then can react with each other, with other water molecules, or with macromolecules within the cell. Reactive oxygen species (ROS) such as superoxide, hydroperoxy radical, hydroxyl radical, and hydrogen peroxide, are formed and can cause general oxidative damage to cellular macromolecules, including DNA. Ionizing radiation has been known for many years to be mutagenic and carcinogenic.

8.1.10   Oncogenes

Certain normal cellular genes, termed proto-oncogenes, appear to be target genes for chemical carcinogens. In normal cells, these genes appear to function in the control of cellular growth and differentiation and have been highly conserved throughout evolution. When altered by a chemical carcinogen or other mutating event,

TABLE 8.4. SOME ONCOGENE PROTEIN PRODUCTS

Oncogene Families	Oncogenes
Growth factors	*sis* (platelet derived growth factor, chain b)
Growth factor receptors	*erb* B (epidermal growth factor receptor)
	met (hepatocyte growth factor receptor)
GTP binding proteins	H-*ras*, K-*ras*, N-*ras*
Tyrosine kinases	*src, fes, abl, trk*
Serine/threonine kinases	*mos, raf*
DNA binding proteins	*myc, fos, myb, jun*

Source: *Smart R: In* Introduction to Biochemical Toxicology, *2nd ed. Hodgson E, Levi PE (eds.). East Norwalk, CT: Appleton & Lange, 1994, p 396.*

these genes, known as oncogenes, have the ability, when activated in cells, to transform the cells from normal to neoplastic.

The various mechanisms by which cellular proto-oncogenes become oncogenes and how these genes effect cell transformation are still not well understood. Some preliminary insights are emerging, however. With some oncogene products, it appears that the formation of an abnormal protein may be a critical factor in the carcinogenic process. In other situations, mutations can turn oncogenes on or off at the wrong time in the cell. The potential for neoplastic behavior appears to exist in all cells and needs only to be activated either directly by a mutation of the cellular oncogene itself, or of a nearby regulatory gene.

Most oncogene protein products appear to function in some aspect of cellular signal transduction. Signal transduction pathways are used by the cells to receive and process information and ultimately effect a biologic response. Alterations in these signal pathways can have very profound effects on cellular growth, differentiation, and gene expression. Some examples of oncogenes and protein products are given in Table 8.4.

8.1.11   Tumor Suppressor Genes

Tumor suppressor genes and the proteins they encode function as negative regulators of cell growth. Their function is in direct contrast to the dominant transforming oncogenes, which act as positive regulators of cell growth. When tumor suppressor genes are lost by deletion or inactivated by point mutation, they are no longer capable of negatively regulating cellular growth. Generally, if one copy of the tumor suppressor gene is inactivated, the cell is normal, but if both copies are inactivated, loss of growth control can occur, playing a critical role in the carcinogenic process.

Whereas oncogenes are positive effectors of cell growth, tumor suppressor genes are negative effectors of cell growth. Oncogenes were originally discovered as transforming sequences contained in retroviruses, whereas tumor suppressor genes were discovered because they were responsible for hereditary predisposition to certain cancers. Oncogenes are generally activated by point mutation, transloca-tion, amplification, or inappropriate expression. Suppressor genes, however, require inactivation and are often associated with chromosome deletion and monosomy, but can also be inactivated by various types of mutations.

Perhaps one of the best known tumor suppressor genes and one that is most frequently mutated in human tumors is *p53*. The protein product of the *p53* gene is involved in the regulation of other genes. Through regulation of these genes, the *p53* protein regulates the progression of cells through the cell cycle late in the G1 phase. Mutated forms of this protein fail to function in regulating the cell cycle, thus cells containing the faulty *p53* gene are not blocked from proliferating and have a selective growth advantage over cells containing a normal *p53* gene.

8.2

MUTAGENESIS

8.2.1 Introduction

Mutations are hereditary changes produced in the genetic information stored in the DNA in all cells. Various physical and chemical agents known to produce such al-terations include ionizing radiation, sulfur and nitrogen mustards, epoxides, ethyl-eneimine, and methylsulfonate.

Such alterations in DNA are not necessarily harmful because mutations are the building blocks for evolutionary change and enable the species to adapt to a changing environment. The danger is that mutations are undirected, and the effects on the indi-vidual organism are usually negative. The harmful effects of mutations include fertil-ity disorders, embryonic and perinatal death, malformations, hereditary diseases, and cancers. Toxicologists working in this area strive to minimize human exposure to ex-ogenous mutagens in order to avoid adding to our existing "genetic load."

In general, the alterations in the genetic material can be divided into two cate-gories: (1) point mutations, which involve a change in a single base such as base–pair exchange or addition or deletion of a base; and (2) chromosomal aberra-tions such as gaps, breaks, translocations, and changes in the number of chromo-somes.

8.2.2 Base–Pair Transformations

The smallest unit of mutation, the transformation of a single base–pair, is called a point mutation. If the replacement involves the same type of base—for example, purine to purine, or pyrimidine to pyrimidine—the mutation is called a base–pair transition. If the change is a purine to pyrimidine replacement, it is termed a

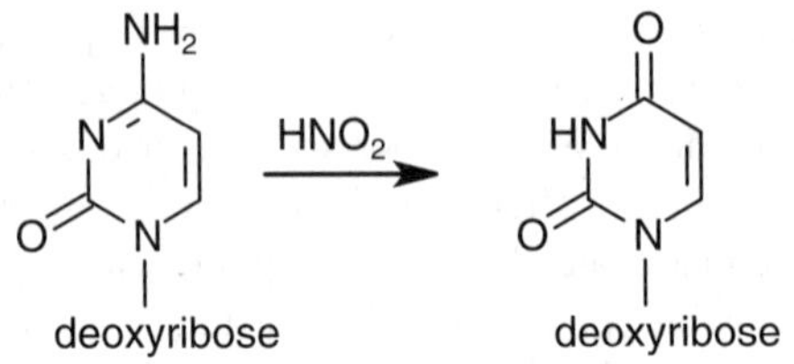

Figure 8.5. Deamination of cytidine to uridine by the action of nitrous acid.

base–pair transversion. These point mutations can be caused in at least three ways: by chemical modification, by incorporation of abnormal base analogs into DNA, and by alkylating agents.

CHEMICAL TRANSFORMATION. An example of chemical transformation of bases is that caused by nitrous acid, HNO_2. This chemical is able to change cytosine to uracil or adenine to hypoxanthine and is known to be mutagenic in phage, bacteria, and fungi. The mechanism for this reaction is shown in Fig. 8.5.

INCORPORATION OF ABNORMAL BASE ANALOGS. Most of the chemicals active in this respect are those developed as drugs for cancer therapy and which owe their effectiveness to their ability to produce lethal mutations in rapidly dividing cancer cells. Some examples of base analogs are 5-bromouracil, 5-fluorodeoxyuridine, 2-aminopurine, and 6-mercaptopurine. The effect of incorporation of abnormal bases and the resulting base transformations is illustrated with 5-bromouracil (Fig. 8.6).

ALKYLATING AGENTS. Alkylating agents are chemicals that can add alkyl groups to DNA. These chemicals yield positively charged carbonium ions (eg, CH_3^+) that combine with the electron-rich bases in the DNA, a classic example of an electrophilic–nucleophilic interaction. Some examples of alkylating agents are shown in Fig. 8.7 A well-known alkylating reaction is that of dimethylnitrosamine, which is illustrated in Fig. 8.8. Alkylation of DNA results both in mispairing of bases and in chromosome breaks.

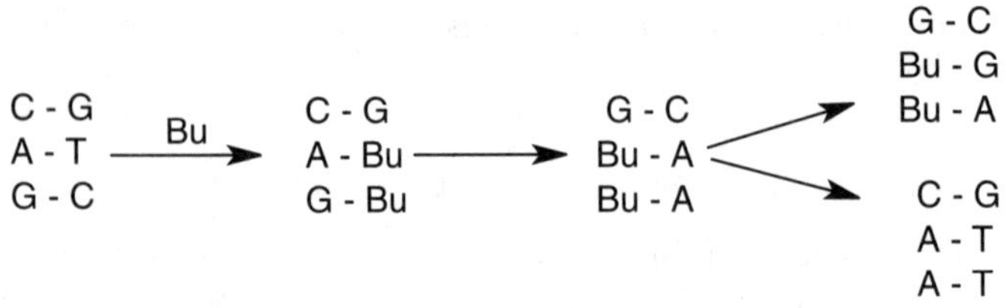

Figure 8.6. Replication of a nucleic acid in the presence of the base analog bromouracil (Bu). This analog will pair with both adenine and guanine. In this case, the result is a transition of G-C to A-T.

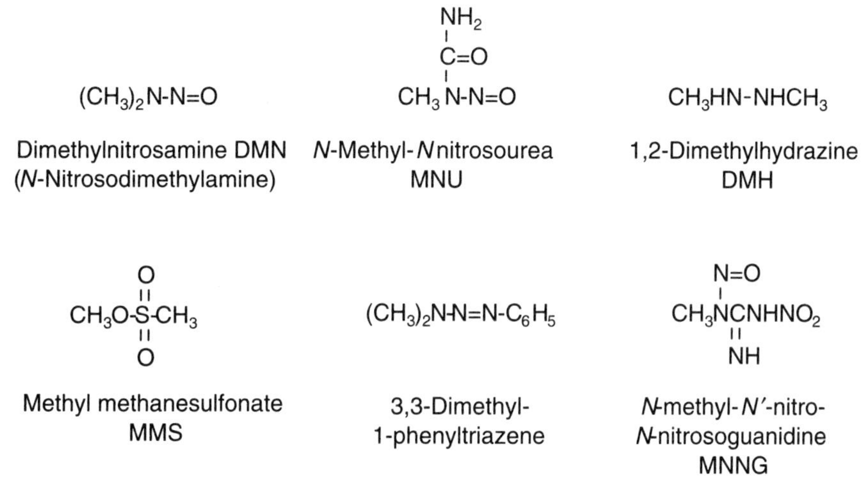

$(CH_3)_2N\text{-}N=O$

Dimethylnitrosamine DMN
(*N*-Nitrosodimethylamine)

$\begin{array}{c} NH_2 \\ | \\ C=O \\ | \\ CH_3\,N\text{-}N=O \end{array}$

N-Methyl-*N*nitrosourea
MNU

$CH_3HN\text{-}NHCH_3$

1,2-Dimethylhydrazine
DMH

$\begin{array}{c} O \\ \| \\ CH_3O\text{-}S\text{-}CH_3 \\ \| \\ O \end{array}$

Methyl methanesulfonate
MMS

$(CH_3)_2N\text{-}N=N\text{-}C_6H_5$

3,3-Dimethyl-
1-phenyltriazene

$\begin{array}{c} N=O \\ | \\ CH_3NCNHNO_2 \\ \| \\ NH \end{array}$

N-methyl-*N*'-nitro-
N-nitrosoguanidine
MNNG

Figure 8.7. Structures of some alkylating carcinogens.

A number of positions in the purine and pyrimidine bases are available for alkylation. For example, adenine can be alkylated at three ring nitrogens: N-1, N-3, or N-7; guanine can undergo alkylation at either N-3, N-7, or O-6; cytosine can be alkylated at N-3 and O-2; and thymine can be alkylated at N-3, O-2, and O-4 (Fig. 8.9). In addition to alkylation of the purine and pyrimidine bases, the phosphates in the DNA may also undergo alkylation.

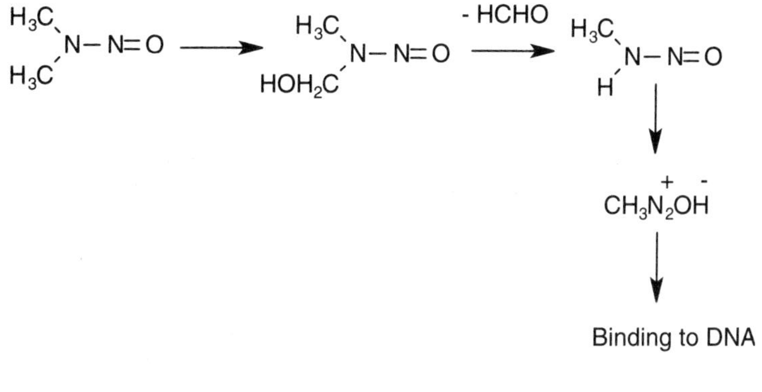

$$\begin{array}{c} H_3C \\ \diagdown \\ N\text{-}N=O \\ \diagup \\ H_3C \end{array} \longrightarrow \begin{array}{c} H_3C \\ \diagdown \\ N\text{-}N=O \\ \diagup \\ HOH_2C \end{array} \xrightarrow{-\,HCHO} \begin{array}{c} H_3C \\ \diagdown \\ N\text{-}N=O \\ \diagup \\ H \end{array}$$

$$\downarrow$$

$$CH_3\overset{+}{N_2}\overset{-}{OH}$$

$$\downarrow$$

Binding to DNA

Figure 8.8. Generation of a methylating agent from dimethylnitrosoamine (DMN). The first step requires metabolic activation to form a highly reactive intermediate that combines nonenezymatically with DNA.

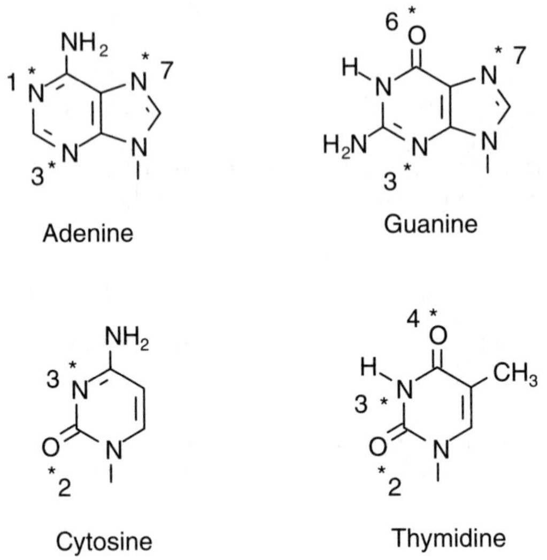

Figure 8.9. Sites of alkylation of DNA under physiological conditions are indicated with an asterisk (*).

8.2.3 Frameshift Mutations

Addition or deletion of a base in the DNA molecule puts the triplet code out of register and results in what is known as a frameshift mutation (Fig. 8.10). If the addition of another base follows in close proximity to a deletion, the production of functional or partially functional proteins may occur. Some chemicals, such as acridine, are known to induce frameshifts. In addition, errors occurring during chromatid crossover may lead to frameshift mutations.

8.2.4 DNA Repair

Fortunately, as stated earlier, cells possess the ability to correct or repair many of the mutations that have occurred to the original DNA molecule. Consequently, fewer mutations are retained in the replicated DNA molecules than occur originally. If the mutation is not recognized and repaired, the incorrect information may be

ACA* AAG AGU CCA UCA

↓

ACA AGA GUC CAU CA

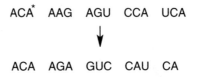

Figure 8.10. Deletion of the base adenine (A*) shifts the reading frame of the triplet code so that different amino acids are coded for in the protein.

transcribed into RNA, and the mutation is then expressed as an altered protein. The change may be critical or insignificant, depending on the position of the amino acid or the amount and function of the protein affected. It is also possible that the mutations may lead to an improvement in the gene product.

The action of several enzymes involved in DNA repair have been characterized. The enzyme that repairs O-6-methylguanine is a methyltransferase that removes the methyl group and restores the DNA structure in a single step. Other enzymes that repair DNA are glycosylases, which split the bond between the N-9 position of the purine and the deoxyribose forming an apurinic site in the DNA. These sites and sites generated by spontaneous hydrolysis of methylated bases are then restored by the action of an endonuclease that breaks the DNA chain, excising 3 to 4 nucleotides, including the damaged site. Subsequently, the gap is filled by nucleotide polymerization by DNA polymerase, followed by closing of the strand by DNA ligase.

8.2.5   Chromosome Aberrations

The term clastogenesis is used to refer to the process resulting in additions, deletions, or rearrangements of parts of the chromosomes that are detectable by light microscopy. Gaps, which are achromatic lesions in a chromosome, may vary in length and are thought to be due to loss of DNA. Breaks are broken ends of chromatids that are dislocated but still contained within the metaphase. Several genetic diseases, such as Bloom's syndrome and Falconi's anemia, are correlated with chromosomal breaks, but it is uncertain whether the breaks are a cause or a symptom of the disease. Many chemicals, as well as ionizing radiation, can cause breakage of chromosomes. Alkylating agents, especially bifunctional chemicals, may cause breaks by cross-linking with DNA.

Chromosomal mutations refer to changes in chromosomes that arise from incorrect reincorporation of broken parts. The main types of change are deletions, translocations, duplications, and inversions. Deletions and translocations are relatively easy to detect by microscopy, and assume more importance in practical mutagenicity testing.

Numeric aberrations are a consequence of unequal division of chromosomes and result in a cell with either more or fewer chromosomes than normal. Such cells may or may not be viable. Several genetic diseases are a result of the unequal division (nondisjunction) of chromosomes. Down syndrome (mongolism) is associated with a trisomy of chromosome 21, and the condition is characterized by a small flattened skull; short, flat-bridged nose; short phalanges; and moderate to severe mental retardation. Two disorders related to nondisjunction of the sex chromosomes are Klinefelter's syndrome (XXY), characterized by small testes with fibrosis and hyalinization of the seminiferous tubules and impairment of function, and Turner's syndrome (XO), characterized by short stature, undifferentiated gonads, and variable abnormalities, including low posterior hairline and cardiac defects.

Several chemicals are known to induce polyploidy. The best known examples are the metaphase poisons, such as colchicine, a specific spindle poison that binds to the spindle protein tubulin and inhibits its polymerization. Thus, colchicine stops mitosis at metaphase, leaving the cell with the doubled quantity of chromosomal material, resulting in a polyploid cell. Other compounds that can cause similar effects are the vinca alkaloids, vincristine and vinblastine, and podophyllotoxin, which binds to the same site as colchicine. Polyploidy is well known in plants and is used extensively in plant breeding; however, polyploidy in animals is not as viable and is generally a lethal mutation.

8.2.6 Mutagenesis and Carcinogenesis

A large body of work on chemical carcinogenesis has now demonstrated that the carcinogenic potency of a compound can often be correlated with its mutagenic ability, suggesting that DNA is the ultimate target of the stage of carcinogenesis known as initiation (Section 8.1.2). In recent years, many chemicals known to be carcinogenic have been found to be mutagenic as well; likewise, many known mutagens have been found to be carcinogenic. Because of the high correlation of mutagenicity of chemicals to carcinogenic potential, the testing of chemicals as mutagens has now become an important screening tool in assessing potential carcinogenic risk of compounds. Short-term tests for genotoxic compounds are discussed in detail in Chapter 11. It must be remembered, however, that many chemicals involved in the development of chemical carcinogenesis, such as promoters, are not usually mutagenic, and therefore other types of tests are needed to assess their toxic potential.

8.3

TERATOGENESIS

8.3.1 Introduction

The word teratogenesis literally means the production of a monstrous or misshapen organism and comes from the Greek *teras* or *teratos,* meaning monster or marvel. At different times in the past and in various cultures, the appearance of unusual or deformed infants was attributed to causes such as hybridization between humans and gods or humans and demons. Among the Ancient Greeks and Romans, there was a tendency to consider monstrous infants divine, and some mythologic figures appear to have been derived from terata. At other times, such as in Europe during the fifteenth and sixteenth centuries, malformations were believed to be the result of association with demons, witches, or other evil creatures, and both the infant and mother were put to death.

Modern experimental teratology gained impetus in the 1940s with the work of Warknay and his colleagues, who demonstrated that environmental factors such as maternal dietary deficiencies and irradiation could affect the intrauterine growth and development of mammals. Earlier studies with fish, amphibians, and chicken embryos had shown them to be very susceptible to adverse conditions, but it was not generally believed that mammals were as vulnerable. Rather, it was widely believed that the mother and ultimately the placenta provided an effective barrier to environmental factors, and that most aspects of abnormal as well as normal development were genetically determined.

In the 1920s, accounts were published of pregnant women who had been exposed to ionizing radiation and who later gave birth to children with CNS and skeletal defects, and in 1941, Gregg reported the association of maternal rubella (German measles) infection while pregnant with death, blindness, and deafness among their offspring. Neither of these reports nor the experiments of Warkany, however, aroused much concern that other extrinsic agents might pose a risk to the developing human fetus. Then, in the late 1950s and early 1960s, the concept of the placental barrier was shattered when thousands of severely malformed infants were born to women who had been taking the presumably harmless sedative thalidomide during their pregnancy. This incident vividly called attention to the fact that human and other mammalian embryos can be highly vulnerable to certain environmental agents, even though these have either negligible or no maternal effects.

For a chemical to be a teratogen, it must increase significantly the occurrence of abnormalities, either structural or functional, in the offspring after being administered to either parent before conception, to the female during pregnancy, or directly to the developing fetus. Many teratologists hold to the idea that any xenobiotic given at a high-enough dose and at the right time can cause some adverse effects in the developing embryo. Therefore, for an agent to be classified as a teratogen, it must produce an adverse effect at an exposure level that does not induce severe toxicity in the mother. Agents that result in the death of the embryo (embryolethality) are referred to as embryotoxic agents rather than teratogens.

8.3.2   General Principles of Teratology

As the science of teratology has expanded, some important generalizations have emerged, been accepted, and modified. Six major generalizations have come to be regarded as fundamental principles of teratology.

GENETIC INFLUENCE. Susceptibility to teratogens depends on the genotype of the organism, including species and strain differences, as well as individual variability. This variation in response may be due in part to differences in maternal metabolism, distribution, or transplacental passage of the compound that results in differential exposure to the ultimate teratogenic agent. For example, rabbits and mice are very susceptible to the induction of cleft palate by cortisone, whereas rats are not. Thalidomide is another teratogen that is very species specific; humans, certain higher primates (macaque monkeys, baboons, and marmosets) and certain white rabbit strains are extremely sensitive to the effects of thalidomide, whereas most other mammals are quite resistant, with only some strains of rats and mice reacting to large doses that must be administered at a very specific time.

CRITICAL PERIODS. The complex process of embryogenesis involves cell proliferation, differentiation, migration, and finally organogenesis, all of which must occur in a precisely timed sequence. The first 2 weeks in human embryonic development is a time of rapid cell proliferation. After fertilization, the cells divide rapidly, forming the blastocyst, with very little morphologic differentiation occurring at this time, except that some cells are on the surface and some are internal. Exposure during this time usually results either in embryolethality, as a result of substantial damage to the undifferentiated embryonic cells, or in survival with no effect.

The time of greatest susceptibility to teratogens, as far as the induction of gross anatomic defects, occurs during the period of germ-layer formation and organogenesis (Fig. 8.11). Although the time span of organ development varies among species (Table 8.5), in all species, organogenesis is the period between germ-layer differentiation and completion of major organ formation. The type of teratogenic response

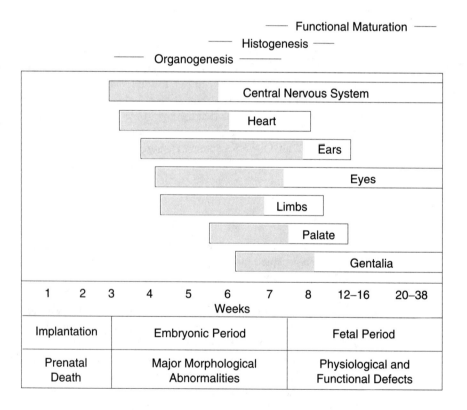

Figure 8.11. Diagram illustrating sequence of events in human development showing sensitive periods for developmental defects. Shaded areas are more sensitive.

TABLE 8.5. COMPARISON OF GESTATION IN SEVERAL SPECIES

Species	Number of Days After Conception		
	Implantation	Embryonic Period[a]	Fetal Period
Human	6–7	20–56	56–280
Rabbit	6–8	8–16	17–34
Rat	6–8	9–17	18–22
Mouse	5–7	7–16	17–20

[a]Period of organogenesis and greatest teratogenic risk.

is determined by the specific developmental stage of the fetus at the time of exposure; that is, there are "critical periods" for the development of the different organ systems. Thus, for a compound to produce a teratogenic effect within a particular organ system, the fetus must be exposed to the compound while the particular organ is being formed. This developmental time is termed the critical period. Because the early events in organ formation are the most sensitive, during testing the teratogen is administered during or just prior to the development of that organ.

Histogenesis and functional development generally begin before organogenesis is completed and continue into the subsequent growth phases. Adverse influences at this time usually do not result in gross malformations but can result in functional abnormalities. This type of physiologic or biochemical defect may be manifested by growth retardation, postnatally persistent functional defects, or the defect may result in fetal death due to interference with some critical biologic function.

INITIATING MECHANISMS. Many different types of compounds frequently cause similar abnormalities if they are administered during the same critical period. This observation has led to the proposal that many teratogenic agents are able to initiate abnormal developments by a number of mechanisms that lead to some common pathogenic responses (Fig. 8.12). The teratogenic agent initiates one or more of these mechanisms, resulting in abnormal embryogenesis. This in turn leads to pathways that seem to be characterized by too few cells or cell products for normal morphogenesis or functional development. This cell death or tissue necrosis is one of the most frequent signs of chemical or physical damage to the developing embryo. Although cell death above normal physiological levels does not inevitably lead to malformation, if a critical mass of cells is destroyed, there may be too few cells or cell products to effect localized morphogenesis or functional developments.

ABNORMAL DEVELOPMENT. There are four manifestations of abnormal development: death, malformation, growth retardation, and functional disorder. Prior to differentiation, the embryo is not usually damaged by most agents; however, a sufficiently high dosage frequently results in the death of the embryo. Xenobiotics that are embryotoxic are not usually called teratogens, but if administered at a lower dose or at a different time period, they may be teratogenic. The time of organogenesis is the most sensitive time for induction of specific malformations, whereas structural de-

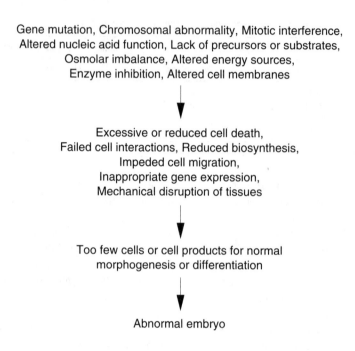

Gene mutation, Chromosomal abnormality, Mitotic interference,
Altered nucleic acid function, Lack of precursors or substrates,
Osmolar imbalance, Altered energy sources,
Enzyme inhibition, Altered cell membranes

Excessive or reduced cell death,
Failed cell interactions, Reduced biosynthesis,
Impeded cell migration,
Inappropriate gene expression,
Mechanical disruption of tissues

Too few cells or cell products for normal
morphogenesis or differentiation

Abnormal embryo

Figure 8.12. Possible sequence of events in the formation of developmental defects.

fects at the tissue level or functional deficits are most likely to occur when damage occurs during the fetal period. Structural defects are usually considered the main criterion in estimating teratologic risks because they are more obvious; however, functional disorders may be as incapacitating and result in as great a mortality rate among offspring as morphologic abnormalities.

ACCESS TO EMBRYO AND FETUS. Only a few agents, such as radiation or ultrasound, can pass directly through the maternal tissue. For chemical compounds and their metabolites, the route of access is by way of the maternal body through fluids surrounding the embryo or by way of the blood after formation of the placenta. Prior to the thalidomide disaster, it was commonly believed that the placental barrier protected the fetus from drugs given to the mother. It is now known, however, that many pharmacologic substances and other chemicals can readily pass from the maternal blood to the fetal blood. Generally, most unbound compounds with a molecular weight of less than 600 and a low ionic charge will readily pass through the placenta by simple diffusion. The most rapid passage occurs with chemicals that are lipophilic and nonionized at physiological pH (see Chapter 2). The chemical half-life of a compound determines whether it can travel from its site of metabolism, usually the maternal liver, to the embryonic tissue; very reactive intermediates will be unstable and react at the site of formation. Other compounds, however, may pass through the maternal blood and be activated by fetoplacental tissue.

DOSE–RESPONSE RELATIONSHIPS. Most teratogens appear to have a threshold or "no-effect" level below which no malformations are observable. Abnormal development frequently seems to depend on the destruction of a critical number of cells above the level that the embryo can restore quickly; destruction of less than this critical mass by a low or moderate dose of teratogen produces no persistent effect, whereas destruction of an excessive number results in fetal death.

8.3.3 Initiating Mechanisms

Because the initiating events of abnormal development usually occur at the subcellular or molecular level, the damage is not readily detected until cell death, morphologic damage, or functional disability is observed. As summarized in Fig. 8.12, probably some eight to ten mechanisms are primarily responsible for the initial molecular damage.

MUTATIONS. It has been estimated that some 20% to 30% of human developmental errors are due to mutations in the germ cells; such changes are hereditary. If the mutations occur in somatic cells, the alteration will be transmitted to all descendants of that cell, but it will not become an inherited change. Somatic mutations in the early embryo may affect enough cells to produce a structural or functional defect, however. Mutagens include such agents as ionizing radiation, chemicals such as nitrous acid, alkylating agents, most carcinogens, and agents that interfere with normal DNA repair mechanisms (see Section 8.2).

CHROMOSOMAL ABNORMALITIES, such as an excess of chromosomes, deficiencies, and rearrangements, may result from nondisjunction or breaks in the chromosomes. These abnormalities probably account for less than 3% of human developmental errors, probably because an excess or deficiency of chromosomal material is usually lethal, the exception being an excess or deficiency of sex chromosomes. Advanced maternal age is known to be a factor in nondisjunction of germ cells, as is aging of germ cells in the genital tract prior to fertilization. Other causes of chromosomal abnormalities include viral infection, irradiation, and chemical agents.

MITOTIC INTERFERENCE. Certain "cytotoxic" chemicals, such as hydroxyurea or irradiation, are known to slow or arrest DNA synthesis, thereby inhibiting mitosis. Other chemicals, such as colchicine and vincristine, interfere with spindle formation and prevent the chromosomes from separating at anaphase. The resulting tetraploid cells usually lead to fetotoxicity. Still other agents such as irradiation or radiomimetic chemicals lead to "stickiness" or "bridges" between chromatids, which prevents proper separation of chromosomes.

INTERFERENCE WITH NUCLEIC ACID FUNCTION. Many antibiotics and antineoplastic drugs are teratogenic by interfering with nucleic acid replication, transcription, or RNA translation. They include cytotoxic chemicals such as cytosine arabinoside, which inhibits DNA polymerase, 5-aza-2'-deoxycytidine, which affects DNA methylation, and 6-mercaptopurine, which blocks incorporation of adenine and guanine into

DNA. Agents that block protein synthesis are generally embryolethal above the no-effect dose; that is, at lower doses some growth retardation occurs, but at higher doses significant blockage of protein synthesis leads to the death of the embryo rather than malformation.

NUTRITIONAL DEFICIENCIES. The lack of precursors or substrates is a well-established mechanism of teratogenesis. Specific dietary deficiencies, especially of vitamins and minerals, are known to be growth inhibiting, teratogenic, and embryolethal. Embryos frequently show teratogenic symptoms before the mother shows signs of deficiencies, contrary to the widespread belief that the embryo will receive nutrients at the mother's expense. A disease in lambs known as "swayback," is primarily due to copper deficiency in pregnant sheep. The disease is characterized by paralysis of the hind limbs, lack of coordination, and in some cases, blindness. The disease can be prevented by giving copper supplements to pregnant ewes.

Endemic cretinism, characterized by mental and physical retardation, pot belly, large tongue, and facial characteristics similar to those of Down syndrome, occurs in areas where the iodine content of the soil is extremely low. The incidence of cretinism has almost been eliminated by addition of iodine to the diet in the form of iodized salt.

Deficiencies can also occur in the presence of analogs or antagonists to vitamins, amino acids, or nucleic acids, which may result in the utilization or the abnormal metabolites in biosynthesis. Other causes of deficiencies may include failure of materials to be absorbed from the maternal digestive system, as with excess zinc or sulfate preventing adequate copper absorption, or the failure of placental transport of essential metabolites as in the teratogenic action of azo dyes in rodents and rabbits, which are dependent for early placental transport of nutrients on the inverted yolk sac placenta.

DEFICIENT OR ALTERED ENERGY SUPPLY. The growth of the embryo requires high levels of energy, and factors that interfere with the energy supply are associated with teratogenesis. These are known to include inadequate glucose supply (dietary deficiency, induced hypoglycemia), interference with glycolysis (iodoacetate, 6-aminonicotinamide), inhibition of the citric acid cycle (riboflavin deficiency, 6-aminonicotinamide), and blockage of the terminal electron transport system (hypoxia, cyanide, dinitrophenol).

CHANGES IN OSMOLARITY. Abnormal fluid accumulations are known to cause tissue distortions sufficient to lead to malformations. For example, hypoxia in chicken embryos leads to edema, hematomas, and blisters, which subsequently give rise to abnormal embryogenesis in eye, brain, and limbs. Agents such as trypan blue, hypertonic solutions, and adrenal hormones are also known to give rise to this "edema syndrome" and the resulting malformations.

CHANGES IN CELL MEMBRANES. Altered membrane permeability can lead to osmolar imbalance and result in changes such as those previously described. It has been suggested that agents such as the solvent dimethylsulfoxide (DMSO) and excess vitamin A may act in this way.

ENZYME INHIBITION. Chemicals that inhibit enzymes, especially those involved in intermediary metabolism, are able to alter fetal growth and development. Other agents are known to be mutagenic and teratogenic agents by inhibiting DNA repair enzymes or by inhibiting polymerases necessary for formation of the mitotic spindle. Some enzyme inhibitors thought to be involved in teratogenesis are: 5-fluorouracil, an inhibitor of thymidylate synthetase; hydroxyurea, an inhibitor of ribonucleoside diphosphate reductase; 5-aza-2′-deoxycytidine, an inhibitor of methyltransferase; and cytosine arabinoside, an inhibitor of DNA polymerase.

8.3.4   Bioactivation of Teratogens

The toxic effects of exogenous compounds often result not from the parent compound per se but from the reactive metabolites formed inside the cell (Chapter 4). The major site of bioactivation of xenobiotics is generally assumed to be the maternal liver. Highly reactive metabolites, however, would be expected to react primarily within the liver or nearby tissue and not survive transport within the circulatory system and passage across the placenta to reach the embryo. Thus, only the more stable and less reactive metabolites would reach embryonic cells. For this reason, it is important to consider the ability of the conceptus to metabolize xenobiotics in situ to potentially toxic compounds.

To date, most activity has focused on P450–catalyzed reactions. The use of in vitro embryonic systems (primarily mouse, rat, and rabbit) has been particularly beneficial for studying activation of teratogens. Activation of several teratogens, including benzo(a)pyrene, diethylstilbestrol (DES), and 2-acetylaminofluorene has been demonstrated using these systems. Thus, it appears likely that although P450 activity may be very low in embryonic tissue as compared to the liver, sufficient quantities of highly reactive intermediates can be generated at the site of action to produce teratogenic effects.

Moreover, conceptual tissue is known to respond to the effects of polycyclic aromatic hydrocarbon (PAH) inducing agents such as 3-methylcholanthrene. Studies of human placentas have established that enzyme activities associated with P450 1A1 are markedly increased in mothers who smoke. Mouse blastocysts exposed to PAH-inducing agents, but not uninduced blastocysts, can activate benzo(a)pyrene. Clearly, more research needs to be done on identifying the P450 isoforms present in conceptual tissue as well as defining P450 regulation during development and by exogenous chemicals.

Other enzymes that are relatively high in embryonic tissue and possess the potential to activate teratogens are the peroxidases, such as those associated with prostaglandin synthetase. It has been suggested that the teratogenic drug phenytoin and similar compounds are activated by a mechanism involving cooxidation by prostaglandin synthetase.

8.3.5   Examples of Human Teratogens

In terms of human developmental abnormality, about 3% to 7% of human babies are born with malformations serious enough to require treatment. Etiologically, these can be divided into several categories: genetic causes (mutant gene), chromosomal abnormalities, environmental agents, multifactorial causes, and unknown (Table 8.6)

FOLIC ACID ANTAGONISTS (aminopterin), known to be embryolethal in laboratory animals, were developed as agents to be used for therapeutic abortions. In the trial tests, however, not all of the fetuses were aborted, and most of those that survived (about 30%) were malformed, being born with hydrocephalus, absent or ossified skull bones, palate defects, and anomalies of the extremities.

ANDROGENIC HORMONES. Progesterone and synthetic progesterones, which were used to treat breast cancers, to prevent spontaneous abortions, and to control bleeding during pregnancy, led to the birth of a number of masculinized female fetuses. This masculinization was due to the androgenic activity of many of the synthetic progestins.

THALIDOMIDE, one of the most potent human teratogens known, was introduced as a sedative–tranquilizer in the former West Germany, England, several other European countries, and Australia in the early 1960s. The drug was effective in producing a teratogenic effect even if taken on only a single day any time from the third to the seventh week of pregnancy. The most pronounced defect was phocomelia—shortening or complete absence of limbs. Altogether, more than 10,000 cases were seen before the drug was withdrawn. The drug was never approved for use in the United States. Thalidomide is very species specific: humans show teratogenic effect at

TABLE 8.6. SOME CAUSES OF HUMAN DEVELOPMENTAL DEFECTS

Known genetic transmission	Drugs and chemicals
Chromosomal aberration	Ethanol
Ionizing radiation	Androgenic hormones
Therapeutic	Phenytoin
Nuclear	Trimethadione
Radioiodine	Cyclophosphamide
Infections	Diethylstilbestrol (DES)
Rubella virus	Thalidomide
Cytomegalovirus (CMV)	Valproic acid
Herpes simplex virus (HSV)	Retinoic acids
Toxoplasmosis	Methotrexate
Syphilis	Cocaine
Maternal metabolic imbalances	Organic mercury
Cretinism	Coumarin anticoagulants
Diabetes	Tetracyclines
Phenylketonuria (PKU)	Folic acid antagonists
Hyperthermia	(Aminopterin)

doses as low as 0.5 to 1.0 mg/kg, whereas there is no or very little effect in most mouse or rat strains at doses as high as 4000 mg/kg. The only animals showing similar responses to humans are certain strains of rabbits and some species of monkeys, baboons, and marmosets.

ALCOHOL. Suspicion that alcohol possessed teratogenic potential stretches back many centuries. During the eighteenth century, England was the scene of what was called the "gin epidemic" as a result of very cheap, readily available gin. In 1736, the following report was submitted to Parliament:

> The contagion has spread even to the female sex. Unhappy mothers habituate themselves to these distilled liquors, whose children are born weak and sickly, and often look shrivel'd and old as though they had numbered many years.

Only recently, however, has the direct involvement of alcohol in abnormal fetal development been firmly established. Fetal alcohol syndrome (FAS) refers to a pattern of defects in children born to alcoholic women. For a diagnosis of FAS to be made, there are three criteria that must be met: (1) prenatal or postnatal growth retardation; (2) characteristic facial anomalies (microcephaly, small eye opening, thinned upper lip); and (3) central nervous system (CNS) dysfunction (mental retardation, developmental delays). If only one or two of these criteria are met, a diagnosis of possible FAS, or fetal alcohol effects (FAE), may be made if the mother is suspected of drinking during pregnancy. Prenatal alcohol exposure is suspected of causing a broad spectrum of effects, ranging from barely perceptible effects to FAS and spontaneous abortion.

One important unanswered question is why some alcoholic women give birth to children with FAS whereas other women who drink the same amount do not. Because it is not known for certain whether the human fetus is at risk from moderate social drinking, the recommendation is that alcohol consumption be reduced to the greatest extent possible during pregnancy.

The overall incidence of FAS among the general population is relatively low; estimates range from 0.4 to 3.1 per 1000; however, if patients showing FAE are included, the incidence is much higher. More importantly, fetal alcohol exposure is a major cause of mental retardation in Western society.

Although there is little doubt that alcohol is a teratogen, the mechanism by which its effects are produced is not known. One of the most likely ways appears to be induced hypoxia to the embryo or fetus, although other mechanisms such as direct toxicity of alcohol or acetaldehyde may also be contributing factors.

METHYL MERCURY. This compound is one of the few environmental contaminants that has been established as an embryotoxic agent in humans. Between 1954 and 1960, at Minamata Bay and elsewhere in Japan, many infants were born with severe neurologic symptoms resembling cerebral palsy. Fetal Minamata disease was traced to the consumption of mercury-contaminated fish by the mothers.

INFECTIOUS DISEASES. In 1941, Gregg first recognized the association between maternal rubella infection (German measles) and infant cataracts. Additional malformations caused by the virus are now known to include eye abnormalities, deafness, cardiac defects, and mental retardation. An epidemic of rubella in 1971 resulted in the birth of more than 20,000 defective children. Other viruses, such as cytomegalovirus (CMV) and herpes simplex, are also known to cause CNS defects. Syphilis during pregnancy is also known to lead to malformations, including hydrocephalus, seizure, and mental retardation due to direct invasion and destruction of fetal tissue by the spirochete, causing syphilis palladiura.

DIETHYLSTIBESTROL (DES). The induction of cancer in the offspring resulting from the exposure of the pregnant female to the teratogenic agent is known as transplacental carcinogenesis. The best known example is the appearance of vaginal cancer in females born to mothers given the drug DES during pregnancy to prevent spontaneous abortion. The carcinogenicity of DES was first recognized because of the occurrence of an unusual type of vaginal adenocarcinoma in young women between 15 and 22 years of age instead of the expected postmenopausal age. The stilbestrols were in widespread use between 1950 and 1970; by 1976, more than 400 cases of DES-related carcinoma of the vagina and cervix had been recorded. Male offspring who were exposed in utero to DES were also affected. Findings included epididymal cysts, hypotropic testes, and poor semen quality. Malignant lesions, however, were not observed in males.

SYNTHETIC RETINOIDS. Isotretinoin (Accutane) is a synthetic retinoid that is highly effective in treating recalcitrant cystic acne. In spite of clear warnings against use during pregnancy, isotretinoin associated defects have been reported each year since its introduction. Isotretinoin is known to be teratogenic in all known laboratory species, as is an excess of retinoic acid (Vitamin A). The important issue is how to make this therapeutically effective drug available to those who can benefit from it while ensuring that exposure during early pregnancy does not occur. As is the case with all human teratogens, a critical question in terms of teratogenic risk is whether pregnancy can be recognized soon enough to avoid exposure to potentially damaging agents. Because organogenesis begins about day 20, many women may not be aware that they are pregnant, especially teenage women with irregular menstrual cycles.

ENVIRONMENTAL CHEMICALS. Recent interest has developed over environmental chemicals that disrupt the endocrine system, behaving like the sex hormones, or disrupting their action. Behavioral and physiological disorders have been observed in wildlife and there is concern that these chemicals may cause similar developmental defects in humans. Chemicals that have the potential to disrupt endocrine function are widespread in the environment and fall into at least three broad classes:

1. Chlorinated hydrocarbons, which include DDT and its breakdown product DDE; hexachlorobenzene; kepone; lindane; triazine herbicides, such as atrazine; certain polychlorinated biphenyls (PCBs) and 2,3,7,8,-tetrachlorodibenzo-p-dioxin (TCDD).

2. Cadmium, lead, and mercury.
3. Naturally occurring chemicals such as phytoestrogens (present in soy products) and mycotoxins.

8.3.6   Future Considerations

The study of teratology has evolved from an area concerned primarily with experimentations and descriptions of malformations to a science concerned with understanding the mechanisms of normal as well as abnormal development. In addition, demands are being placed on toxicologists to predict the risk of xenobiotic exposure on the outcome of human pregnancy, especially in the aftermath of events such as the thalidomide and DES incidents. Generally, federal agencies have focused on acute toxic effects and gross birth defects when assessing human health risks rather than more subtle developmental effects. Research is now increasingly directed toward gaining a better understanding of how xenobiotics are absorbed, distributed, accumulated, and biotransformed by pregnant mammals and their conceptus. Ultimately, however, we will also need a better understanding of the basic processes of development.

Suggested Further Reading

Carcinogenesis

Butterworth BE, Slaga TJ (eds.): *Nongenotoxic Mechanisms in Carcinogenesis,* 25th Banbury Report, Cold Spring Harbor, NY: Cold Spring Harbor Laboratory, 1987.

Floyd RA: Role of oxygen free radicals in carcinogenesis and brain ischemia. *FASEB J* **4:**2587–2597, 1990.

Friedberg EC: DNA repair: looking back and peering forward. *Bioessays* **16:**645–649, 1994.

Green S: Nuclear receptors and chemical carcinogenesis. *Trends Pharm Sci* **13:**251–255, 1992.

Hartwell LH, Kastan MB: Cell cycle control and cancer. *Science* **266:**1821–1827, 1994.

Marshall CJ: Tumor suppressor genes. *Cell* **64:**313–326, 1991.

National Research Council. *Carcinogens and Anticarcinogens in the Human Diet.* Washington, DC: National Academy Press, 1996.

Pitot HC, Dragan YP: Chemical carcinogenesis. In *Casarett & Doull's Toxicology, the Basic Science of Poisons*, Klaassen CD (ed.). New York: McGraw-Hill, 1996, pp 201–267.

Pitot HC, Dragan YP: Facts and theories concerning the mechanisms of carcinogenesis. *FASEB J* **5:**2280–2286, 1991.

Pitot HC: Endogenous carcinogenesis: the role of tumor promotion. *Proc Soc Exp Biol Med* **198:**661–666, 1991.

Pitot HC: The molecular biology of carcinogenesis. *Cancer* **72**(suppl):962–970, 1993.

Ragsdale NH, Menzer RE (eds.). *Carcinogenicity and Pesticides: Principles, Issues, and Relationships.* Washington, DC: American Chemical Society, 1989.

Savitz DA, Chen J: Parental occupation and childhood cancer: review of epidemiologic studies. *Environ Health Perspec* **88:**325–337, 1990.

Smart RC: Carcinogenesis. In *Introduction to Biochemical Toxicology,* 2nd edition. Hodgson E, Levi PE (eds.). Norwalk, CT: Appleton & Lange, 1994.

Tennant RW, Margolin BH, Shelby MD, et al: Prediction of chemical carcinogenicity in rodents from in vitro genetic toxicity assays. *Science* **236:**933–941, 1987.

Mutagenesis

Allen JW, Liang JC, Carrano AV, Preston RJ: Review of literature on chemical-induced aneuploidy in mammalian germ cells. *Mutat Res* **167:**123–137, 1986.

Cole J, Skopek TR: Somatic mutant frequency, mutation rates and mutational spectra in the human population in vivo. *Mutat Res* **304:**33–105, 1990.

Hoffmann GR: Genetic Toxicology. In *Casarett & Doull's Toxicology, the Basic Science of Poisons*, Klaassen CD (ed.). New York: McGraw-Hill, 1996, pp 269–300.

Li AP, Heflick RH (eds.): *Genetic Toxicology*. Boca Raton, FL: CRC Press, 1991.

National Research Council, Committee on the Biological Effects of Ionizing Radiations: *Health Effects of Exposure to Low Levels of Ionizing Radiation: BEIR V*. Washington, DC: National Academy Press, 1990.

Tennant RW, Margolin BH, Shelby MD, et al: Prediction of chemical carcinogenicity in rodents from in vitro genetic toxicity assays. *Science* **236:**933–941, 1987.

Teratogenesis

Barrow MV: A brief history of teratology to the early 20th century. *Teratology* **4:**119–130, 1971.

Brent RL, Beckman DA: Environmental teratogens. *Bull NY Acad Med* **66:**123–163, 1990.

Colin CF: Male mediated teratogenesis. *Repro Toxicol* **7:**3–9, 1993.

Farrar HC, Blumer JL: Fetal effects of maternal drug exposure. *Ann Rev Pharmacol Toxicol* **31:**525–547, 1991.

Fraser FC: Thalidomide retrospective: what did we learn? *Teratology* **38:** 201–202, 1988.

Juchau MR, Lee QP, Fantel AG: Xenobiotic biotransformation/bioactivation in organogenesis-stage conceptal tissues: Implications for embryotoxicity and teratogenesis. *Drug Metabol Rev* **24:**195–238, 1992.

Kimmel CA, Generoso WM, Thomas RD, Bakshi KS: Contemporary issues in toxicology: a new frontier in understanding the mechanisms of developmental abnormalities. *Toxicol Appl Pharmacol* **119:**159–165, 1993.

Kolbe VM (ed.): *Teratogens—Chemicals Which Cause Birth Defects*. Amsterdam: Elsevier, 1993.

Lenz W: A short history of thalidomide embryopathy. *Teratology* **38:**203–215, 1988.

Rogers JM, Kavlock RJ: Developmental Toxicology. In *Casarett & Doull's Toxicology, the Basic Science of Poisons*, Klaassen CD (ed.). New York: McGraw-Hill, 1996, pp 301–331.

Schardein JL: *Chemically Induced Birth Defects*, 2nd ed. New York: Marcel Dekker, 1993.

Tyl RW. Developmental toxicology. In *General and Applied Toxicology*. Ballantyne B, Marrs T, Turner P (eds.). London: Macmillan Press Ltd, 1995, pp 957–982.

TARGET ORGAN TOXICITY

PATRICIA E. LEVI

PATRICIA E. LEVI

9.1

HEPATOTOXICITY

9.1.1 Susceptibility of the Liver

The liver, the largest organ in the body, is often the target organ for chemically induced injuries. Several important factors are known to contribute to the liver's susceptibility. First, most xenobiotics enter the body through the gastrointestinal (GI) tract and, after absorption, are transported by the hepatic portal vein to the liver; thus, the liver is the first organ perfused by chemicals that are absorbed in the gut. A second factor is the high concentration in the liver of xenobiotic-metabolizing enzymes, primarily, the cytochrome P450–dependent monooxygenase system. Although most biotransformations are detoxication reactions, many oxidative reactions produce reactive metabolites (Chapter 4) that can induce lesions within the liver. Often areas of damage are in the centrilobular region, and this localization has been attributed, in part, to the higher concentration of cytochrome P450 in that area of the liver.

9.1.2 Liver Physiology

The basic structure of the liver consists of rows of hepatic cells (hepatocytes or parenchymal cells) perforated by specialized blood capillaries called sinusoids (see Chapter 5, Fig. 5.2). The sinusoid walls contain phagocytic cells called Kupffer cells whose role is to engulf and destroy materials such as solid particles, bacteria, dead blood cells, and so on. The main blood supply comes to the liver from the intestinal vasculature. These vessels, along with those from the spleen and the stomach, merge with each other to form the portal vein (see Chapter 5, Fig. 5.3). On entering the liver, the portal vein subdivides and drains into the sinusoids. The blood then perfuses the liver and exits by the hepatic veins that merge into the inferior vena cava and return blood to the heart. The hepatic artery supplies the liver with oxygenated arterial blood.

Other materials, such as bile acids and many xenobiotics, move from the hepatocytes into the bile-carrying canaliculi, which merge into larger ducts that follow the portal vein branches. The ducts merge into the hepatic duct from which bile drains into the upper part of the small intestine, the duodenum. The gall bladder serves to hold bile until it is emptied into the intestine.

In the liver three main functions occur: storage, metabolism, and biosynthesis. Glucose is converted to glycogen and stored; when needed for energy, it is converted back to glucose. Fat, fat-soluble vitamins, and other nutrients are also stored in the liver. Fatty acids are metabolized and converted to lipids, which are then conjugated with proteins synthesized in the liver and released into the bloodstream as lipoproteins. The liver also synthesizes numerous functional proteins, such as enzymes and blood-coagulating factors. In addition, the liver, which contains numerous xenobiotic-metabolizing enzymes, is the main site of xenobiotic metabolism.

9.1.3 Types of Liver Injury

The type of injuries to the liver depend on the type of toxic agent, the severity of intoxication, and the type of exposure, whether acute or chronic. The main types of liver damage are discussed briefly in this section. Whereas some types of damage—for example, cholestasis—are liver specific, others such as necrosis and carcinogenesis are more general phenomena.

FATTY LIVER refers to the abnormal accumulation of fat in hepatocytes. At the same time, there is a decrease in plasma lipids and lipoproteins. Although many toxicants may cause lipid accumulation in the liver (Table 9.1), the mechanisms may be different. Basically, lipid accumulation is related to disturbances in either the synthesis or the secretion of lipoproteins. Excess lipid can result from an oversupply of free fatty acids from adipose tissues or, more commonly, from impaired release of triglycerides from the liver into the plasma. Triglycerides are secreted from the liver as lipoproteins (very low density lipoprotein [VLDL]). As might be expected, there are a number of points at which this process can be disrupted. Some of the more important ones are as follows:

- Interference with synthesis of the protein moiety
- Impaired conjugation of triglyceride with lipoprotein
- Interference with transfer of VLDL across cell membranes
- Decreased synthesis of phospholipids
- Impaired oxidation of lipids by mitochondria
- Inadequate energy (adenosine triphosphate [ATP]) for lipid and protein synthesis

The role that fatty liver plays in liver injury is not clearly understood, and fatty liver in itself does not necessarily mean liver dysfunction. The onset of lipid accu-

TABLE 9.1. EXAMPLES OF HEPATOTOXIC AGENTS AND ASSOCIATED LIVER INJURY

Necrosis and Fatty Liver

Carbon tetrachloride	Dimethylnitrosamine	Phosphorous
Chloroform	Cyclohexamide	Beryllium
Trichloroethylene	Tetracycline	Allyl alcohol
Tetrachloroethylene	Acetaminophen	Galactosamine
Bromobenzene	Mitomycin	Azaserine
Thioacetamide	Puromycin	Aflatoxin
Ethionine	Tannic acid	Pyrrolizidine alkaloids

Cholestasis (drug-induced)

Chlorpromazine	Imipramine	Carbarsone
Promazine	Diazepam	Chlorthiazide
Thioridazine	Methandrolone	Methimazole
Mepazine	Mestranol	Sulfanilamide
Amitriptline	Estradiol	Phenindione

Hepatitis (drug-induced)

Iproniazid	Methoxyfluorane	Halothane
Isoniazid	Papaverine	Zoxazolamine
Imipramine	Phenyl butazone	Indomethacin
6-Mercaptopurine	Cholchicine	Methyldopa

Carcinogenesis (experimental animals)

Aflatoxin B$_1$	Dimethylbenzanthracene	Acetylaminofluorene
Pyrrolizidine alkaloids	Dialkyl nitrosamines	Urethane
Cycasin	Polychlorinated biphenyls	
Safrole	Vinyl chloride	

mulation in the liver is accompanied by changes in blood biochemistry, and for this reason blood chemistry analysis can be a useful diagnostic tool.

NECROSIS. Cell necrosis is a degenerative process leading to cell death. Necrosis, usually an acute injury, may be localized and affect only a few hepatocytes (focal necrosis) or it may involve an entire lobe (massive necrosis). Cell death occurs, along with rupture of the plasma membrane, and is preceded by a number of morphologic changes such as cytoplasmic edema, dilation of the endoplasmic reticulum, disaggregation of polysomes, accumulation of triglycerides, swelling of mitochondria with disruption of cristae, and dissolution of organelles and nucleus. Biochemical events that may lead to these changes include binding of reactive metabolites to proteins and unsaturated lipids (inducing lipid peroxidation and subsequent membrane destruction), disturbance of cellular Ca^{+2} homeostasis, interference with metabolic pathways, shifts in Na^+ and K^+ balance, and inhibition of protein synthesis. Changes in blood chemistry resemble those seen with fatty liver, except they are quantitatively larger. Because of the regenerating capability of the liver, necrotic lesions are not necessarily critical. Massive areas of necrosis, however, can lead to severe liver damage and failure.

APOPTOSIS is a controlled form of cell death that serves as a regulation point for biologic processes and can be thought of as the counterpoint of cell division by mitosis.

This selective mechanism is particularly active during development and senescence. Although apoptosis is a normal physiological process, it can also be induced by a number of exogenous factors, such as xenobiotic chemicals, oxidative stress, anoxia, and radiation. (A stimulus that induces a cell to undergo apoptosis is known as an *apogen*.) If, however, apoptosis is suppressed in some cell types, it can lead to accumulation of these cells. For example, in some instances, clonal expansion of malignant cells and subsequent tumor growth results primarily from inhibition of apoptosis.

Apoptosis can be distinguished from necrosis by morphologic criteria, using either light or electron microscopy. Toxicants, however, do not always act in a clear-cut fashion, and some toxicants can induce both apoptosis and necrosis either concurrently or sequentially.

CHOLESTASIS is the suppression or stoppage of bile flow, and may have either intrahepatic or extrahepatic causes. Inflammation or blockage of the bile ducts results in retention of bile salts as well as bilirubin accumulation, an event that leads to jaundice. Other mechanisms causing cholestasis include changes in membrane permeability of either hepatocytes or biliary canaliculi. Cholestasis is usually drug induced (Table 9.1) and is difficult to produce in experimental animals. Again, changes in blood chemistry can be a useful diagnostic tool.

CIRRHOSIS is a progressive disease that is characterized by the deposition of collagen throughout the liver. In most cases, cirrhosis results from chronic chemical injury. The accumulation of fibrous material causes severe restriction in blood flow and in the liver's normal metabolic and detoxication processes. This situation can, in turn, cause further damage and eventually lead to liver failure. In humans, chronic use of ethanol is the single most important cause of cirrhosis, although there is some dispute as to whether the effect is due to ethanol alone or is also related to the nutritional deficiencies that usually accompany alcoholism.

HEPATITIS. Hepatitis is an inflammation of the liver and is usually viral in origin; however, certain chemicals, usually drugs, can induce a hepatitis that closely resembles that produced by viral infections (Table 9.1). This type of liver injury is not usually demonstrable in laboratory animals and is often manifest only in susceptible individuals. Fortunately, the incidence of this type of disease is very low.

CARCINOGENESIS. The most common type of primary liver tumor is hepatocellular carcinoma; other types include cholangiocarcinoma, angiosarcoma, glandular carcinoma, and undifferentiated liver cell carcinoma. Although a wide variety of chemicals are known to induce liver cancer in laboratory animals (Table 9.1), the incidence of primary liver cancer in humans in the United States is very low. Some naturally occurring liver carcinogens are aflatoxin, cycasin, and safrole. A number of synthetic chemicals have been shown to cause liver cancer in animals, including the dialkylnitrosamines, dimethylbenzanthracene, aromatic amines such as 2-naphthylamine and acetylaminofluorene, and vinyl chloride. The structure and activation of these compounds can be found in Chapter 4. In humans, the most noted case of occupation-related liver cancer is the development of angiosarcoma, a rare malignancy of blood vessels, among workers exposed to high levels of vinyl chloride in manufacturing plants. For a discussion of chemical carcinogenesis, see Chapter 8, Section 8.1.

9.1.4 Biochemical Mechanisms

Chemically induced cell injury can be thought of as involving a series of events occurring in the affected animal and often in the target organ itself:

1. The chemical agent is activated to form the initiating toxic agent;
2. The initiating toxic agent is either detoxified or causes molecular changes in the cell;
3. The cell recovers or there are irreversible changes;
4. Irreversible changes may culminate in cell death.

Cell injury can be initiated by a number of mechanisms, such as inhibition of enzymes, depletion of cofactors or metabolites, depletion of energy (ATP) stores, interaction with receptors, and alteration of cell membranes. In recent years, attention has focused on the role of biotransformation of chemicals to highly reactive metabolites that initiate cellular toxicity. Many compounds, including clinically useful drugs, can cause cellular damage through metabolic activation of the chemical to highly reactive compounds, such as free radicals, carbenes, and nitrenes (Chapter 4).

These reactive metabolites can bind covalently to cellular macromolecules such as nucleic acids, proteins, cofactors, lipids, and polysaccharides, thereby changing their biologic properties. The liver is particularly vulnerable to toxicity produced by reactive metabolites because it is the major site of xenobiotic metabolism. Most activation reactions are catalyzed by the cytochrome P450 enzymes, and agents that induce these enzymes, such as phenobarbital and 3-methylcholanthrene, often increase toxicity. Conversely, inhibitors of cytochrome P450, such as SKF-525A and piperonyl butoxide, frequently decrease toxicity.

Mechanisms such as conjugation of the reactive chemical with glutathione are protective mechanisms that exist within the cell for the rapid removal and inactivation of many potentially toxic compounds. Because of these interactions, cellular toxicity is a function of the balance between the rate of formation of reactive metabolites and the rate of their removal. Examples of these interactions are presented in the following discussions of specific hepatotoxicants.

9.1.5 Examples of Hepatotoxicants

CARBON TETRACHLORIDE has probably been studied more extensively, both biochemically and pathologically, than any other hepatotoxicant. It is a classic example of a chemical activated by cytochrome P450 to form a highly reactive free radical (Fig. 9.1). First, CCl_4 is converted to the trichloromethyl radical ($CCl_3\bullet$) and then to the trichloromethylperoxy radical ($CCl_3O_2\bullet$). Such radicals are highly reactive and gen-

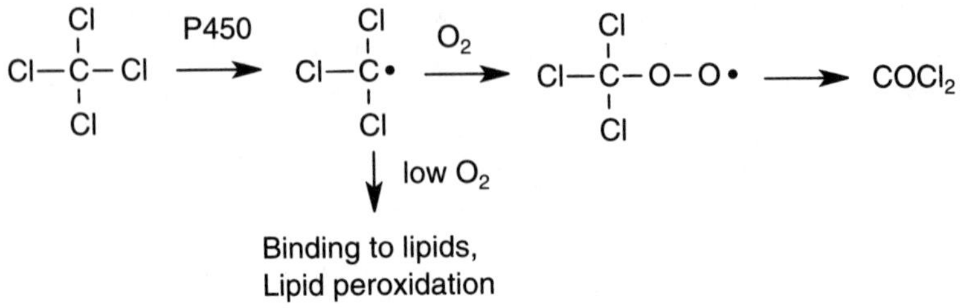

$$\underset{\substack{\text{Cl} \\ | \\ \text{Cl}}}{\text{Cl}-\overset{\text{Cl}}{\underset{|}{\text{C}}}-\text{Cl}} \xrightarrow{\text{P450}} \underset{\substack{\text{Cl} \\ | \\ \text{Cl}}}{\text{Cl}-\overset{\text{Cl}}{\underset{|}{\text{C}}\bullet}} \xrightarrow{\text{O}_2} \underset{\substack{\text{Cl} \\ | \\ \text{Cl}}}{\text{Cl}-\overset{\text{Cl}}{\underset{|}{\text{C}}}-\text{O}-\text{O}\bullet} \longrightarrow \text{COCl}_2$$

low O₂ → Binding to lipids, Lipid peroxidation

Figure 9.1. Metabolism of carbon tetrachloride and formation of reactive metabolites.

erally have a small radius of action. For this reason the necrosis induced by CCl_4 is most severe in the centrilobular liver cells that contain the highest concentration of the P450 isozyme responsible for CCl_4 activation.

Typically, free radicals may participate in a number of events (Fig. 9.2), such as covalent binding to lipids, proteins, or nucleotides as well as lipid peroxidation. It is now thought that $CCl_3\bullet$, which forms relatively stable adducts, is responsible for covalent binding to macromolecules, and the more reactive $CCl_3O_2\bullet$, which is formed when $CCl_3\bullet$ reacts with oxygen, is the prime initiator of lipid peroxidation.

Lipid peroxidation (Fig. 9.3) is the initiating reaction in a cascade of events, starting with the oxidation of unsaturated fatty acids to form lipid hydroperoxides, which then break down to yield a variety of end products, mainly aldehydes, which can go on to produce toxicity in distal tissues. For this reason, cellular damage results not only from the breakdown of membranes such as those of the endoplasmic reticulum, mitochondria, and lysosomes, but also from the production of reactive aldehydes that can travel to other tissues. It is now thought that many types of tissue injury, including inflammation, may involve lipid peroxidation.

BROMOBENZENE is a toxic industrial solvent that is known to produce centrilobular hepatic necrosis through the formation of reactive epoxides. Figure 9.4 summarizes the major pathways of bromobenzene metabolism. Both bromobenzene 2,3-epoxide and bromobenzene 3,4-epoxide are produced by P450 oxidations. The 2,3-epoxide, however, is the less toxic of the two species, reacting readily with cellular water to

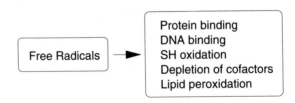

Figure 9.2. Summary of some toxic effects of free radicals.

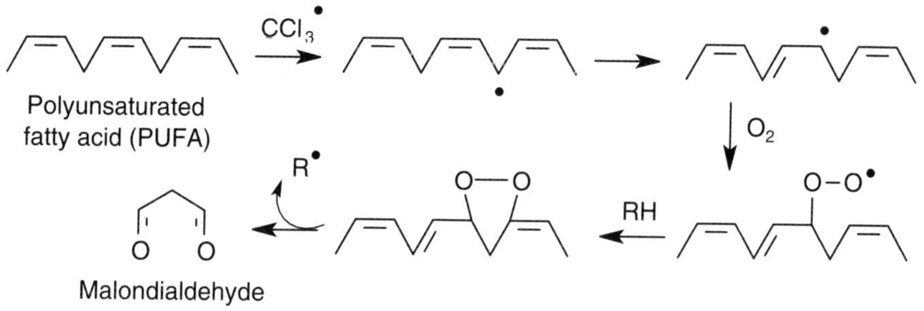

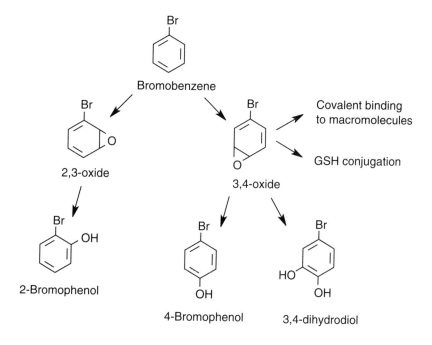

Figure 9.3. Schematic illustrating lipid peroxidation and destruction of membranes.

form the nontoxic 2-bromophenol. The more stable 3,4-epoxide is the form most responsible for covalent binding to cellular proteins. A number of pathways exist for detoxication of the 3,4-epoxide: rearrangement to the 4-bromophenol, hydration to the 3,4-dihydrodiol catalyzed by epoxide hydrolase, or conjugation with glutathione. When more 3,4-epoxide is produced than can readily be detoxified, cell injury increases.

Figure 9.4. Metabolism of bromobenzene.

Pretreatment of animals with inhibitors of cytochrome P450 is known to decrease tissue necrosis by slowing down the rate of formation of the reactive metabolite, whereas pretreatment of animals with certain P450 inducers can increase the toxicity of bromobenzene (eg, the P450 inducer phenobarbital increases hepatotoxicity by inducing a P450 isozyme that preferentially forms the 3,4-epoxide). However, pretreatment with another P450 inducer, 3-methylcholanthrene, decreases bromobenzene hepatotoxicity by inducing a form of P450 that produces primarily the less toxic 2,3-epoxide.

ACETAMINOPHEN is a widely used analgesic that is normally safe when taken at therapeutic doses. Overdoses, however, may cause an acute centrilobular hepatic necrosis that can be fatal. Although acetaminophen is eliminated primarily by formation of glucuronide and sulfate conjugates, a small proportion is metabolized by cytochrome P450 to a reactive electrophilic intermediate believed to be a quinoneimine (see Chapter 4, Fig. 4.4). This reactive intermediate is usually inactivated by conjugation with reduced glutathione and excreted. Higher doses of acetaminophen will progressively deplete hepatic glutathione levels, however, resulting in extensive covalent binding of the reactive metabolite to liver macromolecules with subsequent hepatic necrosis. The early administration of sulfhydryl compounds such as cysteamine, methionine, and N-acetylcysteine is very effective in preventing the liver damage, renal failure, and death that would otherwise follow an acetaminophen overdose. These agents are thought to act primarily by stimulating glutathione synthesis.

In laboratory animals, the formation of the acetaminophen-reactive metabolite, the extent of covalent binding, and the severity of hepatotoxicity can be influenced by altering the activity of various P450 isozymes. Induction of P450 isozymes with phenobarbital, 3-methylcholanthrene, or ethanol increases toxicity, whereas inhibition of P450 with piperonyl butoxide, cobalt chloride, or metyrapone decreases toxicity. Consistent with these effects in animals, it appears that the severity of liver damage after acetaminophen overdose is greater in chronic alcoholics and patients taking drugs that induce the levels of the P450 isozymes responsible for the activation of acetaminophen.

9.1.6 Activation and Toxicity

Studies of liver toxicity caused by bromobenzene, acetaminophen, and other compounds have led to some important observations concerning tissue damage:

- Toxicity may be correlated with the formation of a minor but highly reactive intermediate
- A threshold tissue concentration of the reactive metabolite must be attained before tissue injury occurs
- Endogenous substances, such as glutathione, play an essential role in protecting the cell from injury by removing chemically reactive intermediates and by keeping the sulfhydryl groups of proteins in the reduced state

- Pathways such as those catalyzed by glutathione transferase and epoxide hydrolases play an important role in protecting the cell
- Agents that selectively induce or inhibit the xenobiotic metabolizing enzymes may alter the toxicity of xenobiotic chemicals

These same principles are applicable to the toxicity caused by reactive metabolites in other organs, such as kidney and lung as will be illustrated in the following sections.

9.2

NEPHROTOXICITY

9.2.1   Susceptibility of the Kidney

The kidney appears to be particularly sensitive to a variety of chemical toxicants. Although several factors are involved in this sensitivity (Table 9.2), perhaps the most important is the high renal blood flow. Although the two kidneys comprise less than 1% of the total body mass, they receive approximately 25% of the cardiac output. Because of this high blood flow to the kidneys, any drug or chemical in the systemic circulation will be delivered to the kidney in significant amounts.

A second factor affecting the kidney's sensitivity to chemicals is its ability to concentrate substances. First, as salt and water are reabsorbed from the glomerular filtrate, the substances remaining in the tubular fluid become more concentrated. Thus, a nontoxic concentration in the plasma may reach toxic concentrations in the tubular fluid. Second, the transport characteristics of the kidney also contribute to its ability to concentrate xenobiotic substances within the cells. If the chemical is actively secreted from the blood into the tubular urine, it will be accumulated initially within the cells of the proximal tubules or, if the substance is readsorbed from the urine, it will pass through the epithelial cells in a relatively high concentration.

Another key element in nephrotoxicity is the biotransformation of the parent compound to a toxic metabolite. Although the kidney does not possess the high levels of xenobiotic metabolizing enzymes that are found in the liver, many of these same enzymatic reactions occur in the kidney, and some regions of the kidney contain appreciable levels of xenobiotic metabolizing enzymes. The levels of P450 are highest in the cells of the pars recta of the proximal tubule, an area that is particularly susceptible to toxic damage. Considering the unstable nature of many reactive

TABLE 9.2. FACTORS INFLUENCING SUSCEPTIBILITY OF THE KIDNEY TO TOXICANTS

High renal blood flow
Concentration of tubular fluid and chemicals in fluid
Renal transportation of chemicals into tubular cells
Biotransformation of parent compound to toxic metabolite

metabolites, it seems most likely that covalent binding to tissue macromolecules is in close proximity to the site of activation. Thus, chemicals that exert their toxicity by a reactive intermediate are probably activated directly in the kidney rather than in the liver. As with hepatotoxicity, an important determinant in kidney toxicity is the balance between the rate of generation of reactive metabolites and the rate of their removal. The high levels of glutathione in renal tissue play an important role in the detoxication process.

9.2.2 Renal Physiology and Function

The kidney is an extremely complex organ, in terms of both anatomy and physiology. The primary function of the kidney is the excretion of waste products (see Chapter 5 for a discussion of kidney function). The kidney also plays a significant role in regulation of body homeostasis, regulating extracellular fluid volume and electrolyte balance. Other functions include formation of hormones that influence metabolic functions—for example, 25-hydroxy-vitamin D_3 is metabolized to the active 1,25-dihydroxy-vitamin D_3; renin, involved in the formation of angiotensin and aldosterone, is formed in the kidney; and several prostaglandins are produced here. Thus, toxicity to the kidney could affect any of these functions. Generally, the effects used clinically to diagnose kidney damage are reflective of excretory function damage, such as an increase in blood urea nitrogen (BUN) or an increase in plasma creatinine.

9.2.3 Examples of Nephrotoxicants

METALS. Many heavy metals are potent nephrotoxicants, and relatively low doses can produce toxicity characterized by glucosuria, aminoaciduria, and polyuria. As the dose level increases, renal necrosis, anuria, increased BUN, and death will occur. Several mechanisms appear to protect the kidney from heavy metal toxicity. After low-dose exposure, significant concentrations of metal can be found in renal lysosomes prior to signs of toxicity developing. This binding of metals by lysosomes may result from one of several mechanisms including lysosomal endocytosis of a metal–protein complex, autophagy of metal-damaged organelles such as mitochondria or binding of the metal to lipoproteins within the lysosome. Exposure to high concentrations, however, may overwhelm these mechanisms, resulting in tissue damage. (Metal toxicity is discussed also in Chapter 10, Section 10.6.)

Cadmium. In humans, exposure to cadmium is primarily through food or industrial exposure to cadmium dust. In Japan, a disease called Itai-itai Byo is known to occur among women who eat rice grown in soils with a very high cadmium content. The disease is characterized by anemia, damage to proximal tubules, and severe bone and mineral loss. Cadmium is excreted in the urine mainly as a complex with the protein metallothionein (CdMT). Metallothionein is a low molecular weight protein synthesized in the liver and contains a large number of sulfhydryl groups that bind certain metals. The binding of cadmium by metallothionein appears to protect certain organs such as the testes from cadmium toxicity. At the same time, however, the complex may enhance kidney toxicity because the complex is taken up more readily by the kidney than is the free ion. Once inside the cell, it is thought that the cadmium is released, presumably by decomposition of the complex within the lysosomes. Cadmium has a long biologic half-life, 10 to 20 years in humans; thus, low levels of chronic exposure will eventually result in accumulation to toxic levels.

Lead. Lead, as Pb^{2+}, is taken up readily by proximal tubule cells, where it damages mitochondria and inhibits mitochondrial function, thus altering the normal absorptive functions of the cell. Complexes of lead with acidic proteins appear as inclusion bodies in the nuclei of the tubular epithelium cells. These bodies, which are formed before signs of lead toxicity occur, appear to serve as a detoxication mechanism.

Mercury. Mercury exerts its principle toxic effect on the membrane of the proximal tubule cell. In low concentrations, Hg^{2+} binds to the sulfhydryl groups of membrane enzymes and thus acts as a diuretic by inhibiting sodium reabsorption. Organomercurial diuretics were introduced in the 1920s, and were used clinically into the 1960s. In spite of their widespread acceptance as effective therapeutic agents, it was known that there were problems of severe kidney toxicity. In the absence of other drugs that were as effective, however, the organomercurials proved to be valuable, even life-saving, therapeutic agents. More recently, organic mercury, as an environmental pollutant, has been responsible for renal damage in humans and animals.

Uranium. About 50% of plasma uranium is bound, as the uranyl ion, to bicarbonate, which is filtered by the glomerulus. As a result of acidification in the proximal tubule, the bicarbonate complex dissociates, followed by reabsorption of the HCO_3^- ion; the released UO_2^{2+} then becomes attached to the membrane of the proximal tubule cells. Loss of cell function follows, as evidenced by increased concentration of glucose, amino acids, and proteins in the urine.

AMINOGLYCOSIDES. Certain antibiotics, most notably the aminoglycosides, are known to be nephrotoxic in humans, especially in high doses or after prolonged therapy. This group of compounds includes the drugs streptomycin, neomycin, kananycin, and gentamicin. Aminoglycosides are polar cations that are filtered by the glomerulus and excreted unchanged into the urine. In the proximal tubule, the aminoglycosides are reabsorbed by binding to anionic membrane phospholipids, followed by endocytosis and sequestration in lysosomes (Fig. 9.5). It is thought that when a threshold concentration is reached, the lysosomes rupture, releasing hydrolytic enzymes that cause tissue necrosis.

AMPHOTERICIN B. With some drugs, the damage may be related to the drug's biochemical mechanism of action. For example, the polymycins, such as amphotericin B, are surface-active agents that bind to membrane phospholipids, disrupting the integrity of the membrane and resulting in leaky cells.

REACTIVE METABOLITES. Still other nephrotoxicants are activated in the kidney by xenobiotic metabolizing enzymes to produce strong electrophiles or free radicals that can cause cell necrosis by binding to cell macromolecules or by initiating lipid peroxi-

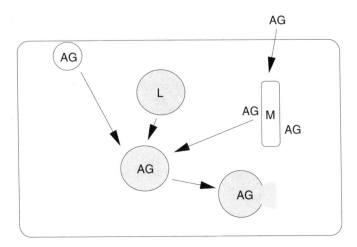

Figure 9.5. Illustration of possible cellular interactions of aminoglycosides.

dation. Many of these toxicants are the same as those that are activated in the liver, such as acetaminophen, bromobenzene, chloroform, and carbon tetrachloride (see Section 9.1.5), resulting in hepatotoxicity.

HEXACHLOROBUTADIENE (HCBD) is a widespread environmental contaminant that is a relatively specific and potent nephrotoxicant. Hexachlorobutadiene first forms the glutathione (GSH) conjugate, which is further metabolized by the mercapturic acid pathway to a cysteine conjugate (see Chapter 3 for a discussion of glutathione conjugation and mercapturic acid formation). In the kidney, the cysteine conjugate is cleaved to a reactive intermediate by the action of the kidney enzyme cysteine-conjugate ß-lyase.

TETRAFLUROETHYLENE. A mode of action similar to that of HCBD is responsible for the nephrotoxicity of this haloalkene. Tetrafluroethylene (TFE) is first metabolized in the liver to the GSH conjugate, which is subsequently converted to the cysteine S-conjugate (TFEC), a substrate for the kidney enzyme cysteine-conjugate ß-lyase. As in the case of HCBD, a reactive product is formed that is capable of binding to cellular macromolecules.

9.3

PULMONARY TOXICITY

9.3.1   Susceptibility of the Lung

The principal function of the lungs is gas exchange, providing O_2 to the tissues and removing CO_2. Because the lung has a large surface area and exchanges a significant volume of air (10,000-20,000 L/day for the average adult), the lung is the major interface between an organism, the environment, and any toxicants present in the air. (The structure and function of the respiratory system are discussed in more detail in Chapter 2, Section 2.7.3.)

Pulmonary diseases caused by agents in the environment have been known for centuries and have been associated with occupations such as stone quarrying, coal mining, and textiles. The problem is more complex and widespread today because new agents are constantly being added to our environments, including gasoline additives and exhaust particles, pesticides, plastics, solvents, deodorant and cosmetic sprays, and construction materials. Table 9.3 lists some important industrial lung toxicants, the exposure sources, and associated injuries.

In addition to being in direct contact with airborne toxicants, the entire body blood volume passes through the lung one to five times a minute, exposing the lung to toxicants and drugs within the systemic circulation. Thus, the possibility of damage from both inhaled and circulating agents is clearly enormous.

TABLE 9.3. SOME IMPORTANT INDUSTRIAL LUNG TOXICANTS AND ASSOCIATED INJURY

Toxicant	Source	Damage
Aluminum dust	Ceramics, paints, fireworks, electrical goods	Fibrosis
Ammonia	Manufacture of fertilizers, explosives, ammonia	Irritation
Arsenic	Manufacture of pesticides, glass, pigments, alloys	Lung cancer, bronchitis
Asbestos	Mining, construction, shipbuilding	Asbestosis, lung cancer
Berryllium	Ore extraction, ceramics, alloys	Fibrosis, lung cancer
Cadmium oxide	Welding, smelting, manufacture of electronics, alloys, pigments	Emphysema
Chlorine	Manufacture of pulp and paper, plastics, chlorinated chemicals	Irritation
Chromium	Manufacture of Cr compounds, paint pigments	Lung cancer
Coal dust	Coal mining	Fibrosis
Hydrogen fluoride	Manufacture of chemicals, plastics, photographic film, solvents	Irritation, edema
Iron oxides	Welding, steel manufacturing, mining, foundry work	Fibrosis
Nickel	Nickel extraction and smelting, electroplating	Nasal cancer, lung cancer, edema
Nitrogen oxides	Welding, explosive manufacturing	Emphysema
Ozone	Welding, bleaching, deodorizing	Emphysema
Phosgene	Production of pesticides, plastics	Edema
Silica	Mining, quarrying, farming	Fibrosis (silicosis)
Sulfur dioxide	Bleaching, refrigeration, fumigation coal combustion	Irritation
Talc	Rubber industry, cosmetics	Fibrosis
Tetrachloroethylene	Dry cleaning, metal degreasing	Edema

As with the liver and kidney, the lungs also possess significant levels of many xenobiotic metabolizing enzymes and thus can play an active role in activation and detoxication of exogenous chemicals.

9.3.2   Types of Toxic Responses

Although many different agents may damage the lung, the patterns of cellular injury and repair are relatively constant, and most fall into one or more of the categories described as follows.

IRRITATION. Perhaps one of the most obvious and familiar chemical effects is irritation caused by volatile compounds, such as ammonia or chlorine gas. Such irritation, especially if severe or persistent, results in constriction of the airways. Edema and secondary infection frequently follow severe or prolonged irritation. Such damage is known to result from exposure to agents such as ozone, nitrogen oxides, and phosgene. (See also Air Pollutants in Chapter 10, Section 10.1.)

CELL NECROSIS. Severe damage to the cells lining the airways can result in increased cell permeability, followed by cell death.

FIBROSIS, or formation of collagenous tissue, was perhaps one of the earliest recognized forms of occupational diseases. *Silicosis,* resulting from inhalation of silica (SiO_2), is thought to involve first the uptake of the particles by macrophages and lysosomal incorporation, followed by rupture of the lysosomal membrane and release of lysosomal enzymes into the cytoplasm of the macrophages. Thus, the macrophage is digested by its own enzymes. After lysis, the free silica is released to be ingested by fresh macrophages, and the cycle continues. It is also thought that the damaged macrophages release chemicals that are instrumental in initiating collagen formation in the lung. Fibrosis may become massive and impair the respiratory function of the lung significantly. *Asbestosis* was recognized as long ago as 1907; however, the magnitude of the risk has become apparent only recently, primarily due to the increased incidence of lung cancer among asbestosis sufferers, especially those who are also cigarette smokers. Both silicosis and asbestosis are thought to be premalignant conditions.

EMPHYSEMA is characterized by an enlargement of the airspaces with destruction of the gas-exchanging surface area. The result is a distended lung that no longer effectively exchanges O_2 and CO_2 because of loss of tissue and air-trapping capacity. Although cigarette smoking is the major cause of emphysema, other toxicants can also cause this condition.

ALLERGIC RESPONSES. Numerous agents, including microorganisms, spores, dust, and chemicals, are known to elicit allergic responses resulting in constriction of the airways. Several diverse examples are farmer's lung from the spores of a mold that grows on damp hay; maple bark stripper's disease from spores of a fungus growing on maple trees; cheese washer's lung from penicillin spores; and mushroom picker's lung from the mushroom spores. Byssinosis comes from the inhalation of cotton, flax, or hemp dusts. This condition, however, does not seem to result from bacterial or fungal exposure but from an apparent toxicant or allergen associated with the plant dusts.

CANCER. Perhaps the most severe response of the lung to injury is cancer, with the primary cause of lung cancer being cigarette smoking. Cigarette smoke contains many known carcinogens as well as lung irritants. Many of the polycyclic aromatic hydrocarbons, such as benzo(a)pyrene, can be metabolized in the lung by pulmonary P450 enzymes to reactive metabolites capable of initiating cancer. In addition, cigarette smoke contains numerous compounds that can act as tumor promoters. Asbestos is associated with two forms of cancer—lung cancer and malignant mesothelioma, a tumor of the cells covering the surface of the lung and the adjacent body wall.

9.3.3 Examples of Lung Toxicants Requiring Activation

The activation of pulmonary toxicants falls into three main categories or mechanisms, depending either on the site of formation of the activated compound or on the nature of the reactive intermediate.

1. The parent compound may be activated in the liver, with the reactive metabolite then transported by the circulation to the lung. As would be expected, the activated compounds may lead to covalent binding and damage to both liver and lung tissues.
2. A toxicant entering the lung, either from inhaled air or the circulatory system, may be metabolized to the ultimate toxic compound directly within the lung itself. Although the total concentration of P450 is less in the lung than in the liver, the concentration varies considerably in the different cell types, with the highest concentration being found in the nonciliated bronchiolar epithelial (Clara) cells of the terminal bronchioles. Because of this, the Clara cells are often a primary target for the effects of activated chemicals.
3. Another means of metabolic activation is the cyclic reduction/oxidation of the parent compound, resulting in high rates of consumption of NADPH and production of superoxide anion. Either the depletion of NADPH and/or the formation of reactive oxygen radicals could lead to cellular injury.

The following three chemicals serve to illustrate these three mechanisms of activation.

MONOCROTALINE. The pyrrolizidine alkaloids (PA), found in the genus *Senecio* and a number of other plant genera, are plant toxins of environmental interest that have been implicated in a number of livestock and human poisonings. Grazing animals may be poisoned by feeding on PA-containing pastures, and human exposure may occur through consumption of herbal teas and contaminated grains and milk. The chemical structure for monocrotaline (MCT) is shown in Chapter 1, Fig. 1.8.

Monocrotaline, found in the leaves and seeds of the plant *Crotalaria spectabilis,* has been the most extensively studied of the pyrrolizidine alkaloids. When MCT is given to rats and other animals at high doses, a pronounced liver injury occurs, and animals usually die of acute effects, presumably liver failure. Lower doses, however, that are only mildly hepatotoxic result in lung injury that is associated with pulmonary hypertension and usually death in several weeks. It is thought that activation of MCT to pyrrolic metabolites occurs in the liver and is mediated by cytochrome P450. Even though monocrotaline acts as a pneumotoxicant, several lines of evidence indicate that the lung is incapable of activating MCT or can do so only at very low levels. Furthermore, the main site of pulmonary injury occurs in the endothelial cells, a target site consistent with a reactive metabolite being absorbed from the circulatory system.

IPOMEANOL. One of the best known examples of a toxic compound being activated in the lung is 4-ipomeanol (Fig. 9.6). This naturally occurring furan is produced by the mold *Fusarium solani* that infects sweet potatoes. Lung edema in cattle is known to be associated with the ingestion of mold-damaged sweet potatoes. A similar pulmonary lesion can be produced in a number of species regardless of the route of administration. Pulmonary injury by 4-ipomeanol is caused, not by the parent compound, but by a highly reactive alkylating metabolite produced in the lung by lung-specific P450 isozymes. In addition, these isozymes are highly concentrated in the Clara cells, which are most affected by 4-ipomeanol toxicity. Although the reactive metabolite has not been identified unambiguously, considerable data suggest a reactive epoxide. Other toxic lung furans, such as the atmospheric contaminants 2-methylfuran and 3-methylfuran, may exert their toxicity through the formation of reactive metabolites, probably reactive aldehydes.

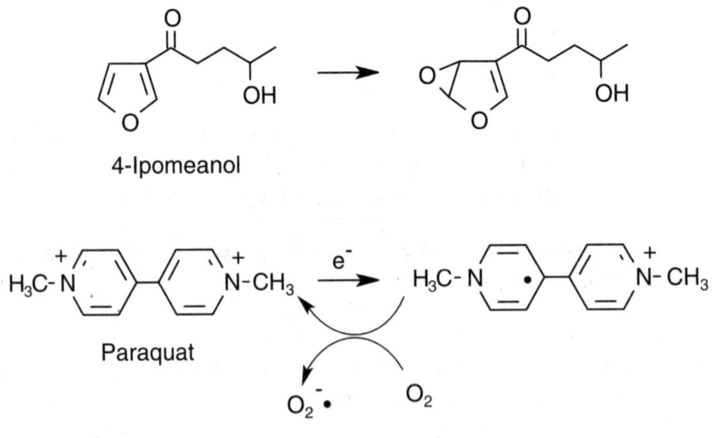

4-Ipomeanol

Paraquat

Figure 9.6. Activation of the pulmonary toxicants 4-ipomeanol and paraquat.

PARAQUAT. Systemic administration of compounds such as the herbicide paraquat (Fig. 9.6), bleomycin (a cancer therapeutic agent), and nitroflurantoin (an antibiotic used for urinary tract infections) initiate a progression of degenerative and potentially lethal lesions in the lung by a mechanism known as *redox cycling*. These compounds are reduced by cytochrome P450 reductase and NADPH, forming a free radical. Although the free radical could potentially react with tissue macromolecules, this mechanism does not appear to be the primary cause of toxicity. Instead, the free radical is oxidized by oxygen, forming the original oxidized species. In the process, one molecule of oxygen is reduced to superoxide that can then be converted to other toxic oxygen species. These reactive compounds may cause peroxidation of cellular membranes. The specific toxicity of paraquat to the lung results from the uptake of this compound by the polyamine transport system in the lung as well as from the high pulmonary oxygen tension. Nitrofurantoin, however, is not actively accumulated in the lung, and its tissue specificity probably results from the high pulmonary oxygen tension.

9.4

NERVOUS SYSTEM TOXICITY

9.4.1 Nervous System Structure and Function

The nervous system, a complex system involved in intercellular communication, is comprised of the brain, spinal cord, and a vast array of nerves and sensory organs that control major body functions. Movement, thought, vision, hearing, speech, heart function, respiration, and numerous other physiological processes are controlled by this complex network of nerve processes, transmitters, hormones, receptors, and channels.

ORGANIZATION. The nervous system is anatomically separated into two major divisions: the central nervous system (CNS) and the peripheral nervous system (PNS). The CNS encompasses the brain and spinal cord, and the PNS includes the nerves that travel to and from the spinal cord, sense organs, glands, blood vessels, and muscles.

CELL TYPES IN THE NERVOUS SYSTEM. Neurons (Fig. 9.7) are the only cells in the nervous system capable of neurotransmission. These elongate cells may extend more than a meter in length. The cell body contains a nucleus and ribosomes for protein synthesis. Clusters of ribosomes, located in the cell body and known as Nissl substance, are found only in neurons. Neurons may have one or more processes extending from them—dendrites, which are branched structures for receiving information coming into the neuron, and axons, which are straight, unbranched structures for conducting information away from the neuron. Whereas a neuron may have numerous dendrites, there is only one axon per neuron. Structural proteins of the axon, especially neurofilaments and microtubules, are frequent targets for toxicants.

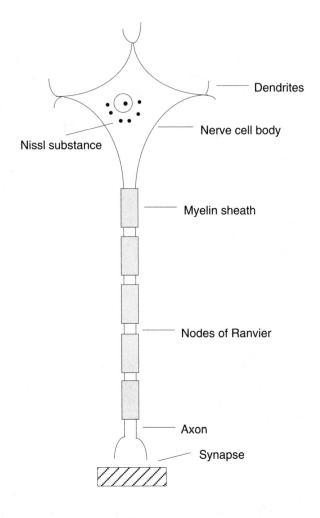

Figure 9.7. Diagram of a neuron.

SUPPORTING CELLS (GLIAL CELLS). Myelin is a specialized membrane structure responsible for isolating axons from one another, thus preventing "cross talk" in the nervous system. In addition, myelin increases the speed of impulses traveling along an axon. In the CNS, myelin is formed by the oligodendroglial cells, and in the PNS it is formed by the Schwann cells. Both oligodendroglial and Schwann cells form myelin by the progressive wrapping of their cytoplasmic processes around the axon in successive loops, resulting in the formation of a concentric lipid-rich structure. This high lipid content aids in the passage of highly lipophilic compounds from the bloodstream into the nervous system. Other supporting cell types include the microglia, which are phagocytic cells of the CNS, and the astrocytes, which are the cells responsible for the blood–brain barrier.

SYNAPSE. Intercellular communication in the nervous system occurs through the synapse—the space between an axon and some target—for example, another nerve cell, a muscle, or a gland. Messages are transmitted chemically at synapses by means of chemicals called neurotransmitters. The neurotransmitters released from the axon travel across the synapse and bind to the postsynaptic receptor in the target cell, leading to a response in the cell. In the case of neuromuscular transmission, acetylcholine crosses the synaptic cleft to bind to the cholinergic receptor of the muscle cell, causing changes in the cell that result in muscle contraction. Commonly recognized neurotransmitters include dopamine, serotonin, acetylcholine, and glutamate. A variety of therapeutic drugs target the process of neurotransmission, and numerous toxic compounds can interfere with transmission of impulses across the synapse.

BLOOD–BRAIN BARRIER. The nervous system is protected from the entry of many potential toxicants by the blood–brain barrier. Foot processes of the astrocytes form tight junctions with the endothelial cells in the brain to prevent passage of large or charged molecules from the bloodstream into the brain. Much of the brain, spinal cord, and PNS, however, lack this barrier, and thus are not protected. In the immature brain, the barrier is generally not as well developed, and toxic doses of some compounds may accumulate in the CNS of children and not in adults.

9.4.2   Vulnerability of the Nervous System

The nervous system is particularly vulnerable to toxic substances for a number of reasons:

- Nerve cells, or neurons, normally cannot regenerate once lost, and for this reason toxic damage to the nervous system is usually permanent.
- Toxic damage may progress with aging because nerve cell loss and other changes in the nervous system occur progressively in the second half of life.
- Many neurotoxic chemicals can cross the blood–brain barrier easily, and other regions of the nervous system lack the barrier.
- The long processes of nerve cells provide a large surface area for chemical attack.
- The delicate electrochemical balance necessary for proper communication provides numerous opportunities for foreign chemicals to interfere with normal function.
- Minor changes in structure or function can have profound consequences for neurologic, behavioral, and related body functions.

9.4.3   What Is Neurotoxicity?

Neurotoxicity is defined as an adverse change in either the *structure* or *function* of the nervous system following exposure to a chemical agent. At the molecular level a substance might interfere with protein synthesis, leading to reduced production of a neurotransmitter and brain dysfunction. Alternatively, a substance might alter the

TABLE 9.4. EXAMPLES OF TOXIC EFFECTS FOLLOWING EXPOSURE TO NEUROTOXICANTS

Motor effects	Cognitive effects
Convulsions	Memory problems
Weakness	Confusion
Tremor, twitching	Speech impairment
Lack of coordination	Learning impairment
Paralysis	**Sensory effects**
Reflex abnormalities	Vision disorders
Mood and personality effects	Auditory disorders
Sleep disturbances	Pain disorders
Excitability	**General effects**
Depression	Narcosis
Irritability	Fatigue
Restlessness	Loss of appetite
Delirium, hallucinations	Stupor
Nervousness, tension	

flow of sodium or potassium across membranes and thereby disrupt transmission of nerve impulses.

Substances that affect sensory or motor function adversely, disrupt learning and memory processes, or cause detrimental behavioral effects are neurotoxic, even if the underlying molecular and cellular effects on the nervous system have not been identified. For example, exposure of children to lead can result in learning deficits, although the mechanisms by which this occurs are not understood. Examples of toxic effects that may occur following exposure to neurotoxic chemicals are given in Table 9.4.

Sometimes defining an adverse effect can be difficult. Some effects are clearly adverse (eg, hallucinations, convulsions, loss of memory); others are more difficult to define (eg, temporary drowsiness, brief headache).

9.4.4   Who Is at Risk?

Although everyone is at risk, individuals in certain age groups, states of health, and occupations face a greater probability of adverse effects from neurotoxic chemicals. Fetuses, children, the elderly, workers in occupations involving exposure to relatively high levels of neurotoxicants, and persons who abuse psychoactive drugs are among those in high-risk groups.

The developing nervous system is particularly vulnerable to some neurotoxicants. It is actively growing and establishing networks, the blood–brain barrier is not yet completely formed, and detoxication systems are not fully developed.

The elderly are more susceptible to certain neurotoxic substances for several reasons. The ability to respond and compensate for toxic effects declines with age and aging may reveal adverse effects masked at a younger age. Moreover, older adults are more likely to be taking multiple drugs that may interact to affect the nervous system adversely.

Workers in industry and agriculture are often exposed to greater quantities of certain substances than are the general population. Pesticides and solvents, both of which have neurotoxic effects, are common sources of exposure in the workplace.

Persons who abuse psychoactive drugs may face particularly severe neurotoxic effects. Some drugs can damage the nervous system permanently. Damage may be so severe as to cause personality changes, neurologic disease, mental illness, and death. Abuse of psychoactive drugs by pregnant women poses a major risk to the developing nervous system of the fetus—for example, both alcohol and cocaine are significant contributors to mental problems in children.

9.4.5 Toxic Effects

STRUCTURAL CHANGES. Toxic substances can alter both the structure and function of cells. Structural alterations include changes in the morphology of the cell and the subcellular structures within it or destruction of cells. At the morphologic level, toxic substances seem to act selectively on the various components of the nervous system, damaging the neuron cell body, the axons (axonopathy), the myelin sheaths (myelinopathy), or the receptor molecules at synapses. Because of the relative inability of the nervous system to repair itself, exposure to chemicals may produce a delayed and progressive deterioration. Examples of specific toxicants and their targets in the nervous system are given in Table 9.5.

Neurons require relatively large quantities of oxygen because of their high metabolic rate and are more susceptible than other cells to anoxia or oxygen deprivation. Thus, any chemical that disrupts the oxygen supply to the nervous system may result in neurotoxic effects, even though the nervous system is not the target organ. For example, carbon monoxide which binds to hemoglobin and prevents the transport of oxygen, can result in neurotoxic effects as a result of a decrease in oxygen reaching the nervous system.

TABLE 9.5. SOME TOXICANTS AND THEIR TARGETS IN THE NERVOUS SYSTEM

Nerve cell body toxicants	Axonal toxicants
Mercury compounds	n-Hexane
Manganese	Carbon disulfide
Aluminum	Taxol
Glutamate	Colchicine
Cyanide	Acrylamide
Domoic acid	Pyrethroids
MPTP	**Neurotransmitter toxicants**
Lead	Nicotine
Myelin toxicants	Organophosphorus compounds
Hexachlorophene	Carbamate insecticides
Triethyl tin (TET)	Amphetamines
Lead	Cocaine
Tellurium	Excitatory amino acids

FUNCTIONAL CHANGES. Toxic chemicals can induce functional changes that involve modifications of motor and sensory activities, emotional states, and integrative capabilities such as learning and memory. Numerous systems can be adversely affected (eg, sight, hearing, touch, pain). Motor and sensory functions may also be affected, leading to muscle weakness, lack of control of movements, and paralysis.

BEHAVIORAL EFFECTS. Behavioral changes may be the first indications of damage to the nervous system. An individual exposed to a toxic substance may initially experience vague feelings of anxiety or nervousness. This situation may progress to depression, difficulty in sleeping, memory loss, confusion, loss of appetite, or speech impairment. In severe cases, a person may exhibit bizarre behavior, delirium, and hallucinations.

9.4.6 Examples of Neurotoxicants

LEAD is one of the oldest and perhaps most ubiquitous of the neurotoxic substances. Although some of the toxic effects of lead were known in earlier times (Dioscorides stated in the second century BC that "Lead makes the mind give way."), lead has been widely used throughout history. Lead is mentioned in ancient Egyptian manuscripts; Egyptians used it in cosmetics; Egyptians and Romans used lead in cooking tools and vessels; and the Romans used it as a sweetener and preservative in wine and ciders.

Lead is a widely distributed metal. Major sources of exposure include water, food, beverages, soil, industrial emissions, and lead-based paints. Lead has profound effects on the nervous system, and even at relatively low levels can cause learning disorders. In children, brain damage resulting from exposure to lead can range in severity from inhibited muscular coordination to stupor, coma, and convulsions. In spite of years of research and considerable regulatory action, lead poisoning in children remains a major public health problem.

MERCURY compounds are potent neurotoxic substances and have caused a number of human poisonings worldwide. Common symptoms of exposure include lack of coordination, speech impairment, and vision problems. In the mid-1950s, a chemical plant near Minamata Bay, Japan, discharged mercury into the bay as part of its waste sludge. Contaminated fish and shellfish were consumed by the local population, resulting in mercury poisonings and severe neurotoxicologic and developmental effects. In another episode, mercury was used as a fungicide in treating seed grain and resulted in serious poisoning in Iraq in 1971 when the grain was used as food. (For additional discussion on lead and mercury, see Chapter 10, Section 10.6, "Metals.")

• PESTICIDES are one of the most commonly encountered neurotoxic substances. The organophosphorus insecticides have neurotoxic properties, as do other classes of pesticides, including the carbamate and organochlorine insecticides.

Organophosphorus (OP) and carbamate insecticides inhibit acetylcholinesterase (AChE), an enzyme responsible for the breakdown of the neurotransmitter acetylcholine (ACh). As a result of this enzyme inhibition, ACh accumulates in the synapses between nerves and muscles, leading to overstimulation of ACh receptor sites, including those that control muscle movement, some organ systems, and thought and emotional processes. In fact, it is this property of OP compounds that led to their development and use as "nerve gases." Acute human poisoning from OP compounds can cause muscle weakness, paralysis, disorientation, and death from paralysis of respiratory muscles. (For a more detailed discussion of cholinesterase inhibition by OP and carbamate compounds see Chapter 7, Section 7.2.1.)

In addition to the acute effects of OP compounds, some OP compounds may also cause a severe delayed distal axonopathy, known as organophosphorus induced delayed neuropathy (OPIDN) in which the degeneration of axons does not commence immediately after acute organophosphorus exposure but is delayed for 7 to 10 days. An OPIDN epidemic of massive proportion occurred in the 1930s during Prohibition in the United States when a popular alcoholic drink, Ginger Jake (so named because it was derived from a Jamaican ginger tonic), was contaminated with tri-*ortho*-cresyl phosphate (TOCP). The contaminated drink caused axonal degeneration in neurons of the CNS and PNS, with symptoms ranging from temporary numbness and tingling in the extremities to permanent partial paralysis. Human cases of paralysis have also occurred after exposure to the agricultural chemicals EPN and leptophos. Because of this property, OP compounds are required to undergo special testing for delayed neurotoxicity.

SOLVENTS. Organic solvents are a class of industrial chemicals that have the potential for significant human exposure. In part, this is because of their volatility. Exposures may be accidental, as often occurs in industrial or household settings, or deliberate, as in glue-sniffing. Many solvents, including ethers, hydrocarbons, ketones, alcohols, and combinations of these, have caused neurologic and behavioral problems in the workplace.

Most solvents are soluble in varying degrees in fat and will, at some level of exposure, produce effects on the lipid-rich CNS. Short-term exposures at low toxicity may produce mucous membrane irritation, nasal irritation, headache, and nausea. With repeated inhalation of high levels, a state of severe narcosis may be produced, whereas at lower levels the effects resemble those of alcohol. Initially there may be euphoria, loquaciousness, and excitement, followed by confusion, dizziness, headache, lack of motor coordination, unconsciousness, and even death.

Other effects may be specific to individual solvents or classes of solvents. For example, neuropathies may result from chronic exposure to hexane, methyl-*n*-butyl ketone, and related solvents. This disorder, sometimes referred to as hexacarbon neuropathy, is characterized by numbness in the hands and feet and may progress to muscle weakness, lack of coordination, or even paralysis.

Some solvents may cause emotional disorders. Carbon disulfide can produce a raging mania and has been associated with increased risk of suicide. Other disorders associated with exposure to solvents include sleep disturbances, nightmares, and insomnia. There is some evidence that toxic encephalopathy (wasting of brain matter leading to expansion of fluid-filled brain cavities) may be caused by chronic exposure to high levels of some organic solvents. Trichloroethylene or its contaminants may damage facial nerves and produce facial numbness. (See also Chapter 10, Section 10.7, "Solvents.")

DRUGS. Although therapeutic drugs often alter the function of the nervous system in a desirable manner (eg, drugs that treat anxiety or depression), such drugs can also have undesirable effects on the brain. In addition, drugs that are used to treat illnesses unassociated with the nervous system may have neurotoxic side effects. (See also Chapter 10, Section 10.8, "Drugs.")

Persons who abuse drugs are often not aware of, or do not take seriously, the adverse health effects of these substances. Although the adverse effects of drugs are often short-lived, effects can be prolonged or permanent. In some cases, damage is so severe that it can cause personality changes, neurologic disease, mental illness, or death. A contaminant of "synthetic heroin," MPTP (1-methyl-4-phenyl-1,2,3,6-tetrahydropyridine), causes irreversible brain damage and symptoms characteristic of Parkinson's disease among users of this illegal drug. In fact, the observation of this neurologic lesion has lead to the suggestion that some cases of Parkinson's disease may result in part from exposure to neurotoxic environmental chemicals.

9.4.7 Testing for Neurotoxicity

The effects of toxic substances on the nervous system may be evaluated through animal tests, cell and tissue culture (in vitro) tests, and human tests. Core neurotoxicologic tests used in initial screening for toxicity include the functional observational battery (FOB) (a series of rapid neurologic tests to evaluate toxic effects on animals), tests of motor activity, and neuropathologic examinations. Additional tests that may be used include schedule-controlled operant behavior tests, acute and subchronic delayed neurotoxicity tests for OP substances, and developmental examinations. Neurophysiological evaluations are also useful in identifying and evaluating neurotoxic substances. Human tests include neurobehavioral evaluations and neurophysiological tests. (Testing is discussed in Chapter 11.)

9.5

REPRODUCTIVE SYSTEM TOXICITY

9.5.1 Introduction

Reproductive toxicity can be defined as a dysfunction of the reproductive system induced by chemical agents and includes effects on any of the processes, from the earliest stages to implantation of the conceptus in the endometrium to parturition and lactation. Because of the complicated biologic interactions on which the mammalian reproductive system depends, there are many targets available for toxic chemicals. In order to understand the basis of reproductive toxicity, the entire spectrum of reproductive processes that must function properly in order to produce healthy offspring must be examined. At this point, it is important to note that reproductive toxicity involves both the male and the female.

The toxic effects of drugs and environmental chemicals on the human reproductive system are of major health concern, and incidents of chemically induced germ-cell damage and sterility appear to be on the increase. Of particular focus in recent years has been environmental chemicals that mimic the female sex hormone estrogen or that are antagonistic to the male sex hormone androgen. Reproductive effects in wildlife, as dramatic as hermaphroditic fish and reduction of penis size in alligators, have been noted in areas of high contamination with chemicals such as DDT, DDE, and Dicofol (see Chapter 15 for a discussion of these interactions). The significance of these effects and, in particular, the potential for adverse effects on human reproduction, is not yet known.

9.5.2 Reproductive Processes

9.5.2.a Development

The development of the reproductive system includes events from embryonic development through mature functioning of the reproductive organ systems. The developing gonads are particularly sensitive to chemical insult, with some cells being more susceptible to chemical toxicity than are others. During the process of genital organogenesis, critical molecular and cellular processes must respond to a variety of hormones and other growth factors to ensure normal postnatal function. Thus, during fetal development, there is considerable potential for environmental chemicals to affect the development of normal reproductive capacity.

9.5.2.b Male Reproduction

TESTICULAR FUNCTION. There are several populations of cell types in the mammalian testes, all of which play important roles in the reproductive process and any of which may be targets for chemical damage (Table 9.6). Spermatogenesis, or the production of sperm, starts at puberty and continues throughout most of the male life span. The

TABLE 9.6. SOME TARGET SITES IN THE MALE REPRODUCTIVE SYSTEM

Target	Chemical
Spermatogonia	Busulfan, procarbazine
Spermatocytes	2-Methoxyethanol, procarbazine
Spermatids	Methyl chloride
Sertoli cells	Dinitrobenzene, hexanedione
Leydig cells	Ethane dimethanesulfonate, imidazoles
Epididymus	Chlorohydrin, methyl chloride, sulfasalazine ethane dimethanesulfonate
Accessory sex glands	Imidazoles

primitive male germ cells are the spermatogonia and are situated next to the basement membrane of the seminiferous tubules. Following birth, spermatogonia are dormant until puberty, when proliferative activity begins again. The onset of spermatogenesis accompanies functional maturation of the testes. Associated testicular cells are the Sertoli cells, which secrete a number of hormones and proteins and the Leydig or interstitial cells, which are the primary site of testosterone synthesis.

POST-TESTICULAR PROCESSES. Maturation changes occur in the immature sperm as they move through the testes and epididymides, where they mature and become more motile. A number of secretory processes exist that control fluid production and ion composition, and secretory organs (prostate and seminal vesicle) contribute to the chemical composition of the semen. For the reproductive act to be completed, the processes of erection and ejaculation in the male must also function normally.

9.5.2.c   Female Reproduction

For successful reproductive function, the hypothalamic–pituitary–gonadal–reproductive axis must be intact so that the appropriate signals and responses will occur to produce ovulation. In addition, the environment of the uterus and fallopian tubes must be conducive to fertilization and continued growth of the embryo. The CNS–gonadal–reproductive tract axis can be disrupted by toxicants as well as by alterations in the levels of endogenous hormones such as estrogens. Normally, three levels of control exist for the female reproductive system: (1) the hypothalamic–pituitary axis; (2) the ovary with its endocrine and ovulatory functions; and (3) the reproductive tract.

HYPOTHALAMUS–PITUITARY. The female reproductive process requires the cyclical production of gonadotropins, such as follicle-stimulating hormone (FSH), luteinizing hormone (LH), and prolactin by the pituitary. Feedback loops among the hypothalamus, pituitary, and ovary control the release of these hormones. Thus, chemicals that disrupt these pathways can alter fertility, either in a reversible or irreversible manner. Therapeutic drugs such as anesthetics, sedatives, analgesics, and tranquilizers, as well as drugs of abuse, such as marijuana, are known to cause temporary disruption in fertility by affecting in the normal pattern of gonadotropic secretions.

OVARIAN FUNCTION. Oogenesis is the production of the ovum or egg. In humans females, around 400,000 follicles are present in each ovary at birth. From birth onward, the number of follicles continuously declines, and only about one-half of the oocytes present at birth remain at puberty. Thus any agent that damages the oocytes will hasten this reduction and can lead to reduced fertility in females. The susceptibility of the ovary to permanent injury is age dependent. Prior to puberty, the ovaries are more resistant to chemical damage, whereas women in their late twenties and older have an increased risk of ovarian failure following exposure to cancer chemotherapeutic drugs.

The ovary also controls the proliferation of the endometrium in the uterus and the function of the fallopian tube. Estrogens and progesterone synthesized by the ovary interact with the CNS to help determine ovulation and prepare the female accessory sex organs to receive the sperm.

FEMALE ACCESSORY SEX ORGANS. The female sex organs that serve to bring together the egg and sperm are the oviducts, uterus, cervix, and vagina. Fertilization—that is, penetration of the egg by sperm and the coming together of the respective DNA material—occurs in the oviduct. Sperm penetration requires only a few minutes, although the time from sperm penetration to first cleavage is around 12 hours. The developing embryo moves down the oviduct into the uterus, where it becomes implanted in the endometrium or uterine lining. Embryonic and maternal tissue combine to become the placenta.

9.5.3   Examples of Reproductive Toxicants

As might be expected a wide variety of chemicals and drugs can affect the reproductive system adversely (Tables 9.7 and 9.8). Not only is there much diversity in the chemical nature of the toxicants, but the sites of action and the mechanisms can also be quite different. Toxicants may act directly on either the gonads or the supporting organs, or toxicants may affect reproduction indirectly by acting on the endocrine sys-

TABLE 9.7. EXAMPLES OF AGENTS AFFECTING THE MALE REPRODUCTIVE SYSTEM

Alcohol
Alkylating agents (nitrogen mustards, ethylenimines, procarbazine)
Analgesics (phenacetin)
Anesthetic gases (halothane, nitrous oxide, methoxyflurane)
Anticonvulsants (phenytoin)
Anti-infective agents (amphotericin, nitrofurans)
Antimetabolites (5-bromodeoxyuridine, 5-fluorouracil, 6-mercaptopurine)
Antiparasitic drugs (quinine, chloroquine)
Antiparkinson drugs (levodopa)
Antitumor antibiotics (actinomycin D, adriamycin)
Appetite suppressants
Caffeine
Diuretics (thiazides, aldactone)
Drugs of abuse (marijuana, cocaine, anabolic steroids)
Food addtives and contaminants (aflatoxin, DES, gossypol, monosodium glutamate)
Fungicides, fumigants (captan, dibromochloropropane [DBCP], ethylene dibromide)
Herbicides (2,4-D; 2,4,5-T; diquat; paraquat)
Histamines, histamine antagonists (cimetidine)
Industrial chemicals (PCBs; TCDD; PAHs; eg, benzo(*a*)pyrene, hydrazines)
Insecticides (DDT, methoxychlor, chlordane, dichlorvos, chlordecone)
Metals (alumininum, cadmium, lead, mercury)
Narcotic analgesics (opioids)
Physical factors (heat, light, altitude)
Radiation
Rodenticldes (fluoroacetamide)
Solvents (benzene, carbon disulfide, glycol ethers, hexane, toluene, xylene)
Steroids (natural and synthetic androgens, estrogens, and progestins)
Tobacco smoking
Tranquilizers (phenothiazines, monoamine oxidase inhibitors)
Vinblastine, vincristine

TABLE 9.8. EXAMPLES OF AGENTS AFFECTING THE FEMALE REPRODUCTIVE SYSTEM

Alkylating agents (cyclophosphamide, busulfan)
Anesthetic gases (enflurane, halothane, methoxyflurane)
Aniline dyes
Antiparkinson drugs (levodopa)
Appetite suppressants
Chlorinated hydrocarbons (PCBs, chloroform, trichloroethylene)
Drugs of abuse (nicotine, ethanol, marijuana, cocaine, heroin)
Epinephrine, norepinephrine, amphetamines
Flame retardants (TRIS, polybrominated biphenyls)
Folic acid antagonists (methotrexate)
Food additives and contaminants (DES, nitrosamines, monosodium glutamate)
Formaldehyde
Herbicides (2,4-D; 2,4,5-T)
Insecticides (lindane, DDT, methoxychlor, chlordane, parathion, chlordecone)
Metals (arsenic, lead, lithium, mercury, selenium, thallium)
Narcotic and nonnarcotic analgesics (opioids)
Neuroleptics (phenothiazines, imipramine, and amitriptyline)
Plasticizers (phthalic acid ester [DEHP])
Serotonin
Solvents (benzene, carbon disulfide, hexane, toluene, glycol ethers)
Steroids (natural and synthetic androgens, estrogen, and progestins)
Tranquilizers (phenothiazines, reserpine, monoamine oxidase inhibitors)

tem. For example, chemicals acting on the CNS that lead to changes in the secretion of hypothalamic-releasing hormones and/or gonadotropins may inhibit ovulation.

The gonads are targets for many drugs and chemicals, particularly cancer therapeutic agents and alkylating agents that interfere with cell division and, thus, also block spermatogenesis. Agents known to be gonadotoxic in humans include busulfan, chlorambucil, cyclophosphamide, nitrogen mustard, and vinblastin.

The fungicide dibromochloropropane (DBCP) can cause human infertility, apparently by acting on the Sertoli cells in males. DBCP appears to be sex specific because it does not cause comparable toxicity in female laboratory animals. The Sertoli cell also appears to be the main target for both dinitrobenzene and dinitrotoluene.

9.5.4   Testing for Reproductive Toxicity

A number of tests have been developed to assess male and female reproductive capacity. Endpoints that are potentially useful in assessing reproductive capacity are discussed in Chapter 11.

Suggested Further Reading

Hepatotoxicity

Corcoran GB, Fix L, Jones DP, Moslen MT, Nicotera P, Oberhammer FA, Buttyan R: Apoptosis: molecular control point in toxicity. *Toxicol Appl Pharmacol* **128:**169–181, 1994.

Ernster L, Hochstein P: Membrane lipid peroxidation: Cellular mechanisms and toxicological implications. In *Methods in Toxicology, Vol 1B.* New York: Academic Press, 1994, pp 33–44.

Krell H, Metz J, Jaeschke H, et al: Drug-induced intrahepatic cholestasis: characterization of different pathomechanisms. *Arch Toxicol* **60**:124–130, 1987.
Kulkarni AP, Byczkowski JZ: Hepatotoxicity. In *Introduction to Biochemical Toxicology,* 2nd ed. Hodgson E, Levi PE, (eds.). Norwalk, CT: Appleton & Lange, 1994, pp 459–490.
Lieber CS: Alcohol and the liver: 1994 update. *Gastroenterology* **106**:1085–1105, 1994.
Meeks RG, Harrison SD, Bull RJ: *Hepatotoxicology.* Boca Raton, FL: CRC Press, 1991.
Moslen MT: Toxic responses of the liver. In *Casarett & Doull's Toxicology, the Science of Poisons,* 5th ed., Klaassen CD (ed.). New York: McGraw-Hill, pp 403–416, 1996.
Reed DJ: Mechanisms of chemically induced injury and cellular protection mechanisms. In *Introduction to Biochemical Toxicology,* 2nd ed. Hodgson E, Levi PE (eds.). Norwalk, CT: Appleton & Lange, 1994, pp 265–294.

Nephrotoxicity
Ballatori N: Mechanisms of metal transport across liver cell plasma membrane. *Drug Metab Rev* **23**:83–132, 1991.
Chen Q, Jones TW, Brown PC, Stevens JL: The mechanism of cysteine conjugate cytotoxicity in renal epithelial cells. *J Biol Chem* **265**:21603–21611, 1990.
Commandeur JNM, Vermeulen NPE: Molecular and biochemical mechanisms of chemically induced nephrotoxicity: a review. In *Frontiers in Molecular Toxicology,* Marnett LJ (ed.). Washington, DC: American Chemical Society, 1992, pp 73–96.
Goldstein RS, Schnellmann RG: Toxic responses of the kidney. In *Casarett & Doull's Toxicology, the Science of Poisons,* 5th ed. Klaassen CD (ed.). New York: McGraw-Hill, 1996, pp 417–442.
Hook JB, Goldstein RS, (eds.). *Toxicology of the Kidney,* 2nd ed. New York: Raven Press, 1993.
Murray MD, Brater DC: Renal toxicity of the nonsteroidal anti-inflammatory drugs. *Ann Rev Pharmacol Toxicol* **32**:435–465, 1993.
Tarloff JB, Goldstein RS: Biochemical mechanisms of renal toxicity. In *Introduction to Biochemical Toxicology,* 2nd ed. Hodgson E, Levi PE (eds.). Norwalk, CT: Appleton & Lange, 1994, pp 519–546.

Pulmonary Toxicity
Bond, JA: Metabolism and elimination of inhaled drugs and airborne chemicals from the lungs. *Pharmacol Toxicol* **72**:36–47, 1993.
Cho M, Chichester C, Plopper C, Buckpitt A: Biochemical factors important in Clara cell selective toxicity in the lung. *Drug Metabol Rev* **27**:369–386, 1995.
Dahl AR, and Lewis JL: Respiratory tract uptake of inhalants and metabolism of xenobiotics. *Ann Rev Pharmacol Toxicol* **32**:383–407, 1993.
Foth H: Role of the lung in accumulation and metabolism of xenobiotic compounds–implications for chemically induced toxicity. *Crit Rev Toxicol* **25**:165–205, 1995.
Sabourin, PJ: Pulmonary toxicity. In *Introduction to Biochemical Toxicology,* 2nd ed. Hodgson E, Levi PE (eds.). Norwalk, CT: Appleton & Lange, 1994, pp 491–517.
Wheeler CW, Guenthner TM: Cytochrome P450-dependent metabolism of xenobiotics in human lung. *J Biochem Toxicol* **6**:163–169, 1991.
Witschi HR, Last JA: Toxic responses of the respiratory system. In *Casarett & Doull's Toxicology, the Science of Poisons,* 5th ed. Klaassen CD (ed.). New York: McGraw-Hill, 1996, pp 443–462.

Nervous System Toxicity

Abel EL, Jacobson S, Sherwin BT: In utero alcohol exposure: Functional and structural brain damage. *Neurobehav Toxicol Teratol* **5**:363–366, 1983.

Abou-Donia MB (ed): *Neurotoxicology*. Boca Raton, FL: CRC Press, 1992.

Abou-Donia MB, Lapadula DM: Mechanisms of organophosphorus ester-induced delayed neurotoxicity: Type I and Type II. *Ann Rev Pharmacol Toxicol* **30**:405–440, 1990.

Anthony DC, Montine TJ, Graham DC: Toxic responses of the nervous system. In *Casarett & Doull's Toxicology, the Science of Poisons,* 5th ed. Klaassen CD (ed.). New York: McGraw-Hill, 1996, pp 463–486.

Atchison WD, Hare MF: Mechanisms of methylmercury-induced neurotoxicity. *FASEB J* **8**: 622–629, 1994.

Chambers JE, Levi PE (eds.): *Organophosphates. Chemistry, Fate, and Effects*. San Diego: Academic Press, 1992.

Dawson R Jr, Beal MF, Bondy SC, DiMonte DA, Isom GE: Excitotoxins, aging, environmental neurotoxins: implications for understanding human neurodegenerative diseases. *Toxicol Appl Pharmacol* **134**:1–17, 1995.

Ecobichon DJ, Joy RM: *Pesticides and Neurological Diseases,* 2nd ed. Boca Raton, FL: CRC Press, 1994.

Mailman R, Lawler CP, Martin P: Biochemical toxicology of the central nervous system. In *Introduction to Biochemical Toxicology,* 2nd ed. Hodgson E, Levi PE (eds.). Norwalk, CT: Appleton & Lange, 1994, pp 431–457.

Morell P, Goodrum JF, Bouldin TW: Biochemical toxicology of the peripheral nervous system. In *Introduction to Biochemical Toxicology,* 2nd ed. Hodgson E, Levi PE (eds.). Norwalk, CT: Appleton & Lange, 1994, pp 415–429.

National Institutes of Health. Risk assessment for neurobehavioral toxicity. *Environ Health Perspect Suppl* **104**:Suppl 2, 1996.

Neurotoxicity, Identifying and Controlling Poisons of the Nervous System. Congress of the United States Office of Technology Assessment (OTA). Superintendent of Documents, Washington, DC: US Government Printing Office, 1990.

Reproductive System Toxicity

Bosland MC: Male reproductive system. *Carcinogenesis* **15**:339–402, 1994.

Carlsen E, Giwercman A, Keiding N, Skakkebaek NE: Evidence for decreasing quality of semen during past 50 years. *BMJ* **305**:609–612, 1992.

Colborn T, vom Saal FS, Soto AM: Developmental effects of endocrine-disrupting chemicals in wildlife and humans. *Environ Health Perspect* **101**(5):378–384, 1993.

Cummings AM. Toxicological mechanisms of implantation failure. *Fund Appl Toxicol* **15**: 571–579, 1990.

Fabrio S: On predicting environmentally-induced human reproductive hazards: an overview and historical perspective. *Fund Appl Toxicol* **5**:609–614, 1985.

Miller RK, Kellog CD, Saltzman RA: Reproductive and perinatal toxicology. In *Toxicology,* Haley TJ, Berndt WO (eds.). Washington, DC: Hemisphere, 1987, pp 195–309.

Schrag SD, Dixon RL: Occupational exposure associated with male reproductive dysfunction. *Ann Rev Pharmacol Toxicol* **25**:567–592, 1985.

Thomas JA: Toxic responses of the reproductive system. In *Casarett & Doull's Toxicology, the Basic Science of Poisons,* 5th ed. Klaassen CD (ed.). New York: McGraw-Hill, pp 547–581.

CLASSES OF TOXIC CHEMICALS 10

PATRICIA E. LEVI

Chemical toxicants may be classified in various ways depending on interest and need. In previous chapters, toxic chemical agents were discussed in terms of their effects (acute toxicity, carcinogenicity, hepatotoxicity, etc.). In this chapter, chemical toxicants are examined according to exposure or specific use categories. Of major concern today are toxic chemicals found in air, soil, water, food, and the workplace, as well as chemicals encountered in specific use categories such as pesticides, drugs, and solvents.

10.1

AIR POLLUTANTS

10.1.1 History

Air pollution probably occurred as soon as humans started to use wood fires for heat and cooking, and for centuries fire was used in such a way that living areas were filled with smoke. After the invention of the chimney, combustion products and cooking odors were removed from living quarters and vented outside. Later, when soft coal was discovered and used for fuel, coal smoke became a problem in the cities. By the thirteenth century, records show that coal smoke had become a nuisance in London, and in 1273 Edward I made the first antipollution law, one that prohibited the burning of coal while Parliament was in session: "Be it known to all within the sound of my voice, whosoever shall be found guilty of burning coal shall suffer the loss of his head." In spite of this and various other royal edicts, however, smoke pollution continued in London.

Increasing domestic and industrial combustion of coal caused air pollution to get steadily worse, particularly in large cities. During the twentieth century, the most significant change was the rapid increase in the number of automobiles, from almost none at the turn of the century to millions within only a few decades. During this time, few attempts were made to control air pollution in any of the industrialized countries until after World War II. Action was then prompted, in part, by two acute pollution episodes in which human deaths were caused directly by high levels of pollutants. One incident occurred in 1948 in Donora, a small steel mill town in western Pennsylvania. In late October, a heavy smog settled in the area, and a weather inversion prevented the movement of pollutants out of the valley. Twenty-one deaths were attributed directly to the effects of the smog. The "Donora episode" helped focus attention on air pollution in the United States.

In London in December 1952, the now infamous "Killer Smog" occurred. A dense fog at ground level coupled with smoke from coal fireplaces caused a severe smog lasting more than a week. The smog was so heavy that daylight visibility was only a few meters, and bus conductors had to walk in front of the buses to guide the drivers through the streets. Two days after the smog began, the death rate began to climb, and between December 5 and December 9, there were an estimated 4000 deaths above normal. The chief causes of death were bronchitis, pneumonia, and associated respiratory complaints. This disaster resulted in the passage in Britain of the Clean Air Act in 1956.

In the United States, the smog problem also began to occur in large cities across the country, becoming especially severe in Los Angeles. In 1955, federal air pollution legislation was enacted, providing federal support for air pollution research, training, and technical assistance. Responsibility for the administration of the federal programs lies with the United States Environmental Protection Agency (EPA). Technological interest since the mid-1950s has centered on automobile air pollution, pollution by oxides of sulfur and nitrogen, and the control of these emissions. Attention is also being directed toward the problems that may be caused by a possible "greenhouse effect" resulting from increased concentrations of carbon dioxide (CO_2) in the atmosphere, possible depletion of the stratospheric ozone layer, long-range transport of pollution, and acid deposition.

10.1.2 Types of Air Pollutants

What is clean air? Unpolluted air is a concept of what the air would be if humans and their works were not on earth, and if the air were not polluted by natural point sources such as volcanoes, forest fires, and so on. The true composition of "unpolluted" air is unknown because humans have been polluting the air for thousands of years. In addition, there are many natural pollutants such as terpenes from plants, smoke from forest fires, fumes and smoke from volcanoes, and so on. Table 10.1 lists the components that, in the absence of such pollution, are thought to constitute clean air.

GASEOUS POLLUTANTS include substances that are gases at normal temperature and pressure as well as vapors evaporated from substances that are liquid or solid. Among pollutants of greatest concern are carbon monoxide (CO), hydrocarbons, hydrogen sulfide (H_2S), nitrogen oxides (N_xO_y), ozone (O_3) and other oxidants, sulfur oxides

TABLE 10.1. GASEOUS COMPONENTS OF NORMAL DRY AIR

Compound	Percent by Volume	Concentration (ppm)
Nitrogen	78.09	780,900
Oxygen	20.94	209,400
Argon	0.93	9,300
Carbon dioxide	0.0325	325
Neon	0.0018	18
Helium	0.0005	5.2
Methane	0.0001	1.1
Krypton	0.0001	1.0
Nitrous oxide		0.5
Hydrogen		0.5
Xenon		0.008
Nitrogen dioxide		0.02
Ozone		0.01–0.04

(S_xO_y), and CO_2. Pollutant concentrations are usually expressed as micrograms per cubic meter ($\mu g/m^3$) or for gaseous pollutants as parts per million (ppm) by volume in which 1 ppm = 1 part pollutant per million parts (10^6) of air.

PARTICULATE POLLUTANTS consist of fine solids or liquid droplets suspended in air. Some of the different types of particulates are defined as follows:

- *Dust*—relatively large particles about 100 μm in diameter that come directly from substances being used (eg, coal dust, ash, sawdust, cement dust, grain dust).
- *Fumes*—suspended solids less than 1 μm in diameter usually released from metallurgical or chemical processes, (eg, zinc and lead oxides).
- *Mist*—liquid droplets suspended in air with a diameter less than 2.0 μm, (eg, sulfuric acid mist).
- *Smoke*—solid particles (0.05–1.0 μm) resulting from incomplete combustion of fossil fuels.
- *Aerosol*—liquid or solid particles (< 1.0 μm) suspended in air or in another gas.

10.1.3   Sources of Air Pollutants

NATURAL POLLUTANTS. Many pollutants are formed and emitted through natural processes. An erupting volcano emits particulate matter as well as gases such as sulfur dioxide, hydrogen sulfide, and methane; such clouds may remain airborne for long periods of time. Forest and prairie fires produce large quantities of pollutants in the form of smoke, unburned hydrocarbons, CO, nitrogen oxides, and ash. Dust storms are a common source of particulate matter in many parts of the world, and oceans produce aerosols in the form of salt particles. Plants and trees are a major source of hydrocarbons on the planet, and the blue haze that is so familiar over forested mountain areas is mainly from the atmospheric reactions of the volatile organics produced by the trees. Plants also produce pollen and spores, which cause respiratory problems and allergic reactions.

ANTHROPOGENIC POLLUTANTS, come primarily from three sources: (1) combustion sources that burn fossil fuel for heating and power, or exhaust emissions from transportation vehicles that use gasoline or diesel fuels; (2) industrial processes; and (3) mining and drilling.

The principal pollutants from combustion are fly ash, smoke, sulfur, and nitrogen oxides, as well as CO and CO_2. Combustion of coal and oil, both of which contain significant amounts of sulfur, yields large quantities of sulfur oxides. One effect of the production of sulfur oxides is the formation of acidic deposition, including acid rain. Nitrogen oxides are formed by thermal oxidation of atmospheric nitrogen at high temperatures; thus, almost any combustion process will produce nitrogen oxides. Carbon monoxide is a product of incomplete combustion; the more efficient the combustion, the higher the ratio of CO_2 to CO.

Transportation sources, particularly automobiles, are a major source of air pollution and include smoke, lead particles from tetraethyl lead additives, CO, nitrogen oxides, and hydrocarbons. Since the mid-1960s, there has been significant progress in reducing exhaust emissions, particularly with the use of low-lead or no-lead gasolines as well as the use of oxygenated fuels—for example, fuels containing ethanol or MTBE (methyl *t*-butyl ether).

Industries may emit various pollutants relating to their manufacturing processes—acids (sulfuric, acetic, nitric, and phosphoric); solvents and resins; gases (chlorine and ammonia); and metals (copper, lead, and zinc).

INDOOR POLLUTANTS. In general, the term "indoor air pollution" refers to home and non-factory public buildings (eg, office buildings, hospitals). Pollution can come from heating and cooking, pesticides, tobacco smoking, radon, gases, and microbes from people and animals.

Although indoor air pollution has increased in developed nations because of tighter building construction and the use of building materials that may give off gaseous chemicals, indoor air pollution is a particular problem in developing countries. Wood, crop residues, animal dung, and other forms of biomass are used extensively for cooking and heating—often in poorly ventilated rooms. For women and children in particular, this leads to high exposures to air pollutants such as CO and polycyclic aromatic hydrocarbons.

10.1.4 Examples of Air Pollutants

Most of the information on the effects of air pollution on humans comes from acute pollution episodes such as the ones in Donora and London. Illnesses may result from chemical irritation of the respiratory tract, with certain sensitive subpopulations being more affected: (1) very young children, whose respiratory and circulatory systems are poorly developed; (2) the elderly, whose cardiorespiratory systems

TABLE 10.2. PRINCIPAL AIR POLLUTANTS, SOURCES, AND EFFECTS

Pollutant	Sources	Significance
Sulfur oxides, particulates	Coal and oil power plants Oil refineries, smelters Kerosene heaters	Main component of acid deposition Damage to vegetation, materials Irritating to lungs, chronic bronchitis
Nitrogen oxides	Automobile emissions Fossil fuel power plants	Pulmonary edema, impairs lung defenses Important component of photochemical smog and acid deposition
Carbon monoxide	Motor vehicle emissions Burning fossil fuels Incomplete combustion	Combines with hemoglobin to form carboxyhemoglobin, poisonous Asphyxia and death
Carbon dioxide	Product of complete combustion	May cause "greenhouse effect"
Ozone (O_3)	Automobile emissions Photochemical smog	Damage to vegetation Lung irritant
Hydrocarbons, C_xH_y	Smoke, gasoline fumes Cigarette smoke, industry Natural sources	Contributes to photochemical smog Polycyclic aromatic hydrocarbons; lung cancer
Radon	Natural	Lung cancer
Asbestos	Asbestos mines Building materials Insulation	Asbestosis Lung cancer, mesothelioma
Allergens	Pollen, house dust Animal dander	Asthma, rhinitis
Arsenic	Copper smelters	Lung cancer

function poorly; and (3) people with cardiorespiratory diseases such as asthma, emphysema, and heart disease. Heavy smokers are also affected more adversely by air pollutants. In most cases, the health problems are attributed to the combined action of particulates and sulfur dioxides (SO_2); no one pollutant appears to be responsible. Table 10.2 summarizes some of the major air pollutants and their sources and effects.

CARBON MONOXIDE. Carbon monoxide combines readily with hemoglobin (Hb) to form carboxyhemoglobin (COHb), thus preventing the transfer of oxygen to tissues. The affinity of hemoglobin for CO is approximately 210 times its affinity for oxygen. A blood concentration of 5% COHb, equivalent to equilibration at approximately 45 ppm CO, is associated with cardiovascular effects. Concentrations of 100 ppm can cause headaches, dizziness, nausea, and breathing difficulties. An acute concentration of 1000 ppm is invariably fatal. Carbon monoxide levels during acute traffic congestion have been known to be as high as 400 ppm; in addition, people who smoke elevate their total body burden of CO as compared with nonsmokers. The effects of low concentrations of CO over a long period are not known, but it is possible that heart and respiratory disorders are exacerbated.

SULFUR OXIDES. Sulfur dioxide is a common component of polluted air that results primarily from the industrial combustion of coal, with soft coal containing the highest levels of sulfur. The sulfur oxides tend to adhere to air particles and enter the inner respiratory tract, where they are not effectively removed. In the respiratory tract, SO_2 combines readily with water to form sulfurous acid, resulting in irritation of mucous membranes and bronchial constriction. This irritation in turn increases the sensitivity of the airway to other airborne toxicants.

NITROGEN OXIDES. Nitrogen dioxide (NO_2), a gas found in photochemical smog, is also a pulmonary irritant and is known to lead to pulmonary edema and hemorrhage. The main issue of concern is its contribution to the formation of photochemical smog and ozone, although nitrogen oxides also contribute to acid deposition.

OZONE, a highly irritating and oxidizing gas formed by photochemical action of ultra-violet (UV) light on nitrogen dioxide in smog. The resulting ozone can produce pulmonary congestion, edema, and hemorrhage.

$$NO_2 + UV \text{ light} \longrightarrow NO + O^{\bullet}$$
$$O^{\bullet} + O_2 \longrightarrow O_3$$

At this point, it is worth distinguishing between "good" and "bad" ozone. *Tropospheric ozone* occurs from 0 to 10 miles above the earth's surface and is harmful. *Stratospheric ozone*, located about 30 miles above the earth's surface, is responsible for filtering out incoming UV radiation and thus is beneficial. It is the decrease in the stratospheric ozone layer that has been of much concern recently. It is estimated that a 1% decrease in stratospheric ozone will increase the amount of UV radiation reaching the earth's surface by 2% and cause a 10% increase in skin cancer. Major contributors to damage to stratospheric ozone are thought to be the chlorofluorocarbons (CFCs). Chlorine is removed from the CFC compounds in the upper atmosphere by reaction with UV light and is then able to destroy the stratospheric ozone through self-perpetuating free radical reactions.

$$Cl + O_3 \longrightarrow ClO + O_2$$
$$ClO + O \longrightarrow Cl + O_2$$

Before being inactivated by nitrogen dioxide or methane, each chlorine atom can destroy up to 10,000 molecules of ozone. Use of CFC compounds is now being phased out by international agreements.

HYDROCARBONS (HCs) OR VOLATILE ORGANIC COMPOUNDS (VOCs) are derived primarily from two sources: approximately 50% are derived from trees as a result of the respiration process (biogenic); the other 45% to 50% comes from the combustion of fuel and from vapor from gasoline. Many gasoline pumps now have VOC recovery devices to reduce pollution.

LEAD. One of the most familiar of the particulates in air pollutants is lead, with young children and fetuses being the most susceptible. Lead can impair renal function, interfere with the development of red blood cells, and impair the nervous system, leading to mental retardation and even blindness. The two most common routes of exposure to lead are inhalation and ingestion. It is estimated that approximately 20% of the total body burden of lead comes from inhalation.

SOLID PARTICLES, such as dust and fibers from coal, clay, glass, asbestos, and minerals, can lead to scarring or fibrosis of the lung lining. Pneumoconiosis, or dust disease (silicosis), and asbestosis are all well-known industrial pollution diseases.

10.1.5   Environmental Effects

VEGETATION may be visibly injured by pollutants as shown by bleaching, other color changes, and necrosis, or by more subtle changes such as alterations in growth or reproduction. Table 10.3 lists some of the more common visual effects of air pollutants on vegetation. Air pollution can also result in measurable effects on forest ecosystems, such as reduction in forest growth, change in forest species, and increased susceptibility to forest pests. High-dose exposure to pollutants, which is associated with point source emissions such as smelters, frequently results in complete destruction of trees and shrubs in the surrounding area.

DOMESTIC ANIMALS. Although domestic animals can be affected directly by air pollutants, the main concern is chronic poisoning as a result of ingestion of forage that has been contaminated by airborne pollutants. Pollutants important in this connection are arsenic, lead, and molybdenum. Fluoride emissions from industries producing phosphate fertilizers and derivatives have damaged cattle throughout the world. The raw material, phosphate rock, can contain up to 4% fluoride, some of which is released into the air and water. Farm animals, particularly cattle, sheep, and swine, are susceptible to fluoride toxicity (fluorosis), which is characterized by mottled and soft teeth, and osteofluoritic bone lesions which lead to lameness and, eventually, death.

MATERIALS AND STRUCTURES. Building materials have become soiled and blackened by smoke, and damage by chemical attack from acid gases in the air has led to the deterioration of many marble statues in western Europe. Metals are also affected by air pollution; for example, SO_2 causes many metals to corrode at a faster rate. Ozone is known to oxidize rubber products, and one of the effects of Los Angeles smog is cracking of rubber tires. Fabrics, leather, and paper are also affected by SO_2 and sulfuric acid, causing them to crack, become brittle, and tear more easily.

TABLE 10.3. EXAMPLES OF AIR POLLUTION INJURY TO VEGETATION

Pollutant	Symptoms
Sulfur dioxide	Bleached spots, interveinal bleaching
Ozone	Flecking, stippling, bleached spotting
Peroxyacetylnitrate (PAN)	Glazing, silvering, or bronzing on lower leaf surface
Nitrogen dioxide	White or brown collapsed lesion near leaf margins
Hydrogen fluoride	Tip and margin burns, dwarfing

ATMOSPHERIC EFFECTS. The presence of fine particles (0.1–1.0 mm in diameter) or NO_2 in the atmosphere can result in atmospheric haze or reduced visibility due to light scattering by the particles. The major effect of atmospheric haze has been a degradation in visual air quality and is of particular concern in areas of scenic beauty, including most of the major national parks such as Grand Canyon, Yosemite, and Zion Park.

There is also concern over the increase in CO_2 in the atmosphere because CO_2 absorbs heat energy strongly and retards the cooling of the earth. This is often referred to as the "greenhouse effect"; theoretically, an increase in CO_2 levels would result in a global increase in air temperatures. In addition to CO_2, other gases contributing to the greenhouse effect include methane, CFCs, nitrous oxide, and ozone.

ACIDIC DEPOSITION. Acidic deposition is the combined total of wet and dry deposition, with wet acidic deposition being commonly referred to as acid rain. Normal uncontaminated rain has a pH of about 5.6, but acid rain usually has a pH of less than 4.0. In the eastern United States, the acids in acid rain are approximately 65% sulfuric, 30% nitric, and 5% other; whereas in the western states, 80% of the acidity is due to nitric acid.

Many lakes in northeastern North America and Scandinavia have become so acidic that fish are no longer able to live in them. The low pH not only directly affects fish, but also contributes to the release of potentially toxic metals, such as aluminum, from the soil. The maximum effect occurs when there is little buffering of the acid by soils or rock components. Maximum fish kills occur in early spring due to the "acid shock" from the melting of winter snows. Much of the acidity in rain may be neutralized by dissolving minerals in the soil, such as aluminum, calcium, magnesium, sodium, and potassium, which are leached from the soil into surface waters. The ability of the soil to neutralize or buffer the acid rain is very dependent on the alkalinity of the soil. Much of the area in eastern Canada and the northeastern United States is covered by thin soils with low neutralizing capacity. In such areas, the lakes are more susceptible to the effects of acid deposition leading to a low pH and high levels of aluminum, a combination toxic to many species of fish.

A second area of concern is that of reduced tree growth in forests. The leaching of nutrients from the soil by acid deposition may cause a reduction in future growth rates or changes in the type of trees to those able to survive in the altered environment. In addition to the change in soil composition, there are the direct effects on the trees from sulfur and nitrogen oxides as well as ozone.

10.2

SOIL AND WATER POLLUTANTS

With three quarters of the Earth's surface covered by water and much of the remainder covered by soil, it is not surprising that water and soil serve as the ultimate sinks for most anthropogenic chemicals. Until recently, the primary concern with water pollution was that of health effects due to pathogens and, in fact, this is still the case in most developing countries. In the United States and other developed countries, however, treatment methods have largely eliminated bacterial disease organisms from the water supply, and attention has been turned to chemical contaminants.

10.2.1 Sources of Soil and Water Pollutants

Surface water can be contaminated by point or nonpoint sources. A runoff pipe from an industrial plant or a sewage-treatment plant is a point source; a field from which pesticides and fertilizers are carried by rainwater into a river is a nonpoint source. Industrial wastes probably constitute the greatest single pollution problem in soil and water. These contaminants include organic wastes, inorganic wastes, such as chromium and mercury, and many unknown chemicals. Contamination of soil and water results when by-product chemicals are not properly disposed of or conserved. In addition, industrial accidents may lead to severe local contamination. For a more in-depth discussion of sources and movements of water pollutants, see Chapter 16.

Domestic and municipal wastes, both from sewage and from disposal of chemicals, are another major source of chemical pollutants. At the turn of the twentieth century, municipal wastes received no treatment but were discharged directly into rivers or oceans. Even today, many older treatment plants do not provide sufficient treatment, especially plants in which both storm water and sewage are combined. In addition to organic matter, pesticides, fertilizers, detergents, and metals are significant pollutants discharged from urban areas.

Contamination of soil and water also results from the use of pesticides and fertilizers. Persistent pesticides applied directly to the soil have the potential to move from the soil into the water and thus enter the food chain from both soil and water. In a similar manner, fertilizers leach out of the soil and into the natural water systems.

Pollution from petroleum compounds has been a major concern since the mid-1960s. In 1967, the first major accident involving an oil tanker occurred. The *Torrey Canyon* ran onto rocks in the English Channel, spilling oil that washed onto the shores of England and France. It is estimated that at least 10,000 serious oil spills occur in the United States each year. In addition, flushing of oil tankers plays a major role in marine pollution. Other sources, such as improper disposal of used oil by private car owners and small garages, also contribute to oil pollution.

10.2.2 Examples of Pollutants

METALS that are of environmental concern fall into three classes; (1) metals that are suspected carcinogens, (2) metals that move readily in soil, and (3) metals that move through the food chain.

LEAD. The heavy metals of greatest concern for health with regard to drinking water exposure are lead and arsenic. The sources of lead in drinking water that are most important are from lead pipes and lead solder. Also of concern is the seepage of lead from soil contaminated with the fallout from leaded gasoline and seepage of lead from hazardous-waste sites. Lead and associated toxic effects are discussed more fully in Section 10.6.

ARSENIC. Drinking water is at risk for contamination by arsenic from the leaching of inorganic arsenic compounds formerly used in pesticide sprays, from the combustion of arsenic-containing fossil fuels, and from the leaching of mine tailings and smelter runoff. Chronic high-level exposures can cause abnormal skin pigmentation, hyperkeratosis, nasal congestion, and abdominal pain. At lower levels of exposure, cancer is the major concern. Epidemologic studies have linked chronic arsenic exposure to various cancers, including skin, lungs, and lymph glands.

CADMIUM. One of the most significant effects of metal pollution is that aquatic organisms can absorb and accumulate metals in their tissues, leading to increasing concentrations in the food chain. Concern about long-term exposure to cadmium intensified after recognition of the disease Itai-Itai (painful-painful) in certain areas of Japan. The disease is a combination of severe kidney damage and painful bone and joint disease and occurs in areas where rice is contaminated with high levels of cadmium. This contamination resulted from irrigation of the soil with water containing cadmium released from industrial sources. Cadmium toxicity in Japan has also resulted from consumption of cadmium-contaminated fish taken from rivers near the smelting plants.

MERCURY. In Japan in the 1950s and 1960s, wastes from a chemical and plastics plant containing mercury were drained into Minamata Bay. The mercury was converted to the readily absorbed methylmercury by bacteria in the aquatic sediments. Consumption of fish and shellfish by the local population resulted in numerous cases of mercury poisoning, or Minamata disease. By 1970, at least 107 deaths had been attributed to mercury poisoning, and 800 cases of Minamata disease were confirmed. Even though the mothers appeared healthy, many infants born to these mothers who had eaten contaminated fish developed cerebral palsy–like symptoms and mental deficiency.

PESTICIDES are also a major source of concern as soil and water pollutants. Because of their stability and persistence, the most hazardous pesticides are the organochlorine compounds such as DDT, aldrin, dieldrin, and chlordane. Persistent pesticides can accumulate in food chains; for example, shrimp and fish can concentrate some pesticides as much as 1000- to 10,000-fold. This bioaccumulation has been well documented with the pesticide DDT, which is now banned in many parts of the world. In contrast to the persistent insecticides, the organophosphorus (OP) pesticides, such as malathion, and the carbamates, such as carbaryl, are short-lived and generally persist for only a few weeks to a few months. Thus, these compounds do not usually represent as serious a problem as the earlier insecticides. Herbicides, because of the large quantity used, are also of concern as potential toxic pollutants. Peticides are discussed in more detail in Section 10.5.

NITRATES AND PHOSPHATES are two important nutrients that have been increasing markedly in natural waters since the mid-1960. Sources of nitrate contamination include fertilizers, discharge from sewage treatment plants, and leachate from septic systems and manure. Nitrates from fertilizers leach readily from soils, and it has been estimated that up to 40% of applied nitrates enter water sources as runoff and leachate. Fertilizer phosphates, however, tend to be adsorbed or bound to soil particles, so that only 20% to 25% of applied phosphate is leached in water. Phosphate detergents are another source of phosphate, one that has received much media attention in recent years.

The increase in these nutrients, particularly phosphates, is of environmental concern because excess nutrients can lead to "algal blooms" or eutrophication, as it is known, in lakes, ponds, estuaries, and very slow moving rivers. The algal bloom reduces light penetration and restricts atmospheric reoxygenation of the water. When the dense algal growth dies, the subsequent biodegradation results in anaerobic conditions and the death of many aquatic organisms. High phosphate concentrations and algal blooms are not a problem in moving streams, because such streams are continually flushed out and algae do not accumulate.

There are two potential adverse health effects from nitrates in drinking water: (1) nitrosamine formation and (2) methemoglobinemia. Ingested nitrates can be converted to nitrites by intestinal bacteria. After entering the circulatory system, nitrite ions combine with hemoglobin to form methemoglobin, thus decreasing the oxygen-carrying capacity of the blood and resulting in anemia or blue-baby disease. It is particularly severe in young babies who consume water and milk–formula prepared with nitrate-rich water. Older children and adults are able to detoxify the methemoglobin as a result of the enzyme methemoglobin reductase, which reverses the formation of methemoglobin. In infants, however, the enzyme is not fully functional. Certain nitrosamines are known carcinogens.

OILS AND PETROLEUM are ever-present pollutants in the modern environment, whether from the used oil of private motorists or spillage from oil tankers. At sea, oil slicks are responsible for the deaths of many birds. Very few birds that are badly contaminated recover, even after de-oiling and hand feeding. Oil is deposited on rocks and sand as well, thus preventing the beaches from being used for recreation until after costly clean up. Shore animals, such as crabs, shrimp, mussels, and barnacles, are also affected by the toxic hydrocarbons they ingest. The subtle and perhaps potentially more harmful long-term effects on aquatic life are not yet understood.

VOLATILE ORGANIC COMPOUNDS (VOCs). Other common groundwater contaminants include halogenated solvents and petroleum products, collectively referred to as VOCs. Both groups of compounds are used in large quantities by a variety of industries, such as degreasing, dry cleaning, paint, and the military. Historically, protroleum products have been stored in underground tanks that would erode, or were spilled onto soil surfaces. The EPA's National Priority List includes 11 VOCs: trichloroethylene; toluene; benzene; chloroform; tetrachloroethylene; 1,1,1-trichloroethane;

ethylbenzene; trans-1,2-dichloroethane; xylene; dichloromethane; and vinyl chloride.

The physical and chemical properties of VOCs permit them to move rapidly into groundwater, and almost all of the previously mentioned chemicals have been detected in groundwater near contaminant sites. High levels of exposure can cause headache, impaired cognition, and kidney toxicities. At levels of exposure most frequently encountered, cancer and reproductive effects are of most concern, particularly childhood leukemia.

LOW MOLECULAR WEIGHT CHLORINATED HYDROCARBONS are a by-product of the chlorination of municipal water. Chlorine reacts with organic substances commonly found in water to generate trihalomethanes (THMs), such as chloroform. The main organics that have been detected are chloroform, bromodichloromethane, dibromochloromethane, bromoform, carbon tetrachloride, and 1,2-dichloroethane. These compounds are associated with an increased risk of cancer. Studies in New Orleans in the mid-1970s showed that tap water in New Orleans contained more chlorinated hydrocarbons than did untreated Mississippi River water or well water. In addition, chlorinated hydrocarbons, including carbon tetrachloride, were detected in blood plasma from volunteers who drank treated tap water. Epidemiologic studies indicated that the cancer death rate was higher among white males who drank tap water than among those who drank well water.

RADIOACTIVE CONTAMINATION. Although some background radiation from natural sources, such as radon, occurs in some regions of the world, there is particluar concern over the contamination of surface water and groundwater by radioactive compounds generated by the production of nuclear weapons and by the processing of nuclear fuel. Many of these areas have remained unrecognized because of government secrecy.

ACIDS, present in rain or drainage from mines, are major pollutants in many freshwater lakes. Because of their ability to lower the pH of the water to toxic levels and release toxic metals into solution, acids are considered particularly hazardous (see Section 10.1.5).

PCBs. The number of organic compounds found as soil and water contaminants continues to grow each year. They include polychlorinated biphenyls (PCBs), phenols, cyanides, plasticizers, solvents, and numerous industrial chemicals. PCBs are by-products of the plastic, lubricant, rubber, and paper industries. They are stable, lipophilic, and break down only slowly in tissues. Because of these properties, they accumulate to high concentrations in waterfowl; in 1969, PCBs were responsible for the death of thousands of birds in the Irish Sea.

DIOXIN. Large areas of water and soil have been contaminated with the extremely toxic TCDD (2,3,7,8-tetrachlorodibenzo-p-dioxin) through industrial accidents and through widespread use of the herbicide 2,4,5-T, which contained small amounts of TCDD as a contaminant in herbicide manufacturing (see Section 10.5.6 and Fig. 10.8). The US Army used this herbicide, known as Agent Orange, extensively as a defoliant in Vietnam. TCDD is one of the most toxic synthetic substances known for laboratory animals: LD50 for male rats, 0.022 mg/kg; LD50 for female rats, 0.045 mg/kg; LD50 for female guinea pigs (the most sensitive species tested), 0.0006 mg/kg. In addition, it is fetotoxic to pregnant rats at a dose of only 1/400 of the LD50, and has been shown to cause birth defects at levels of 1–3 ng/kg. TCDD is a proved carcinogen in both mice and rats, with the liver being the primary target. Although TCDD does not appear to be particularly acutely toxic to humans, chronic low-level exposure is suspected of contributing to reproductive abnormalities and carcinogenicity.

10.3

FOOD ADDITIVES AND CONTAMINANTS

Direct, or intentional, food additives are natural or synthetic compounds added deliberately to make some change in the food product; for example, to add color, to preserve, or to provide a nutritional supplement. Indirect, or unintentional, additives are chemicals or compounds that are present but have not been added deliberately. They may include chemicals such as pesticides or chemicals derived from packaging materials.

Food additives are almost as old as humans, being first added to food by fire and smoke when meats were cooked, and as salts and spices later added to foods for flavor. The Egyptians were known to have used food colorings as early as 3500 years ago.

The Food Additive Amendment of 1958 (an amendment to the Food, Drug and Cosmetic Act of 1938) provides that any substance added to food must be proved safe by the manufacturer before it is offered for sale, except for those additives generally recognized as safe (the GRAS list), based on past experience and conditions of intended use. The Color Additive Amendment (1960) required colorings to be reexamined, and those found to cause cancer in laboratory animals were banned while establishing use limits for others (certified colors). Colorings currently in use, however, are permitted to remain in use as "uncertified" colors until scientific tests are completed.

10.3.1 Types of Food Additives

Food additives are used by the food industry for four primary reasons: nutrition, freshness, sensory effects, and processing.

- Nutritive additives are used to prevent or eliminate nutritional deficiencies, such as the addition of iodine to table salt to prevent goiter, or to replace nutrients lost in processing—for example, thiamine, which is lost in processing wheat and rice.

- Antioxidants, preservatives, sequestrants, and stabilizers are the main types of chemicals used to extend the shelf life of food by maintaining freshness and retarding spoilage.
- Sensory additives are compounds used to change or maintain aroma, flavor, texture, or the color of foods. All of these components affect the acceptability and thus the marketability of food.
- Processing aids, such as bleaching agents, help make processing of food faster or simpler.

Table 10.4 gives a partial listing of the many use categories of food additives and some examples of each. Only a few of these additives are discussed in detail.

FOOD COLORINGS are added to enhance the visual appeal of food products. Colors may be derived from natural compounds, such as carotene and chlorophyll, or they may be synthetic. The synthetic dyes currently in use are all water soluble and almost all are insoluble in organic solvents. Some of these are listed in Table 10.5. FD&C lakes, derivatives of the dye, are insoluble pigments made by adsorbing the dye onto aluminum hydroxide. These pigments color the food by dispersion. The only fat-soluble colors are found among the natural dyes. Among the natural coloring agents, the carotenoids are the most widespread, occurring in numerous fruits and vegetables such as carrots, tomatoes, apricots, and oranges. These colors are essen-

TABLE 10.4. TYPES OF FOOD ADDITIVES AND EXAMPLES

Types of Additives	Examples
Anticaking agents	Calcium silicate, magnesium carbonate
Antioxidants	Ascorbic acid, BHT, BHA
Bleaching agents	Benzoylperoxide
Colors	Synthetic and natural
Curing and pickling agents	Nitrites, nitrates, salt, sodium triphosphate
Emulsifiers	Lecithin, cholic acid
Firming agents	Alum in pickles
Flavor enhancers	Monosodium glutamate (MSG)
Flavorings	Natural (spices) and synthetic (aldehydes)
Humectants	Sorbitol, propylene glycol
Leavening	Baking powder
Nutrient supplements	Vitamins and minerals
pH agents	Acids (acetic, tartaric), bases (sodium bicarbonate), buffers (sodium citrate)
Preservatives	Calcium propionate, sodium benzoate
Propellants	Nitrogen gases, carbon dioxide
Sequesterants	Calcium acetate, sodium citrate, EDTA
Stabilizers	Starches and gums
Surfactants	Vegetable gums, monoglycerides, diglycerides
Sweeteners (nonsugar)	Saccharin, aspartame, acetsulfam
Texturizers	Starches

TABLE 10.5. EXAMPLES OF CERTIFIED SYNTHETIC COLORS

Official Name	Common Name
FD&C Blue No. 1[a]	Brilliant Blue FCF
FD&C Blue No. 2	Indigo Carmine
FD&C Green No. 3	Fast Green FCF
FD&C Red No. 3	Erythrosine
FD&C Red No. 40	Allura Red AC
FD&C Yellow No. 5	Tartrazine
FD&C Yellow No. 6	Sunset Yellow FCF
Citrus Red No. 2	Solvent Red 80
Orange B	Acid Orange 137

[a] FD&C = Food, Drug and Cosmetic Act.

tial in situations in which oil-soluble food colors are deemed necessary. Annatto colors are extracted from the seeds of the tropical tree, *Bixa orellana*; the extract, bixin, which is oil soluble, is used to color butter, margarine, popcorn oil, and salad dressings. Titanium dioxide (TiO_2), a white pigment, is used primarily in icings or is mixed with sugar syrup as a coating for pharmaceutical tablets.

A common assumption is that the "artificial" colors are more hazardous than "natural" or "vegetable" dyes. In fact, the artificial dyes are purified synthetic compounds whose toxicology has been studied in detail, whereas the natural dyes are often complex mixtures whose only toxicologic assessment is that humans have used them with apparent safety for many years.

Many of the synthetic dyes have been banned in the United States because of problems associated with use (for example, overuse of FD&C Orange No. 1 and FD&C Red No. 3 in candy and popcorn led to cases of diarrhea in children) or because of the results from chronic toxicity testing. Amaranth, FD&C Red No. 2, is now banned because studies carried out by the US Food and Drug Administration (FDA) suggested that it was embryotoxic in the rat. Another controversy is that certain food dyes, particularly Yellow No. 5 (Tartrazine) may cause hyperactivity in children; however, animal studies to date have failed to confirm this. A greater problem, however, may be the allergic reactions that many people have to this dye.

ANTIOXIDANTS. Lipids in foods can undergo oxidative degradation that results in off-flavors and off-odors. The use of food antioxidants are effective in preventing or retarding certain oxidation reactions, such as lipid oxidation of unsaturated fatty acids, which produces a "rancid" flavor. Some antioxidants are also added to fruits and vegetables to prevent enzymatic browning. Most of the naturally occurring antioxidants, as well as the synthetic antioxidants used in foods, are phenols (Fig. 10.1). The commonly used phenols include butylated hydroxyanisole (BHA), butylated hydroxytoluene (BHT), various gallates, ascorbic acid, and α-tocophenol.

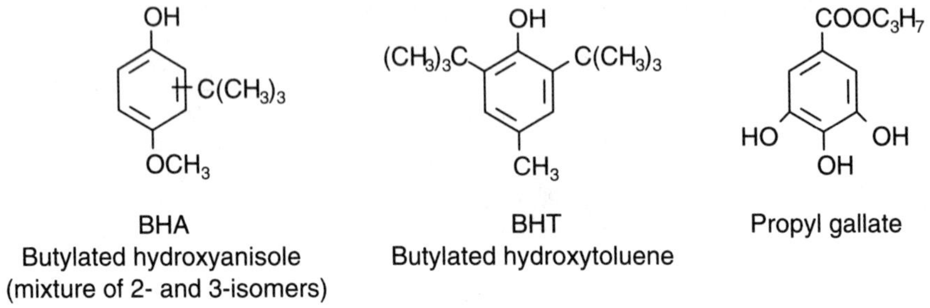

Figure 10.1. Structures of some commonly used antioxidants.

Recent interest has centered on the potential protective role of these compounds as anticarcinogens by virtue of their role as antioxidants and free-radical scavengers.

PRESERVATIVES are added to prolong the shelf life of foods by preventing or inhibiting microbial growth. Table 10.6 lists some of the approved antimicrobial agents and uses. Structures of some of the more common ones are given in Fig. 10.2. Benzoic acid and sodium benzoate have been used for many years as antimicrobial agents in foods. Because they are most active at pH less than 4.0, they have been used widely in carbonated drinks, fruit juices, and pickles. Sodium benzoate is considered to be most active against yeasts and bacteria. Benzoate is readily excreted from the body, being conjugated with either glycine or glucuronic acid, and eliminated through the urine. The alkyl esters (methyl, ethyl, propyl, and butyl) of *p*-hydroxybenzoic acid (parabens) are similar in structure to benzoic acid, but are effective at a higher pH, primarily against molds and yeasts. Hydrolysis of the esters and conjugation constitute the chief route of elimination in mammals.

Sorbic acid and its sodium and potassium salts are particularly effective against molds and yeasts, and for this reason have found extensive use in foods and

TABLE 10.6. SOME ANTIMICROBIAL AGENTS USED IN THE UNITED STATES

Preservative	Important Uses
Benzoic acid, sodium benzoate	Beverages, margarine, pickles
Ethyl and propyl paraben	Beverages, beer, pastries, dried fruit
Sorbates	Beverages, wine, cheese, pastries, dried fruits, processed meats
Propionates	Cheese, baked goods
Sulfides	Beverages, wines, pickles, dried fruits
Acetates, diacetates	Baked goods, salad dressings, pickles
Nitrite, nitrate	Processed meat
Ethylene and propylene oxide	Spices, nuts, glazed fruit
Diethylpyrocarbonate	Wine

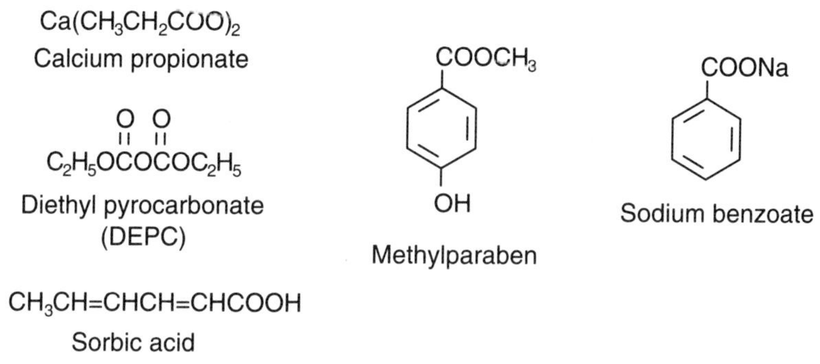

$Ca(CH_3CH_2COO)_2$
Calcium propionate

$$\underset{C_2H_5OCOCOC_2H_5}{\overset{\displaystyle O\ \ O}{\overset{\displaystyle ||\ \ ||}{}}}$$

Diethyl pyrocarbonate
(DEPC)

$CH_3CH=CHCH=CHCOOH$
Sorbic acid

COOCH₃ (Methylparaben structure with OH)

Methylparaben

COONa (Sodium benzoate structure)

Sodium benzoate

Figure 10.2. Structures of some preservatives used in food.

on food wrappers—especially for cheese products and baked goods. Sorbic acid has very low toxicity, probably because it is metabolized in the same way as other fatty acids. Both sodium and calcium propionates are more active against bread molds than is sodium benzoate. The calcium salt is preferred in bread because the calcium also contributes to nutritive value. The sodium salt is used in cakes and other baked goods in which the calcium ion can interfere with chemical leavening. No known mammalian toxicity is associated with the propionates.

Sulfur dioxide has been used for centuries in the wine-making industries, and the sulfides, sodium and potassium salts, are used extensively in the drying of fruits and vegetables. The use of sulfides is limited by the fact that, at levels below 500 ppm, the disagreeable taste becomes noticeable. Acetic acid (vinegar) and its salts are effective antimicrobials, especially at an acidic pH when the salts are dissociated to form the free acid. Vinegar is used in such foods as catsup, mayonnaise, pickles, and salad dressings, whereas the acetate salts are used in baked goods.

Nitrates and nitrites are used in the curing of meats to develop and fix the color; the nitrites decompose to NO, which then reacts with heme pigments to form nitrosomyoglobin, imparting the characteristic pink color to processed meats. Nitrites, in conjunction with the added sodium chloride, also provide antimicrobial action. Controversy in recent years has centered on the role nitrites might play in carcinogenesis. Most N-nitroso compounds, such as dimethylnitrosamine (DMN), are carcinogenic in a wide range of animal species. Some nitroso compounds are found in preserved meats as a result of interaction of nitrites and secondary or tertiary amines; in addition, the stomach provides favorable conditions for the generation of nitrosamines from nitrites and amines. At a low pH, nitrite is protonated to nitrous acid, a very reactive nitrosating and oxidizing agent. Although the carcinogenicity of nitroso compounds has been demonstrated in animals, epidemiologic studies have not yet established a valid association between cancer and exposure to nitrates and nitrites in humans.

Ethylene and propylene oxides are used as fumigants on dry foods such as spices and nutmeats. Both are broad-range microbiocides and ethylene oxide is effective against viruses. Diethylpyrocarbonate (DEPC) permits "cold sterilization" of foods, especially wines, in which it kills yeasts. DEPC is rapidly hydrolyzed to ethanol and CO_2, leaving only trace residues and no taste or odor.

FLAVORS AND FLAVOR ENHANCERS. Flavor additives constitute the largest group of additives used in foods, with the most commonly used ones numbering about 150. Of these, about half are natural, and the remainder are synthetic. Most of the additives are on the GRAS list; thus, their safety is subject to review. Frequently used natural flavorings are derived from spices and fruits (basil, clove, ginger, lemon, pepper, vanilla, etc.), whereas many synthetic flavors are esters, aldehydes, and ketones. Flavor enhancers, such as monosodium glutamate (MSG), enhance the flavor of foods to which they have been added.

NONNUTRITIVE SWEETENERS. The need for low-calorie or nonnutritive sweeteners has been recognized for the control of diabetes and for others wishing to restrict sugar intake. Saccharin (Fig. 10.3), discovered accidentally in 1879, has been used by diabetics for many years. Other sweeteners have been introduced by the soft-drink industry, with one of the most successful being sodium cyclamate because it did not leave the bitter aftertaste characteristic of saccharin. Chronic testing of these sweeteners has yielded conflicting results. Early tests indicated that cyclamate alone did not possess carcinogenic activity, but a subsequent test, using a combination of cyclamate and saccharin, produced bladder tumors in rats. Initially, cyclamate was implicated and banned from use in the United States. Later studies showed that saccharin alone in very high doses could produce bladder tumors, and as a result, saccharin was banned in Canada and cyclamates were permitted. In the United States a moratorium was placed on a proposed saccharin ban in the United States because of public reaction and the fact that saccharin was the only artificial sweetener in use at that time. Products containing saccharin, however, are required to carry a label warning of its potential carcinogenicity.

A more recent sugar substitute is aspartame (Nutrasweet), composed of two naturally occurring amino acids, aspartic acid and phenylalanine. Extensive toxicologic testing to date has not shown any carcinogenic potential. Because it does not leave a bitter aftertaste, aspartame is frequently preferred to saccharin and most diet soft drinks in the United States are now sweetened with aspartame.

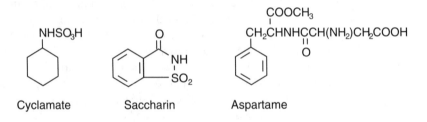

Figure 10.3. Chemical structures of three widely used artificial sweeteners.

There is, however, a problem with use of aspartame for people with the disease phenylketonuria (PKU). This condition, caused by a mutant recessive gene, results in the absence of the enzyme phenylalanine hydroxylase, which converts phenylalanine to tyrosine; about 1 in every 10,000 persons develops PKU. In the absence of phenylalanine hydroxylase, a minor pathway, little used in normal individuals, becomes prominent; this path converts phenylalanine to phenylpyruvic acid, which accumulates in the blood and is excreted in the urine. In childhood, excess circulating phenylpyruvate impairs normal brain development, causing mental retardation. PKU was among the first genetic defects of metabolism recognized in humans, and the urine of infants is tested routinely for the disease. Restriction of dietary phenylalanine reduces the blood level of phenylpyruvic acid and prevents the mental retardation. For this reason, people with PKU are advised not to use products sweetened with aspartame, and products containing aspartame carry a warning label for consumers.

10.3.2 Unintentional Additives and Contaminants

Unintentional, or indirect, additives and contaminants are agents that accidentally or incidentally find their way into the finished food product. Table 10.7 lists some of these agents and the point at which they may contaminate foods. These contaminants include such diverse pollutants as insect parts, pesticides, phytotoxins, mycotoxins, and antibiotics. Examples of some common types of contaminants of concern to toxicologists are in the following list and many of these are discussed in detail in other sections of this text:

- Metals (selenium, lead, mercury)
- Pathogens such as bacteria (*Clostridium botulinium, Salmonella* spp), mycotoxins (aflatoxins), viral infections (raw shellfish from waters contaminated by sewage)

TABLE 10.7. SOURCES AND TYPES OF UNINTENTIONAL FOOD ADDITIVES

During Production
  Antibiotics
  Growth-promoting substances
  Parasites and microorganisms
  Pesticides
  Metals
  Radioactive compounds
During Processing
  Microorganisms and toxins
  Processing residues
  Radionucleotides
  Miscellaneous foreign objects
During Packaging and Storage
  Labeling and stamping materials
  Packaging material chemicals
  Microorganisms
  Chemicals from external sources

- Organic compounds (PCBs, polybrominated biphenyls [PBBs])
- Pesticides
- Antibiotic residues
- Hormone residues
- Packaging materials

The most important of the indirect additives are anabolic agents and antibiotics used in raising animals used for food as well as ingredients of packaging material that may migrate into food.

PACKAGING MATERIALS. Conventional packing materials such as paper and wood are considered safe, whereas more recent synthetic materials made of polymeric materials may need more careful evaluation. The polymers themselves are generally inert, but the monomers, residual reactants, intermediates, solvents, and so on, may migrate into the food. Some of these chemicals, such as vinyl chloride and acrylonitrile, have been shown to be carcinogenic, but because of the exceedingly low levels of exposure, their continued use is permitted. Packaging dyes may also leach onto foods from containers.

DRUG RESIDUES. Drugs may present a problem related not only to the parent chemical, but also to its metabolite. Antibiotics are usually added to feeds both to prevent disease and to promote growth. Because residues are generally very low they are not expected to cause toxicity. However, there is concern relating to the emergence of resistant strains of pathogenic organisms and to hypersensitivity reactions in people taking the same antibiotic for medical reasons. Anabolic agents are growth promoting substances and are usually implanted subcutaneously in a part of the animal that is not eaten, such as the ear. Residue levels in meat are generally low enough to be free of toxic effects, although there is concern over potential carcinogenicity even at very low levels. Anabolic agents include natural or endogenous compounds such as estradiol, progesterone, and testosterone, or synthetic compounds, such as trenbolone acetate and zeranol.

MYCOTOXINS. Aflatoxins, produced by the mold *Aspergillus flavus*, occur on nuts and grains, especially in warm, humid conditions. The aflatoxins exist as a mixture of toxins, with aflatoxin B_1 being the most potent carcinogen. In addition, a positive correlation has been noted between aflatoxin intake and liver cancer incidence in some regions of Africa and Thailand (see Fig. 4.2 for the bioactivation of aflatoxin). Other micotoxins include the trichothecenes from *Fusarium* spp and *Trichoderm* spp, ochratoxins from *Aspergillus* and *Penicillium*, and ergot from *Claviceps purpurea*.

METALS. Among the metals that have caused most concern are mercury, lead, and cadmium. A number of poisoning episodes have resulted from mercury compounds that were used as fungicides on seed grain. The poisonings occurred either from improper application or from the use of the seed grain as food. Other cases of mercury toxicity have occurred as a result of eating fish contaminated with methyl mercury.

Lead is a widespread contaminant as it has been used in the past as a fuel additive, in paints, pipes, batteries, canning, and so on. Humans are exposed to this metal from air, water, and food sources. Another source of lead is from improperly fired ceramic eating containers. The lead is released from the glaze and may contaminate food in contact with the containers. Although glazes and pottery in the United States are generally safe, pottery from developing countries, especially from small shops, are more likely to be a source of lead contamination.

Cadmium is released into the environment from industrial sources and may enter the food chain through contaminated soil and water. In Japan the disease Itai-Itai that affects bones, joints, and kidneys results from eating rice grown in areas contaminated with cadium.

ORGANIC COMPOUNDS. Among organic chemicals that have raised concern are organochlorine insecticides, PCBs, and dioxin and related chemicals. Although use of these compounds has declined because of their persistence in the environment, they are still present in foods in trace amounts.

10.4

OCCUPATIONAL TOXICANTS

Assessment of hazards in the workplace is a concern of occupational/industrial toxicology and has a history that dates back to ancient civilizations. The Greek historian Strabo, who lived in the first century AD, gave a graphic description of the arsenic mines in Pantus: "The air in mines is both deadly and hard to endure on account of the grievous odor of the ore, so that the workmen are doomed to a quick death." With the coming of the industrial revolution in the nineteenth century, industrial diseases increased, and new ones, such as chronic mercurialism caused by exposure to mercuric nitrate used in "felting" animal furs, were identified. Hatmakers, who were especially at risk, frequently developed characteristic tremors known as "hatters' shakes," and the expression "mad as a hatter" was coined. In recent years, concern has developed over the carcinogenic potential of many workplace chemicals.

10.4.1 Regulation of Exposure Levels

The goal of occupational toxicology is to ensure work practices that do not entail any unnecessary health risks. To do this, it is necessary to define suitable permissible levels of exposure to industrial chemicals, using the results of animal studies and epidemiologic studies. These levels can be expressed by the following terms for allowable concentrations.

THRESHOLD LIMIT VALUES (TLVs) refer to airborne concentrations of substances and represent conditions under which it is believed that nearly all workers may be repeatedly exposed day after day without adverse effect. Because of wide variation in individual susceptibility, a small percentage of workers may experience discomfort from some substances at or below the threshold limit; a smaller percentage may be affected more seriously by aggravation of a preexisting condition or by development of an occupational illness. Threshold limits are based on the best available information from industrial experience, from experimental human and animal studies, and, when possible, from a combination of the three. The basis on which the values are established may differ from substance to substance; protection against impairment of health may be a guiding factor for some, whereas reasonable freedom from irritation, narcosis, nuisance, or other forms of stress may form the basis for others. Three categories of TLVs follow.

THRESHOLD LIMIT VALUE–TIME-WEIGHTED AVERAGE (TLV–TWA) is the TWA concentration for a normal 8-hour workday or 40-hour workweek to which nearly all workers may be repeatedly exposed, day after day, without adverse effect. Time-weighted averages allow certain permissible excursions above the limit provided they are compensated by equivalent excursions below the limit during the workday. In some instances, the average concentration is calculated for a workweek rather than for a workday.

THRESHOLD LIMIT VALUE–SHORT-TERM EXPOSURE LIMIT (TLV–STEL) is the maximal concentration to which workers can be exposed for a period up to 15 minutes continuously without suffering from (1) irritation, (2) chronic or irreversible tissue change, or (3) narcosis of sufficient degree that would increase accident proneness, impair self-rescue, or materially reduce work efficiency, provided that no more than four excursions per day are permitted, with at least 60 minutes between exposure periods, and provided that the daily TLV–TWA is not exceeded.

THRESHOLD LIMIT VALUE–CEILING (TLV–C) is the concentration that should not be exceeded even instantaneously. For some substances—for instance, irritant gases—only one category, the TLV ceiling, may be relevant. For other substances, two or three categories may be relevant.

BIOLOGIC LIMIT VALUES (BLVs) represent limits of amounts of substances (or their affects) to which the worker may be exposed without hazard to health or well-being as determined by measuring the worker's tissues, fluids, or exhaled breath. The biologic measurements on which the BLVs are based can furnish two kinds of information useful in the control of worker exposure: (1) measure of the worker's overall exposure, and (2) measure of the worker's individual and characteristic response. Measurements of response furnish a superior estimate of the physiological status of the worker, and may consist of: (1) changes in amount of some critical biochemical constituent, (2) changes in activity or a critical enzyme, and (3) changes in some physiological function. Measurement of exposure may be made by (1) determining in blood, urine, hair, nails, or body tissues and fluids, the amount of substance to which the worker was exposed; (2) determinating the amount of the metabolite(s) of the substance in tissues and fluids; and (3) determinating the amount of the substance in the exhaled breath. The biologic limits may be used as an adjunct to the TLVs for air, or in place of them.

IMMEDIATELY DANGEROUS TO LIFE OR HEALTH (IDLH). Conditions that pose an immediate threat to life or health or conditions that pose an immediate threat of severe exposure to contaminants, such as radioactive materials, that are likely to have adverse cumulative or delayed effects on health are termed IDLH. Two factors are considered when establishing IDLH concentrations. The worker must be able to escape: (1) without loss of life or without suffering permanent health damage within 30 minutes; and (2) without severe eye or respiratory irritation or other reactions that could inhibit escape. If the concentration is above the IDLH, only highly reliable breathing apparatus is allowed.

10.4.2 Routes of Exposure

The principal routes of industrial exposure are dermal and inhalation. Occasionally toxic agents may be ingested if food or drinking water is contaminated. Exposure to the skin often leads to localized effects known as "occupation dermatosis" caused by either irritating chemicals or allergenic chemicals. Such effects include scaling, eczema, acne, pigmentation changes, ulcers, and neoplasia. Some chemicals may also pass through the skin; these include aromatic amines such as aniline and solvents such as carbon tetrachloride and benzene.

Toxic or potentially toxic agents may be inhaled into the respiratory tract where they may cause localized effects such as irritation (eg, ammonia, chlorine gas), inflammation, necrosis, and cancer. Chemicals may also be absorbed by the lungs into the circulatory system, thereby leading to systemic toxicity (eg, CO, lead).

10.4.3 Examples of Industrial Toxicants

CARCINOGENS. Aside from exposure to carcinogens due to lifestyle, such as cigarette smoking, occupation is an important source of exposure to carcinogens. Table 10.8 lists some occupational chemical hazards and the cancers associated with them.

CADMIUM is a very cumulative toxicant with a biologic half-life of more than 10 years in humans. More than 70% of the cadmium in the blood is bound to red blood cells; accumulation occurs mainly in the kidney and the liver, where cadmium is bound to metallothionein. In humans, the critical target organ after long-term exposure to cadmium is the kidney, with the first detectable symptom of kidney toxicity being an increased excretion of specific proteins.

CHROMIUM toxicity results from compounds of hexavalent chromium that can be readily absorbed by the lung and gastrointestinal (GI) tract and to a lesser extent by the skin. Occupational exposure to chromium (Cr^{6+}) causes dermatitis, ulcers on the hands and arms, perforation of the nasal septum (probably caused by chromic acid), inflammation of the larynx and liver, and bronchitis. Chromate is a carcinogen causing bronchogenic carcinoma; the risk to chromate plant workers for lung cancer is 20 times greater than that for the general population. Compounds of trivalent chromium are poorly absorbed. Chromium is not a cumulative chemical and, once absorbed, it is rapidly excreted into the urine.

LEAD is a ubiquitous toxicant in the environment, and consequently the normal body concentration of lead is dependent on environmental exposure conditions. Approximately 50% of lead deposited in the lung is absorbed, whereas usually less than 10% of ingested lead passes into the circulation. Lead is not a major occupational

TABLE 10.8. SOME OCCUPATIONAL HAZARDS AND ASSOCIATED CANCERS

Agent	Tumor Sites	Occupation
Asbestos	Lung, pleura, peritoneum	Miners, manufacturers, users
Arsenic	Skin, lung, liver	Miners and smelters, oil refinery workers, pesticide workers
Benzene	Hemopoietic tissue	Process workers, textile workers
Cadmium	Lung, kidney, prostate	Battery workers, smelters
Chloroethers	Lung	Chemical plant workers, process workers
Chromium	Lung, nasal cavity, sinuses	Process and production workers, pigment workers
Mustard gas	Bronchi, lung, larynx	Production workers
Naphthylamines	Bladder	Dyestuff makers and workers, chemical workers, printers
Nickel	Lung, nasal sinuses	Smelters and process workers
Polycyclic hydrocarbons	Respiratory system, bladder	Furnace, foundry, shale, and gas workers; chimney sweeps
Radon, radium, uranium	Skin, lung, bone tissue, bone marrow	Medical and industrial chemists, miners
UV radiation	Skin	Outdoor exposure
X-rays	Bone marrow, skin	Medical and industrial workers

problem today, but environmental pollution is still widespread. Lead interferes in the biosynthesis of porphyrins and heme, and several screening tests for lead poisoning make use of this interaction by monitoring either inhibition of the enzyme δ-aminolevulinic acid dehydratase (ALAD) or appearance in the urine of aminolevulinic acid (ALA) and coproporphorin (UCP). The metabolism of inorganic lead is closely related to that of calcium and excess lead can be deposited in the bone, where it remains for years. Inorganic lead poisoning can produce fatigue, sleep disturbances, anemia, colic, and neuritis. Severe exposure, mainly of children who have ingested lead, may cause encephalopathy, mental retardation, and occasionally, impaired vision.

Organic lead has an affinity for brain tissue; mild poisoning may cause insomnia, restlessness, and GI symptoms, whereas severe poisoning results in delirium, hallucinations, convulsions, coma, and even death.

MERCURY is widely used in scientific and electrical apparatus, with the largest industrial use of mercury being in the chlorine–alkali industry for electrolytic production of chlorine and sodium hydroxide. Worldwide, this industry has been a major source of mercury contamination. Most mercury poisoning, however, has been due to methyl mercury, particularly as a result of eating contaminated fish. Inorganic and organic mercury differ in their routes of entry and absorption. Inhalation is the principal route of uptake of metallic mercury in industry, with approximately 80% of the mercury inhaled as vapor being absorbed; metallic mercury is less readily absorbed by the GI route. The principal sites of deposition are the kidney and brain after exposure to mercury vapor and the kidney after exposure to inorganic mercury salts. Organic mercury compounds are readily absorbed by all routes. Industrial mercurialism produces features such as inflammation of the mouth, muscular tremors (hatters' shakes), psychic irritation, and a nephrotic syndrome characterized by proteinuria. Overall, however, occupational mercurialism is not a significant problem today.

BENZENE was used extensively in the rubber industry as a solvent for rubber latex in the latter half of the nineteenth century. The volatility of benzene, which made it so attractive to the industry, also caused high atmospheric levels of the solvent. Benzene-based rubber cements were used in the canning industry and in the shoe manufacturing industry. Although cases of benzene poisoning had been reported as early as 1897 and additional reports and warnings were issued in the 1920s, the excellent solvent properties of benzene resulted in its continued extensive use. In the 1930s, cases of benzene toxicity occurred in the printing industry in which benzene was used as an ink solvent. Today, benzene use exceeds 11 billion gallons per year.

Benzene affects the hematopoietic tissue in the bone marrow and also appears to be an immunosuppressant. There is a gradual decrease in white blood cells, red blood cells, and platelets, and any combination of these signs may be seen. Continued exposure to benzene results in severe bone marrow damage and aplastic anemia. Benzene exposure has also been associated with leukemia.

ASBESTOS AND OTHER FIBERS. Asbestos is a general name for a group of naturally occurring silicates that will separate into flexible fibers. Chrysotile is the most important commercially and represents about 90% of the total used. Use of asbestos has been extensive, especially in roofing and insulation, asbestos cements, brake linings, electrical appliances, and coating materials. Asbestosis, a respiratory disease, is characterized by fibrosis, calcification, and lung cancer. In humans, not only is there a long latency period between exposure and development of tumors, but other factors also influence the development of lung cancer. Cigarette smoking, for example, enhances tumor formation. Recent studies have shown that stomach and bowel cancers occur in excess in workers (such as insulation workers) exposed to asbestos. Other fibers have been shown to cause a similar disease spectrum, for instance, zeolite fibers.

10.5

PESTICIDES

Pesticides are unusual among environmental pollutants in that they are used deliberately for the purpose of killing some form of life. The ideal situation, of course, is that pesticides be highly selective, destroying target organisms while leaving nontarget organisms unharmed. In reality, most pesticides are not so selective. In considering the use of pesticides, the benefits must be weighed against the risk to human health and environmental quality. Among the benefits of pesticides are control of vectorborne diseases, increased agricultural productivity, and control of urban pests. A major risk is environmental contamination, especially translocation within the environment where pesticides may enter both food chains and natural water systems. Factors to be considered in this regard are persistence in the environment and potential for bioaccumulation.

10.5.1   Organochlorine Insecticides

The chlorinated hydrocarbon insecticides include DDT, methoxychlor, chlordane, hepatochlor, aldrin, dieldrin, endrin, toxaphene, mirex, kepone, strobane, pentac, and lindane. The structures of several of the most familiar ones are shown in Fig. 10.4. The chlorinated hydrocarbons are neurotoxicants and cause acute effects by interfering with the transmission of nerve impulses along the axons. DDT apparently changes the transport of sodium and potassium across the axon membranes so that normal polarization is not restored.

Structure	Name	LD50
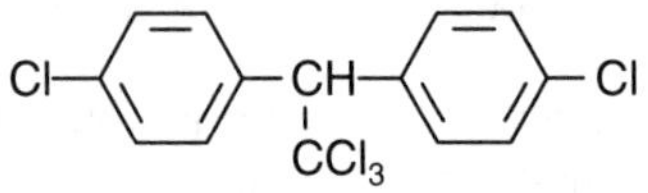	DDT	113
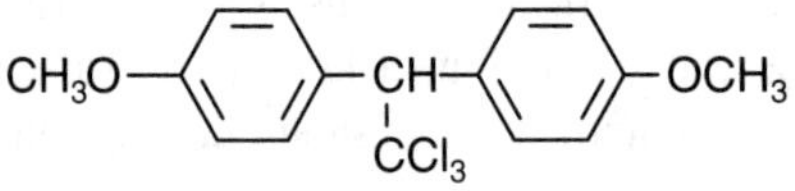	Methoxychlor	5000
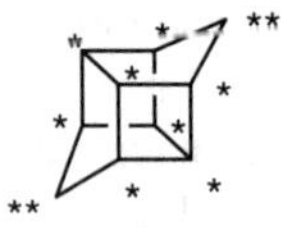	Mirex	600
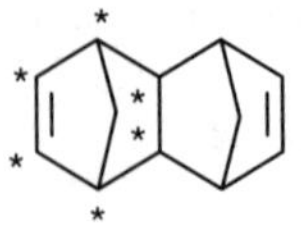	Aldrin	55
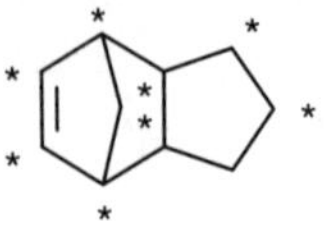	Chlordane	343
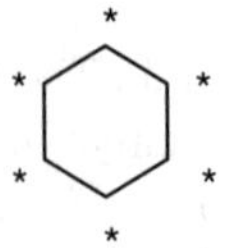	Lindane	88

Figure 10.4. Structures of some organochlorine insecticides. LD50, orally in rats, mg/kg.

Although DDT was synthesized in 1874, its insecticidal properties were not noted until 1939, when Dr. Paul Mueller, a Swiss chemist, discovered its effectiveness as an insecticide. In 1948, he was awarded a Nobel prize for his work. During World War II, the United States used large quantities of DDT to control vectorborne diseases, such as typhus and malaria, to which US troops were exposed. After the war, DDT use became widespread in agriculture, public health, and households. One of the characteristics that contributed to the popularity of DDT, its persistence, later became the basis for public concern over the use of this chemical. Although some warnings were raised early over the hazards of DDT, it was the publication of Rachel Carson's book *Silent Spring* in 1962 that stimulated public concern and eventually led to the ban of DDT in the United States in 1972.

DDT, as well as other organochlorines, were used extensively from the 1940s through the 1960s in agriculture and mosquito control, particularly in the World Health Organization (WHO) malaria control programs. Because of their persistence in the environment, potential for bioaccumulation through the food chain, injury to wildlife, contamination of the human food supply, and suspected carcinogenicity, many organochlorine insecticides have now been phased out and replaced by more biodegradable insecticides. Two organochlorine insecticides with relatively low persistence, toxaphene and methoxychlor, are still widely used.

10.5.2   Organophosphorus Insecticides

Organophosphorus pesticides (OPs) are phosphoric acid esters or thiophosphoric acid esters (Fig. 10.5) and are among the most widely used pesticides for insect control. In Germany in the 1930s and 1940s, Gerhard Schrader and coworkers began investigating OP compounds. They realized the insecticidal properties of these compounds and by the end of the war had made many of the insecticidal phosphates in use today, such as dimefax in 1940, schradan (as it is now called, after its discoverer) in 1942, and parathion in 1944. The first OP insecticide in wide use was tetraethylpyrophosphate (TEPP), which was approved in Germany in 1944 and marketed as a substitute for nicotine against aphids. Because of its high mammalian toxicity and rapid hydrolysis in water, TEPP was replaced by other OP insecticides. Parathion soon became a widely used insecticide due to its stability in aqueous solutions and its broad range of insecticidal activity. Because it has high mammalian toxicity by all routes of exposure, however, other less hazardous compounds are now often used.

Malathion, in particular, has low mammalian toxicity because mammals possess certain enzymes, the carboxylesterases, which readily hydrolyze the carboxyester link, detoxifying the compound. Insects, by contrast, do not readily hydrolyze this ester, and the result is its selective insecticidal action.

OP compounds are toxic because of their inhibition of the enzyme acetylcholinesterase found in the nervous system (see Section 7.2.1, Cholinesterase inhibitors, and Fig. 7.1). This enzyme inhibition results in the accumulation of acetylcholine in nerve tissue and effector organs, with the principal site of action being the peripheral nervous system (PNS). Symptoms of OP poisoning from cholinesterase inhibition include tightness in the chest due to bronchoconstriction and increased bronchial secretions, increased salivation, lacrimation, sweating, nausea, vomiting, diarrhea, and constriction of the pupils. Muscular effects include fatigue, weakness, and cramps. In fatal OP poisoning, the immediate cause of death is respiratory failure. In agricultural and public health usage exposure is primarily dermal, whereas the oral route of exposure occurs with accidental poisoning, homocide, and suicide. Treatment of OP poisoning is covered in Chapter 14.

In addition to acute effects, some OP compounds have been associated with delayed neurotoxicity, known as organophosphorus-induced delayed neuropathy (OPIDN). The characteristic clinical sign is bilateral paralysis of the distal muscles, predominantly of the lower extremities, occurring some 7 to 10 days following ingestion. Histologic studies of nerve tissue from animal experiments show extensive damage to the myelin sheath, suggesting demyelination as a primary mechanism. Not all OP compounds cause delayed neuropathy. Among the pesticides associated with OPIDN are leptophos, mipafox, EPN, DEF, and trichlorofon. Testing is now required for OP substances prior to their use as insecticides. The best experimental animal for OPIDN is the chicken. The usual laboratory species, including the rat, mouse, rabbit, and hamster are much less susceptible to OPIDN. Additional information on delayed toxicity can be found in Section 9.4.6.

Structure	Name	LD50
$(C_2H_5O)_2\overset{S}{\overset{\|\|}{P}}-O-\langle C_6H_4 \rangle-NO_2$	Parathion	3–13
$(C_2H_5O)_2\overset{S}{\overset{\|\|}{P}}-O-$ pyrimidine with $CH(CH_3)_2$ and CH_3	Diazinon	250–285
$(C_2H_5O)_2\overset{S}{\overset{\|\|}{P}}-S(CH_2)_2SC_2H_5$	Disulfoton	2–7
$(CH_3O)_2\overset{S}{\overset{\|\|}{P}}-SCHCOOC_2H_5$ $\quad\quad\quad CH_2COOC_2H_5$	Malathion	1000–1375

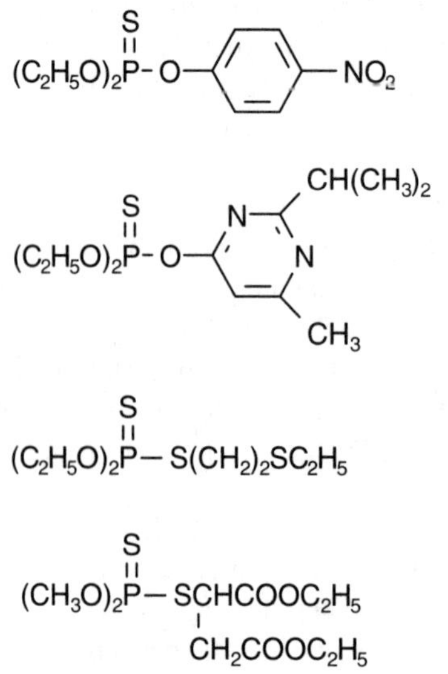

Figure 10.5. Structures of some organophosphorus insecticides. LD50, orally in rats, mg/kg.

The OP and carbamate insecticides are relatively nonpersistent in the environment. They are applied to the crop or directly to the soil as systemic insecticides, and they generally persist from only a few hours to several months. Thus, these compounds, in contrast to the organochlorine insecticides, do not represent a serious problem as contaminants of soil and water and rarely enter the human food chain. Being esters, the compounds are susceptible to hydrolysis, and their breakdown products are generally nontoxic. Direct contamination of food by concentrated compounds has been the cause of poisoning episodes in several countries.

10.5.3 Carbamate Insecticides

The carbamate insecticides are esters of *N*-methyl (or occasionally *N,N*-dimethyl) carbamic acid (NH_2COOH). The toxicity of the compound varies according to the phenol or alcohol group (Fig. 10.6). For example, aldicarb (Temik) is extremely toxic by both oral and dermal routes, and for this reason is recommended only for limited use. Like the OP insecticides, the mode of action of the carbamates is inhibition of acetylcholinesterase. The important difference, however, is that with carbamates the inhibition is more rapidly reversed than with OP compounds.

10.5.4 Botanical Insecticides

Nicotine (see Fig. 1.3) is an alkaloid occurring in a number of plants and was first used as an insecticide in 1763. Nicotine is quite toxic orally as well as dermally. The acute oral LD50 of nicotine sulfate for rats is 83 mg/kg and the dermal LD50 is

Structure	Name	LD50
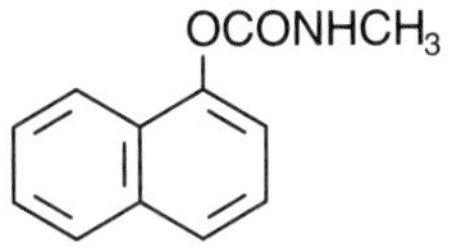 $OCONHCH_3$ (naphthyl)	Carbaryl (Sevin)	250–550
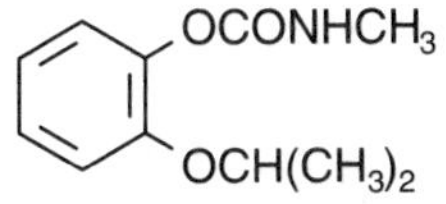 $OCONHCH_3$, $OCH(CH_3)_2$ (phenyl)	Propoxur (Baygon)	100
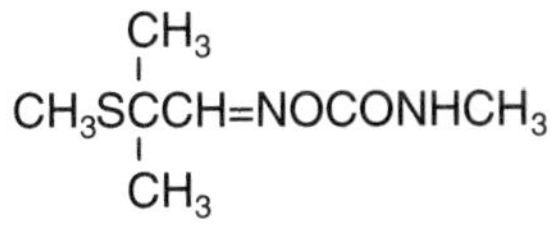 $CH_3SC(CH_3)_2CH=NOCONHCH_3$	Aldicarb (Temik)	~1

Figure 10.6. Structures of some carbamate insecticides. LD50, orally in rats, mg/kg.

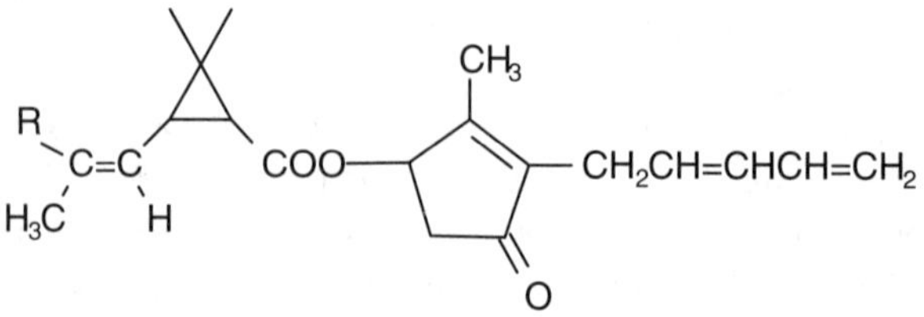

Pyrethrin I   (R=CH$_3$)   LD50 800–1500
Pyrethrin II   (R=COOCH$_3$)

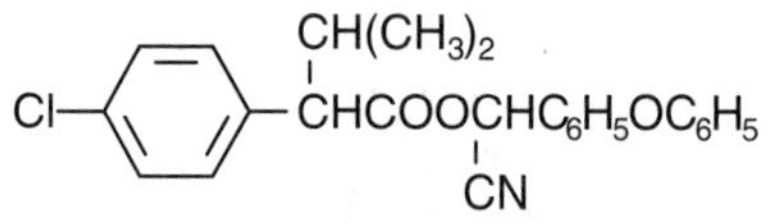

Fenvalerate   LD50 450

Figure 10.7. Structure of pyrethrins I and II, two of the six pyrethrins in natural pyrethrum, and fenvalerate, one of the synthetic pyrethroids. LD50, orally in rats, mg/kg.

285 mg/kg. Symptoms of acute nicotine poisoning occur rapidly, and death may occur with a few minutes. In serious poisoning cases, death results from respiratory failure due to paralysis of respiratory muscles. In therapy, attention is focused primarily on support of respiration.

Pyrethrum (Fig. 10.7), which is extracted from several types of chrysanthemum, is one of the oldest insecticides used by humans. Pyrethrins are used in many household insecticides because of their quick "knockdown" action. Although pyrethrins are used to control several agricultural pests, their rapid degradation by heat and sunlight limits their usefulness.

Mammalian toxicity to pyrethrins is very low, apparently due to its rapid breakdown by liver microsomal enzymes and esterases. The acute LD50 to rats is about 1500 mg/kg. The most frequent reaction to pyrethrins is contact dermatitis and allergic respiratory reactions, probably as a result of other constituents in the extract; about 50% of patients who are sensitive to ragweed show cross-reactivity to pyrethrum. Many of the synthetic pyrethrins, known as pyrethroids, have greater insecticidal activity and are more photostable than pyrethrum, especially those containing the α cyano group, such as fenvalerate (Fig. 10.7). Pyrethrins affect nerve membranes by modifying the sodium and potassium channels, resulting in depolarization of the membranes. Formulations of these insecticides frequently contain the insecticide synergist piperonyl butoxide, which acts to increase the efficacy of the insecticide by inhibiting the cytochrome P450 enzymes responsible for the breakdown of the insecticide. This mechanism is discussed in Chapter 3, Section 3.2.2.4 under Methylenedioxy Ring Cleavage and is illustrated in Fig. 3.8.

10.5.5   Herbicides

Phenolic compounds, such as dinitrophenol, dinitro-orthocresol, and penta-chlorophenol, are used as contact herbicides; the chlorophenols are also used as fungicides, especially for the preservation of wood products. The mode of action is the uncoupling of oxidative phosphorylation, increasing O_2 consumption and heat production, leading to hyperthermia (see Section 7.4, Uncouplers of oxidative phos-phorylation, and Fig. 7.3).

The chlorophenoxy herbicides such as 2,4-D and 2,4,5-T (Fig. 10.8) are sys-temic herbicides for broadleaf plants that act as growth hormones. The oral toxici-ties of these compounds is low. The major toxicological concern of the chlorophen-oxy herbicides results from the presence of the contaminant TCDD (Fig. 10.8), which is formed during the manufacturing process. TCDD is one of the most toxic synthetic substances known in laboratory animals. The LD50 for male rats is 0.022 mg/kg, and for female guinea pigs (the most sensitive species tested) the LD50 is 0.0006 mg/kg. In addition, it is fetotoxic to pregnant rats at a dose of only 1/400 of the LD50, and has been shown to cause birth defects at levels of 1 to 3 ng/kg. TCDD is a proven carcinogen in both mice and rats, with the liver being the pri-mary target. This chemical has also been shown to alter the immune system and de-crease immunocompetence in exposed animals. A mixture of 2,4-D and 2,4,5-T, known as Agent Orange, was used by the US military as a defoliant during the Viet-nam conflict, and much controversy has arisen over claims by military personnel of long-term health effects.

Paraquat is a very water-soluble contact herbicide that is active against a broad range of plants and is used as a defoliant on many crops. Most poisoning cases, which are often fatal, are due to accidental or deliberate ingestion of paraquat. Toxi-city results from lung injury resulting from both the preferential uptake of paraquat by the lungs and the redox cycling mechanism (see Section 9.3.3, Pulmonary toxic-ity, and Fig. 9.6).

The triazines and triazoles are cyclic nitrogen compounds and have a low acute mammalian toxicity. The major concern with these types of compounds is their car-cinogenic effects. Atrazine (see Fig. 1.4), one of the most widely used of the tri-azine herbicides, is a frequently found contaminant of groundwater.

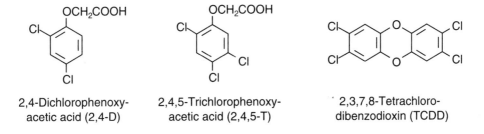

2,4-Dichlorophenoxy-
acetic acid (2,4-D)   2,4,5-Trichlorophenoxy-
acetic acid (2,4,5-T)   2,3,7,8-Tetrachloro-
dibenzodioxin (TCDD)

Figure 10.8. Chlorophenoxy herbicides and the toxic contaminant TCDD.

10.5.6   Fungicides

Fungicides include such compounds as mercury fungicides, used to treat seed grains; pentachlorophenol (see Fig. 7.3), used as a wood preservative; and dithiocarbamates (maneb, zineb, and nabam), used widely in agriculture. The dithiocarbamates, in general, have a low acute toxicity. Recent concern has surfaced concerning the potential of fungicides, such as vinclozolin, to affect reproductive processes.

10.5.7   Rodenticides

The main toxicological problem associated with rodenticides results from accidental or suicidal ingestion of the compounds. Fluoroacetate (compound 1080) and fluoroacetamide (compound 1081) are highly toxic compounds (see Section 7.5 and Fig. 7.4), and their use is restricted to pest control operators. Other rodenticides are warfarin (an anticoagulant, see Fig. 1.4), red squill (cardiac poison), ANTU (α-naphthylthiourea), strychnine, and thallium salts.

10.5.8   Fumigants

Fumigants are gases used to protect stored produce, especially grains, and to kill soil nematodes. They present a special hazard due to inhalation exposure and rapid diffusion into the pulmonary blood. Most are also extremely toxic. Commonly used fumigants include methylbromide, carbon tetrachloride, acrylonitrite, carbon disulfide, ethylene dibromide, ethylene oxide, hydrogen cyanide, formaldehyde, acrolein, chloropicrin, and phosphine. The use of many of these (eg, ethylene dibromide) is now being restricted or banned, particularly in the United States.

10.6

METALS

Although most metals occur in nature in rocks, ores, soil, water, and air, levels are usually low and widely dispersed. In terms of human exposure and toxicological significance, it is anthropogenic activities that are most important because they increase the levels of metals at the site of human activities.

Metals have been used throughout much of human history to make utensils, machinery, and so on, and mining and smelting supplied metals for these uses. These activities increased environmental levels of metals. More recently, metals have found a number of uses in industry, agriculture, and medicine. These activities have increased exposure not only to metal-related occupational workers, but also to consumers of the various products.

In spite of the wide range of metal toxicity and toxic properties, there are a number of toxicological features that are common to many metals. Some of the more important aspects are discussed briefly in the following sections. For a metal to exert its toxicity it must cross the membrane and enter the cell. If the metal is in a lipophilic form such as methyl mercury, it readily penetrates the membrane; when bound to proteins such as cadmium–metallothionein, the metal is taken into the cell by endocytosis; other metals (eg, lead) may be absorbed by passive diffusion. The toxic effects of metals usually involve interaction between the free metal and the cellular target. These targets tend to be specific biochemical processes and/or cellular and subcellular membranes.

10.6.1   Common Toxic Mechanisms

ENZYME INHIBITION. A major site of action of metals is interaction with enzymes resulting in enzyme inhibition. Two mechanisms are of particular importance in this regard. Inhibition may occur as a result of interaction between the metal and sulfhydryl (SH) groups on the enzyme or the metal may displace an essential metal cofactor of the enzyme. For example, lead may displace zinc in the zinc-dependent enzyme δ-aminolevulinic acid dehydratase (ALAD), thereby inhibiting the synthesis of heme, an important component of hemoglobin and heme-containing enzymes, such as the various cytochromes.

SUBCELLULAR ORGANELLES. Toxic metals may disrupt the structure and function of a number of organelles. For example, enzymes associated with the endoplasmic reticulum may be inhibited; metals may be accumulated in the lysosomes; respiratory enzymes in the mitochondria may be inhibited by metals; and metal inclusion bodies may be formed in the nucleus.

CARCINOGENICITY. A number of metals have been shown to be carcinogenic in humans or animals. Arsenic, certain chromium compounds, and nickel are known human carcinogens; beryllium, cadmium, and cisplatin are probable human carcinogens. The carcinogenic action, in some cases, is thought to result from the interaction of the metallic ions with DNA.

KIDNEY. Because the kidney is the main excretory organ of the body, it is a common target organ for metal toxicity. Cadmium and mercury in particular are potent nephrotoxicants and are discussed more fully in the following sections on cadmium and mercury and in the earlier chapter on organ toxicity (Section 9.2, Nephrotoxicity).

NERVOUS SYSTEM. The nervous system is also a common target of toxic metals, particularly organic metal compounds (see Section 9.4, Neurotoxicity). For example, methyl mercury, because it is very lipophilic, readily crosses the blood–brain barrier and enters the nervous system. By contrast, inorganic mercury compounds, which are more water soluble, are less likely to enter the nervous system and are primarily nephrotoxicants. Likewise, organic lead compounds are mainly neurotoxicants, whereas the first site of action of inorganic lead is enzyme inhibition (eg, enzymes involved in heme synthesis).

RESPIRATORY SYSTEM. Occupational exposure to metals in the form of metal dust makes the respiratory system a likely target. Acute exposure may cause irritation and inflammation of the respiratory tract, whereas chronic exposure may result in fibrosis (aluminum) or carcinogenesis (arsenic, chromium, nickel).

ENDOCRINE AND REPRODUCTIVE EFFECTS. Because the male and female reproductive organs are under complex neuroendocrine and hormonal control, any toxicant that alters any of these processes can affect the reproductive system. In addition, metals can act directly on the sex organs. Cadmium is known to produce testicular injury after acute exposure, and lead accumulation in the testes is associated with testicular degeneration, inhibition of spermatogenesis, and Leydig-cell atrophy.

METAL-BINDING PROTEINS. The toxicity of many metals such as cadmium, lead, and mercury depends on their transport and intracellular bioavilability. This availability is regulated to a degree by high-affinity binding to certain cytosolic proteins. Such ligands usually posess numerous SH binding sites that can outcompete other intracellular proteins and thus mediate intracellular metal bioavailability and toxicity. These intracellular "sinks" are capable of partially sequestering toxic metals away from sensitive organelles or proteins until their binding capacity is exceeded by the dose of the metal.

METALLOTHIONEIN (MT) is a low molecular weight protein (approximately 7000 Da), that is particularly important in regulating the intracellular bioavailability of cadmium, zinc, mercury, silver, copper, and bismuth. For example, in vivo exposure to cadmium results in the transport of cadmium in the blood by various high molecular weight proteins and uptake by the liver, followed by hepatic induction of MT. Subsequently, cadmium can be found in the circulatory system bound to MT as the cadmium–metallothionein complex (CdMT).

10.6.2 Lead

Because lead has had widespread use both historically and industrially, it is among one of the most ubiquitous of the toxic metals. Exposure may be through air, water, or food sources. In the United States the major industrial uses, such as fuel additives and lead pigments in paints, have been phased out, but other uses, such as in batteries, have not been reduced. Other sources of lead include lead from pipes and glazed ceramic food containers.

Inorganic lead may be absorbed through the GI tract, the respiratory system, and the skin. Ingested inorganic lead is absorbed more efficiently from the GI tract of children than that of adults, readily crosses the placenta, and in children penetrates the blood–brain barrier. Initially, lead is distributed in the blood, liver, and kidney; after prolonged exposure, as much as 95% of the body burden of lead is found in bone tissue.

The main targets of lead toxicity are the hematopoietic system and the nervous system. Several of the enzymes involved in the synthesis of heme are sensitive to inhibition by lead. The two most susceptible enzymes are ALAD and heme synthetase (HS). Although clinical anemia occurs only after moderate exposure to lead, biochemical effects can be observed at lower levels. For this reason, inhibition of ALAD or appearance in the urine of ALA can be used as an indicator of lead exposure.

The nervous system is another important target tissue for lead toxicity, especially in infants and young children in whom the nervous system is still developing (Section 9.4). Even at low levels of exposure, children may show hyperactivity, decreased attention span, mental deficiencies, and impaired vision. At higher levels, encephalopathy may occur in both children and adults. Lead damages the arterioles and capillaries, resulting in cerebral edema and neuronal degeneration. Clinically, this damage manifests itself as ataxia, stupor, coma, and convulsions.

Another system affected by lead is the reproductive system. Lead exposure can cause male and female reproductive toxicity, miscarriages, and degenerate offspring.

10.6.3   Mercury

Mercury exists in the environment as both inorganic and organic compounds, with inorganic mercury occurring as elemental mercury as well as mercurous (Hg^+) and mercuric (Hg^{2+}) salts. Elemental mercury, in the form of mercury vapor, is almost completely absorbed by the respiratory system, whereas ingested elemental mercury is not readily absorbed and is relatively harmless. Once absorbed, elemental mercury can cross the blood–brain barrier into the nervous system. Most exposure to elemental mercury tends to be from occupational sources.

Of more concern from environmental contamination is exposure to organic mercury compounds. Inorganic mercury may be converted to organic mercury through the action of anaerobic bacteria, especially to produce methyl mercury, a form readily absorbed across membranes. Several large episodes of mercury poisoning have resulted from consuming seed grain treated with mercury fungicides or from eating fish contaminated with methyl mercury. In Japan in the 1950s and 1960s, wastes from a chemical and plastics plant containing mercury were drained into Minamata Bay. The mercury was converted to the readily absorbed methyl mercury by bacteria in the aquatic sediments. Consumption of fish and shellfish by the local population resulted in numerous cases of mercury poisoning or Minamata disease. By 1970, at least 107 deaths had been attributed to mercury poisoning, and 800 cases of Minamata disease were confirmed. Even though the mothers appeared healthy, many infants born to mothers who had eaten contaminated fish developed cerebral palsy–like symptoms and mental deficiency. Organic mercury primarily affects the nervous system, with the fetal brain being more sensitive to the toxic effects of mercury than adults.

Inorganic mercury salts, however, are primarily nephrotoxicants, with the site of action being the proximal tubular cells. Mercury binds to SH groups of membrane proteins, affecting the integrity of the membrane and resulting in aliguria, anuria, and uremia.

10.6.4   Cadmium

Cadmium occurs in nature primarily in association with lead and zinc ores and is released near mines and smelters processing these ores. Industrially, cadmium is used as a pigment, in electroplating, and making alloys and alkali storage batteries. Environmental exposure to cadmium is mainly from contamination of groundwater from smelting and industrial uses as well as the use of sludge as a food-crop fertilizer. Grains and cereal products usually constitute the main source of cadmium in food. Reference has already been made to the disease Itai-Itai resulting from consumption of cadmium-contaminated rice in Japan (see Section 9.2.3).

Acute effects of exposure to cadmium result primarily from local irritation. After ingestion, the main effects are nausea, vomiting, and abdominal pain. Inhalation exposure may result in pulmonary edema and chemical pneumonitis.

Chronic effects are of particular concern because cadmium is very slowly excreted from the body, with a half-life of about 30 years. Thus, low levels of exposure can result in considerable accumulation of cadmium. The main organ of damage following long-term exposure is the kidney, with the proximal tubules being the primary site of action. Cadmium is present in the circulatory system bound primarily to the metal-binding protein, metallothionein, produced in the liver. Following glomerular filtration in the kidney, CdMT is readsorbed efficiently by the proximal tubule cells, where it accumulates within the lysosomes. Subsequent degradation of the CdMT complex releases Cd^{+2}, which inhibits lysosomal function, resulting in cell injury (see Section 9.2).

10.6.5   Chromium

Because chromium occurs in ores, environmental levels are increased by mining, smelting, and industrial uses. Chromium is used in making stainless steel, various alloys, and pigments. The levels of this metal are generally very low in air, water, and food, and the major source for human exposure is occupational. Chromium occurs in a number of oxidation states from $^{+2}$ to $^{+6}$, but only the trivalent (Cr^{+3}) and the hexavalent (Cr^{+6}) are of biologic significance. Although the trivalent compound is the most common form found in nature, the hexavalent form is of greater industrial importance. In addition, hexavalent chromium, which is not water soluble, is more readily absorbed across cell membranes than is trivalent chromium. In vivo the hexavalent form is reduced to the trivalent form, which can complex with intracellular macromolecules, resulting in toxicity. Chromium is a known human carcinogen and induces lung cancers among exposed workers. The mechanism of chromium (Cr^{+6}) carcinogenicity in the lung is believed to be its reduction to Cr^{+3} and generation of reactive intermediates, leading to bronchogenic carcinoma.

10.6.6   Arsenic

In general, the levels of arsenic in air and water are low, and the major source of human exposure is food. In certain parts of Taiwan and South America, however, the water contains high levels of this metalloid, and the inhabitants often suffer from dermal hyperkeratosis and hyperpigmentation. Higher levels of exposure result in a more serious condition; gangrene of the lower extremities or "blackfoot disease." Cancer of the skin also occurs in these areas.

Approximately 80% of arsenic compounds are used in pesticides. Other uses include glassware, paints, and pigments. Arsine gas in used in the semiconductor industry. Arsenic compounds occur in three forms: (1) pentavalent, As^{+5}, organic or arsenate compounds (eg, alkyl arsenates); (2) trivalent, As^{+3}, inorganic or arsenite compounds (eg, sodium arsenite, arsenic trioxide); and (3) arsine gas, AsH_3, a colorless gas formed by the action of acids on arsenic. The most toxic form is arsine gas with the TLV–TWA of 0.05 ppm.

Microorganisms in the environment convert arsenic to dimethylarsenate, which can accumulate in fish, providing a source for human exposure. Arsenic compounds can also be present as contaminants in well water. Arsenite (As^{+3}) compounds are lipid soluble and can be absorbed following ingestion, inhalation, or skin contact. Within 24 hours of absorption arsenic distributes over the body, where it binds to SH groups of tissue proteins. Only a small amount crosses the blood–brain barrier. Arsenic may also replace phosphorus in bone tissue and be stored for years.

After acute poisoning, severe GI gastrointestinal symptoms occur within 30 minutes to 2 hours. These include vomiting; watery, bloody diarrhea; severe abdominal pain; and burning esophageal pain. Vasodilation, myocardial depression, cerebral edema, and distal peripheral neuropathy may also follow. Later stages of poisoning include jaundice and renal failure. Death usually results from circulatory failure within 24 hours to 4 days.

Chronic exposure results in nonspecific symptoms such as diarrhea, abdominal pain, hyperpigmentation, and hyperkeratosis. A symmetrical sensory neuropathy often follows. Late changes include gangrene of the extremities, anemia, and cancer of the skin, lung, and nasal tissue.

10.6.7   Treatment of Metal Poisoning

Treatment of metal exposure to prevent or reverse toxicity is by chelating agents or antagonists. Chelation is the formation of a metal ion complex, in which the metal ion is associated with an electron donor ligand. Metals may react with O-, S-, and N-containing ligands (eg, -OH, -COOH, -S-S-, and -NH$_2$). Chelating agents need to be able to reach sites of storage, form nontoxic complexes, not readily bind essential metals (eg, calcium, zinc), and be easily excreted.

One of the first clinically useful chelating drugs was British antilewisite (BAL [2,3-dimercaptopropanol]), which was developed during World War II as an antago-

TABLE 10.9. EXAMPLES OF CHELATING DRUGS USED TO TREAT METAL TOXICITY

British antilewisite (BAL[2,3-dimercaptopropanol]), dimercaprol
DMPS (2,3-dimercapto-1-propanesulfonic acid)
DMSA (meso-2,3-dimercaptosuccinic acid), succimer
EDTA (ethylenediaminetetraacetic acid, calcium salt)
DTPA (diethylenetriaminepentaacetic acid, calcium salt)
DTC (dithiocarbamate)
Penicillamine (β-β-dimethylcysteine), hydrolytic product of penicillin

nist to arsenical war gases. BAL is a dithiol compound with two sulfur atoms on adjacent carbon atoms that compete with critical binding sites involved in arsenic toxicity. Although BAL will bind a number of toxic metals, it is also a potentially toxic drug with multiple side effects. In response to BAL's toxicity, several analogs have now been developed. Table 10.9 lists some of the more common chelating drugs in therapeutic use. Treatment of metal toxicity is discussed in more detail in Chapter 14.

10.7

SOLVENTS

Organic solvents and their vapors are commonly encountered in our modern environment—in industries in which large quantities may be used in manufacturing and processing and in the home as a result of exposure to materials such as gasoline vapors, aerosol sprays, and paint removers.

10.7.1 Aliphatic Hydrocarbons

Methane and ethane are the gases present in natural gas; they are not usually associated with systemic effects, but are asphyxiants when the concentration is high enough to reduce oxygen levels in inhaled air. Propane and butane (bottled gas) are highly volatile liquids, and inhalation of the vapors produces central nervous system (CNS) depression, resulting in dizziness and incoordination. Many commercial products and solvents contain mixtures of the higher molecular weight hydrocarbons—pentane, hexane, heptane, and octane, including both straight-chain and branched-chain compounds. Inhalation of vapors from products containing these hydrocarbons produces CNS depression. Gasoline and kerosene are mixtures of hydrocarbons that contain both aromatic and aliphatic hydrocarbons. In normal exposure, such as the vapors encountered by gas station attendants, toxic effects do not normally occur.

A significant source of poison deaths, however, is ingestion of petroleum products by children, especially children younger than 5 years of age; such ingestion accounts for up to 25% of all poison deaths in this age group. The most commonly ingested hydrocarbons, in order of frequency, are kerosene, mineral oil preparations, turpentine, gasoline, lighter fluids, and pesticides with a petroleum base. An important factor in ingestion by children is that these compounds, such as kerosene, are often placed in soft-drink bottles or other unlabeled containers and left within easy access of children. The acute toxicity of these compounds is quite low, but significant damage can occur as a result of small quantities entering the lung, where a thin layer spreads rapidly over the moist lung surfaces, causing edema and hemorrhage due to damage of the pulmonary membranes. For this reason, it is wise not to induce vomiting.

10.7.2   Aliphatic Halogenated Hydrocarbons

Because of their excellent solvent properties, low flammability, and relative chemical stability, the aliphatic halogenated hydrocarbons are among the compounds most widely used as industrial solvents. Halogenated hydrocarbons tend to be well absorbed through the skin, lungs, and GI tract. A common physiological property associated with these compounds is CNS depression. They may also be associated with damage to the heart, liver, and/or kidney; at least one compound, vinyl chloride, is carcinogenic in humans.

CHLOROFORM ($CHCl_3$) was once used extensively as a clinical anaesthetic but because of liver injury and to a lesser extent cardiac sensitization, it is no longer used for this purpose. It is widely used in industry and in the laboratory as a chemical intermediate and solvent. Because chloroform has been established as a carcinogen in laboratory animals, its use is no longer permitted as a component in drugs. High concentrations of chloroform or repeated exposure may lead to liver and kidney damage. Chloroform is metabolized by cytochrome P450 isozymes to produce chloromethanol, which rapidly and spontaneously dechlorinates to yield HCl and the toxic compound phosgene (Fig. 10.9).

CARBON TETRACHLORIDE (CCl_4) has been widely used as a dry-cleaning chemical, degreasing agent, and fire extinguisher. At one time it was used as a clinical drug for control of hookworm. Recent FDA regulations have now restricted its use to industry and laboratories. Carbon tetrachloride has anesthetic properties similar to those

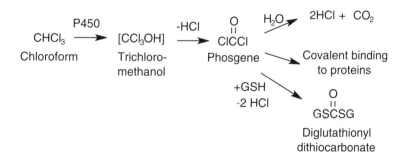

Figure 10.9. Metabolism of chloroform.

of chloroform, but is less potent. In addition, it causes marked hepatic and renal toxicity, and even low concentrations cause fatty degeneration in the liver (see Hepatotoxicity, Section 9.1).

METHYLENE CHLORIDE (CH_2Cl_2) is a common ingredient in paint removers and is a solvent in aerosol products. Due to its extreme volatility, high concentrations may occur readily in poorly ventilated areas. Following inhalation, methylene chloride is metabolized by P450 to CO_2 and CO. Significant levels of COHb may occur due to CO binding to hemoglobin in the blood. In common with other low molecular weight halogenated hydrocarbons, methylene chloride is a CNS depressant. Initial signs of inhalation are dizziness and numbness; other symptoms that have been reported are tingling of the extremities, fatigue, and nausea. Severe or prolonged exposure may lead to respiratory depression and death. If high COHb levels are present, the symptoms of acute CO poisoning will also occur.

METHYL CHLORIDE (CH_3Cl) is a colorless gas used as a chemical intermediate, particularly in methylating reactions. Occasionally, it is used as a blowing agent in molding polystyrene and polyurethane. Following acute exposure, patients feel inebriated and develop nausea, abdominal pains, and diarrhea. Chronic industrial exposure has led to confusion, blurring of vision, slurred speech, and staggering gait.

TRICHLOROETHYLENE $(Cl_2C=CHCl)$ and tetrachloroethylene $(CCl_2=CCl_2)$ are both used widely as industrial degreasing solvents and in the dry-cleaning industry. Overexposure by inhalation results in CNS depression, confusion, incoordination, nausea, and irritation of the eyes and nose. At high concentrations, these compounds may be fatal.

VINYL CHLORIDE $(CH_2=CHCl$ [monochloroethylene]) is a colorless gas that is highly flammable and explosive and is usually handled as a liquid under pressure. In this form, it polymerizes readily at temperatures between 40° and 70°C to form polyvinylchloride (PVC). Epidemiologic studies of autoclave cleaners in PVC plants showed a high incidence of a rare tumor, angiosarcoma of the liver. The main route of absorption of vinyl chloride is through the lungs, although some skin penetration does occur. Metabolism of vinyl chloride to the reactive metabolite occurs through the hepatic P450 enzymes (Fig. 10.10). The epoxide, thought to be the ultimate carcinogen, binds covalently to DNA, RNA, and protein, and chloroacetaldehyde is a known mutagen. Detoxication of these metabolites occurs mainly by conjugation with glutathione.

10.7.3 Alcohols

The aliphatic alcohols have wide application as industrial solvents and, of this series, only ethanol has the physiological effects and low toxicity that has resulted in its use as an alcoholic beverage. The other alcohols, especially methanol, are characterized by considerable toxicity.

METHANOL $(CH_3OH$ [methyl alcohol or wood alcohol]) is a widely used commercial solvent and is a solvent in paints, varnishes, and shellacs. It is commonly used in

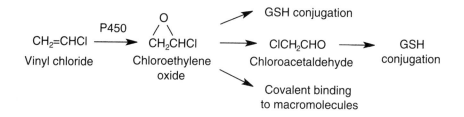

Figure 10.10. Metabolism of vinyl chloride.

windshield wiping fluids and in formulations as a liquid fuel for small engines. Because methanol resembles ethanol in odor and taste and is tax-free and less expensive than ethanol, it has sometimes been used as an adulterant in alcoholic beverages, and "epidemics" of methanol poisoning are not uncommon. Although toxicity may occur from skin absorption or inhalation, the main route of uptake is ingestion. In poisoning, about 30% of the dose is excreted as methanol by the respiratory tract (the main mode of excretion of unchanged methanol); the remainder of the methanol is converted, principally in the liver, by alcohol dehydrogenase to formaldehyde and then to formic acid by aldehyde dehydrogenase. The local production of formaldehyde in the retina is thought to be responsible for the production of the retinal edema and blindness characteristic of methanol poisoning.

Symptoms of methanol poisoning may be delayed for 6 to 18 hours due to the delayed metabolism of methanol to the toxic products, formaldehyde and formic acid. The initial symptoms are a minor CNS intoxication similar to ethyl alcohol, followed by a mild drowsiness. This is followed by an asymptomatic period (6–30 hours) and then the characteristic symptoms and signs of methanol poisoning (Table 10.10). In severe cases, delirium may be a marked feature, and death may be either rapid or occur many hours after the onset of the coma. Ethanol is adminis-

TABLE 10.10. MAJOR SIGNS AND SYMPTOMS OF METHANOL INTOXICATION

Early
 Inebriation
 Drowsiness
Delayed (6–30 h)
 Dizziness
 Abdominal pain, vomiting
 Breathing difficulty
 Blurred vision
 Dilated pupils
 Blindness
 Urinary formaldehyde smell

tered immediately to act as a competitive substrate for alcohol dehydrogenase and thus reduce the conversion of methanol to formaldehyde. This is followed by hemodialysis to remove the methanol, formic acid, and formaldehyde.

ISOPROPYL ALCOHOL is an important alcohol used in industry and in medicine as rubbing alcohol. In the home, isopropyl alcohol may be found in rubbing alcohol, aftershave lotions, and window-cleaning solutions. As with methanol, isopropyl alcohol is sometimes ingested mixed with or in place of ethanol. Isopropyl alcohol is more toxic than ethanol but less toxic than methanol. The signs and symptoms are similar to those of ethanol toxicity; acute ingestion may be followed by a deep coma and respiratory arrest, all occurring within a few hours.

HIGHER SATURATED ALCOHOLS. These compounds also have some toxicity. The butyl alcohols are generally less toxic than the amyl alcohols, but are more toxic than isopropanol. *n*-Butanol vapors have produced conjunctivitis and keratitis, and inhalation may produce pulmonary injury. In general, however, toxicity is not a problem with the higher alcohols.

10.7.4 Glycols and Derivatives

Glycols (Fig. 10.11) have general use as heat exchangers, antifreeze formulations, hydraulic fluids, chemical intermediates, solvents for pharmaceuticals, food additives, and cosmetics. Because of their low volatility, the glycols have little vapor hazard at ordinary temperatures.

ETHYLENE GLYCOL is a major component in antifreeze. Ingestion results in serious and dramatic poisoning. As with methanol and isopropanol, ethylene glycol has been ingested in place of or mixed with ethanol. Initially, the user appears to be drunk, but without an alcohol smell on the breath; this is followed by nausea, coma, seizure, respiratory failure, and cardiovascular collapse. Toxicity results from ethylene gly-

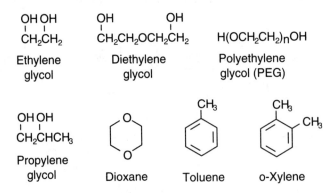

Figure 10.11. Structures of some glycols and aromatic hydrocarbons.

col's metabolites: aldehydes, glycolate, oxalate, and lactate. Survivors of the acute phase experience renal failure caused by deposition of calcium oxalate crystals in the renal tubules and severe acidosis due to aldehyde, glycolate, and lactate production. Hypocalcemia also occurs as a result of calcium chelation by oxalate. The metabolism of ethylene glycol depends on hepatic alcohol dehydrogenase and, as in methanol poisoning, ethanol is administered to act as a preferential substrate for the enzyme. During subsequent hemodialysis, ethanol is commonly added to the dialysate to maintain plasma levels of ethanol.

PROPYLENE GLYCOL is relatively nontoxic and is used in cosmetics, foods, and as a solvent for certain drugs; for example, it is a major part of the solvent composition for the intravenous (IV) preparation of phenytoin and, if injected too rapidly, can cause cardiac arrhythmias. Most of the higher molecular weight glycols are also of very low toxicity.

GLYCOL ETHERS are both water soluble and soluble in organic solvents, and thus are used in many oil–water combinations. Toxicity from these compounds generally occurs by inhalation of the vapors, which have been known to cause bone marrow depression and kidney damage.

10.7.5   Aromatic Hydrocarbons

BENZENE, the simplest of the aromatic hydrocarbons, has excellent solvent properties and high volatility. Because it dries rapidly, it has been a solvent of choice in certain industries such as printing. In addition, it has widespread use as starting material for the synthesis of various aromatic products. Benzene is toxic to hematopoietic tissues and is known to cause leukemia. The toxicity of benzene is also discussed in Section 10.4.3.

TOLUENE (Fig. 10.11) is a colorless liquid used extensively as a solvent in the chemical, rubber, paint, and pharmaceutical industries, but with much lower volatility than benzene. Toluene is a narcotic; acute symptoms from inhalation include euphoria, excitement, dizziness, headache, and nausea. Extreme acute exposure can result in coma and even death. Because toluene is a solvent for glue, it is frequently one of the solvents associated with "glue sniffing." Chronic exposure to toluene, however, does not involve the hematologic effects that characterize benzene exposure.

XYLENE (Fig. 10.11) is another aromatic hydrocarbon that is widely used as a solvent in paints, lacquers, pesticides, adhesives, and the paper-coating industry. Inhalation may lead to dizziness, excitement, drowsiness, and lack of coordination.

10.8

DRUGS

10.8.1 Therapeutic Drugs

In the medical use of drugs, a narrow dose range often separates the clinically desired effect from a harmful or toxic manifestation of the drug. Many factors, both endogenous and exogenous, can alter the metabolism of a drug, thus affecting its efficacy as well as its toxicity. Such factors include genetic polymorphisms in drug metabolizing enzymes and drug interactions leading to inhibition and/or induction of enzymes. Examples of these interactions are discussed in Chapter 6.

Other problems associated with therapeutic drugs occur due to accidental acute intoxication by children and deliberate suicidal and homicidal overdose by adults. The opportunities for these events are numerous in a drug-oriented society. Drug abuse, drug addiction, adverse drug effects, and chronic drug intoxications all contribute to serious health problems as well as to increased medical costs. Examples of some of these types of toxicities are discussed briefly in the following sections. Examples of toxic mechanisms of several drugs are also discussed in other chapters (Acetaminophen, Section 4.5.3; Nephrotoxic antibiotics, Section 9.2.3).

BARBITURATES are derivatives of barbituric acid (Fig. 10.12) and, depending on the compound, have a wide range of duration of activity from less than 1 hour to as much as 12 hours. In recent years, the death rate from overuse of barbiturates has declined because of a decrease in prescriptions by doctors together with the intro-

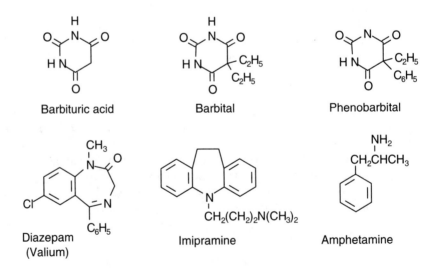

Figure 10.12. Structures of some common tranquilizers, antidepressants, and stimulants.

duction of safer drugs, such as the benzodiazepines. Barbiturates are legally available only on prescription, but the street use of "downers" continues. Barbiturates are administered orally and most are metabolized by the liver, with some metabolism in the kidney and other tissues. The desired CNS effect is mild sedation to general anesthesia; in addition, some have anticonvulsant activity and lessen anxiety. Tolerance to barbiturates develops very rapidly, so that increasing doses are necessary to be effective, often by as much as six times. Although barbiturates induce the liver microsomal enzymes that metabolize them, the level of tolerance is more than can be accounted for by induction of the microsomal enzymes. Induction of P450 by barbituates causes a significant increase in the elimination of other drugs such as dicumarol, digoxin, tetracycline, oral contraceptives, and hormones. Most cases of barbiturate poisoning are suicide attempts, but accidental poisonings are more common with children and those who abuse and/or are addicted to drugs ("street users"). The characteristic signs and symptoms of barbiturate poisoning are depression of the CNS and cardiovascular systems. Severe intoxication produces coma and may progress to death, frequently due to cardiorespiratory arrest. The simultaneous ingestion of other drugs such as alcohol may contribute to CNS depression.

BENZODIAZEPINES (Fig. 10.12) are nonbarbiturate compounds that possess CNS-depressant properties and are often described as hypnotics, sedatives, depressants, tranquilizers, or relaxants. These drugs have largely replaced the barbiturates for this use. In the 1970s, diazepam (Valium) was the most widely prescribed drug in the United States. Benzodiazepines are popular because of their efficacy as well as their safety. They are relatively safe in overdose and not associated with serious addiction, abstinence syndrome, tolerance development, or microsomal enzyme induction. The most frequent side effect of therapeutic doses is drowsiness; in some cases, dizziness and weakness occurs. The usual result of benzodiazepine overdose is sleep induction and occasionally coma; in most overdose fatalities involving benzodiazepines, other drugs were also ingested. Benzodiazepines alone rarely cause respiratory or circulatory depression. It has been suggested that there is a risk of teratogenicity when the drugs are used during the first trimester, but epidemiologic studies have not confirmed this association.

TRICYCLIC ANTIDEPRESSANTS (Fig. 10.12) are important drugs used to treat endogenous depression. Because they are given to patients who are often suicidal, they are a major cause of toxic overdose in clinical use. The parent compound, usually a tertiary amine, and its metabolite, a secondary amine, are responsible for both the antidepressant and the toxic effects. Side effects of use are tiredness, dizziness, blurred vision, and urinary retention. The CNS effects of overdose include confusion, agitation, and finally, coma; anticholinergic effects include flushing, dry mouth, and dilated pupils. The cardiotoxic effects, arrhythmias and hypotension, are the cause of death, however.

AMPHETAMINES. Amphetamine (Fig. 10.12) was first synthesized in 1887 and marketed in the United States in 1932 as a nasal inhalant and decongestant. It is a CNS stimulant, and during World War II was widely used to combat battle fatigue and domestically to increase production among workers. In the 1950s, amphetamines were popular with college students and cross-country truckers. Abuse became a serious problem, however, and legal use became more tightly controlled. Until recently, amphetamines were used to treat obesity as a major component of "diet pills"; today, medical use is restricted to treatment of narcolepsy and hyperkinetic behavior in children.

Although no longer as readily available, amphetamines are easily synthesized from commercially available starting materials and have widespread street use. Symptoms of overdose are restlessness, irritability, tremor, confusion, and sweating in mild cases, to delirium, arrhythmias, convulsions, coma, and occasionally death in severe overdose. Birth defects, including limb deformities, have been associated with amphetamine use during the first trimester, and neonatal withdrawal symptoms also occur.

NARCOTIC ANALGESICS (OPIATES). The word narcotic comes from the Greek *narkoun*, which means to be numb or in a stupor; generally, the term narcotic is used to refer to compounds with sedative, mood-altering, analgesic properties and includes the drugs most often prescribed for relief of intense pain, such as opium and its derivatives. Opiates include drugs derived from opium, synthesized from opium, or wholly synthetic drugs (Fig. 10.13).

Heroin is prepared by acetylation of the hydroxyl groups of morphine, resulting in the ethyl ester of both hydroxyl groups; codeine is the methyl ester of the hydroxyl at the C-3 position. The effects of the opiates on the CNS are a combination of depression and stimulation and include increased pain tolerance, suppression of

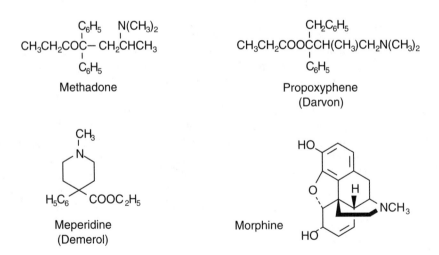

Figure 10.13. Structures for several opiates and synthetic narcotic analgesics.

anxiety, and sedation. Higher doses result in drowsiness, mood changes, mental clouding, nausea, and respiratory depression. The major complications of chronic clinical opiate use are development of tolerance, psychological dependence, and physical dependence. Opiate poisoning occurs most commonly following IV heroin administration or oral methadone overdose by addicts or nontolerant infrequent users. Severe overdose is characterized by apnea, circulatory collapse, convulsions, cardiac arrest, and death.

PHENYTOIN (Dilantin) is the preferred drug in the treatment of epilepsy and in the control of arrhythmias from intoxication by other drugs such as digitalis and tricyclic antidepressants. There have been very few reported deaths from either acute or chronic overdoses, and most deaths have been due to hypersensitivity of patients already intoxicated from other drugs. Phenytoin, however, has been associated with a wide range of congenital abnormalities in infants of mothers taking the drug for control of epilepsy. These effects, known as the fetal hydantoin syndrome, include cleft palate, hydrocephalus, microcephalus, broad nose, digital thumbs, short neck, and various heart defects.

ISONIAZID (INH) is an antimicrobial that has been used in the treatment of tuberculosis (TB) since 1952 and has proved to be very effective with a relatively low toxicity. In the United States, however, the incidence of acute INH toxicity is especially high in certain populations, such as Native Americans and Eskimos. In sensitive individuals, therapeutic doses of INH lead to liver injury due to a reactive intermediate formed from the INH metabolite acetylisoniazid (Fig. 10.14), and occurs most often in patients who are genetically fast acetylators, thus metabolizing INH more

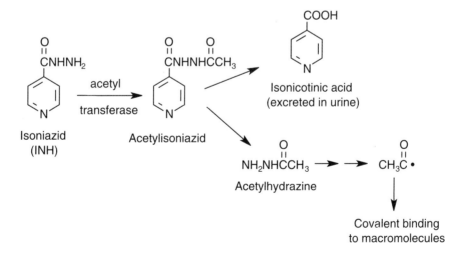

Figure 10.14. Metabolism of isoniazid showing formation of a reactive metabolite that can bind covalently to macromolecules, resulting in liver necrosis.

rapidly than do slow acetylators. Among both Caucasian and African Americans, about 50% of the population are fast acetylators, whereas more than 95% of the Eskimo population are fast acetylators. The Japanese are also rapid acetylators, with about 88% of the population being rapid acetylators, whereas among Egyptians, only 18% are rapid acetylators.

LITHIUM. The use of lithium carbonate has become an indispensable tool in the psychiatric treatment of manic-depressive illness. Lithium was first used to treat mania in 1949; prior to that time, lithium carbonate had been used as a "salt" substitute and was added to mineral waters, such as "lithia water." Lithium has a narrow therapeutic window, and slight elevations of serum levels result in toxicity. For this reason, patients on therapy must be monitored closely. A gradual onset of intoxication is more common than an acute overdose; the early symptoms include drowsiness, lethargy, slurred speech, muscle twitching, vomiting, and diarrhea. Extremely high serum lithium levels may lead to life-threatening toxicity.

10.8.2   Drugs of Abuse

COCAINE has probably been used for more than 2,000 years as a stimulant. Cocaine (see Fig. 1.1) is an alkaloid from the plant *Erythroxylon coca,* which grows extensively in the Andes Mountains of South America; its leaves contain from 1% to 2% cocaine. The Indians living in the region chew the leaves to offset fatigue and hunger and, as a result of the drug's stimulant effect, are able to work for long hours. People of the ancient Inca civilization regarded the coca plant as a gift from the gods.

In the late nineteenth and early twentieth centuries, cocaine from the coca leaves was a major ingredient in many popular beverages, such as Mariani Coca Wine. Coca-Cola was first marketed as an elixir containing cocaine from the coca leaf and caffeine from the African kola nut; hence the name Coca-Cola. In 1906, after public pressure, Coca-Cola agreed to use decocainized coca leaves. Cocaine came under strict control with the passage of the Harrison Narcotics Act of 1914, and was seen by many legislators as the major drug problem at that time. Use of cocaine diminished and became insignificant from the 1930s to the 1950s. Starting in the 1960s, however, an explosion in use occurred. In clinical use, cocaine is an excellent local anaesthetic and vasoconstrictor of mucous membranes. For these reasons, it is used in nasal surgery, rhinoplasty, and emergency nasotracheal intubation.

Nonmedicinal cocaine is brought into this country illegally from South America—mainly from Columbia, Peru, Bolivia, and Ecuador—where it is extracted and refined to form the hydrochloride salt. The cocaine is then "cut" with mannitol, lactose, glucose, or cornstarch. The most common route of use is by inhalation, after which the onset of action is rapid, occurring within 5 to 10 minutes, with a duration of about 60 minutes.

Cocaine is a powerful CNS stimulant, and occasional users experience euphoria, stimulation, reduced fatigue, garrulousness, a joyous feeling, increased energy, confidence, and a sensation of mastery and competence. The cocaine high is extremely pleasurable; laboratory animals will give up food for self-administered

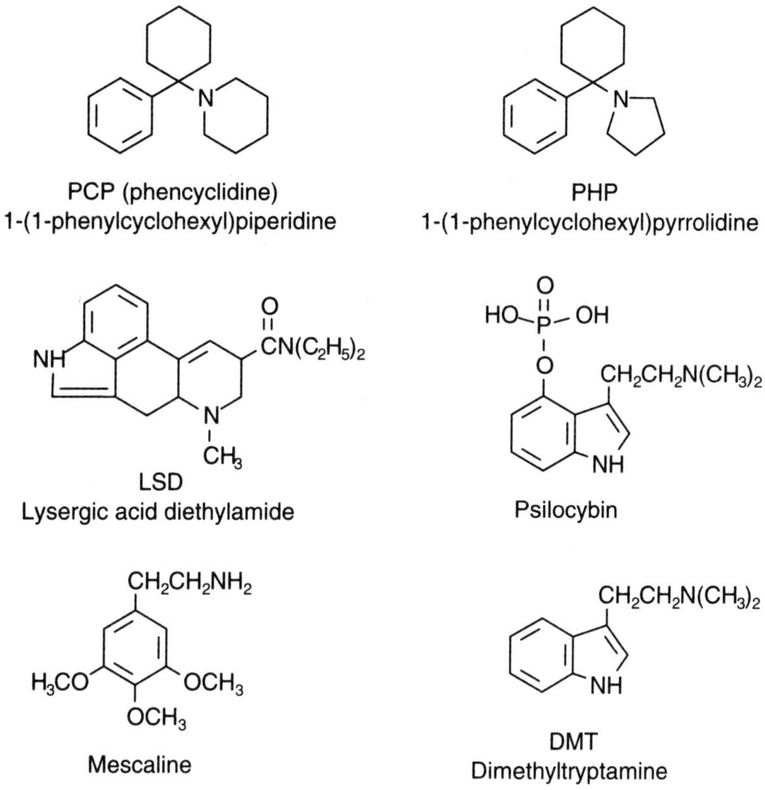

PCP (phencyclidine)
1-(1-phenylcyclohexyl)piperidine

PHP
1-(1-phenylcyclohexyl)pyrrolidine

LSD
Lysergic acid diethylamide

Psilocybin

Mescaline

DMT
Dimethyltryptamine

Figure 10.15. Structures of some common hallucinogens.

doses of cocaine and will even starve to death to continue receiving the drug. Heavy regular use generates a number of unpleasant side effects, however: insomnia, anxiety, paranoia, and hallucinations. A common occurrence is "cocaine bugs"—the sensation of bugs crawling under the skin. Cocaine does not produce physical addiction but does become psychologically addictive. Acute overdoses are most common when users inject cocaine by IV or use freebase; toxicological symptoms include seizures, cardiac arrhythmias, and respiratory arrest.

PHENCYCLIDINE (PCP) was marketed in 1958 for experimental use in humans as a general anaesthetic under the trade-name Scrnyl (Fig. 10.15). It was a superior anaesthetic in that it was nonnarcotic and did not depress respiration, but its use was discontinued because of adverse side effects, including extreme agitation, delirium, disorientation, and hallucinations. In 1967, it was reintroduced as a veterinary anesthetic, Sernylan, and was used until 1978 when it was voluntarily withdrawn. By the early and mid-1970s, PCP had appeared on the streets. PCP can be taken by mouth, inhalation (smoking), or snorting; rarely is it used IV. Phencyclidine has more than 30 chemical analogs, many of which produce similar effects. For example, the compound PHP contains pyrrolidine rather than piperidine (Fig. 10.15) and is a common substitute for PCP. Users of low doses frequently feel inebriated and disoriented and experience a kind of "numbness," progressing to inability to feel pain. Nystagmus, or involuntary movement of the eyeballs, is frequently seen with PCP use and is characteristic of that drug. Moderate to high doses usually result in the user becoming comatose—most often for only a few hours, but occasionally as long as 6 to 10 days. Deaths from PCP intoxication are usually the result of accidents related to delirium of the user (eg, drownings, automobile accidents, fires, street fights, and other dangers); PCP itself is relatively nontoxic.

LYSERGIC ACID DIETHYLAMIDE (LSD) (Fig. 10.15) is a very potent and widely used hallucinogen. LSD was synthesized by Swiss chemist Albert Hoffman in 1938. LSD is an abbreviation of the German lyserg saure diethylamid. Its potent psychoactive properties were discovered by Hoffman in 1943 when he accidently inhaled a minute quantity of the drug. He later described his experience: " . . . fantastic visions of extraordinary vividness accompanied by a kaleidoscopic play of intense coloration continuously swirled around me. After 2 hours this condition subsided." In the middle to late 1950s, LSD was used widely by psychiatrists in diverse clinical investigations, most frequently to increase insight and resurrect repressed material. Because efficacy was inconsistent and it was not superior to other forms of psychotherapy, however, its use declined. Because of its extremely high potency, an ounce of uncut LSD will provide up to 150,000 doses of 200 mg each. LSD is available in tablet or powder and occasionally it is placed on sugar cubes, chewing gum, crackers, or as colored dots of LSD on aspirin. LSD is almost always taken orally, rather than IV or by smoking. It is rapidly absorbed from the GI tract, producing effects within 30 minutes, with peak activity in 1 to 2 hours. At times, the psychic effects last for 10 to 12 hours. The effects of visual illusions and altered perceptions of color and distances are frequent. Time sense is lost, and concentration is attenuated; many users believe that they can think "more deeply" and may become engrossed in philosophical or ethical issues that to an "outsider," make little or no sense. The most common adverse reaction to LSD results from a bad trip associated with frightening illusions, and the user develops a panic state, fearing insanity. Other phenomena of LSD use are flashbacks, or spontaneous recurrences of the trip; these may occur several times a day and sometimes up to 18 months after use. These flashbacks occur most frequently in chronic LSD users and may be pleasant or unpleasant. LSD is most often implicated in accidental deaths (for example, users who believe they can fly) and suicides. Several investigations of the ability of LSD to cause teratogenesis or chromosome breaks have proved inconclusive.

MESCALINE (Fig. 10.15), named after the Mascalero, an Apache tribe, is the major active psychedelic alkaloid in the peyote cactus, which grows in Mexico and the southwestern United States. Mescaline was first isolated in 1896 and was successfully synthesized in 1918. Today, it is available for street use as either peyote extracts or from synthesis. The term peyote refers to the unmodified cactus, usually chewed in the form of a dried "button," which may contain as much as 6% mescaline. Peyote was used in Mexico by the Aztecs in religious ceremonies for centuries, and peyote cults became established in this country in the late nineteenth century as a result of raids into Mexico. Peyote use in Indian religious ceremonies became widespread, and the Native American Church was founded in 1918 as a defense against antipeyote legislation. When used as a religious sacrament, peyote use is legal in the United States.

PSILOCYBIN. The ancient Aztec rituals included not only the use of peyote cactus, but also morning glory seeds (which have psychedelic properties) and the "sacred" mushroom, teonanacatl, containing at least 20 hallucinogenic mushroom species. The active ingredient is psilocybin (Fig. 10.15), a derivative of dimethyltryptamine. Psilocybin is shorter acting, but with similar effects to LSD.

DIMETHYLTRYPTAMINE (DMT) (Fig. 10.15) is representative of many of the hallucinogenic tryptamine derivatives. DMT was first isolated from hallucinogenic snuffs used by the native Indians of the Caribbean and South America. DMT is inactive when ingested orally, so it is usually inhaled either by sniffing the powder or by smoking tobacco or marijuana previously soaked in it. DMT and diethyltryptamine (DET) have effects similar to those of LSD, but the "high" lasts for only 30 to 60 minutes.

MARIJUANA is a commonly used illegal drug in America. Although there are fads in illegal drug use, the use of marijuana has remained consistently high. *Cannabis sativa* is a hemp plant that has been used for centuries, not only for its psychoactive resin, but also for production of hemp fiber and rope. The cannaboid delta-9-tetrahydrocannabinol (THC) is the principal active ingredient in the plant (see Fig. 1.1). Depending on cultivation, the concentration of THC can range from 0.4% to 5%. Marijuana generally refers to tobacco-like preparations of leaves and flowers, whereas hashish is the resin extracted from the tops of the flowering plants and may contain up to 10% THC.

Smoking the cigarette or "joint" is the most common method of use of marijuana in the United States, and effective brain levels are rapidly achieved. Users of low to moderate doses generally report a feeling of well-being, a state of pleasant relaxation, a heightening of their senses (for example, clearer perception of music), and an alteration of time and space perception. Most describe their use in favorable terms and enjoy their experiences. However, while intoxicated, users may have poor cognitive functions and difficulty with motor functions. The chronic effects of marijuana remain controversial; although there is no direct evidence that smoking marijuana correlates with lung cancer, evidence does indicate that daily use of marijuana can lead to lung damage similar to that seen in cigarette smokers. Studies on reproductive effects have also been inconclusive. Although decreases in sperm count and motility have been found, there is usually a return to normal when marijuana use is discontinued.

Suggested Further Reading

Air Pollutants

Christiani DC: Urban and transboundary air pollution: human health consequences. In *Critical Condition. Human Health and the Environment*. Chivian E, McCally M, Hu H, Haines A, (eds.). Cambridge, MA: MIT Press, 1993, pp 13–30.

Costa DL, Amdur MO: Air pollution. In *Casarett & Doull's Toxicology, the Basic Science of Poisons,* 5th ed. Klaassen CD (ed.). New York: McGraw-Hill, 1996, pp 857–882.

Dockers DW, Pope CA: Acute respiratory effects of particulate air pollution. *Rev Public Health* **15:**107–132, 1994.

Freemantle M: The acid test for Europe. *Chemical and Engineering News*, May 1, 1995, pp 10–17.

Gardner DE, Gardner SCM: Toxicology of air pollution. In *Basic Environmental Toxicology,* Cokerham LG, Shane BS (eds.). Boca Raton, FL: CRC Press, 1994, pp 287–319.

Kaiser J: Acid rain's dirty business: stealing minerals from soil. *Science* **272:**198, 1996.

Landis WG, Yu M-H: Inorganic gaseous pollutants. In *Introduction to Environmental Toxicology.* Boca Raton, FL: Lewis Publishers, 1995, pp 135–158.

Leaf A: Loss of stratospheric ozone and health effects of increased ultraviolet radiation. In *Critical Condition. Human Health and the Environment.* Chivian E, McCally M, Hu M, Haines A (eds.). Cambridge, MA: MIT Press, 1993, pp 139–150.

Mlot, C: A clearer view of why plants make haze. *Science* **268:**641–642, 1995.

Samet JM, Marbury MC, Spengler JD: Health effects and sources of indoor air pollution. Part I. *American Review of Respiratory Diseases* **137:**221–242, 1988.

Spengler JD, Sexton K: Indoor air pollution: a public health perspective. *Science* **221:**9–17, 1983.

Thurston GD, et al: Reexamination of London, England, mortality in relation to exposure to acidic aerosols during 1963–71 winters. *Environ Health Perspect* **79:**73–82, 1989.

Soil and Water Pollutants

Bates MN, Smith AH, Hopenhayn-Rich C: Arsenic ingestion and internal cancers: a review. *Am J Epidemiol* **135:**462–476, 1992.

Centers for Disease Control. *Preventing Lead Poisoning in Young Children.* US Department of Health and Human Services, 1991.

Egboka BC, et al: Principles and problems of environmental pollution of groundwater resources with case examples from developing countries. *Environ Health Perspect* **83:**39–68, 1989.

Environmental Protection Agency, Office of Drinking Water Health Advisories. Nitrate and nitrite. *Rev Environ Contamin Toxicol* **107:**1988.

Forman D: Are nitrites a significant risk factor in human cancer? *Canc Surv* **8:**443–458, 1989.

Hu H, Kim NK: Drinking-water pollution and human health. In *Critical Condition. Human Health and the Environment.* Chivian E, McCally M, Hu H, Haines A (eds.). Cambridge, MA: MIT Press, 1993, pp 31–48.

Igbedioh SO: Effects of agricultural pesticides on humans, animals, and higher plants in developing countries. *Arch Environ Health* **46:**218–223, 1991.

Johnson CJ, Kross BD: Continuing importance of nitrate contamination of groundwater and wells in rural areas. *Am J Ind Med* **18:**449–456, 1990.

National Academy of Sciences. *The Health Effects of Nitrate, Nitrite, and* N-*Nitroso Compounds.* 1981.

NIH:NIEHS (National Institutes of Health: National Institutes of Environmental Health): Health Effects of Toxic Wastes. *Environ Health Perspect* **48:**1–145,1983.

Nriagu JO, Pacyna JM: Quantitative assessment of worldwide contamination of air, water, and soils by trace metals. *Nature* **333:**134–139, 1988.

Ritter, WF: Pesticide contamination of groundwater in the United States—a review. *J Environ Sci Health* **25:**1–29, 1990.

Food Additives and Contaminants

Ames BN, Profet M, Gold LS: Dietary pesticides (99.989% all natural). *Proc Natl Acad Sci* **87:**7777–7781, 1990.

Archer MC: Mechanisms of action of *N*-nitroso compounds. *Canc Surv* **8:**241–250, 1989.

Bowen, EL, Hu H: Food contamination due to environmental pollution. In *Critical Condition. Human Health and the Environment.* Chivian E, McCally M, Hu H, Haines A (eds.). Cambridge, MA: MIT Press, 1993, pp 49–69.

Concon J: *Food Toxicology.* New York: Marcel Dekker, 1988.

Ellwein LB, Cohen SM: The health risks of saccharin revisited. *Crit Rev Toxicol* **20:**311–326, 1990.

Ferrer A, Cabral JPR: Epidemics due to pesticide contamination of food. *Food Additives and Contaminants* **6:**(Suppl1):S95–S98, 1989.

Institute of Medicine. *Seafood Safety.* Washington, DC: National Academy Press, 1991.

Kotsonis FN, Burdock GA, Flamm WG: Food toxicology. In *Casarett & Doull's Toxicology. The Basic Science of Poisons,* 5th ed. Klaassen CD (ed.). New York: McGraw-Hill, 1996, pp 909–949.

National Academy of Sciences. *Health Effects of Nitrate, Nitrite and N-Nitroso Compounds.* Washington, DC: National Academy Press, 1981.

National Research Council. *Carcinogens and Anticarcinogens in the Human Diet.* Washington, DC: National Academy Press, 1996.

National Research Council. *Diet, Nutrition and Cancer.* Washington, DC: National Academy Press, 1982.

National Research Council. *Pesticides in the Diets of Infants and Children.* Washington, DC: National Academy Press, 1982.

Shank FR, Carson KL: What is safe food? In *Food Safety Assessment,* Finley JW, Robinson SF, Armstong DJ (eds.). Washington, DC: American Chemical Society, 1992, pp 26–35.

Tanner CM, Langston JW: Do environmental toxins cause Parkinson's disease? A critical review. *Neurology* **40:**17–30, 1990.

Verhagen H, Schilderman PA, Kleinjans, JC: Butylated hydroxyanisole in perspective. *Chem Biol Interact* **89:**109–134, 1991.

Occupational Toxicants

American Conference of Governmental Industrial Hygienists: *TLVs, Threshold Limit Values for Chemical Substances and Physical Agents and Biological Exposure Indices (BEIs).* Cincinnati, OH: American Conference of Governmental Industrial Hygienists, 1995–1996.

Albertson TE, Cross CE: Pesticides in the workplace: a worldwide issue. *Arch Environ Health* **48:**364–365, 1993.

Baker DB, Landregan PJ: Occupational exposure and human health. *In Critical Condition. Human Health and the Environment.* Chivian E, McCally M, Hu H, Haines A (eds.). Cambridge, MA: MIT Press, 1993, pp 71–91.

International Agency for Research on Cancer. *IARC Monographs on the Evaluation of the Carcinogenic Risk of Chemicals to Humans: Some Industrial Chemical Dyestuffs.* Lyons, France: International Agency for Research on Cancer, 1982.

Lauwerys R, Hoet P: *Industrial Chemical Exposure: Guidelines for Biological Monitoring,* 2nd ed. Boca Raton, FL: Lewis, 1993.

Lauwerys RR: Occupational toxicology. In *Casarett & Doull's Toxicology. The Basic Science of Poisons,* 5th ed. Klaassen CD (ed.). New York: McGraw-Hill, 1996, pp 987–1009.

Levy BS, Wegman DH (eds.): *Occupational Health—Recognizing and Preventing Work-Related Diseases,* 2nd ed. New York, NY: Brown & Co., 1988.

O'Donoghue JL (ed.): *Neurotoxicity of Industrial and Commercial Chemicals.* Vols. 1, 2. Boca Raton, FL: CRC Press, 1985.

Snyder R: The benzene problem in historical perspective. *Fund Appl Toxicol* **4:**692–699, 1984.

Pesticides

Abou-Donia MB, Lapadula D: Mechanisms of organophosphorus ester-induced delayed neurotoxicity: type I and type II. *Ann Rev Pharmacol Toxicol* **30:**405–440, 1990.

Abou-Donia MB: Pesticides. In *Neurotoxicology.* Abou-Donia, MB (ed.). Boca Raton, FL: CRC Press, 1992, pp 437–478.

Ames BN, Profet M, Gold LS: Dietary pesticides (99.989% all natural). *Proc Nat Acad Sci* **87:**7777–7781, 1990.

Baker SR, Wilkinson CF (eds.): *The Effects of Pesticides on Human Health. Advances in Modern Environmental Toxicology,* Vol XVIII, Princeton, NJ: Princeton Scientific, 1990.

Chambers JE, Levi PE (eds.): *Organophosphates. Chemistry, Fate and Effects.* New York: Academic Press, 1992.

Ecobichon DJ, Joy RM (eds.): *Pesticides and Neurological Diseases,* 2nd ed. Boca Raton, FL: CRC Press, 1994.

Ecobichon DJ: Toxic effects of pesticides. In *Casarett & Doull's Toxicology. The Basic Science of Poisons,* 5th ed. Klaassen CD (ed.). New York: McGraw-Hill, 1996, pp 643–689.

Igbedioh SO: Effects of agricultural pesticides on humans, animals, and higher plants in developing countries. *Arch Environ Health* **46:**218–223, 1991.

Marrs, TC: Organophosphate poisoning. *Pharmacol Ther* **58:**51–66, 1993.

National Research Council. *Pesticides in the Diets of Infants and Children.* Washington, DC: National Academy Press, 1982.

Onyeama HP, Oehme FW: A literature review of paraquat toxicity. *Vet Hum Toxicol* **26:**494–502, 1984.

Ragsdale NN, Menzer RE: *Carcinogenicity and Pesticides: Principles, Issues, and Relationships.* Washington, DC: American Chemical Society, 1989.

Ritter WF: Pesticide contamination of groundwater in the United States—a review. *J Environ Sci Health* **25:**1–29, 1990.

Winter CK: Dietary pesticide risk assessment. *Rev Environ Contam Toxicol* **127:**23–67, 1992.

Wolff MS: Blood levels of organochlorine residues and risk of breast cancer. *J Natl Cancer Inst* **85:**648–652, 1993.

Metals

Abou-Donia MB: Metals. In *Neurotoxicology.* Abou-Donia MB (ed.). Boca Raton, FL: CRC Press, 1992, pp 363–393.

Bates MN, Smith AH, Hopenhayn-Rich C: Arsenic ingestion and internal cancers: a review. *AJ Epid* **135:**462–476, 1992.

Centers for Disease Control. *Preventing Lead Poisoning in Young Children.* US Department of Health and Human Services, No 99-2230, Washington, DC: US Government Printing Office, 1991.

Chen CL, Kuo TL, Wu MM: Arsenic and cancers. *Lancet* **1:**414–415, 1988.

Cohen AJ, Rose FJ: Review of lead toxicology relevant to the safety assessment of lead acetate as a hair colouring. *Food Chem Toxicol* **29:**485, 1991.

Fitzgerald WF, Clarkson TW: Mercury and monomethylmercury: present and future concerns. *Environ Health Perspect* **96:**159–166, 1991.

Goyer RA: Toxic effects of metals. In *Casarett & Doull's Toxicology. The Basic Science of Poisons,* 5th ed. Klaassen CD (ed.). New York: McGraw-Hill, 1996, pp 691–736.

Hernandez-Avila M, et al: Lead-glazed ceramics as major determinants of blood lead levels in Mexican women. *Environ Health Perspect* **94:**117–120, 1991.

Hostynek JJ, Hinz RS, Lorence CR, Price M, Guy RH: Metals and the skin. *Crit Rev Toxicol* **23:**171–235, 1993.

Nakagawa H, et al: High mortality and shortened life-span in patients with Itai-Itai disease and subjects with suspected disease. *Arch Environ Health* **45:**283–287. 1990.

Needleman HL, et al: The long-term effects of exposure to low doses of lead in children. *N Engl J Med* **322:**83–88, 1990.

Philipp R: Arsenic exposure: health effects and the risk of cancer. *Rev Environ Health* **5:**27, 1985.

Ruff HA, et al: Declining blood lead levels and cognitive changes in moderately lead-poisoned children. *JAMA* **269:**1641–1646, 1993.

Tseng WP: Effects and dose–response relationship of skin cancer and Blackfoot disease with arsenic. *Environ Health Perspect* **19:**109–199, 1977.

Solvents

Abou-Donia MB: Solvents. In *Neurotoxicology.* Abou-Donia MB (ed.). Boca Raton, FL: CRC Press, 1992, pp 395–421.

Beauchamp RO Jr, Bus JS, Popp JA, et al: A critical review of the literature on carbon disulfide toxicity. *CRC Crit Rev Toxicol* **11:**169–278, 1983.

Benignus VA: Neurobehavior effects of toluene: a review. *Neurobehav Toxicol Teratol* **3:**407–415, 1981.

Linz DH, deGarmo PL, Morton WE, et al: Organic solvent–induced encephalophy in industrial painters. *J Occup Med* **28:**119–125, 1986.

Morton HG: Occurrence and treatment of solvent abuse in children and adolescents. *Pharmacol Ther* **33:**449–469, 1987.

National Institutes of Health: National Institute of Environmental Health (NIH:NIEH). Toxic Effects of Glycol Ethers. *Environ Health Perspect* **57:**1–278, 1984.

Pohl LR: Biochemical toxicology of chloroform. In *Reviews in Biochemical Toxicology 1.* Hodgson E, Bend JR, Philpot RM (eds.). New York: Elsevier, 1979, pp. 79–107.

Reese E, Kimbrough RD: Acute toxicity of gasoline and some additives. *Environ Health Perspect* **101**(Suppl 6):115–131, 1993.

Snyder R, Kalf GF: A perspective on benzene leukemogenesis. *Crit Rev Toxicol* **24:**177–209, 1994.

Snyder R, Andrews LS: Toxic effects of solvents and vapors. In *Casarett & Doull's Toxicology. The Basic Science of Poisons,* 5th ed. Klaassen CD (ed.). New York: McGraw-Hill, 1996, pp 737–771.

Snyder R, Witz G, Goldstein BD: The toxicology of benzene. *Environ Health Perspect* **100**:293–306, 1993.

Drugs

Abou-Donia MB: Drugs of abuse. In *Neurotoxicology.* Abou-Donia MB (ed.). Boca Raton, FL: CRC Press, 1992, pp 497–499.

Frommer DA, Kulig KW, Marx JA, Rumack B: Tricyclic antidepressant overdose: a review. *JAMA* **257**:521–526, 1987.

Haddad LM, Winchester JF (eds.). *Clinical Management of Poisoning and Drug Overdose.* Philadelphia: WB Saunders, 1983.

Martin WR: Pharmacology of opioids. *Pharmacol Rev* **35**:285–323, 1984.

Pentel P: Toxicity of over-the-counter stimulants. *JAMA* **252**:1898–1903, 1984.

Smith EA, Meloan CE, Pickell JA, et al: Scopolamine poisoning from homemade "Moon Flower" wine. *J Anal Toxicol* **15**:216–219, 1991.

Stollard D, Edes TE: Muscarinic poisoning from medications and mushrooms. *Postgrad Med* **85(1)**:341–345, 1989.

Temple AR: Acute and chronic effects of aspirin toxicity and their treatment. *Arch Intern Med* **141**:364–369, 1981.

TOXICITY TESTING AND RISK ASSESSMENT

11

ERNEST HODGSON

11.1

INTRODUCTION

Although testing for toxicity, usually for the purposes of risk assessment, might be expected to be one of the more routine aspects of toxicology, it is actually one of the more controversial. Among the many areas of controversy are the use of animals for testing and the welfare of the animals used; choice of animals and genetic strains; extrapolation from experimental animals to humans; extrapolation from high-dose to low-dose effects; and the increasing cost and complexity of testing protocols relative to the benefits expected. New tests are constantly being devised and are often added to testing requirements already in existence.

Most testing can be subdivided into in vivo tests for acute, subchronic, or chronic effects and in vitro tests for genotoxicity or cell transformation, although other tests are used and are described in this chapter. Any chemical that has been introduced into commerce or that is being developed for possible introduction into commerce is subject to toxicity testing to satisfy the regulations of one or more regulatory agencies. Furthermore, compounds produced as waste products of industrial processes (eg, combustion products) are also subject to testing.

Toxicity assessment is the determination of the potential of any substance to act as a poison, the conditions under which this potential will be realized, and the characterization of its action. *Risk assessment*, however, is a quantitative assessment of the probability of deleterious effects under given exposure conditions. Both are involved in the regulation of toxic chemicals. *Regulation* is the control, by statute, of the manufacture, transportation, sale, or disposal of chemicals deemed to be toxic after testing procedures or according to criteria laid down in the law in question.

Testing in the United States is carried out by many groups: industrial, governmental, academic, and others (Table 11.1). Regulation, however, is carried out by a

TABLE 11.1. SOME EXAMPLES OF ORGANIZATIONS INVOLVED IN TOXICITY TESTING IN THE UNITED STATES

Industry (in-house or through contract laboratories)
Nongovernment institutes
   Chemical Industries Institute for Toxicology (CIIT)
Contract laboratories
   Hazleton Laboratories
   Research Triangle Institute
   SRI International
Federal agencies (often through contract laboratories)
   Environmental Protection Agency (EPA)
   Food and Drug Agency (FDA)
   National Toxicology Program (NTP)
   National Cancer Institute (NCI)
   National Center for Toxicological Research (NCTR)
   Occupational Safety and Health Administration (OSHA)
Academic institutions (usually involved only in specific parts of the overall testing program or in methods development)

narrow range of governmental agencies, each charged with the formulation of regulations under a particular law or laws and the administration of those regulations. Regulations for the United States are shown in Table 11.2. Other industrialized countries have counterpart laws and agencies for the regulation of toxic chemicals.

Although the objective of much, but by no means all, toxicity testing is the elimination of potential risks to humans, most of the testing is carried out on experimental animals. This is necessary because our current knowledge of quantitative structure activity relationships (QSAR) does not permit accurate extrapolation to new compounds. Human data is difficult to obtain experimentally for ethical reasons, but is necessary for such deleterious effects as irritation, nausea, allergies, odor evaluation, and some higher nervous system functions. Some insight may be obtained in certain cases from occupational exposure data, although this tends to be

TABLE 11.2. AGENCIES AND STATUTES INVOLVED IN REGULATION OF TOXIC CHEMICALS IN THE UNITED STATES

Food and Drug Administration (FDA)
   Food, Drug and Cosmetic Act
Labor Department
   Occupational Safety and Health Act
Consumer Products Safety Commission

Environmental Protection Agency (EPA)
   Federal Insecticide, Fungicide and Rodenticide Act
   Clean Air Act
   Federal Water Pollution Control Act
   Safe Drinking Water Act
   Toxic Substances Control Act
   Resource Conservation and Recovery Act

State governments
   Various state and local laws
   Enforcement of certain aspects of federal law delegated to states

irregular in time and not clearly defined as to the composition of the toxicant or the exposure levels, because multiple exposure is common. Clearly, any experiments involving humans must be carried out under carefully defined conditions after other testing is complete.

Although extrapolation from experimental animals to humans presents problems due to differences in metabolic pathways, penetration, mode of action, and so on, experimental animals present numerous advantages in testing procedures. These advantages include the possibility of clearly defined genetic constitution and their amenity to controlled exposure, controlled duration of exposure, and the possibility of detailed examination of all tissues following necropsy.

Although not all tests are required for all potentially toxic chemicals, any of the tests shown in Table 11.3 may be required by the regulations imposed under a

TABLE 11.3. A SUMMARY OF TESTS FOR TOXICITY

I. Chemical and physical properties
   For the compound in question, probable contaminants from synthesis as well as intermediates and waste products from synthetic processes.
II. Exposure and environmental fate
   A. Degradation studies—hydrolysis, photodegradion, etc.
   B. Degradation in soil, water, etc., under various conditions
   C. Mobility and dissipation in soil, water, and air
   D. Accumulation in plants, aquatic animals, wild terrestrial animals, food plants and animals, etc.
III. In vivo tests
   A. Acute
      1. LD50 and/or LC50—oral, dermal, or inhaled
      2. Eye irritation
      3. Dermal irritation
      4. Dermal sensitization
   B. Subchronic
      1. 90-day feeding
      2. 30- to 90-day dermal or inhalation exposure
   C. Chronic
      1. Chronic feeding (including oncogenicity tests)
      2. Teratogenicity
      3. Reproduction (more than one generation)
   D. Special tests
      1. Neurotoxicity (delayed neuropathy)
      2. Potentiation
      3. Metabolism
      4. Pharmacodynamics
      5. Behavioral
IV. In vitro tests
   A. Mutagenicity—prokaryote (Ames test)
   B. Mutagenicity—eukaryote (*Drosophilia,* mouse, etc.)
   C. Chromosome aberration (*Drosophilia,* sister chromatid exchange, etc.)
V. Effects on wildlife
   Selected species of wild mammals, birds, fish, and invertebrates: acute toxicity, accumulation, and reproduction in laboratory simulated field conditions or actual field conditions.

particular law. The particular set of tests required depends on the predicted or actual use of the chemical, the predicted or actual route of exposure, and the chemical and physical properties of the chemical.

11.2

EXPERIMENTAL ADMINISTRATION OF TOXICANTS

Regardless of the chemical tested and whether the test is for acute or chronic toxicity, all in vivo testing requires the administration of a known dose of the chemical under test that is applied in a reproducible manner, which is generally related to the expected route of exposure of humans to the chemical in question. The nature and degree of toxic effect may or may not be affected by the route of administration (Table 11.4). This may be related to differences at the portals of entry or to effects on pharmacokinetic processes. In the latter case, one route may give rise to a concentration high enough to saturate some rate-limiting process, whereas another may distribute the dose over a longer time and avoid such saturation. Another key question is that of appropriate experimental controls. To identify effects of handling and other stresses as well as the effects of the solvents or other carriers, it is usually better to compare treated animals with both solvent-treated and untreated or possibly sham-treated controls.

ORAL. Oral administration is often referred to as administration per os (PO). Compounds can be administered mixed in the diet, dissolved in drinking water, by gastric gavage, by controlled-release capsules, or by gelatin capsules. In the first two cases, either a measured amount can be provided or access can be ad libitum, with the dose estimated from consumption measurements. In the last case, controls should be pair-fed, that is, permitted only the amount of food consumed by treated

TABLE 11.4. VARIATION IN TOXICITY BY ROUTE OF EXPOSURE

Chemical	Species/Gender	Route	LD50 (mg/kg)
N-Methyl-N-(1-naphthyl) fluoracetamide[a]	Mouse/M	Oral	371
		Dermal	402
		Subcutaneous	250
N-Methyl-N-(1-naphthyl) fluoracetamide[a]	Rat/M	Oral	115
		Dermal	300
		Subcutaneous	78
Chlordane[b]	Rat/M	Oral	335
		Dermal	840
Endrin[b]	Rat/M	Oral	18
		Dermal	18

[a] Data from Hashimoto Y, et al.: Toxicol Appl Pharmacol 12:536–547, 1968.
[b] Data from Allen JR, et al.: Pharmacol Ther 7:513–547, 1979.

animals, and, in any case, it is essential to consider possible nutritional effects caused by reduction of food intake due to distasteful or repellent test materials. In the case of gastric gavage, the test material is administered through a stomach tube or gavage needle; if a solvent is necessary, it is administered also to control animals.

DERMAL. Dermal administration is required for estimation of toxicity of chemicals that may be taken up through the skin, as well as for estimation of skin irritation and photosensitization. Compounds are applied, either directly or in a suitable solvent, to the shaved skin of experimental animals. Frequently, the animals must be under restraint to prevent licking, and hence oral uptake, of the material. Solvent and restraint controls are necessary because considerable stress is involved. Skin irritancy tests may be conducted on humans, using volunteer test panels.

INHALATION. The respiratory system is an important portal of entry and, for evaluation purposes, animals must be exposed to atmospheres containing potential toxicants. The generation and control of the physical characteristics of such contaminated atmospheres is technically complex and expensive in practice. The alternative—direct instillation into the lung through the trachea—presents problems of reproducibility and stress and for these reasons is generally unsatisfactory.

Inhalation toxicity studies are conducted in inhalation chambers. The complete system contains an apparatus for the generation of aerosol particles, dusts or gas mixtures of defined composition and particle size, a chamber for the exposure of experimental animals, and a sampling apparatus for the determination of the actual concentration within the chamber. All these devices present technical problems that are difficult to resolve.

Animals are normally exposed for a fixed number of hours each day and a fixed number of days each week. Exposure may be head only, in which the head of the animal, wearing an airtight collar, is inserted into the chamber; or whole body, in which the animal is placed inside the chamber. In the latter case, variations due to unequal distribution are minimized by rotation of the position of the cages in the chamber during subsequent exposures. Figure 11.1 shows a typical inhalation system and supporting equipment.

INJECTION. Except in the case of certain pharmaceuticals and drugs of abuse, injection (parenteral administration) does not correspond to any of the expected modes of exposure. It may be useful, however, in studies of mechanism or in QSAR studies in order to bypass absorption and permit rapid action. Methods of injection include intravenous (IV), intramuscular (IM), intraperitoneal (IP), and subcutaneous (SC); infusion of toxicants over an extended period is also possible. Again, both solvent controls and untreated controls are necessary for proper interpretation of the results.

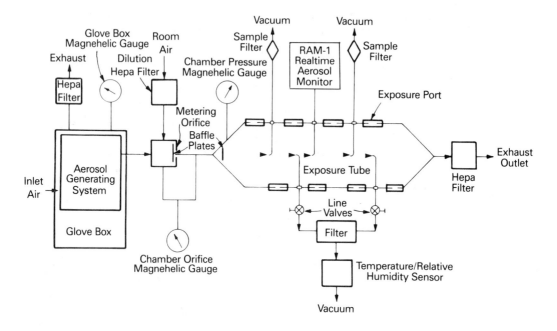

Figure 11.1. An inhalation exposure system. *(Source: Modified from Adkins et al: Am Int Hyg Assoc J **41**:494, 1980.)*

11.3

CHEMICAL AND PHYSICAL PROPERTIES

Although the determination of chemical and physical properties of known or potential toxicants does not constitute a test for toxicity, it is an essential preliminary for such tests. The information obtained can be used as follows:

- For structure activity comparisons with other known toxicants, which may indicate the most probable hazards.
- As an aid in identification in subsequent poisoning episodes.
- In determining stability to light, oxidizing or reducing agents, heat, and so on that, may enable preliminary estimates of persistence in the environment as well as indicate the most likely breakdown products that may also require testing for toxicity.
- In establishing such properties as the lipid solubility or octanol/water partition coefficient, which may enable preliminary estimates of rate of uptake

and persistence in living organisms. Vapor pressure may indicate whether the respiratory system is a probable route of entry.

• In acquiring knowledge of the chemical and physical properties needed to develop analytical methods for the measurement of the compound and its degradation products.

• If the chemical is being produced for commercial use, similar information is needed on intermediates in the synthesis or by-products of the process because both are possible contaminants in the final product.

11.4

EXPOSURE AND ENVIRONMENTAL FATE

Data on exposure and environmental fate are needed, not to determine toxicity, but to provide information that may be useful in the prediction of possible exposure in the event that the chemical is toxic. Primarily useful for chemicals released into the environment such as pesticides, these tests include the rate of breakdown under aerobic and anaerobic conditions in soils of various types, the rates of leaching into surface water from soils of various types, or the rate of movement toward groundwater. The effect of physical factors on degradation through photolysis and hydrolysis studies and the identification of the products formed can indicate the rate of loss of the hazardous chemical or the possible formation of hazardous degradation products. Tests for accumulation in plants and animals and movement within the ecosystem are considered in Section 11.7.

11.5

IN VIVO TESTS

Traditionally, the basis for the determination of toxicity has been administration of the suspected compound, in vivo, to one or more species of experimental animal, followed by examination for mortality in acute tests, or by pathological examination for tissue abnormalities in chronic tests. Such results are then used, by a variety of extrapolation techniques, to estimate hazard to humans. These techniques, which still offer many advantages and are widely used, are summarized in the remainder of this section. They suffer from a number of disadvantages: They require large numbers of animals, numbers deemed unnecessary by both animal rights and animal welfare advocates; they are extremely expensive to conduct; and they are time consuming. As a result, they have been supplemented by many specialized in vitro tests, some of which are summarized in Section 11.6.

11.5.1   Acute Toxicity

Acute toxicity is usually concerned with lethality through the estimation of the median lethal dose (LD50) or the median lethal concentration (LC50), although other acute effects, such as eye or skin irritation, are also subject to such tests.

11.5.1.1   LD50 and LC50

The LD50 is the estimated dose that, when the toxicant is administered directly to experimental test animals, results in the death of 50% of the population so exposed under the defined conditions of the test. The LC50 is the estimated concentration, in the environment to which animals are exposed, that will kill 50% of the population so exposed under the defined conditions of the test. The LD50 concept was developed by Trevan in 1927. The values are usually presented as an estimate with confidence limits, derived from treating several groups of animals with different doses. The simplest method for the determination of LD50 and LC50, with confidence limits, is a graphic one and is based on the assumption that the effect is a quantal one (all or none), that the percentage responding in an experimental group is dose-related, and that the cumulative effect follows a normal distribution.

Data from a typical example (Fig. 11.2) can be plotted against the log dose to give either a normal distribution (frequency or mortality of one dose minus that of the lower dose) or a sigmoid curve (percentage of mortality at each dose). If the distribution is normal, the point of inflection is the LD50 and the extrapolated doses at 16% and 84% mortality are equal to ±1 standard deviation (SD). The sigmoid curve causes problems of extrapolation and slope determination, however, and methods have been developed to linearize mortality plots. The one described is used almost exclusively and involves the transformation of the percentage of mortality figure to probits, units based on normal distribution statistics. This is done graphically by plotting the data on log/probit graph paper on which the mortality scale is derived so that the divisions marked as percentages are in fact probit units (Fig. 11.2); thus, percentage data are plotted directly as probits. Similarly, the dose scale is a logarithmic scale; by plotting the raw data on such a scale, a log transformation is obtained without calculation.

CRITICISM OF THE LD50 TEST. The LD50 test has been the subject of much recent controversy, being criticized on various grounds, including:

- Used uncritically, it is an expression of lethality only, not reflecting other acute effects.
- It requires large numbers of experimental animals to obtain statistically acceptable values. Moreover, the results of LD50 tests are known to vary with species, strain, sex, age, and so on (Table 11.5); thus, the values are seldom closely similar from one laboratory to another, in spite of the numbers used.
- Because, for regulatory purposes, the most important information needed concerns chronic toxicity, little useful information is derived from the LD50

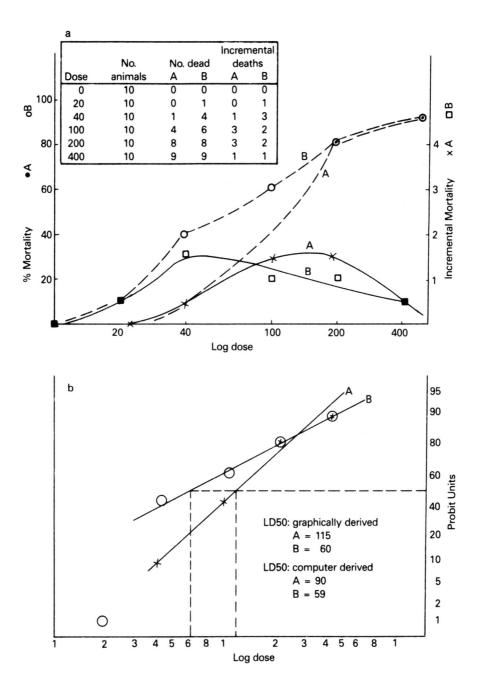

Figure 11.2. Data from an LD50 experiment plotted as percentage of mortality at each dose (graph a) or with the percentages expressed as probit units (graph b).

TABLE 11.5. FACTORS CAUSING VARIATION IN LD50 VALUES

Species	Health	Temperature
Strain	Nutrition	Time of day
Age	Gut contents	Season
Weight	Route of administration	Human error
Gender	Housing	

test. The small amount of information that is acquired could be acquired as well from an approximation requiring only a small number of animals.

- Extrapolation to humans is difficult.

SUPPORT OF THE LD50 TEST. Continued use of the test has been advocated, however, on the grounds that it is of use in the following ways:

- Properly conducted, acute toxicity tests yield not only the LD50, but also information on other acute effects such as cause of death, time of death, symptomatology, nonlethal acute effects, organs affected, and reversibility of nonlethal effects.
- Information concerning mode of action and metabolic detoxication can be inferred from the slope of the mortality curve.
- The results can form the basis for the design of subsequent subchronic studies.
- The test is useful as a first approximation of hazards to workers.
- The test is rapidly completed.

For the previously listed reasons, there has been a concerted effort in recent years to modify the concept of acute toxicity testing as it is embodied in the regulations of many countries and to substitute more meaningful methods that use fewer experimental animals. The article by Zbinden and Flury-Roversi is an excellent summary of the factors affecting LD50 determinations, the advantages and disadvantages of requiring such tests, and the nature and value of the information derived. It concludes that the acute toxicity test (single-dose toxicity) is still of considerable importance for the assessment of risk posed by new chemical substances, and for a better control of natural and synthetic agents in the human environment. It is not permissible, however, to regard a routine determination of the LD50 in various animal species as a valid substitute for an acute toxicity study.

SUGGESTED ALTERNATIVES. The summary of suggested alternatives that follows owes much to the previously cited review:

- All regulations and guidelines should make clear that the classic LD50 test is not identical to the modern acute toxicity test.
- LD50 tests on animals of large size should be abandoned, and comprehensive acute toxicity tests using only small numbers of such animals should be substituted. These tests should include detailed observations of symptoms and physiological measurements such as blood pressure, body temperature,

TABLE 11.6. TOXICITY CLASSES

Class		LD50 (mg/kg)	Example
I	Extremely toxic	≤1	TCDD
II	Highly toxic	1–50	Picrotoxin
III	Moderately toxic	50–500	Phenobarbital
IV	Slightly toxic	500–5000	Morphine sulfate
V	Practically nontoxic	5000–15,000	Ethanol

Source: Modified after Zbindon G, Flury-Reversi M: Significance of the LD50-test for the toxicological evaluation of chemical substances. Arch Toxicol **47**:*77–99, 1981. Based on Loomis TA, Hayes AW: Loomis's Essentials of Toxicology, 4th ed. San Diego: Academic Press, 1996, pp 24–25.*

reflex activity, electrocardiogram (ECG), electroencephalogram (EEG), food and water intake, respiration, behavior, and so on. Chemical determinations such as blood chemistry and urinalysis should also be made, as well as measurement of excretion of the parent compounds and its possible metabolites, Finally, gross and microscopic pathology should be determined.

- Alternatives to the classic LD50 tests, even in those cases in which a numerical value is essential, should be used. They include the approximate lethal dose method of Deichman and Le Blanc, the moving average method of Thompson, the up and down method of Dixon and Mood, or the method recently proposed by Molinengo based on the relationship between dose and survival time. All these methods use small numbers of animals; the details of their use may be found in Hayes (Section 11.10).

- For many regulatory purposes, it is valuable to classify chemicals into toxicity classes (Table 11.6). This can be done by treating small numbers of animals with doses that represent the upper limit of the class, starting with the lowest dose and stopping the test with the dose at which 50% or more of the animals die.

- LD50 tests should never be carried out on pharmacologically inert compounds. It is sufficient to know, for exmple, that a single oral dose of 5 g/kg or a single parenteral dose of 2 g/kg causes neither death nor acute symptoms.

11.5.1.2   Eye Irritation

Because of the prospect of permanent blindness, ocular toxicity has long been a subject of both interest and concern. Although all regions of the eye are subject to systemic toxicity, usually chronic but sometimes acute, the tests of concern in this section are tests for irritancy of compounds applied topically to the eye. The tests used are all variations of the Draize test, and the preferred experimental animal is the albino rabbit.

The test consists of adding the material to be tested directly into the conjunctival sac of one eye of each of several albino rabbits, with the other eye serving as the control. The lids are held together for a few seconds, and the material is left in the eye for at least 24 hr. After that time it may be rinsed out, but in any case, the eye is graded after 1, 2, and 3 days. Grading is subjective and based on the appearance of the cornea, particularly as regards opacity; the iris, as regards both appearance and reaction to light; the conjunctiva, as regards redness and effects on blood vessels; and the eyelids, as regards swelling. Fluorescein may be used to assist visual examination because the dye is more readily absorbed by damaged tissues, which then fluoresce when the eye is illuminated. Each item in the evaluation is scored on a numerical scale and chemicals are compared on this basis. Although each regulatory agency may require a slightly different evaluation protocol, all are variations of those as described here.

This test is probably the most criticized by advocates of animal rights and animal welfare, primarily on the grounds that it is inhumane. It has also been criticized on narrower scientific grounds in that both concentration and volumes used are unrealistically high, and that the results, because of high variability and the greater sensitivity of the rabbit eye, may not be applicable to humans. It is clear, however, that because of great significance of visual impairment, tests for ocular toxicity will continue.

Attempts to solve the dilemma have taken two forms: to find substitute in vitro tests and to modify the Draize test so that it becomes not only more humane but also more predictive for humans. Substitute tests consist of attempts to use cultured cells or eyes from slaughtered food animals, but neither method is yet acceptable as a routine test. Modifications consist primarily of using smaller volumes and lower concentrations of test materials. This appears to reduce variability and should probably be adopted.

11.5.1.3   Dermal Irritation and Sensitization

There are tests for dermal irritation caused by topical application of chemicals. These fall into four general categories: primary irritation, cutaneous sensitization, phototoxicity, and photosensitization. Because many foreign chemicals come into direct contact with the skin, including cosmetics, detergents, bleaches, and many others, these tests are considered essential to the proper regulation of such products. Less commonly, dermal effects may be caused by systemic toxicants.

In the typical primary irritation test, the backs of albino rabbits are clipped free of hair and two areas of about 5 cm^2 on each rabbit are used in the test. One such area is lightly abraded; both areas are then treated with either 0.5 mL or 0.5 g of the compounds to be tested and are covered with a gauze pad. The entire trunk of the rabbit is wrapped with an impervious material that is held in place with adhesive tape. After 23 hr, the tape and gauze are removed; after another hour, the treated areas are evaluated for erythematous lesions (redness of the skin produced by congestion of the capillaries) and edematous lesions (accumulation of excess fluid in SC tissue), each of which is expressed on a numerical scale. After an additional 48 hr, the treated areas are again evaluated.

Some tests are simply variants of those described and are the most frequently used tests for evaluation of primary skin irritation. Other tests such as the mouse ear test and the guinea pig immersion test are also available, but are used much less frequently.

Skin sensitization tests are designed to test the ability of chemicals to affect the immune system in such a way that a second contact causes a more severe reaction. This latter may be elicited at a much lower concentration and in areas beyond the area of initial contact. The antigen involved is presumed to be formed by the binding of the chemical to body proteins, the ligand–protein complex then being recognized as a foreign protein to which antibodies can be formed. Subsequent exposure may then give rise to an allergic reaction. The test animal commonly used in skin sensitization tests is the guinea pig; animals are treated with the test compound in a suitable vehicle, with the vehicle alone, or with a positive control such as 2,4-dinitrochlorobenzene in the same vehicle. During the induction phase, the animals are treated for each of 3 days evenly spaced during a 2-week period. This is followed by a 2-week rest period, followed by the challenge phase of the test. This consists of a 24-hr topical treatment carried out as described for primary skin irritation tests. The lesions are scored on the basis of severity and the number of animals responding (incidence).

Other test methods include those in which the induction phase is conducted by intradermal injection together with Freund's adjuvant (a chemical mixture that enhances the antigenic response) and the challenge by dermal application, or tests in which both induction and challenge doses are topical but the former is accompanied by intradermal injections of Freund's adjuvant. It is important that compounds that cause primary skin irritation be tested for skin sensitization at concentrations low enough that the two effects are not confused.

Phototoxicity tests are designed to evaluate the combined dermal effects of light (primarily ultra violet [UV] light) and the chemical in question. Tests have been described for both phototoxicity and photoallergy. In both cases, the light energy is believed to cause a transient excitation of the toxicant molecule, which, on returning to the lower energy state, generates a reactive, free-radical intermediate. In phototoxicity, these organic radicals act directly on the cells to cause lesions, whereas in photoallergy they bind to body proteins. These modified proteins then stimulate the immune system to produce antibodies, because the modifications cause them to be recognized as foreign or "nonself" proteins. These tests are basically modifications of the tests for primary irritation and sensitization except that, following application of the test chemical, the treated area is irradiated with UV light. The differences between the animals treated and irradiated and those treated and not irradiated is a measure of the phototoxic effect.

These dermal tests have all been criticized on various grounds. They can cause discomfort and are, to some extent, inhumane. The data generated are hard to extrapolate to humans; some tests (for example, those involving intradermal injection) are considered unrealistic. However, none of the in vitro tests investigated as alternatives have yet proved applicable, nor have they been accepted by regulatory agencies.

Much knowledge in these areas was previously obtained using human test panels. Objections to this on ethical grounds have been almost as numerous as objections to animal studies. At the same time, in view of the large number of chemicals to which human skin is exposed, it is difficult to foresee a time when some form of testing for dermal toxicity will not be required.

11.5.2 Subchronic Tests

Subchronic tests examine toxicity caused by repeated dosing over an extended period, but not one that is so long as to constitute a significant portion of the expected life span of the species tested. A 90-day oral study in the rat or dog would be typical of this type of study, as would a 30-day dermal application study or a 30- to 90-day inhalation study. Such tests provide information on essentially all types of chronic toxicity other than carcinogenicity and are usually believed essential for establishing the dose regimens for prolonged chronic studies. They are frequently used as the basis for the determination of the no-observable-effect level (NOEL). This value is often defined as the highest dose level at which no deleterious or abnormal effect can be measured, and is often used in risk assessment calculations. Subchronic tests are also useful in providing information on target organs and on the potential of the test chemical to accumulate in the organism.

11.5.2.1 Ninety-Day Feeding Tests

Chemicals are usually tested by administration in the diet, less commonly in the drinking water, and only when absolutely necessary by gavage, because the last process involves much handling and subsequent stress. The complexity of these tests is such that absolute care and attention must be paid at all times. Numerous experimental variables must be controlled and biologic variables evaluated. In addition, the number of endpoints that can be measured is also large and, as a consequence, record keeping and data analysis present problems. If all is done with care, however, much may be learned from such tests.

EXPERIMENTAL (NONBIOLOGIC) VARIABLES. Several environmental variables may affect toxicity evaluations, some directly and others by their effects on animal health. Major deviations from the optimum temperature and humidity for the species in question can cause stress reactions. Stress can also be caused by housing more than one species of experimental animal in the same room. Many toxic or metabolic effects show diurnal variations that are related to photoperiod. Cage design and the nature of the bedding have also been shown to affect the toxic response. Thus, the optimum housing conditions are clean rooms, each containing a single species, with the temperature, humidity, and photoperiod being constant and optimized for the species in question. Cages should be the optimum design for the species, bedding should be inert (not cause enzyme induction or other metabolic effect), and cages should not be overcrowded, with individual caging whenever possible.

Dose selection, preparation, and administration are all important variables. Subchronic studies are usually conducted using three (less often, four) dose levels. The highest should produce obvious toxicity but not high mortality and the lowest only slight or no mortality, whereas the intermediate dose(s) should give effects clearly intermediate between these two extremes. Although the doses can be extrapolated from acute tests, such extrapolation is difficult, particularly in the case of compounds that accumulate in the body; frequently, a 14-day range finding study is made. Although the route of administration should ideally mimic the expected route of exposure in humans, in practice the chemical is usually administered ad libitum in the diet, because this is, on average, most appropriate. Measurement of food consumption and pair-feeding with controls is recommended. In cases in which accurate measurement of consumption is an important factor in the experimental design, the animals may be fed by gavage or with capsules containing the toxicant.

To avoid effects from nonspecific variations on the diet, enough feed from the same batch should be obtained for the entire study. Part is set aside for the controls, and the remainder is mixed with the test chemical at the various dose levels. Care should be taken to store all food in such a way that not only does the test chemical remain stable, but the nutritional value is also maintained. The identity and concentration of the test chemical should be checked periodically by chemical analysis.

Subchronic studies are usually conducted with 10 to 20 males and 10 to 20 females of a rodent species at each dose level and 4 to 8 of each sex of a larger species, such as the dog, at each dose level. Animals should be drawn from a larger group and assigned to control or treatment groups by some random process, but the larger group should not vary so much that the mean weights and ages of the subgroups vary significantly at the beginning of the experiment.

BIOLOGIC VARIABLES. Subchronic studies should be conducted on two species, ideally a rodent and a nonrodent. Although the species chosen should be those with the greatest pharmacokinetic and metabolic similarity to humans for the compound in question, this information is seldom available. In practice, the most common rodent used is the rat, and the most common nonrodent used is the dog. It has long been held that inbred rodent strains should be used to reduce variability. This and the search for strains that were sensitive to chemical carcinogenesis but did not have an unacceptably high spontaneous tumor rate led to widespread use of the F344 rat and the B6C3F$_1$ mouse.

Although ideally the age should be matched to the expected exposure period in terms of the stage of human development, this is not often done. Young adult or adolescent animals that are still growing are preferred in almost all cases, and both sexes are routinely used.

Good animal care is critical at all times, becaue toxicity has been shown to vary with diet, disease, and environmental factors. Animals should be quarantined for some time before being admitted to the test area, their diet should be optimum for the test species, and the facility should be kept clean at all times. Regular inspection by a veterinarian is essential, and any animals showing unusual symptoms not related to the treatment (eg, in controls or in low-dose but not high-dose animals), should be removed from the test and autopsied.

RESULTS. Although the information required from subchronic tests varies somewhat from one regulatory agency to another, the requirements are basically similar (Table 11.7).

TABLE 11.7. SUMMARY OF SUBCHRONIC TEST GUIDELINES

			Regulatory Agency			
Character of tests	EPA Pesticide Assessment Guidelines (1982)	FDA "Red Book" (1982)	FDA IND/NDA Pharmacology Review Guidelines (1981)	OECD (1981)	EPA Health Effects Test Guidelines (1982)	NTP (1976)
Purpose	Pesticide registration support	Food and color additives; safety assessment	IND/NDR pharmacology review guidelines (1981)	Assessment and evaluation of toxic characteristics	Select chronic dose levels	Predict dose range for chronic study
	No-observed-effect level	No observed adverse effects, no-effect level	Characterize pharmacology, toxicology, pharmacokinetics, and metabolism of drugs for precautionary clinical decisions	Select chronic dose levels	Establish safety criteria for human exposure	
				Useful information and permissible human exposure	No-observed-effect level	
Species	Rat, dog	Rat, dog	Rat, mouse, other rodents, dog, monkey, other non-rodents	Rat, dog	Rat, dog	Fischer 344 rats, B6C3F₁ mice
Doses	Three dose levels	Three dose levels	Three dose levels	Three dose levels	Three dose levels	Five dose levels
Endpoints	Ophthalmology Hematology Clinical chemistry Histopathology rat, dog Target organs	Ophthalmology Hematology Clinical chemistry Histopathology rat Target organs	Ophthalmology Hematology Clinical chemistry Histopathology Target organs, behavioral and pharmacological effects	Ophthalmology Hematology Clinical chemistry Histopathology Target organs	Ophthalmology Hematology Clinical chemistry Histology Target organs	Weight loss, histopathology Target organs

EPA, Environmental Protection Agency; FDA, Food and Drug Administration; IND/NDA, investigative new drug/new drug assessment; OECD, Organization for Economic Cooperation and Development; NTP, National Toxicology Program.
Source: From the National Toxicology Program: Report of the NTP ad hoc panel on chemical carcinogenesis testing and evaluation, Washington, DC: Department of Health and Human Services, 1984.

While in practice, the data collected may be limited to those required for regulatory purposes, a great deal of additional information can be obtained from a complete test. In either case, the data are of two types: that which can be obtained from living animals during the course of the test and that which is obtained from animals sacrificed either during or at the end of the test period. Many of the tests performed on living animals can be carried out first before the test period begins to provide a baseline for comparison to subsequent measurement. A group of treated animals should be removed from the treated food at the end of the test period and returned to the control diet for 21 to 28 days while the various endpoints are followed. This is necessary to establish whether any effects noted are reversible. Autopsies should be performed on all animals found dead or moribund during the course of the test. The following is a list of tests that may be carried out during a 90-day oral toxicity study.

A. Interim Tests. Interim tests are carried out at intervals before the study, to establish baselines at intervals during the study, and at the end of the study, prior to killing the animals.
   1. *Appearance*—Mortality and morbidity as well as the condition of the skin, fur, mucous membranes, and orifices should be checked at least daily. Presence of palpable masses or external lesions should be noted.
   2. *Eyes*—Ophthalmologic examination of both cornea and retina should be carried out at the beginning and at the end of the study.
   3. *Food consumption*
   4. *Body weight*
   5. *Neurologic response*
   6. *Behavioral abnormalities*
   7. *Respiration*—Rate, regularity, and so on, should be assessed.
   8. *ECG*—Particularly with larger animals.
   9. *EEG*—Particularly with larger animals.
   10. *Hematology*—Assessment should be made prior to chemical administration (pretest) and monthly thereafter. Hemoglobin, hematocrit, RBC and WBC and differential counts, platelets, reticulocytes, and clotting parameters should be assessed.
   11. *Blood Chemistry*—Pretest and monthly tests should be done. Electrolytes and electrolyte balance; acid–base balance; glucose; urea nitrogen; serum lipids; serum proteins (albumin–globulin ratio); enzymes indicative of organ damage such as transaminases and phosphatases; also, plasma and RBC cholinesterase levels and toxicant and metabolite levels should be assessed.
   12. *Urinalysis*—Pretest and monthly tests should be done. Microscopic appearance (sediment, cells, stones, etc.); pH; specific gravity; chemical analysis for reducing sugars, proteins, ketones, bilirubin, and so on; and toxicant and metabolite levels should be assessed.
   13. *Fecal Analysis*—Occult blood, fluid content, and toxicant and metabolite levels should be assessed.

B. Termination Tests. Because the number of tissues that may be sampled is large (Table 11.8) and the number of microscopic methods is also large, it is necessary to consider all previous results before carrying out the pathological examination. For example, clinical tests or blood chemistry analyses may implicate a particular target organ that can then be examined in greater detail. All control and high-dose animals are examined in detail. If lesions are found, the next lowest dose group is examined for these lesions, and this method continues until a no-effect group is reached.

Because pathology is largely a descriptive science with a complex terminology that varies from one practitioner to another, it is critical that the terminology be defined at the beginning of the study and that the same pathologist examine the slides from both treated and control animals. Pathologists are not in agreement on the necessity or the wisdom of coding slides so that the assessor is not aware of the treatment given the animal from which a particular slide is derived. Such coding, however, eliminates unintentional bias, a hazard in a procedure that depends on subjective evaluation. Other items of utmost importance are quality control, slide identification, and data recording. Many tissues may be examined; consequently, an even larger number of tissue blocks must be prepared. Because each of these may yield many slides to be stained, comparable quality of staining and the accurate correlation of a particular slide with its parent block, tissue, and animal is critical.

1. *Necropsy*—This must be conducted with care to avoid postmortem damage to the specimens. Tissues are removed, weighed and examined closely for gross lesions, masses, etc. Tissues are then fixed for subsequent histologic examination in neutral buffered formalin or Millonigs phosphate-buffered formalin.

2. *Histology*—The tissues listed in Table 11.8 plus any lesions, masses, or abnormal tissues are embedded, sectioned, and stained for light microscopy. Parafin embedding and stained with hemotoxylin and eosin are the preferred

TABLE 11.8. TISSUES AND ORGANS TO BE EXAMINED HISTOLOGICALLY IN CHRONIC AND SUBCHRONIC TOXICITY TESTS

Adrenals	Larynx	Salivary gland
Bone and bone marrow	Liver	Sciatic nerve
Brain	Lungs and bronchi	Seminal vesicles
Cartilage	Lymph nodes	Skin
Cecum	Mammary glands	Spinal cord
Colon	Mandibular lymph node	Spleen
Duodenum	Mesenteric lymph node	Stomach
Esophagus	Nasal cavity	Testes
Eyes	Ovaries	Thigh muscle
Gallbladder	Parathyroids	Thymus
Ileum	Pituitary	Urinary bladder
Jejunum	Prostate	Uterus
Kidneys	Rectum	

routine methods, but special stains may be used for particular tissues or for a more specific examination of certain lesions. Electron microscopy is also used for more specific examination of lesions or cellular changes after their initial localization by more routine methods.

11.5.2.2   Thirty-Day Dermal Tests

Thirty-day dermal tests are particularly important when the expected route of human exposure is by contact with the skin, as is the case with many industrial chemicals, pesticides, and so on. Compounds to be tested are usually applied weekly to shaved or clipped areas on the back of the animal, either undiluted or in a suitable solvent. In the latter case, the solvent is applied alone to the controls. Selection of a suitable solvent is difficult because many affect the skin, causing either drying or irritation, whereas others may markedly affect the rate of penetration of the test chemical. Corn oil, ethanol, or carboxylmethyl cellulose are preferred to dimethyl sulfoxide (DMSO) or acetone. It should also be considered that some of the test chemical may be ingested as a result of grooming by the animal, although this can be controlled to some extent by use of restraining collars.

The criteria for environment, dose selection, species selection, and so on are not greatly different to the criteria used for 90-day feeding tests, nor are the endpoints to be examined. It is necessary, however, to pay close attention to the skin at the point of application, because local effects may be as important as systemic ones.

11.5.2.3   Thirty-Day to Ninety-Day Inhalation Tests

Inhalation studies are indicated whenever the route of exposure is expected to be through the lungs. Animals are commonly exposed for 6 to 8 hr each day, 5 days each week, in chambers of the type previously discussed. Even in those cases in which the animals are maintained in the inhalation chambers during nonexposure hours, food is always removed during exposure. In spite of this, exposure tends to be in part dermal and, due to grooming of the fur, in part oral. Environmental and biologic parameters are the same as for other subchronic tests, as are the routine endpoints to be measured before, during, and after the test period. Particular attention must be paid, however, to effects on the tissues of the nasal cavity and the lungs, because these are the areas of maximum exposure.

11.5.3   Chronic Tests

Chronic tests are those conducted over the greater part of the life span of the test animal or, in some cases, over more than one generation. The most important tests of this type are chronic toxicity, carcinogenicity, teratogenicity, and reproduction.

11.5.3.1   Chronic Toxicity and Carcinogenicity

Descriptions of tests for both chronic toxicity and carcinogenicity are included here because the design is similar—so similar in fact that they can be combined into one test, although this is not usually done. If they were combined, the length of time and the number of animals involved, as well as the many endpoints to be examined, would require a complex and difficult protocol. This is avoided, to some extent, by conducting the tests separately. In the latter case, differences between the test protocols can also be permitted.

Chronic toxicity tests are designed to discover any of numerous toxic effects and to define safety margins to be used in the regulation of chemicals. As with subchronic tests, two species are usually used, one of which is either a rat or a mouse strain, in which case the tests are run for 2 to 2.5 yr or 1.5 to 2.0 yr, respectively. The nonrodent species, if used, may be the dog, a nonhuman primate, or a small carnivore such as the ferret. Chronic toxicity tests may involve administration in the food, in the drinking water, by gavage, or by inhalation, the first being the most common. The dose used is the maximum tolerated dose (MTD) and usually two lower doses, 0.25 MTD and 0.125 MTD.

MTD. The MTD has been defined for testing purposes by the US Environmental Protection Agency (EPA) as:

> The highest dose that causes no more than a 10% weight decrement, as compared to the appropriate control groups; and does not produce mortality, clinical signs of toxicity, or pathologic lesions (other than those that may be related to a neoplastic response) that would be predicted to shorten the animals' natural life span.

This dose is determined by extrapolation from subchronic studies.

The requirements for animal facilities, housing, and environmental conditions are as described for subchronic studies. Special attention must be paid to diet formulation, becaue it is impractical to formulate all of the diets for 2-yr or more study from a single batch. In general, semisynthetic diets of specified components should be formulated regularly and analyzed before use.

The endpoints used in these studies are those described for the subchronic study: appearance, ophthalmology, food consumption, body weight, clinical signs, behavioral signs, hematology, blood chemistry, urinalysis, fecal analysis, organ weights, and histology. Some animals may be killed at fixed intervals during the test (eg, 6, 12, or 18 months) for histologic examination. Particular attention is paid to any organs or tests that showed compound-related changes in the subchronic tests.

Carcinogenicity tests have many requirements in common (physical facilities, diets, etc.) with both chronic and subchronic toxicity tests as previously described; these requirements are not repeated. Because of the numbers and time required, most tests are carried out using rats and/or mice, but in some cases an additional nonrodent species may also be used. The chemical under test may be administered in the food, by gavage, in the drinking water, by dermal application, or by inhalation, the first two methods being the most common. Because the oncogenic potency of chemicals varies through extreme limits, the purity of the test chemical is of great concern. A 1% contaminant need only be 100 times as potent as the test chemical to have an equivalent effect, and differences of this magnitude and greater are not uncommon.

Dosing is carried out over the major part of the life span (1.5–2.0 yr for mice, $\geq$ 2.0 yr or more for rats) beginning at weaning. The highest dose used is the MTD, together with one lower dose, usually 0.5 MTD. The principal endpoint is tumor incidence as determined by histologic examination. The statistical problem of distinguishing between spontaneous tumor occurrence in the controls and chemical-related tumor incidence in the treated animals is great; for that reason, large numbers of animals are used. A typical test involves 50 or more rats or mice of each sex in each treatment group. Thus, a typical one-species test will include 300 animals: 50 males and 50 females at the MTD, 50 males and 50 females at 0.5 MTD; and 50 males and 50 females as controls. Some animals are necropsied at intermediate stages of the test (eg, at 12 months), as are any animals found dead or moribund; all surviving animals are necropsied at the end of the test.

Tissues to be examined are listed in Table 11.8, with particular attention being paid to abnormal masses, lesions, and so on.

11.5.3.2   Reproductive Toxicity and Teratogenicity

The task of presenting a brief but instructive account of toxicity testing in this area is difficult, primarily because there appears to be little unanimity between either experts in the area or between regulatory agencies. The result is that many complex protocols exist, with little available objective criteria to facilitate a preference for any one over the others. Additional problems exist in that the terminology used in teratology is extensive, highly specialized, and varies from one research group to another. The following description represents an attempt to embody the general features of the most common protocols and, where necessary, to comment on additional features of protocols not described. The subject is divided into four areas:

1. Fertility and general reproductive performance—single generation tests
2. Fertility and general reproductive performance—multigeneration tests
3. Teratology
4. Effect of chemicals in late pregnancy and lactation (perinatal and postnatal effects)

In all these descriptions, the principles of animal husbandry as they apply to facilities, cages, environmental controls, diet, and so on should be adhered to closely, as mentioned in the previous sections on acute, subchronic and chronic testing.

FERTILITY AND GENERAL REPRODUCTIVE PERFORMANCE: SINGLE-GENERATION TESTS. Single-generation tests for fertility and general reproductive performance are usually carried out on rats (Fig. 11.3); in typical tests, 20 males are treated with the test compound for 60 days prior to mating, and 20 females are treated for 14 days prior to mating. These treatment times are selected to coincide with the times during which spermatogenesis and ovulation occur. After mating, treatment of the females is continued through pregnancy and until the pups are weaned.

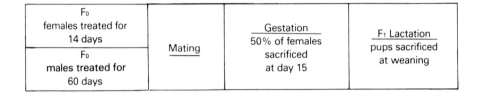

Figure 11.3. Abbreviated protocol for a one-generation reproductive toxicity test.

The test compound is administered either in the feed, in the drinking water, or by gavage. The high dose is variously described as that which causes some, but not excessive, maternal toxicity or that which just fails to cause maternal toxicity. The low dose should either be that to which humans are expected to be exposed or a dose that gives measurable tissue levels but no measurable toxicity. Because the effects in question generally vary linearly when plotted against the logarithm of the dose, the intermediate dose(s) should be evenly spaced, on a logarithmic scale, between the low and high doses. The rats are placed in cohabitation, with one male and one female caged together. Mating is confirmed by the appearance of spermatozoa in the daily vaginal smear for rats or by the appearance of a copulatory (vaginal) plug in mice. Day 1 of gestation is the day insemination is confirmed. Half of the females are killed at midgestation and examined for preimplantation and postimplantation lethality, the other half are permitted to bear and nurse their pups, the litters being culled to a constant number (usually 10), after 3 to 4 days. At weaning, the pups are killed and autopsied for gross and internal abnormalities.

Because both males and females are treated, it is not possible to distinguish between maternal and paternal effects in the subsequent performance. To permit this separation, it is necessary to treat additional animals to the stage of mating and then to outcross them to untreated members of the opposite sex. Subsequent examination of the females may be carried out as in the combined tests. Similarly, with effects seen at weaning, it is not possible to distinguish between effects mediated in utero or mediated by lactation. This distinction can be made by "cross-fostering" the offspring of treated females to untreated females and vice versa.

The endpoints observed are as follows:

1. Preimplantation death, or the number of corpora lutea in the ovaries relative to the number of implantation sites
2. Postimplantation deaths, or the number of resorption sites in the uterus relative to the number of implantation sites
3. Gross effects on male or female reproductive system
4. Duration of gestation
5. Litter size and condition, number of dead and live pups, weight of pups, gender of pups, gross morphological variation in pups

6. Subsequent survival and performance of dam and pups, weight gain, mortality, etc.
7. Gross and visceral abnormalities in weanlings

Detailed examination of the pups is possible, but is better done under the protocol described for teratology testing. A number of variations of this test have been proposed. For example, it has been suggested that a number of weanlings be left to develop and be tested later for behavioral and/or physiological defects.

FERTILITY AND GENERAL REPRODUCTIVE PERFORMANCE: MULTIGENERATION TESTS. Multigeneration tests for fertility and general reproductive performance (Fig. 11.4) are also carried out with rodents, usually rats. The test compound is administered to males and females

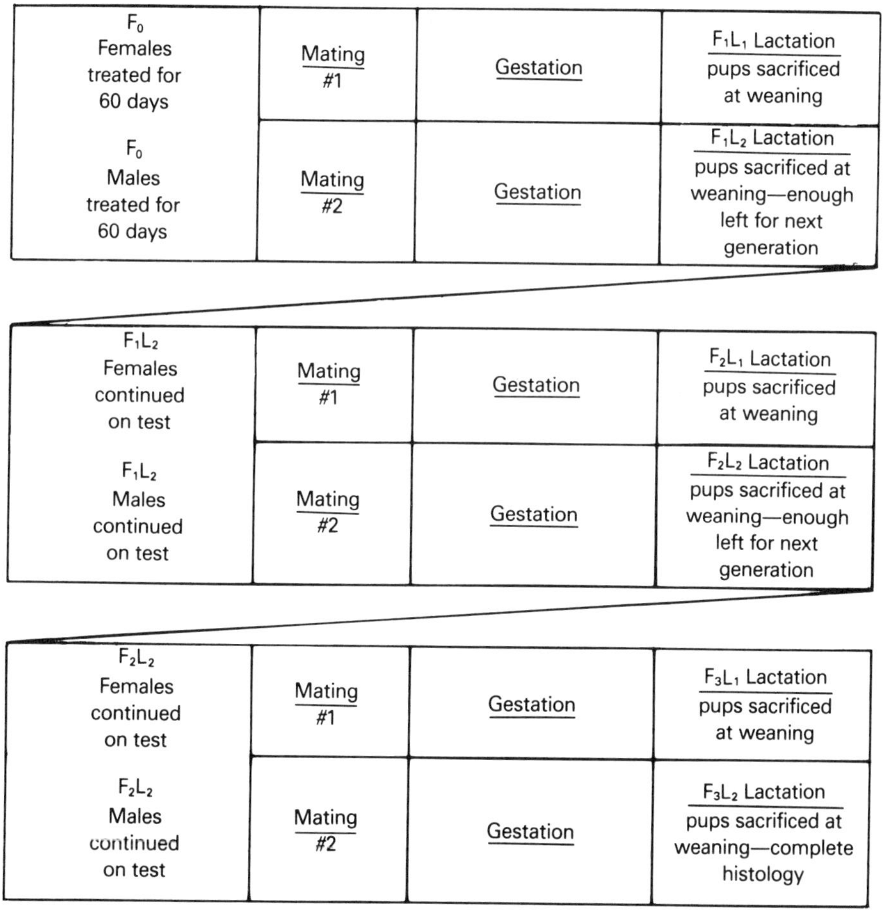

| F_0 Females treated for 60 days | Mating #1 | Gestation | F_1L_1 Lactation pups sacrificed at weaning |
| F_0 Males treated for 60 days | Mating #2 | Gestation | F_1L_2 Lactation pups sacrificed at weaning—enough left for next generation |

| F_1L_2 Females continued on test | Mating #1 | Gestation | F_2L_1 Lactation pups sacrificed at weaning |
| F_1L_2 Males continued on test | Mating #2 | Gestation | F_2L_2 Lactation pups sacrificed at weaning—enough left for next generation |

| F_2L_2 Females continued on test | Mating #1 | Gestation | F_3L_1 Lactation pups sacrificed at weaning |
| F_2L_2 Males continued on test | Mating #2 | Gestation | F_3L_2 Lactation pups sacrificed at weaning—complete histology |

Figure 11.4. Abbreviated protocol for a multigeneration reproductive toxicity test.

from weaning of the F_0 generation and throughout the test, which is carried out for up to three generations. The test compound is administered in the food or drinking water, usually at three levels. The high level is approximately one-tenth of the LD50, the low dose is one that subchronic studies indicate should not cause toxic effects in either dams or fetuses of the F_1 generation, and the intermediate dose (or doses) should be equally spaced on a logarithmic scale between the low and high doses. Enough females from the F_0 groups and enough survivors of the F_1 and F_2 groups are provided so that each generation has 20 pregnant females per dose level (including controls).

After males and females of the initial group have been treated for 60 days, they are mated to produce the first F_1 litter (F_1L_1). After birth, the pups are weighed, differentiated by sex, and examined for external abnormalities, after which the litters are culled to a constant number of pups (usually 10). Pup weight and survival are followed to weaning; the pups are killed and necropsied to detect internal abnormalities, obtain organ weights, and so on. The parents are permitted to mate again after the first litter is weaned, to produce the second litter (F_1L_2). The pups of the second litter are treated in the same way as the first except that enough are permitted to survive to produce the 20 or more males and females for the next generation. Again each pair is allowed to produce two litters (F_2L_1 and F_2L_2), which are treated in the same way as those of the first generation, setting aside enough animals to produce the two litters of the third generation (F_3L_1 and F_3L_2). Because this is the final generation, all weanlings are examined as previously described except that a selected number are used in a complete histologic examination. As with other tests, all animals that die or become moribund during the course of the test are given a complete necropsy. The following endpoints are evaluated:

1. Fertility index, the number of pregnancies relative to the number of matings
2. The number of live births, relative to the number of total births
3. Gender and initial weight of pups
4. Growth rate of pups
5. Survival of pups relative to number born (or relative to the number to which litters are culled)
6. Gross deformities at birth
7. Internal abnormalities at weaning
8. Histologic changes at weaning (third generation only)

With this test, as with the single-generation test, males or females of any question can be mated to unmated individuals of the opposite sex to determine the sex specificity of any effect observed. It has been suggested that modification of the test would permit delayed effects on physiological or behavioral parameters to be assessed. This may be useful for low-dose studies of these parameters but high-dose studies would have to be carried out as separate one-generation studies. Similarly, modifications to permit detailed teratologic evaluation have been proposed, but again, these would be optimal if conducted as separate one-generation studies including higher dose levels.

TERATOLOGY. Teratology is the study of abnormal fetal development. In teratogenic testing, exposure to the test chemical may be from implantation to parturition, although it is usually restricted to the period of major organogenesis, the most sensitive period for inducing structural malformations. Observations may be extended throughout life, but usually they are made immediately prior to birth. The endpoints currently observed are mainly morphologic (structural changes and malformations), although embryo–fetal mortality is also used as an endpoint. Although many protocols have been used, a description of the most straightforward follows (Fig. 11.5), with others being commented on as necessary.

Teratogenic studies are carried out in a rodent species (usually the rat), sometimes also in another species (such as the rabbit), but only rarely in species such as nonhuman primates or dogs. Enough females should be used so that, given normal fertility for the strain, there are 20 pregnant females in each dosage group of rodents or 10 pregnant females per dosage group of nonrodents. The test chemical is administered in the diet, in the drinking water, or by gavage, the latter being required by some regulatory agencies. The high-dose level is one at which some maternal toxicity is known to occur, but only that which will cause less than 10% mortality. The low dose should be one at which no maternal toxicity is apparent, and the intermediate dose(s) should be spaced evenly on a logarithmic scale, between the low and high doses.

The timing of compound administration is usually such that the dam is exposed during the period of major organogenesis, that is, days 6 through 15 of gestation in the case if the rat or mouse and days 6 through 18 in the case of the rabbit. Day 1 is the day spermatozoa appear in the vagina or a vaginal plug appears in the case of rats and mice, or the day of mating in the rabbit.

Teratology

| Untreated females | Mating | Gestation
Pregnant females treated on days 6-15. Pups and dams sacrificed day 20 |
| Untreated males | | |

Perinatal/Postnatal

| Untreated females | Mating | Gestation
Pregnant females treated on days 15-21 | Lactation
Females treated to weaning. Pups and dams sacrificed at weaning |
| Untreated males | | | |

Figure 11.5. Abbreviated protocol for a teratology test and for a perinatal/postnatal toxicity test.

The test is terminated by killing and dissection of the dams on the day before normal delivery is expected. The uterus is examined for implantation and resorption sites and for live and dead fetuses and the ovaries for corpora lutea. In rodent studies, one-third of the fetuses are examined for soft tissue malformations, and the remaining two-thirds are examined for skeletal malformations. In nonrodents, all fetuses are examined for both soft tissue and skeletal malformations. The various endpoints that may be examined include maternal toxicity, embryo–fetal toxicity, external malformations, and soft tissue and skeletal malformations.

Maternal toxicity is evaluated from a relatively small number of parameters and is useful in assessing the validity of the high-dose level and the possibility that maternal toxicity is involved in subsequent events. The parameters used include body weight, food consumption, clinical signs, and necroscopy data such as organ weights.

Because exposure starts after implantation, conception and implantation rates should be the same in controls and all treatment levels. If not, the test is suspect, with a possible error in the timing of the dose.

Embryo–fetal toxicity is determined from the number of dead fetuses and resorption sites relative to the number of implantation sites. In addition to the possibility of lethal malformations, such toxicity can be due to maternal toxicity, stress, or direct toxicity to the embryo or fetus that is not related to developmental malformations. A high level of embryo–fetal toxicity may also obscure teratologic effects that could have occurred at a lower dose. In that case, the next lower dose level should be evaluated with care and, if necessary, the study should be repeated with additional dose levels. Fetal weight and fetal size may also be a measure of toxicity but should not be confused with the variations seen as a result of differences in the number of pups per litter.

Anomalies may be regarded either as variations that may not adversely affect the fetus and not have a fetal outcome, or as malformations that are considered to have adverse effects on the fetus. There is little agreement on a precise definition of which anomalies fall in which class and the distinction may be academic, because a dose-related increase, even in a variation known to occur in controls, is still regarded as evidence of teratogenic potential. An example of such a variation is the number of ribs in the rabbit.

Common external anomalies (Table 11.9) are determined by examination of fetuses fixed in Bouin's fixative or by the method of Staples and by hand-sectioning by the method of Wilson. Some common visceral anomalies are listed in Table 11.10.

Skeletal anomalies are examined by first fixing the fetus and then staining the cartilage with Alizarin Red. Numerous skeletal variations occur in controls and may not have an adverse effect on the fetus (Table 11.11). Their frequency of occurrence may, however, be dose related and should be evaluated.

Almost all chemically induced malformations have been observed in control animals, and essentially all such malformations are known to be produced by more than one cause. Thus, it is obvious that great care and a conservative approach are necessary in the interpretation of teratogenic studies.

TABLE 11.9. EXTERNAL MALFORMATIONS COMMONLY SEEN IN TERATOGENICITY TESTS

Brain, cranium, spinal cord
  Encephalocele—protrusion of brain through an opening of the skull. Cerebrum is well formed
    and covered by transparent connective tissue
  Exencephaly—lack of skull with disorganized outward growth of the brain
  Microcephaly—small head on normal-sized body
  Hydrocephaly—marked enlargement of the ventricles of the cerebrum
  Craniorachischisis—exposed brain and spinal cord
  Spina bifida—Nonfusion of spinal processes. Usually ectoderm covering is missing,
    and spinal cord is evident
Nose
  Enlarged naris—enlarged nasal cavities
  Single naris—a single naris, usually median
Eye
  Microphthalmia—small eye
  Anophthalmia—lack of eye
  Open eye—no apparent eyelid; eye is open
Ear
  Anotia—absence of the external ear
  Microtia—small ear
Jaw
  Micrognathia—small lower jaw
  Agnathia—absence of lower jaw
  Aglossia—lack of tongue
  Astomia—lack of mouth opening
  Bifid tongue—forked tongue
  Cleft lip—either unilateral or bilateral cleft of upper lip
Palate
  Cleft palate—a cleft or separation of the median portion of the palate
Limbs
  Clubfoot— foot that has grown in a twisted manner, resulting in an abnormal shape or position.
    It is possible to have a malposition of the whole limb
  Micromelia—abnormal shortness of the limb
  Hemimelia—absence of any of the long bones, resulting in a shortened limb
  Phocomelia—absence of all the long bones of a limb; the limb is attached directly
    to the body

Many variations in teratogenic tests have been suggested, some trivial, others impractical, but some worthy of serious consideration. It has been suggested that dosing be extended to the end of pregnancy, and at least one regulatory agency requires such a protocol, even though this type of procedure may be counterproductive. Of more importance is the suggestion that some of the offspring born to dams treated for teratogenic evaluation should be allowed to survive and be subjected to a variety of behavioral tests as they develop. Such tests would have the potential to detect functional defects that are either not apparent morphologically or that appear later in development. Physiological functions could also be tested postnatally, including growth rate, kidney function, liver function, EEG, and EKG. Such testing is advisable.

TABLE 11.10. SOME COMMON VISCERAL ANOMOLIES SEEN IN TERATOGENICITY TESTS

Intestines
    Umbilical hernia—protrusion of the intestines into the umbilical cord
    Ectopic intestines—extrusion of the intestines outside the body wall
Heart
    Dextrocardia—rotation of the heart axis to the right
    Enlarged heart—either the atrium or the ventricle may be enlarged
Lung
    Enlarged lung—all lobes are usually enlarged
    Small lung—all lobes are usually small. Lobes may appear immature
Uterus/testes
    Undescended testes—testes are located anterior to the bladder instead of lateral; may be bilateral or unilateral
    Agenesis of testes—one or both testes may be missing
    Agenesis of uterus—one or both horns of the uterus may be missing
Kidney
    Hydronephrosis—fluid-filled kidney, often grossly enlarged; may be accompanied by a hydroureter (enlarged fluid-filled ureter)
    Fused—kidneys fused, appearing as one misshapen kidney with two ureters
    Agenesis—one or both kidneys missing
    Misshapen—small, enlarged (normal internally), spherical, or odd-shaped kidneys

EFFECT OF CHEMICALS IN LATE PREGNANCY AND LACTATION (PERINATAL AND POSTNATAL EFFECTS). These tests are usually carried out on rats, and 20 pregnant females per dosage group are treated during the final third of gestation and through lactation to weaning (day 15 of pregnancy through day 21 postpartum) (Fig. 11.5). The duration of gestation, parturition problems, and the number and size of pups in the naturally delivered litter are observed, as is the growth performance of the offspring. Variations of this test are the inclusion of groups treated only to parturition and only postpartum in order to separate prenatal and postnatal effects. Cross-fostering of pups to untreated dams may also be used to the same end. Behavioral testing of the pups has been suggested, and this and other physiological testing is to be recommended.

TABLE 11.11. SKELETAL ABNORMALITIES COMMONLY SEEN IN TERATOGENICITY TESTS

Digits
    Polydactyly—presence of extra digits; in mouse, six or more instead of five
    Syndactyly—fusion of two or more digits
    Oligodactyly—absence of one or more digits
    Brachydactyly—smallness of one or more digits
Ribs
    Wavy—ribs may be any aberrant shape
    Extra—may have extra ribs on either side
    Fused—may be fused anywhere along length of rib
    Branched—single base and branched
Tail
    Short—short tail, usually lack of vertebrae
    Missing—absence of tail
    Corkscrew—corkscrew-shaped tail

11.5.4 Special Tests

This general heading is used to include brief assessments of tests ally required but that may be required in particular cases or have been useful adjuncts to current testing protocols. Many are in areas of toxicology developing rapidly; as a result, no consensus has yet evolved as to the best to sequence of tests, only an understanding that such evaluations may shed light on previously undefined aspects of chemical toxicity.

11.5.4.1 Neurotoxicity (Including Delayed Neuropathy)

The nervous system is complex, both structurally and functionally, and toxicants can affect one or more units of the system in selective fashion. It is necessary, therefore, to devise tests or sequences of tests that measure not only changes in overall function but that also indicate which basic unit is affected and how the toxicant interacts with its target. This is complicated by the fact that the nervous system has a considerable functional reserve, and specific observable damage may not affect overall function until it becomes even more extensive. Types of damage to the nervous system are classified in various ways but include neuronal toxicity, axonopathy, toxic interruption of impulse transmission, myelinopathy, and synaptic alterations in transmitter release or receptor function. With the exception of tests for the delayed neuropathy associated with certain organophosphates, specific tests for neurotoxicity are seldom required by regulatory agencies because neurotoxicity is frequently revealed by the acute, subchronic, chronic, behavioral, and other tests that are required. Neurotoxicity is of great significance in toxicology, however, and tests have been devised to supplement those routinely required.

BEHAVIORAL AND PHARMACOLOGICAL TESTS. Behavioral and pharmacological tests involve the observation of clinical signs and behavior. These include signs of changes in awareness, mood, motor activity, central nervous system (CNS) excitation, posture, motor incoordination, muscle tone, reflexes, and autonomic functions. If these tests so indicate, more specialized tests can be carried out that evaluate spontaneous motor activity, conditioned avoidance responses, operant conditioning, as well as tests for motor incoordination such as the inclined plane or rotarod tests.

Tests for specific classes of compounds include the measurement of transmitter stimulated adenyl cyclase and Na/K–ATPase for compounds that affect receptor function, or cholinesterase inhibition for organophosphates or carbamates. Electrophysiological techniques may detect compounds such as DDT or pyrethroids, which affect impulse transmission.

NEUROPATHOLOGICAL METHODS. It is difficult to carry out routine pathological examination of all parts of a structure as complex as the nervous system, and the routine methods of pathology can, in any case, detect only fairly extensive damage. Recently, however, it has been suggested that, using more sensitive methods and sampling at only two sites—the medulla oblongata and the tibial nerve—can permit detection of distal axonopathies, neuronopathies, and myelinopathies. This technique, said to be sensitive enough to detect early damage, consists of fixation with buffered glu-taraldehyde, postfixation with osmium tetroxide, preparation of thin plastic sec-tions, and staining with a variety of routine stains.

BIOCHEMICAL METHODS. Biochemical methods include the appearance of cholesterol es-ters and the increase in ß-glucuronidase and ß-galactosidase characteristic of Wal-lerian degeneration. The latter two enzymes are easily measured and this technique may prove to be generally applicable to a wide range of toxicants. The measure-ment of cholinesterase (plasma, red blood corpuscle, or brain) is a well-established and easily performed test for cholinesterase inhibitors and is carried out routinely with some categories of pesticides.

DELAYED NEUROTOXICITY (OPIDN). The delayed neurotoxic potential of certain organophos-phates such as tri-o-cresyl phosphate (TOCP) is usually tested for by clinical signs (paralysis of leg muscles in hens) or pathology (degeneration of the motor nerves in hens), but a biochemical test involving the ratio between the ability to inhibit cholinesterase relative to the ability to inhibit an enzyme that has been referred to as the neurotoxic esterase (NTE) has been suggested. The ability of chemicals to cause delayed neuropathy is generally correlated with their ability to inhibit this nonspe-cific esterase, found in various tissues, although the role, if any, of the enzyme in the sequence of events leading to nerve degeneration is not known. The preferred test organism is the mature hen, because the clinical signs are similar to those in hu-mans and such symptoms cannot be readily elicited in the common laboratory ro-dents.

Although in vitro cultivation of nerve cells has been possible for some time, none of the in vitro tests of nerve function have yet been developed to the point at which they may be of practical use in routine toxicity testing.

11.5.4.2   Potentiation

Potentiation and synergism represent interactions between toxicants that are poten-tial sources of hazard because neither humans nor other species are usually exposed to one chemical at a time. The enormous number of possible combinations of chem-icals makes routine screening for all such effects not only impractical, however, but impossible.

One of the classic cases is the potentiation of the insecticide malathion by an-other insecticide, EPN, the LD50 of the mixture being dramatically lower than that of either compound alone. This potentiation can also be seen between malathion and certain contaminants that are formed during synthesis, such as isomalathion. For this reason, quality control during manufacture is essential. This example of po-tentiation involves inhibition, by EPN or isomalathion, of the carboxylesterase re-sponsible for the detoxication of malathion in mammals.

It is practical to test for potentiation only when there has been some prelimi-nary indication that it might occur or when either or both of the compounds belong to chemical classes previously known to cause potentiation. Such a test can be conducted by comparing the LD50, or any other appropriate toxic endpoint, of a mixture of equitoxic doses of the chemicals in question with the same endpoint measured with the two chemicals administered alone.

In the case of synergism, in which one of the compounds is relatively nontoxic when given alone, the toxicity of the toxic compound can be measured when administered alone or after a relatively large dose of the nontoxic compound.

11.5.4.3 Toxicokinetics and Metabolism

Routine toxicity testing without regard to the mechanisms involved is likely to be wasteful of time and of human, animal, and financial resources. A knowledge of toxicokinetics and metabolism can give valuable insights and provide for testing that is both more efficient and more informative. Such knowledge provides the necessary background to make the most appropriate selection of test animal species and of dose levels, and the most appropriate method for extrapolating from animal studies to the assessment of human hazard. Moreover, they may provide information on possible reactive intermediates as well as information on induction or inhibition of the enzymes of xenobiotic metabolism, the latter being critical to an assessment of possible interactions.

The nature of metabolic reactions and their variations between species is detailed in Chapters 3, 4, and 6 with some elementary aspects of toxicokinetics in Chapter 2. The methods used for the measurement of toxicants and their metabolites are detailed in Chapter 12. The present section is not concerned with these aspects but with the general principles, use, and need for metabolic and toxicokinetic studies in toxicity testing.

Toxicokinetic studies are designed to measure the amount and rate of the absorption, distribution, metabolism, and excretion of a xenobiotic. These data are used to construct predictive mathematical models so that the distribution and excretion of other doses can be simulated. Such studies are carried out using radiolabeled compounds to facilitate measurement and total recovery of the administered dose. This can be done entirely in vivo by measuring levels in blood, expired air, feces, and urine; these procedures can be done relatively noninvasively and continuously in the same animal. Tissue levels can be measured by sequential killing and analysis of organ levels. It is important to measure not only the compound administered but also its metabolites, because simple radioactivity counting does not differentiate among them.

The metabolic study, considered separately, consists of treatment of the animal with the labeled compound followed by chemical analysis of all metabolites formed in vivo and excreted via the lungs, kidneys, or bile. Although reactive intermediates are unlikely to be isolated, the chemical structure of the end products may provide vital clues to the nature of the intermediates involved in their formation. The use of tissue homogenates, subcellular fractions, and purified enzymes may serve to clarify events occurring during metabolic sequences leading to the end products.

Information of importance in test animal selection is the similarity in toxicodynamics and metabolism to that of humans. Although all of the necessary information may not be available for humans, it can often be inferred with reference to metabolism and excretion of related compounds, but it is clearly ill advised to use an animal that differs from most others in the toxicokinetics or metabolism of the compound in question or that differs from humans in the nature of the end products. Dose selection is influenced by a knowledge of whether a particular dose saturates a physiological process such as excretion or whether it is likely to accumulate in a particular tissue, because these factors are likely to become increasingly important the longer a chronic study continues.

11.5.4.4   Behavior

Although the primary emphasis in toxicity testing has long been the estimation of morphologic changes, with particular reference to carcinogenesis, much recent interest has focused on more fundamental evaluations. One such aspect has been the evaluation of chemical effects on behavior. For a number of years, behavioral tests had been incorporated as part of the regulatory process in what was the former Soviet Union but not in the United States or Western Europe, and the claim was often made that behavioral tests were more sensitive than pathological tests. This latter is difficult to document, but it is clear that behavior is the functional integration of all of the various activities of the nervous system and even, in part, of some other systems such as the endocrine glands, whose activity affects the nervous system. For this reason alone, behavioral tests are necessary to evaluate toxicity fully.

Many behavioral tests exist, and no particular set or sequence has been prescribed for regulatory purposes. The categories of methods used in behavioral toxicology have been classified by Norton, however. They fall into two principal classes, stimulus-oriented behavior and internally generated behavior. The former includes two types of conditioned behavior: operant conditioning, in which animals are trained to perform a task in order to obtain a reward or to avoid a punishment, and classical conditioning, in which an animal learns to associate a conditioning stimulus with a reflex action. Stimulus-oriented behavior also involves unconditioned responses in which the animal's response to a particular stimulus is recorded.

Internally generated behavior includes observation of animal behavior in response to various experimental situations, and includes exploratory behavior, circadian activity, social behavior, and so on. The performance of animals treated with a particular chemical is compared with that of untreated controls as a measure of the effect of the chemical.

Many of the variables associated with other types of testing must also be controlled in behavioral tests: sex, age, species, environment, diet, and animal husbandry. Behavior may vary with all of these. Norton describes a series of four tests that may form an appropriate series inasmuch as they represent four different types of behavior; the series should therefore reflect different types of nervous system activity. They are as follows:

1. Passive avoidance. This test involves the use of a shuttle box, in which animals can move between a light side and a dark side. After an acclimatization period, in which the animal can move freely between the two sides, it receives an electric shock while in the dark side. During subsequent trials, the time spent in the "safe side" is recorded.
2. Auditory startle. This test involves the response (movement) to a sound stimulus either without, or preceded by, a light-flash stimulus.
3. Residential maze. Movements of animals in a residential maze are automatically recorded during both light and dark photoperiods.
4. Walking patterns. Gait is measured in walking animals, including such characteristics as the length and width of stride and the angles formed by the placement of the feet.

Problems associated with behavioral toxicology include the functional reserve and adaptability of the nervous system. Frequently, behavior is maintained in spite of clearly observable injury. Other problems are the statistical ones associated with multiple tests, multiple measurements, and the inherently large variability in behavior.

The use of human subjects occupationally exposed to chemicals is often attempted, but such tests are complicated by the subjective nature of the endpoints (dizziness, etc.).

11.5.4.5 Covalent Binding

Toxicity has been associated with covalent binding in a number of ways. Organ-specific toxicants administered in vivo bind covalently to macromolecules, usually at a higher level in the target tissues than in nontarget tissues. Examples include acetaminophen in the liver, carbon tetrachloride in the liver, p-aminophenol in the kidney, and ipomeanol in the lung. Similarly, many carcinogens are known to give rise to DNA adducts. In general, covalent binding occurs as a result of metabolism of the toxicant to highly reactive intermediates, usually, but not always, by cytochrome P450. Because these intermediates are highly reactive electrophiles, they bind to many nucleophilic sites on DNA, RNA, or protein molecules, not just the site of toxic action. Thus, measurement of covalent binding may be a measure of toxic potential rather than a specific measurement, related directly to a mechanism of action. The occurrence of covalent binding at the same time as toxicity is so common an occurrence, however, that a measurement of covalent binding of a chemical may be regarded as an excellent although perhaps not infallible indication of potential for toxicity. Although such tests are not routine, considerable interest has been shown in their development.

The measurement of DNA adducts is an indirect indication of genotoxic (carcinogenic) potential, and DNA adducts in the urine are an indication, obtained by a noninvasive technique, of recent exposure. Protein adducts give an integrated measure of exposure because they accumulate over the life span of the protein and, at the same time, indicate possible organ toxicity.

Tissue protein adducts are usually demonstrated in experimental animals following injection of radiolabeled chemicals and, after a period of time, the organs are removed, homogenized and, by rigorous extraction, all the noncovalently bound material is removed. Extraction methods include lipid solvents, acids and bases, concentrated urea solutions, and solubilization and precipitation of the proteins. They tend to underestimate the extent of covalent binding because even covalent bonds may be broken by the rigorous procedures used. Newer methods involving dialysis against detergents will probably prove more appropriate.

Blood proteins, such as hemoglobin, may be used in tests of human exposure because blood is readily and safely accessible. For example, the exposure of mice to ethylene oxide or dimethylnitrosamine was estimated by measuring alkylated residues in hemoglobin. The method was subsequently extended to people exposed occupationally to ethylene oxide by measuring N-3-(2-hydroxyethyl) histidine residues in hemoglobin. Similarly, methyl cysteine residues in hemoglobin can be used as a measure of methylation.

DNA–RNA adducts can also be measured in various ways, including rigorous extraction, separation and precipitation following administration of labeled compounds in vivo, or use of antibodies raised to chemically modified DNA or RNA. Attempts have also been made to measure adducts of DNA degradation products in the urine, a method that should prove valuable in human studies.

Although many compounds of different chemical classes have been shown to bind covalently when activated by microsomal preparations in vitro (eg, aflatoxin, ipomeanol, stilbene, vinyl chloride), these observations have not been developed into routine testing procedures. Clearly, such procedures would be useful in predicting toxic potential.

11.5.4.6   Immunotoxicity

Immunotoxicology comprises two distinct types of toxic effects: the involvement of the immune system in mediating the toxic effect of a chemical and the toxic effects of chemicals on the immune system. The former is shown, for example, in tests for cutaneous sensitization, whereas the latter is shown in impairment of the ability to resist infection.

Tests for immunotoxicity are not yet required by all regulatory agencies, but it is an area of great interest, both in the fundamental mechanisms of immune function and in the design of tests to measure impairment of immune function. As a result of the recent rapid expansion of knowledge in this area, there is no uniform agreement on a test or series of tests. Moreover, there is considerable functional reserve in the immune system, so that the demonstration in vitro of impairment of a particular facet of the system may not be reflected in an impairment of in vivo function.

As indicated previously, many compounds can elicit immune reactions even though they may not be proteins or other macromolecules normally associated with antibody formation. Presumably, this occurs because they or their metabolites interact with endogenous macromolecules to modify them in such a way that the immune system then sees them as "foreign" or "nonself." The result may be allergies, delayed hypersensitivity, and so on. (This aspect is not considered further; the remainder of the section is devoted to impairment of immune function)

The humoral and cell-mediated systems represent the two major parts of the overall immune system (Fig. 11.6), the former involving primarily the B lymphocytes and the latter the T lymphocytes. The humoral system is involved in the production of antibodies that react with foreign material (antigens), whereas the latter involves primarily the mobilization of phagocytic leukocytes to ingest such foreign organisms as bacteria. The two systems function together by complex feedback mechanisms. One of the key characteristics in immune function is the rapid amplification of the number of cells capable of specific reaction to an antigen. This derives from memory cells that were adapted specifically to the antigen at the time of initial exposure.

Tests of the immune system may be divided into three classes:

1. Weight and morphology of the lymphoid organs
2. Capacity to respond to challenges such as those of mitogens, that is, compounds that induce mitosis (phytohemagglutinin, concavalin A, lipopolysaccharide, pokeweed mitogen) or antigens (*Candida*, typhoid)

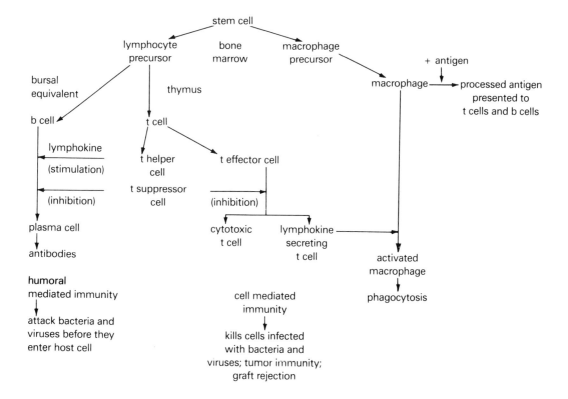

Figure 11.6. Diagrammatic representation of the mammalian immune system.

3. Specific in vitro tests of components of the immune system designed to elicit the mechanism of changes shown in tests in 1 and 2.

The initial examination consists of routine hematology, because changes in blood cells, particularly in the differential WBC count, may be indicative of effects on the immune system. Examination of the weight and pathology of the thymus and spleen are considerably more important, however, because effects noted therein are more specific (although not infallible) indications of immune impairment. For example, atrophy of the thymus usually indicates immunosuppression, although some nonimmunosuppressive chemicals can cause thymus atrophy. Similarly, changes in the bone marrow, lymph nodes, spleen, and thymus may, after treatment with a particular chemical, indicate changes in the immune system such as B or T cell deficiency. B cells and T cells are either formed or reside in particular locations in these organs, and their presence or absence may be indicative of dysfunction.

The second category of tests, those for overall immunocompetence, includes skin tests for antibody-mediated responses and for delayed hypersensitivity. It also

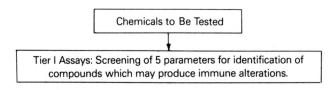

Chemicals to Be Tested

Tier I Assays: Screening of 5 parameters for identification of compounds which may produce immune alterations.

1. Immunopathology—hematology; histology and gross pathology of spleen, thymus, and lymph nodes.

2. Host resistance — susceptibility to transplantable syngeneic tumor.

3. Cell-mediated immunity—response of lymphocytes to mitogens; natural killer cell activity.

4. Humoral-mediated immunity—antibody plaque-forming cell (PFC) response to sheep erythrocytes.

5. Macrophage function—quantitation of cell number, phagocytic activity, and cytolytic activity.

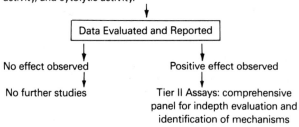

Data Evaluated and Reported

No effect observed   Positive effect observed

No further studies   Tier II Assays: comprehensive panel for indepth evaluation and identification of mechanisms

Figure 11.7. Screening tests for potential immunotoxicity.

includes tests that determine the predisposition of animals for disease, such as infections with *Streptococcus pneumoniae*, and increased susceptibility to cancer and autoallergic effects or autoimmune diseases.

The third category consists of a constantly growing body of tests, each of which examines some narrow aspect of the immune system in great detail. It includes tests for the production of different classes of antibodies as well as tests of leukocyte function and differentiation: macrophage aggregation, inhibition of macrophage migration, lymphocyte transformation by antigens and mitogens, and many others.

It is not yet clear how best to select from the tests available or how these tests can be integrated to provide a coherent picture of immunotoxic effects. It is clear, however, that this is important, and one such attempt is shown in Fig. 11.7.

11.6

IN VITRO AND OTHER SHORT-TERM TESTS

11.6.1 Introduction

The toxicity tests that follow are tests conducted largely in vitro with isolated cell systems. Some are short-term tests carried out in vivo or are combinations of in vivo and in vitro systems. The latter are included because of similarities in approach, mechanism, or intent. In general, these tests measure effects on the genome or on cell transformation; their importance lies in the relationship between such effects and the mechanism of chemical carcinogenesis. Mutagenicity of cells in the germ line is itself an expression of toxicity, however, and the mutant genes can be inherited and expressed in the next or subsequent generations.

The theory that the initiating step of chemical carcinogenesis is a somatic mutation is well recognized, and considerable evidence shows that mutagenic potential is correlated with carcinogenic potential. Thus, the intent of much of this type of testing is to provide early warning of carcinogenic potential without the delay involved in conducting lifetime chronic feeding studies in experimental animals. In spite of the numerous tests that have been devised, regulatory agencies have not yet seen fit to substitute any of them, or any combination of them, for chronic feeding studies. Instead, they have been added as additional testing requirements. One function of such tests should be to identify those compounds with the greatest potential for toxicity and enable the amount of chronic testing to be reduced to more manageable proportions.

11.6.2 Prokaryote Mutagenicity

11.6.2.1 Ames Test

The Ames test, developed by Bruce Ames and his coworkers of the University of California, Berkeley, depends on the ability of mutagenic chemicals to bring about reverse mutations in mutant *Salmonella typhimurium* strains that have defects in the histidine biosynthesis pathway. These strains will not grow in the absence of histidine but can be caused to mutate back to the wild type, which can synthesize histidine and hence can grow in its absence. The postmitochondrial supernatant (S-9 fraction), obtained from homogenates of livers of rats previously treated with PCBs in order to induce certain cytochrome P450 isozymes, is also included to provide the activating enzymes involved in the production of the potent electrophiles often involved in the toxicity of chemicals to animals.

Bacterial tester strains have been developed that can test for either base-pair (eg, strain TA-1531) or frameshift (eg, strains TA-1537, TA-1538) mutations. Other, more sensitive strains such as TA-98 and TA-100 are also used, although they may be less specific with regard to the type of mutation caused.

In brief, the test is carried out (Fig. 11.8) by mixing a suspension of bacterial cells with molten top agar. This also contains cofactors, S-9 fraction, and the material to be tested. The mixture is poured onto Petri plates containing hardened minimal agar. The number of bacteria that revert and acquire the wild-type ability to grow in the absence of histidine can be estimated by counting the colonies that develop on incubation. To provide a valid test, a number of concentrations are tested, and positive controls with known mutagens are included along with negative con-

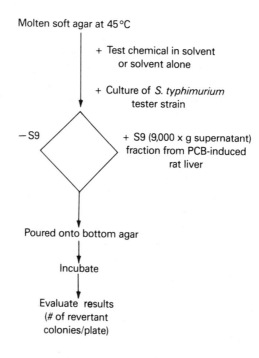

Molten soft agar at 45 °C

+ Test chemical in solvent
 or solvent alone

+ Culture of *S. typhimurium*
 tester strain

− S9

+ S9 (9,000 x g supernatant)
 fraction from PCB-induced
 rat liver

Poured onto bottom agar

Incubate

Evaluate results
(# of revertant
colonies/plate)

Figure 11.8. Protocol for the Ames test for mutagenesis.

trols that lack only the test compound. The entire test is replicated often enough to satisfy appropriate statistical tests for significance. Parallel tests without the S-9 fraction may help distinguish between chemicals with intrinsic mutagenic potential and those that require metabolic activation.

Although several hundred chemicals have been tested by this method, according to McCann et al, only about one-third of these tests were adequate for quantitative analysis. It is clear, however, that the Ames test, if properly conducted, is reproducible and accurate.

The question of correlation between mutagenicity and carcinogenicity is crucial in any consideration of the utility of this or similar tests. In general, this appears to be high, although a small proportion of both false negatives and false positives occurs. For example, certain base analogs and inorganics such as manganse are not carcinogens but are mutagens in the Ames test, whereas diethylstilbestrol (DES) is a carcinogen but not a bacterial mutagen.

11.6.2.2   Related Tests

Related tests include tests based on reverse mutations, as is the Ames test, as well as tests based on forward mutations. Examples include:

1. Reverse mutations in *Escherichia coli*. This test is similar to the Ames test and depends on reversion of tryptophan mutants, which cannot synthesize this amino acid, to the wild type, which can. The S-9 fraction from the liver of induced rats can also be used as an activating system in this test. Other *E coli* reverse-mutation tests utilize nicotinic acid and arginine mutants.
2. Forward mutations in *S typhimurium*. One such assay, dependent on the appearance of a mutation conferring resistance to 8-azaguanine in a histidine revertant strain, has been developed and is said to be as sensitive as the reverse-mutation tests.
3. Forward mutations in *E coli*. These mutations depend on the mutation of galactose-nonfermenting *E coli* to galactose-fermenting *E coli* or the change from 5-methyltryphtophane sensitivity to 5-methyltryptophane resistance.
4. DNA repair. Polymerase-deficient, and thus DNA repair-deficient, *E coli* has provided the basis for a test that depends on the fact that the growth of a deficient strain is inhibited more by a DNA-damaging agent than is that of a repair-competent strain. The recombinant assay using *Bacillus subtilis* is conducted in much the same way, because recombinant deficient strains are more sensitive to DNA-damaging agents.

11.6.3   Eukaryote Mutagenicity

11.6.3.1   Mammalian Cell Mutation

The development of cell culture techniques that permit both survival and replication have led to many advances in cell biology, including the use of certain of these cell lines for detection of mutagens. Although such cells, if derived from mammals, would seem ideal for testing for toxicity toward mammals, there are several problems. Primary cells, which generally resemble those of the tissue of origin, are difficult to culture and have poor cloning ability. Because of these difficulties, certain established cell lines are usually used. These cells, such as Chinese hamster ovary cells and mouse lymphoma cells, clone readily and do not become senescent with passage through many cell generations. Unfortunately, they have little metabolic activity toward xenobiotics and thus do not readily activate toxicants. Moreover, they usually show chromosome changes, such as aneuploidy (ie, more or fewer than the usual diploid number of chromosomes).

The characteristics usually involved in these assays are resistance to 8-azaguanine or 6-thioguanine (the hypoxanthine guanine phosphoribosyl transferase or HGPRT locus), resistance to bromodeoxyuridine or trifluorothymidine (the thymidine kinase or TK locus) or resistance to ouabain (the OU or Na/K-ATPase locus). HGPRT is responsible for incorporation of purines from the medium into the nucleic acid synthesis pathway. Its loss prevents uptake of normal purines and also of toxic purines such as 8-azaguanine or 6-thioguanine, which would kill the cell. Thus, mutation at this locus confers resistance to these toxic purine analogs. Similarly, TK permits pyrimidine transport, and its loss prevents uptake of toxic pyrimidine analogs and confers resistance to them. In the absence of HPGRT or TK, the cells can grow by de novo synthesis of purines and pyrimidines. Ouabain kills cells by combining with the Na/K-ATPase. Mutation at the OU locus alters the ouabain binding site in a way that prevents inhibition and thus confers resistance.

A typical test system is the analysis of the TK locus in mouse lymphoma cells for mutations that confer resistance to bromodeoxyuracil. The tests are conducted with and without the S-9 fraction from induced rat liver because the lymphoma cells have little activating ability. Both positive and negative controls are included, and the parameter measured is the number of cells formed that are capable of forming colonies in the presence of bromodeoxyuridine.

11.6.3.2 *Drosophila* Sex-Linked Recessive Lethal Test

The advantages of *Drosophila* (fruitfly) tests are that they involve an intact eukaryotic organism with all of its interrelated organ systems and activation mechanisms but, at the same time, are fast, relatively easy to perform, and do not involve mammals as test animals. The most obvious disadvantages are that the hormonal and immune systems of insects are significantly different from those of mammals and that the nature, specificity, and inducibility of the cytochrome P450s are not as well understood in insects as they are in mammals.

In a typical test, males that are 2 days postpuparium and that were raised from eggs laid within a short time period (usually 24 hr) are treated with the test compound in water to which sucrose has been added to increase palatability. Males from a strain carrying a gene for yellow body on the X chromosome are used. Preliminary tests determine that the number of offspring of the survivors of the treat-

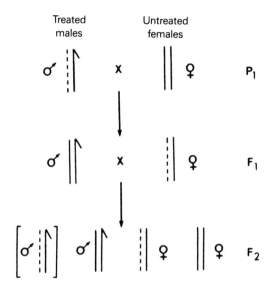

Figure 11.9. The Basc (Muller-5) mating scheme. Dashed lines represent the treated X chromosome of males. Brackets indicate males with yellow bodies, which would be absent if a lethal mutation occurred on the X chromosome of the treated male.

ment doses (usually 0.25 LD50 and 0.5 LD50) are adequate for future crosses. Appropriate controls, including a solvent control (with emulsifier if one was necessary to prepare the test solution), and a positive control, such as ethyl methane sulfonate, are routinely included with each test. Individual crosses of each surviving treated male with a series of three females are made on a 0- to 2-, 3- to 5-, and 6- to 8-day schedule. The progeny of each female is reared separately, and the males and females of the F_1 generation are mated in brother–sister matings. If there are no males with yellow bodies in a particular set of progeny, it should be assumed that a lethal mutation was present on the treated X chromosome. A comparison of the F_2 progeny derived from females inseminated by males at different times after treatment allows a distinction to be made between effects on spermatozoa, spermatids, and spermatocytes

In the Basc (Muller-5) test shown in Fig. 11.9, the strain used for the females in the F_1 cross is a multiple-marked strain that carries a dominant gene for bar eyes and recessive genes for apricot eyes and a reduction of bristles on the thorax (scute gene). (Basc is an acronym for bar, apricot, and scute.)

11.6.3.3   Related Tests

Many tests related to the two types of eukaryote-mutation tests are discussed in Sections 11.6.3.1 and 11.6.3.2, and many of them are simply variations of the tests described. Two distinct classes are worthy of mention: the first uses yeasts as the test organisms, and the second is the spot test for mutations in mice.

One group of tests using yeasts includes tests for gene mutations and strains that can be used to detect forward mutations in genes that code for enzymes in the purine biosynthetic pathway; other strains can be used to detect reversions. Yeasts can also be used to test for recombinant events such as reciprocal mitotic recombination (mitotic crossing over) and nonreciprocal mitotic recombination. *Saccharomyces cerevisiae* is the preferred organism in almost all these tests. Although yeasts possess P450s capable of metabolizing xenobiotics, their specificity and sensitivity are limited as compared with those of mammals, and an S-9 fraction is often included, as in the Ames test, to enhance activation.

The gene mutation test systems in mice include the specific locus test, in which wild-type treated males are crossed with females carrying recessive mutations for visible phenotypic effects. The F_1 progeny have the same phenotype as the wild-type parent unless a mutation, corresponding to a recessive mutant marker, has occurred. Such tests are accurate, and the spontaneous (background) mutation rate is very low, making them sound tests that are predictive for other mammals. Unfortunately, the large number of animals required has prevented extensive use. Similar tests involving the activity and electrophoretic mobility of various enzymes in the blood or other tissues in the F_1 progeny from treated males and untreated females have been developed. In the previously mentioned tests, as with many others, sequential mating of males with different females can provide information about the stage of sperm development at which the mutational event occurred.

11.6.4   DNA Damage and Repair

Many of the endpoints for tests described in this chapter, including gene mutation, chromosome damage, and oncogenicity, develop as a consequence of damage to or chemical modification of DNA. Most of these tests, however, also involve metabolic events that occur both prior to and subsequent to the modification of DNA. Some tests, however, use events at the DNA level as endpoints. One of these, the unscheduled synthesis of DNA in mammalian cells, is described in some detail; the others are summarized briefly.

11.6.4.1   Unscheduled DNA Synthesis in Mammalian Cells

The principle of this test is that it measures the repair that follows DNA damage and is thus a reflection of the damage itself. It depends on the autoradiographic measurement of the incorporation of tritiated thymidine into the nuclei of cells previously treated with the test chemical.

The preferred cells are usually primary hepatocytes in cultures derived from adult male rats, the cells of which are dispersed and allowed to attach themselves to glass coverslips. From this point on, the test is carried out on the attached cells. Both positive controls with agents known to stimulate unscheduled DNA synthesis, such as the carcinogen aflatoxin B_1 or 2-acetylaminofluorene, and negative controls, which are processed through all procedures except exposure to the test compound, are performed routinely with every test. Cells are exposed by replacing the medium for a short time with one containing the test chemical. The dose levels are determined by a preliminary cell viability test (trypan blue exclusion test) and consist of several concentrations that span the range from no apparent loss of viability to almost complete loss of viability. Following exposure, the medium is removed, and the cells are washed by several changes of fresh medium and finally placed in a medium containing tritiated thymidine. The cells are fixed and dried, and the coverslip with the cells attached is coated with photographic emulsion. After a suitable exposure period (usually several weeks), the emulsion is developed and the cells are stained with hemotoxylin and eosin. The number of grains in the nuclear region is corrected by subtracting nonnuclear grains, and the net grain count in the nuclear area is compared between treated and untreated cells.

This test has several advantages in that primary liver cells have considerable activation capacity and the test measures an event at the DNA level. It does not, however, distinguish between error-free repair and error-prone repair, the latter being itself a mutagenic process. Thus, it cannot distinguish between events that might lead to toxic sequelae and those that do not. A modification of this test measures in vivo unscheduled DNA synthesis. In this modification, animals are first treated in vivo, and primary hepatocytes are then prepared and treated as already described.

11.6.4.2   Related Tests

Tests for the measurement of binding of the test material to DNA have already been discussed under covalent binding (Section 11.5.4.5). Another method of assessing DNA damage is the estimation of DNA breakage following exposure to the test chemical; the DNA–strand length is estimated by using alkaline elution or sucrose density gradient centrifugation. This has been done with a number of cell lines and with freshly prepared hepatocytes, in the latter case following treatment either in vivo or in vitro. It may be regarded as promising but not yet fully validated. The polymerase-deficient *E coli* tests as well as recombinant tests using yeasts are also related to DNA repair.

11.6.5   Chromosome Aberrations

Tests for chromosome aberrations involve the estimation of effects on extended regions of whole chromosomes rather than on single or small numbers of genes. Primarily, they concern chromosome breaks and the exchange of material between chromosomes.

11.6.5.1   Sister Chromatid Exchange

Sister chromatid exchange (SCE) occurs between the sister chromatids that together make up a chromosome. It occurs at the same locus in each chromatid and is thus a symmetrical exchange of chromosome material. In this regard, it is not strictly an aberration because the products do not differ in morphology from normal chromosome. SCE, however, is susceptible to chemical induction and appears to be correlated with the genotoxic potential of chemicals as well as with their oncogenic potential. The exchange is visualized by permitting the treated cells to pass through two DNA replication cycles in the presence of 5-bromo-2'-deoxyuridine, which is incorporated in the replicated DNA. The cells are then stained with a fluorescent dye and irradiated with UV light, which permits differentiation between chromatids that contain bromodeoxyuridine and those that do not (Fig. 11.10).

The test can be carried out on cultured cells or on cells from animals treated in vivo. In the former case, the test chemical is usually evaluated in the presence and absence of the S-9 activating system from rat liver. Typically, cells from a Chinese hamster ovary cell line are incubated in a liquid medium and exposed to several concentrations of the test chemical, either with or without the S-9 fraction, for about 2 hr. Positive controls, such as ethyl methane sulfonate (a direct-acting compound) or dimethylnitrosamine (one that requires activation), as well as negative controls are also included. Test concentrations are based on cell toxicity levels determined by prior experiment and are selected in such a way that even at the highest dose excess growth inhibition does not occur. At the end of the treatment period, the cells are washed, bromodeoxyuridine is added, and the cells are incubated for ≥ 24 hr or more. The cells are then fixed, stained with a fluorescent dye, and irradiated with UV light. Second division cells are then scored under the microscope for SCEs (Fig. 11.10).

The test can also be carried out on cells treated in vivo, and analyses have been made of SCEs in lymphocytes from cancer patients, cancer patients treated with chemotherapeutic drugs, smokers, and workers exposed occupationally. In several

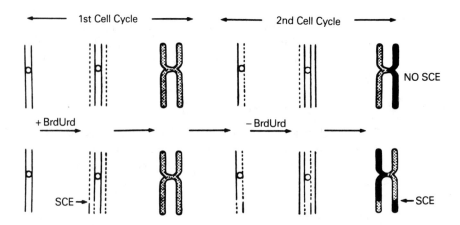

Figure 11.10. Visualization of sister chromatid exchange.

cases, increased incidence of SCEs has been noted. This is a sensitive test for compounds that alkylate DNA, with few false positives. It may also be useful for detecting promoters such as phorbol esters.

11.6.5.2   Micronucleus Test

The micronucleus test is an in vivo test usually carried out in mice. The animals are treated in vivo, and the erythrocyte stem cells from the bone marrow are stained and examined for micronuclei. Micronuclei represent chromosome fragments or chromosomes left behind at anaphase. It is basically a test for compounds that cause chromosome breaks (clastogenic agents) and compounds that interfere with normal mitotic cell division, including compounds that affect spindle fiber function.

Male and female mice from an outbred strain are handled by the best animal husbandry techniques, as described for acute, subchronic, and chronic tests, and are treated either with the solvent, 0.5 LD50, or 0.1 LD50 of the test chemical. Animals are killed at several time intervals up to 2 days; the bone marrow is extracted, placed on microscope slides, dried, and stained. The presence of micronuclei is scored visually under the microscope.

Although the test is relatively simple and treatment is carried out on the intact animal, it is not as sensitive as many other tests, for example, the SCE test.

11.6.5.3   Dominant Lethal Test in Rodents

The dominant lethal test, which is performed using rats, mice, or hamsters, is an in vivo test to determine the germ-cell risk from a suspected mutagen. The test consists of treating males with the test compound for several days, followed by mating to different females each week for enough weeks to cover the period required for a complete spermatogenesis sequence. Animals are maintained under optimal conditions of animal husbandry and are dosed, usually by gavage, with several doses of less than 0.1 LD50. The females are killed after 2 wk of gestation and dissected; corpora lutea and living and dead implantations are counted. The endpoints used to determine the occurrence of dominant lethal mutations in the treated males are the fertility index (ratio of pregnant females to mated females), preimplantation losses (the number of implantations relative to the number of corpora lutea), the number of females with dead implantations relative to the total number of pregnant females, and the number of dead implantations relative to the total number of implantations.

11.6.5.4   Related Tests

Many cells exposed to test chemicals can be scored for chromosome aberrations by staining procedures followed by visual examination with the aid of the microscope. These include Chinese hamster ovary cells in culture treated in a protocol very similar to that used in the test for SCEs, bone marrow cells from animals treated in vivo, or lymphocytes from animals treated in vivo. The types of aberrations evaluated include: chromatid gaps, breaks, and deletions; chromosome gaps, breaks, and deletions; chromosome fragments; translocations; and ploidy.

Heritable translocations can be detected by direct examination of cells from male or female offspring in various stages of development or by crossing the treated animals to untreated animals and evaluating fertility, with males with reduced fertility being examined for translocations, and so on. Progeny from this or other tests, such as those for dominant lethals, can be permitted to survive and then examined for translocations and other abnormalities.

11.6.6   Mammalian Cell Transformation

Most cell transformation assays utilize fibroblast cultures derived from embryonic tissue. The original studies showed that cells from C3H mouse fibroblast cultures developed morphologic changes and changes in growth patterns when treated with carcinogens. Later, similar studies were made with Syrian hamster embryo cells. The direct relationship of these changes to carcinogenesis was demonstrated by transplantation of the cells into a host animal and the subsequent development of tumors. The recent development of practical assay procedures involves two cell lines from mouse embryos, Balb/3T3 and C3H/10T1/2, in which transformation is easily recognized and scored. In a typical assay situation, cells, such as Balb/3T3 mouse fibroblasts, will multiply in culture until a monolayer is formed. At this point, they cease dividing unless transformed. Chemicals that are transforming agents will, however, cause growth to occur in thicker layers above the monolayer. These clumps of transformed cells are known as foci. In spite of many recommended controls, the assay is only semiquantitative. The doses are selected from the results of a preliminary experiment and range from a high dose that reduces colony formation (but not by >50%) to a low dose that has no measurable effect on colony formation. After exposure to the test chemical for 1 to 3 days, the cells are washed and incubation is continued for up to 4 weeks. At that time, the monolayers are fixed, stained, and scored for transformed foci.

Although transformation assays have not been developed to the point of being quantitative, they nevertheless have several distinct advantages. Because transplanted foci give rise to tumors in congenic hosts (those from the same inbred strain from which the cells were derived) whereas untransformed cells do not, cell transformation is believed to be illustrative of the overall expression of carcinogenesis in mammalian tissues. The two cell types used most (Balb/3T3 and C3H/10T1/2) respond to promoters in the manner predicted by the multistage model for carcinogenesis in vivo and may eventually be useful in the development of assays for promotion. Unfortunately, a large number of false-negative results are obtained because these cell lines do not show much activation capacity; it has not proved practical to combine them with the S-9 activation system. Furthermore, the cells are aneuploid and may be preneoplastic in the untreated state. Syrian hamster cells, which do have considerable activation capacity, have proved difficult to use in test procedures and are difficult to score. Other transforming systems are known but have not yet been reduced to practical assay status.

11.6.7   General Considerations and Testing Sequences

Considering all of the tests for acute and chronic toxicity, long and short term, in vivo and in vitro, it is clearly impractical to apply a complete series of tests to all commercial chemicals and all their derivatives in food, water, and the environment. The challenge of toxicity testing is to identify the most effective set or sequence of tests necessary to describe the apparent and potential toxicity of a particular chemical or mixture of chemicals. The enormous emphasis on in vitro or short-term tests that has occurred since the mid-1970s had its roots in the need to find substitutes for lifetime feeding studies in experimental animals or, at the very least, to suggest a sequence of tests that would enable priorities to be set for which chemicals should be subjected to chronic tests. Such tests might also be used to eliminate the need for chronic testing for chemicals that either clearly possessed the potential for toxicity or clearly did not. Although there has been much success in test development, the challenge outlined here has not been met, primarily because of the failure of scientists and regulatory agencies, worldwide, to agree on test sequences or on the circumstances in which short-term tests may substitute for chronic tests. Thus, not only are short-term tests often required, but they also are required in addition to all the other tests required before their development. As an example, the US EPA requirements for the Federal Insecticide, Fungicide, and Rodenticide Act (FIFRA) include, in addition to a full battery of acute, subchronic, and chronic tests, tests to address the following three categories: gene mutations, structural chromosome aberrations, and other genotoxic tests as appropriate (such as DNA damage and repair and chromosome aberrations). It is important, however, that test sequences have been suggested and considered by regulatory agencies. One such sequence is shown in Table 11.12.

TABLE 11.12. A THREE-TIER DECISION POINT PROTOCOL FOR EVALUATING CHEMICALS FOR MUTAGENESIS AND CARCINOGENESIS

A. Structure of chemical

B. In vitro tests
1. Bacterial mutagenesis (Ames test)
2. Mammalian mutagenesis
3. DNA repair
4. Chromosome tests (SCE, micronucleus, etc.)
5. Cell transformation

Decision Point 1
Evaluation of tests from A and B; select appropriate tests for C.

C. In vivo testing—limited bioassays
1. Skin tumor induction in mice
2. Pulmonary tumor induction in mice
3. Breast cancer induction in female rats
4. Altered foci induction in rodent liver
5. Assays for promoters

Decision Point 2
Evaluation of data from tests A–C.

D. Long-term bioassay

Decision Point 3
Final evaluation of all results.

Source: Adapted from Weisburger JH, Williams GM: Science **214:***401–407, 1981.*

11.7

ECOLOGICAL EFFECTS

Tests for ecological effects include those designed to address the potential of chemicals to affect the environment and the occurrence of toxic chemicals in the environment. In addition to potential effects on humans and domestic animals, such tests are designed to estimate the possibility of effects on field populations of vertebrates, invertebrates, and plants.

11.7.1 Laboratory Tests

There are two types of laboratory tests: toxicity determinations on wildlife and aquatic organisms and the use of model ecosystems to measure bioaccumulation and transport of toxicants and their degradation products.

Among the tests included in the first category are the avian oral LD50, the avian dietary LC50, wild mammal toxicity, and avian reproduction. The avian tests are usually carried out on bobwhite quail or mallard ducks, whereas the wild mammals may be species such as the pine mouse, *Paramyscus*. The tests are similar to those described under acute and chronic testing procedures but suffer from some drawbacks; the standards of animal husbandry used with rats and mice are probably unattainable with birds or wild mammals even though bobwhite quail and mallards are easily reared in captivity. The genetics of the birds and mammals used are much more variable than are those of the traditional laboratory rodent strains.

Similar tests can be carried out with aquatic organisms (eg, the LC50 for freshwater fish such as rainbow trout and bluegills), the LC5O for estuarine and marine organisms, the LC50 for invertebrates such as *Daphnia*, and the effect of chemicals on the early stages of fish and various invertebrates.

Model systems, first developed by ecologists to study basic ecological processes, have been adapted to toxicological testing. The models developed by Metcalf have been the most important. These models were developed to determine the movement and concentration of pesticides. Typically, the model has a water phase containing vertebrates and invertebrates, and a terrestrial phase containing at least one plant species and one herbivore species. First, the ^{14}C-labeled pesticide or other environmental contaminant is applied to the leaves of the terrestrial plant, sorghum *(Sorgum halpense)*, then salt marsh caterpillars *(Estigmene acrea)* are placed on the plants. The larvae eat the plants and contaminate the water with feces and their dead bodies. The aquatic food chain is simulated with plankton (diatoms, rotefers, etc.), water fleas *(Daphnia)*, mosquito larvae *(Culex pipiens)*, and fish *(Gambusia affinis)*. From an analysis of the plants, animals, and substrates for the ^{14}C-labeled compound and its degradation products, the biologic magnification or rate of degradation can be calculated.

More complex models involving several compartments, simulated rain, simulated soil drainage, simulated tidal flow, and so on, have been constructed and their properties investigated, but none have been brought to the stage of use in routine testing. Similarly, aquatic models using static, recirculating, and continuous flow have also been used, as have entirely terrestrial models; again, none have been developed for routine testing. The most important feature of any model ecosystem designed for routine testing of environmental contaminants is the ability to measure biologic magnification or the rate of degradation so as to predict the possible fate of the chemical in the environment.

11.7.2   Simulated Field Tests

Simulated field tests may be quite simple, consisting of feeding treated prey to predators and studying the toxic effects on the predator, enabling some predictions concerning effects to nontarget organisms. In general, however, the term is used for greenhouse, small plot, small artificial pond, or small natural pond tests. These serve to test biologic accumulation and degradation under conditions somewhat more natural than the conditions in the artificial ecosystem, and the test compounds are exposed to environmental as well as biologic degradation. Population effects may be noted, but these methods are more useful for soil invertebrates, plants, and aquatic organisms because other organisms are not easily contained in small plots.

11.7.3   Field Tests

In field-test situations, test chemicals are applied to large areas under natural conditions. The areas are at least several acres and may be either natural or part of some agroecosystem. Because the area is large and in the open, radiolabeled compounds cannot be used and it is not possible to obtain a balance between material applied and material recovered.

The effects are followed over a long period of time, and two types of control may be used: first, a comparison with a similar area that is untreated; and second, a comparison with the same area before treatment. In the first case it is difficult, if not impossible, to duplicate exactly a large natural area, and in the second, changes can occur that are unrelated to the test material.

In either case, studies of populations are the most important focus of this type of testing, although the disappearance of the test material, its accumulation in various life forms, and the appearance, accumulation, and disappearance of its degradation products are also important. The population of soil organisms, terrestrial organisms, and aquatic organisms as well as plants all must be surveyed and characterized, both qualitatively and quantitatively. Following application of the test material, the populations can be followed through two or more annual cycles to determine both acute and long-term population effects.

11.8

RISK ANALYSIS

The preceding tests for various kinds of toxicity can be used to measure adverse effects of many different chemical compounds in different species, organs, tissues, cells, or even populations, and under many different conditions. This information can be used to predict possible toxicity of related compounds from QSAR or of the same chemical under different conditions (eg, mutagenicity as a predictor of carcinogenicity). It is considerably more difficult to use this information to predict possible risk to other species, such as humans, because little experimental data on this species is available. Some methods are available to predict risk to humans and to provide the risk factor in the risk benefit assessment that provides the basis for regulatory action, however. The benefit factor is largely economic in nature, and the final regulatory action is not, in the narrow sense, a scientific one. It also involves political and legal aspects and, in toto, represents society's evaluation of the amount of risk that can be tolerated in any particular case.

The estimation of risk may be implicit, as in the process by which an acceptable daily intake (ADI) or threshold limit value (TLV) is established, or explicit, as in calculations that lead to a numerical probability of toxic effect for a given dose or a numerical expression of changes in mortality or morbidity rates in exposed populations.

The ADI is calculated by dividing the NOEL by a safety factor. The NOEL is derived from chronic or subchronic studies and is the highest level tested that did not cause any observable effect related to the test chemical—that is, effects observed at higher doses. For all effects other than cancer, the results of a 6-month study are probably adequate. The traditional safety factor is 100, with 10 representing the potential increased sensitivity of humans and 10 allowing for the genetic diversity of the human population. This presents several problems, the most important of which is the fact that the lower the number of animals tested, the smaller the probability of detecting an adverse effect at a particular dose. Thus, the NOEL and hence the ADI may be unrealistically high if too few animals are used. The regulation of chemicals such as pesticides, which may appear in many different foodstuffs as well as in drinking water, becomes a particularly intractable problem because the ADI must be divided between all of these sources as a maximum permitted residue or tolerance for each one. Because of the many different ethnic groups and diets, meaningful tolerances are difficult to formulate. The safety factor itself lacks any particular scientific rationale, and it should probably be reduced when good epidemiologic data are available and increased when either good epidemiologic data are not available or when the experimental data are not extensive.

The area of risk assessment for chemical carcinogens is one that has attracted the most attention, but it is still far from resolved. The problems include extrapolation to low doses and extrapolation between species.

Low-dose extrapolation, that is, prediction of the effects of expected environmental levels from results obtained at high levels, is complicated by many factors, but the basic difficulty is that the shape of the dose–response curve is unknown at lower doses. The extremely high doses (MTD) used in carcinogenesis assays are unrealistic in that they may cause metabolic and pharmacokinetic effects not seen at lower doses and thus may not even lie on an upward extrapolation from intermediate doses. They may be valuable for demonstrating the potential of the compound for carcinogenesis, but possibly should not be used in extrapolations for the purpose of risk assessment.

In general, models used for low-dose extrapolation fall into the following classes: tolerance distribution; simple linear extrapolation; hit models, such as one-hit and multihit; and time-to-tumor models. The tolerance distribution model assumes a lower threshold for each individual, below which the individual would not be affected and further assumes that the variation in this threshold can be described by a probability distribution function.

The Mantel–Bryan model is a log-probit extrapolation in which a straight line is extrapolated from the measured values to an acceptable level of risk (eg, 10^{-6}). This model has been subjected to a variety of criticisms, not least of which is that it often does not fit even the observed values, and it has been necessary to propose various corrective factors. In spite of the attempted corrections, this type of simple extrapolation is subjected to much criticism, and most risk assessment involves more complex models.

The various hit models assume either a one-hit hypothesis (ie, there is a finite probability of tumor formation if a single target interacts with an effective unit of dose) or a multihit hypothesis, which does not make the single-hit assumption but assumes a more complex set of events prior to tumor formation. This last is probably the most rational but is still problematical.

The most complex of the models based on tumor frequency at different dose levels over the time of the study is the Gamma multihit model of Cornfield and Van Ryzin, which assumes a multihit mechanism and provides a model that can be corrected for spontaneous tumor formation.

Currently, attempts are being made to incorporate time-to-tumor occurrence into predictive models; this shows considerable promise as an improvement in predictability. Even more assurance of accuracy of low-dose predictions should come from the incorporation of pharmacokinetic and metabolic parameters into the model, and much effort is being devoted to this end.

The other major problem with risk assessment is extrapolation from one species (ie, the experimental animal in question) to another species (ie, usually humans). Difficulties arise in part from not knowing how a biologic function may vary with size. Many physiological functions appear to be related to some exponent of body weight, the exponent varying with the function in question. In toxicity studies, the manner in which the dose is expressed becomes critical, and studies have compared such expressions as milligram per kilogram of body weight per day, milligram per square meter of body surface per day, and milligram per kilogram of body weight per lifetime as the basis for extrapolation. The ultimate tests of the utility of such extrapolations to humans are comparisons with actual epidemiologic data, and thus it is a difficult question to decide because little data of this type is available. Milligram per kilogram of body weight per day and milligram per square meter of body surface per day have been said to give more accurate predictions than does milligram per kilogram of body weight per lifetime, however; the use of the most sensitive species has been said to require little correction.

11.9

THE FUTURE OF TOXICITY TESTING

Because of the public awareness of the potentially harmful effects of chemicals, it is clear that toxicity testing will continue to be an important activity and that it will be required by regulatory agencies before the use of a particular chemical is permitted either in commercial processes or for use by the public. Because of the proliferation of testing procedures, the number of experimental species and other test systems available, as well as the high dose rates usually used, it is clear that eventually some expression of some type of toxicity will be obtained for most exogenous chemicals. Thus, the identification of toxic effects with the intent of banning any chemical causing such effects is no longer a productive mode of attack. The aim of toxicity testing should be to identify those compounds that present an unacceptable potential for risk to humans or to the environment and thus ought to be banned, but, at the same time, provide an accurate assessment of the risk to humans and the environment for less toxic compounds so that their use may be regulated.

Subjecting all chemicals to all possible tests is logistically impossible, and the future of toxicity testing must lie in the development of techniques that will narrow the testing process so that highly toxic and relatively nontoxic compounds can be identified early and either banned or permitted unrestricted use without undue waste of time, funds, and human resources. These vital commodities could then be concentrated on compounds whose fate and effects are less predictable.

Such progress will come from further development and validation of the newer testing procedures and the development of techniques to select, for any given chemical, the most suitable testing methods. Perhaps of most importance is the development of integrated test sequences that permits decisions to be made at each step, thereby either abbreviating the sequence or making the next step more effective and efficient. As more data are developed and analyzed, structure activity models should become more predictive. Some current models for predicting the potential for carcinogenesis are accurate in about 90% of cases.

Suggested Further Reading

Balls M, Riddell RJ, Worden AN: *Animals and Alternatives in Toxicity Testing.* London: Academic Press, 1983.
Clark B, Smith DA: Pharmacokinetics and toxicity testing. *CRC Crit Rev Toxicol* **12**:343, 1984.

Couch JA, Hargis WJ, Jr: Aquatic animals in toxicity testing. *J Am Coll Toxicol* **3:**331, 1984.

Dean JH, Luster MI, Murray MJ, Laver LD: Approaches and methodology for examining the immunological effects of xenobiotics. *Immunotoxicology* **7:**205, 1983.

de Serres FJ, Ashby J (eds): *Evaluation of Short Term Tests for Carcinogens.* New York: Elsevier, 1981.

Ecobichon DJ: *The Basis of Toxicity Testing.* Boca Raton, FL: CRC Press, 1992.

Enslein K, Craig PN: Carcinogenesis: a predictive structure-activity model. *J Toxicol Environ Health* **10:**521, 1982.

Gillette JR, Pohl LR: A perspective on covalent-binding and toxicity. *J Toxicol Environ Health* **2:**849, 1977.

Gorrod JW (ed): *Testing for Toxicity.* London: Taylor & Francis, 1981. Relevant chapters include:

Chapter 3. Brown VKH: Acute toxicity testing—a critique.

Chapter 4. Roe FJC: Testing in vivo for general chronic toxicity and carcinogenicity.

Chapter 7. Gorrod JW: Covalent binding as an indicator of drug toxicity.

Chapter 15. Dewar AJ: Neurotoxicity testing—with particular reference to biochemical methods.

Chapter 18. Cobb LM: Pulmonary toxicity.

Chapter 20. Parish WE: Immunological tests to predict toxicological hazards to man.

Chapter 21. Venitt S: Microbial tests in carcinogenesis studies.

Chapter 22. Styles JA: Other short-term tests in carcinogenesis studies.

Gralla EJ (ed): *Scientific Consideration in Monitoring and Evaluating Toxicology Research.* Washington, DC: Hemisphere, 1981.

Hayes AW (ed): *Principles and Methods of Toxicology,* 2nd ed. New York: Raven Press, 1989. This volume contains the following chapters of particular relevance to this chapter:

Chapter 6. Chan PK, Hayes AW: Principles and methods for acute and eye irritancy.

Chapter 7. Mosberg AT, Hayes AW: Subchronic toxicity testing.

Chapter 8. Stevens KR, Gallo MA: Practical considerations in the conduct of chronic toxicity studies.

Chapter 9. Roberts JF, Piegorsch WW, Schueler RL: Methods in testing for carcinogenicity.

Chapter 10. Zenick H, Clegg ED: Assessment of male reproductive toxicology: a risk assessment approach.

Chapter 11. Manson JM, Kang YJ: Test methods for assessing female reproductive and developmental toxicology.

Chapter 12. Kennedy GL, Jr: Inhalation toxicology.

Chapter 13. Patrick E, Maiback HI: Dermatotoxicology.

Chapter 14. Brusick D: Genetic toxicology.

Chapter 17. Burger GT, Miller LC: Animal care and facilities.

Chapter 18. Norton S: Methods for behavioral toxicology.

Chapter 26. Dean JH, et al: Immune system: evaluation of injury.

Chapter 30. Renwick AG: Pharmacokinetics in toxicology.

Chapter 31. Hogan MD, Hoel DG: Extrapolation to man.

Homburger F, Hayes JA, Pelikan EW (eds): *A Guide to General Toxicology.* Basel, New York: Karger, 1983. This volume contains the following chapters of particular relevance to this chapter:

Chapter 4. Wong S, Natarajan C: Immunotoxicology.

Chapter 6. Hayes JA: Inhalational toxicology.

Chapter 11. Homburger F: Carcinogenesis—concepts.

Chapter 15. Rogers AE: Factors influencing the results of animal experiments in toxicology.

Chapter 16. Homburger F: In vivo testing in the study of toxicity and safety evaluation.

Chapter 17. Christian MS, Voytek PE: In vivo reproductive and mutagenicity tests.

Chapter 18. Brusick DJ: Mutagenesis and carcinogenesis in mammalian cells.

Chapter 19. Jagannath DR, Brusick DJ: Mutagens and carcinogens in bacteria.

Jollow DJ, Roberts S, Price V, Longacre S, Smith C: Pharmacokinetic consideration in toxicity testing. *Drug Metab Rev* **13**:983, 1982.

Loomis TA, Hayes AW: *Loomis's Essentials of Toxicology,* 4th ed. San Diego: Academic Press, 1996.

Luotola M: Use of laboratory model ecosystems for the evaluation of environmental contaminants. In Hodgson E (ed): *Reviews in Environmental Toxicology.* Amsterdam: Elsevier Biomedical Press, 1985.

McCann J, Horn L, Koldor J: An evaluation of *Salmonella* (Ames) test data in the published literature: application of statistical procedures and analysis of mutagenic potency. *Mutation Res* **134**:1, 1984.

Mitchell CL, Tilson HA: Behavioral toxicology in risk assessment: problems and research needs. *CRC Crit Rev Toxicol* 265–274, 1982.

National Toxicology Program: Report of the NTP ad hoc panel on chemical carcinogenesis testing and evaluation. Washington, DC: Department of Health and Human Services, 1984.

Parke DV: Significance of the metabolism of xenobiotics for toxicological evaluation. In Bartosek I, et al. (eds): *Animals in Toxicological Research.* New York: Raven Press, 1982, pp 189–201.

Sperling F. (ed): *Toxicity: Principles and Practice.* Vol. 2. New York: Wiley, 1984. Contains the following chapters of relevance to this chapter:

Chapter 1. Sperling F: Toxicokinetics: the determinants of toxicity.

Chapter 6. Swanborg RH: Immune response in toxicology.

Chapter 9. Kirwin CJ, Jr: Eye and skin local toxicity testing.

Chapter 10. Sperling F: Quantitation of toxicity—the dose–response.

WHO–IARC: Monograph Supplement 4 to the monograph series on "The evaluation of the carcinogenic risk of chemicals to humans." Lyons, France: IARC, 1982.

WHO–Geneva: Environmental Health Criteria 6. Principles and methods for evaluating the toxicity of chemicals. Geneva, Switzerland: WHO–GENEVA, 1978.

Zbindon G, Flury-Reversi M: Significance of the LD50-test for the toxicological evaluation of chemical substances. *Arch Toxicol* **47**:77, 1981.

THE MEASUREMENT OF TOXICANTS

ROSS B. LEIDY • ERNEST HODGSON

12.1

INTRODUCTION

Some 200,000 chemicals are synthesized annually worldwide, and the toxicity of most of them is unknown. Few of these chemicals reach the stage of further development and use, but those that do usually find their way into the environment. Some are persistent and remain adsorbed to soil particles or soil organic matter; some find their way into water through soil movement or aerial deposition; others are metabolized by microorganisms into compounds of greater toxicity that move up the food chain. Over time, their accumulation in higher life forms could result in debilitating alterations in metabolism, leading to illness. It might be years before such illness could be attributed to specific compounds because of the difficulty involved in identifying and quantitating them. The concern over the role of persistent organochlorines in the food chain and their possible role as human xenoestrogens is an example. The identification and quantitation of chemicals in both the environment and in living beings relies on the development of analytical techniques and instruments.

Advances in analytical techniques continue to multiply in all fields of toxicology and, as mentioned, many of these focus on the environmental area. Whether looking for new techniques to sample water or for an automated instrument to determine quantities of sulfur-containing compounds in air, such devices are available. In many instances, developments in environmental analyses are adaptable to experimental work related to drug toxicity, or in forensic medicine, to determine the cause of poisoning.

Although new techniques and instruments continue to enter the commercial market, the basic analytical process has not changed: define the research goal(s), develop a sampling scheme to obtain representative samples, isolate the com-

TABLE 12.1. TYPICAL PROTOCOLS FOR ANALYSIS OF TOXICANTS

	Toxicant		
Step	*Arsenic*	*TCDD*	*Chlorpyrifos*
Sampling	Grind solid sample or homogenize tissue to homogeneity; subsample	Grind solid sample or homogenize tissue to homogeneity; subsample	Grind solid sample or homogenize tissue to homogeneity; subsample soxhlet extract with acetone (1:1)
Extraction	Dry ash; redissolve residue; generate arsine and absorb into solution	Extract with ethanol and KOH; remove saponified lipids; column chromatogrphy on H_2SO_4/silica gel followed by basic alumina and then by $AgNO_3$/silica gel followed by basic alumina; reverse-phase HPLC	Remove coextractives on fluorisil using ether; petroleum ether
Analysis	AA spectroscopy	GLC–mass spectrometer	GLC–NPD or FPD

TLC, thin-layer chromatography; HPLC, high-performance liquid chromatography; GLC, gas–liquid chromatography; AA, atomic adsorption; NPD, nitrogen phosphorus detector; FPD, flame photometric detector.

Source: Modified from Everson RJ, Oehme FW: Analytical Toxicology Manual. *Manhattan, KS: American College of Veterinary Toxicologists, 1981.*

pound(s) of interest, remove potential interfering components, and quantitate and evaluate the data in relation to the initial hypothesis. Based on the data generated, many options are available. For example, was the sampling scheme complete? Would further refinement of the analytical procedure be required? Should other sample types be analyzed? Thus, it is obvious that within these general categories particular methods vary considerably depending on the chemical characteristics of the toxicant (Table 12.1).

This chapter is concerned with the sampling, isolation, separation, and measurement of toxicants, including bioassay methods. Bioassay does not measure toxic effects; rather, it is the quantitation of the relative effect of a substance on a test organism as compared with the effect of a standard preparation of a basic toxicant. Although bioassay has many drawbacks, particularly lack of specificity, it can provide a rapid analysis of the relative potency of environmental samples.

12.2

CHEMICAL AND PHYSICAL METHODS

12.2.1 Sampling

Even with the most sophisticated analytical equipment available, the resulting data are only as representative as the samples from which the results are derived. This is particularly true for environmental samples. In this case, care must be taken to assure that the sample is representative of the object of study. Often, special attention to sampling procedures is necessary. Sampling accomplishes a number of objectives, depending on the type of area being studied. In environmental areas (eg, wilderness regions, lakes, rivers) sampling can provide data not only on the concentration of pollutants, but also on the extent of contamination. In urban areas, sampling can provide information on the types of pollutants, to which one is exposed, either by dermal, inhalation, or by ingestion over a given period of time.

In industrial areas, hazardous conditions can be detected and sources of pollution can be identified. Sampling is used in the process of designing pollution controls and can provide a chronicle of the changes in operational conditions as controls are implemented. Another important application of sampling in industrial areas in the United States is the documentation of compliance with existing Occupational Safety and Health Administration (OSHA) and United States Environmental Protection Agency (EPA) regulations. The many methods available for sampling the environment can be divided into categories of air, soil, water, and tissue sampling. The fourth category is of particular interest in experimental and forensic studies.

12.2.1.1   Air

Most pollutants entering the atmosphere come from fuel combustion, industrial processes, and solid waste disposal. Additional miscellaneous sources, such as nuclear explosions, forest fires, solid dusts, volcanoes, natural gaseous emissions, agricultural burning, and pesticide drift, contribute to the level of atmospheric pollution. To affect terrestrial animals and plants, particulate pollutants must be in a size range that allows them to enter the body and remain there; that is, they must be in an aerosol (defined as an airborne suspension of liquid droplets) or on solid particles small enough to possess a low settling velocity. Suspensions can be classified as liquids—including fogs (small particles) and mists (large particles) produced from atomization, condensation, or entrainment of liquids by gases; and solids—including dusts, fumes, and smoke produced by crushing, metal vaporization, and combustion of organic materials, respectively.

At rest, an adult human inhales 6 to 8 L of air each minute ($1 \text{ L} = 0.001 \text{m}^3$) and, during an 8-hour workday, can inhale from 5 to 20 m^3 depending on the level of physical activity. The optimum size range for aerosol particles to get into the lungs and remain there is 0.5 to 5.0 μm. Thus, air samplers have been miniaturized and adsorbents have been developed to collect either particulate matter in the size range most detrimental to humans or to "trap" organic toxicants from air.

An air sampler generally consists of an inlet to direct air through a filter to entrap particles that might be of interest (eg, dust); through the adsorbent, which collects organic vapors, a flowmeter and valve to calibrate airflow and a pump to pull air through the system (Fig. 12.1). Personnel samplers are run by battery power and can be attached to an individual's clothing, thus allowing continual monitoring while performing assigned tasks in the work environment. This allows the estimation of individual exposure.

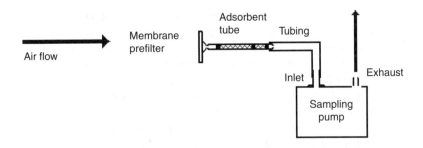

Figure 12.1. Schematic representation of a typical air sampling device.

Many air samplers use various types of filters to collect solid particulate matter, such as asbestos, which is collected on glass fiber filters with pores 20 μm or less in diameter. Membrane filters with pores 0.01 to 10 μm in diameter are used to collect dusts and silica. Liquid-containing collectors called impingers are used to trap mineral dusts and pesticides. Mineral dusts are collected in large impingers that have flow rates of 10 to 50 L of air per minute, and insecticides can be collected in smaller "midget" impingers that handle flows of 2 to 4.5 L of air per minute. Depending on the pollutant being sought, the entrapping liquid might be distilled water, alcohol, ethylene glycol, hexylene glycol, or some other solvent. Because of the ease of handling and the rapid desorption of compounds, polyurethane foam (PUF) has become a popular trapping medium for pesticides and is rapidly replacing the use of midget impingers. A large volume air sampler has been developed by the EPA for detection of pesticides and polychlorinated biphenyls (PCBs): air flows through a PUF pad at a rate of 225.0 L/min, and the insecticides and PCBs are trapped in the foam. Small glass tubes approximately 7.0×0.5 cm in diameter containing activated charcoal are used to entrap organic vapors in air.

A number of specialty companies have and are continuing to develop adsorbents to collect organic molecules from air samples. Industrial chemicals resulting from syntheses or used in production, pesticides, and emissions from exhaust towers are monitored routinely with commercially available adsorbents. Personnel monitoring can be accomplished without a pump using a system composed of a porous membrane through which air diffuses and compounds of interest are collected by an adsorbent.

Minute quantities of gaseous pollutants (eg, CO_2, HNO_3), are monitored with direct reading instruments, using infrared spectroscopy, and have been in use for a number of years. These instruments passively monitor large areas and rely on extensive statistical evaluations to remove substances like water vapor, which can mask the small quantities of these pollutants. Research into the millimeter/submillimeter area of spectroscopy coupled with Russian technologies is leading to the development of a direct reading instrument that will quantitate any atmospheric gas or a mixture of gases containing a dipole moment within 10 seconds, regardless of the presence or quantity of water vapor in the atmosphere. Such devices are expected to be commercially available early in the twenty-first century.

12.2.1.2   Soil

When environmental pollutants are deposited on land areas, their subsequent behavior is complicated by a series of simultaneous interactions with organic and inorganic components, the existing liquid–gas phases, and the living and nonliving components of the soil. Depending on its chemical and physical structure, the pollutant might remain in one location for long or short periods, be absorbed into plant tissue, or move into the soil by diffusion resulting from random molecular motion. Movement is also affected by mass flow as a result of external forces, such as the pollutant being dissolved or suspended in water or adsorbed onto inorganic and organic soil components. Thus, sampling for pollutants in soils can be simple or very difficult.

To obtain representative samples, the chemical and physical characteristics of the sampling site(s) must be considered, as well as possible reactions of the pollutant with soil components and the degree of variability in the sampling area. With these data, the site(s) can then be divided into homogeneous areas and the required number of samples can be collected. The number of samples depends on the functions of variance and the degree of accuracy required. Once the correct procedure has been determined, sampling can proceed by random or systematic means.

Many types of soil samplers are available, but various coring devices are preferred because this method of collection allows determination of a pollutant's vertical distribution. These devices can be either steel tubes, which vary from 2.5 to 7.6 cm in diameter and 60 to 100 cm in length (operated by hand) or large boring tubes that are 1.0×200 cm (operated mechanically). It is possible to sample to uniform depths with such devices, and one can subdivide these cores into specific depths (eg, 0–7.6 cm, 7.6–15.2 cm, etc.) to determine movement. Another type of coring equipment is a wheel to which small tubes are attached so that large numbers of small subsamples can be taken, thus allowing more uniform sampling over a given site. Specialty samplers with large diameters (about 25 cm) incorporate a blade to slice a core of soil after placing the sampler at the desired depth to obtain the sample slice.

12.2.1.3   Water

Many factors must be considered to obtain representative samples of water. The most important are the pollutant and the point at which it entered the aquatic environment. Pollutants can be contributed by agricultural, industrial, municipal, or other sources, such as spills from wrecks or train derailments. The prevailing wind direction and speed, the velocity of stream or river flow, temperature, thermal and salinity stratification, and sediment content are other important factors.

Two questions—where to monitor or sample and what device is best to use to obtain representative samples—are important.

Surface water samples often are collected by automatic sampling devices controlled by a variety of sensors. The simplest method of collecting water is the "grab" technique, whereby a container is lowered into the water, rinsed, filled, and capped. Specialized samplers frequently are used to obtain water at greater depths.

With the implementation in the United States of the Clean Water Act of 1977, continuous monitoring is required to obtain data for management decisions. A number of continuous monitoring wells are in operation. Sampling from potable wells can be accomplished by collecting from an existing tap, either in the home or from an outside fixture. However, multistep processes are required to collect samples from wells used to monitor pollutants. Standing water must be removed after measuring the water table elevation. If wells are used to monitor suspected pollutants, two criteria are used to determine the amount of water removed prior to sampling: conductivity and pH. Removal of a specific number of well volumes by bailers or pumps is done until these are constant. A triple-rinsed bottle is then used to collect the sample.

Because large numbers of samples can be generated by such devices, collectors containing membranes with small pores (about 45.0 μm) to entrap metal-containing pollutants or cartridges containing ion-exchange resins or long-chain hydrocarbons (eg, C_{18}) bonded to silica to bind organic pollutants often are used to diminish the number and bulk of the samples by allowing several liters of water to pass through and leave only the pollutants entrapped in a small cylinder or container. A new technique, using a filter containing a Teflon matrix in which C_{18} hydrocarbon chains are embedded, has been developed to concentrate pollutants by passing water through the membrane and eluting them with suitable solvents.

Once samples have been collected, they should be frozen immediately in solid CO_2 (dry ice) and returned to the laboratory. If they are not analyzed at that time, they should be frozen at temperatures of $-20^\circ C$ or lower to ensure that sufficient head space is available to prevent breakage.

12.2.1.4   Tissues

12.2.1.4a   Environmental Studies

When environmental areas are suspected of being contaminated, surveys of plants and animals are conducted. Many of the surveys, conducted during hunting and fishing seasons by federal and state laboratories, determine the number of animals killed and remove organs and other tissues for analysis of suspected contaminants. Sampling is conducted randomly throughout an area; the analysis can help determine the concentration, extent of contamination within a given species, and areas of contamination.

Many environmental pollutants are known to concentrate in bone, certain organs, or specific tissues (eg, adipose). These organs are removed from recently killed animals for analysis. In many instances, the organs are not pooled with others from the same species but are analyzed separately as single subsamples.

When plant material is gathered for analysis, it is either divided into roots, stems, leaves, and flowers and/or fruit, or the whole plant is analyzed as a single entity. Pooling of samples from a site can also provide a single sample for analysis. The choice depends on the characteristics of the suspected contaminant.

12.2.1.4b   Experimental Studies

Experimental studies, particularly those involving the metabolism or mode of action of toxic compounds in animals (or, less often, plants), can be conducted either in vivo or in vitro. Because organisms or enzyme preparations are treated with known compounds, the question of random sampling techniques does not arise as it does with environmental samples. Enough replication is needed for statistical verification of significance, and it should always be borne in mind that repeated determinations carried out on aliquots of the same preparation do not represent replication of the experiment; at best, they test the reproducibility of the analytical method.

In environmental studies, the analyst is concerned with stable compounds or stable products; in metabolic studies, the question of reactive (therefore unstable) products and intermediates is of critical concern. Thus, the reaction must be stopped, and the sample must be processed using techniques that minimize degradation. This is facilitated by the fact that the substrate is known, and the range of possible products can be the subject of a much-informed hypothesis.

The initial sampling step is to stop the reaction, usually by a protein precipitant. Although traditional compounds such as trichloroacetic acid are effective protein precipitants, they are usually undesirable. Water-miscible organic solvents such as ethanol or acetone are milder, whereas a mixture of a miscible and an immiscible solvent (chloroform/methanol, for example) not only denatures the protein but also effects a preliminary separation into water-soluble and organic-soluble products. Rapid freezing is a mild method of stopping reactions, but low temperature during the subsequent handling is necessary.

In toxicokinetic studies involving sequential killing and tissue examination, it is critical to obtain uncontaminated organ samples. Apart from contamination by blood, suitable samples can be obtained by careful dissection and rinsing of the organs in ice-cold buffer, saline, or other appropriate solution. Blood samples themselves are obtained by cardiac puncture, and blood contamination of organ samples is minimized by careful bleeding of the animal at the time of killing or, if necessary, by perfusion of the organ in question.

12.2.1.4c   Forensic Studies

Because forensic toxicology deals primarily with sudden or unexpected death, the range of potential toxicants is extremely large. The analyst does not usually begin examination of the samples, however, until all preliminary studies are complete, including necropsy and microscopic examination of all tissues. Thus, the analyst is usually able to begin with some working hypothesis of the possible range of toxicants involved.

Because further sampling usually involves exhumation and is therefore unlikely or, in the case of cremation, impossible, adequate sampling and sample preservation is essential. For example, various body fluids must be collected in a proper way: blood by cardiac puncture, never from the body cavity; urine from the urinary bladder; bile collected intact as part of the ligated gallbladder; and so on. Adequate sample size is important. Blood can be analyzed for carbon monoxide, ethanol and other alcohols, barbiturates, tranquilizers, and other drugs; at least 100 mL should be collected. Urine is useful for analysis of both endogenous and exogenous chemicals and the entire content of the bladder is retained. The liver frequently contains high levels of toxicants and/or their metabolites, and it and the kidney are the most important solid tissues for forensic analysis; 100 to 200 g of the former and the equivalent of one kidney usually are retained.

An unusual requirement with important legal ramifications is that of possession. An unbroken chain of identifiable possession must be maintained. All transfers are marked on the samples as to time and date, and all transfers must be signed by both parties. The security of samples during time of possession must be verifiable as a matter of law.

12.2.2   Extraction

In most cases, the analysis of a pollutant or other toxicant depends on its physical removal from the sample medium. In order to ensure that the sample used is homogeneous, it is chopped, ground, or blended to a uniform consistency and then subsampled. This subsample is extracted, which involves bringing a suitable solvent into intimate contact with the sample, generally in a ratio of 5 to 25 volumes of solvent to 1 volume of sample. One or more of four different procedures can be used, depending on the chemical and physical characteristics of the toxicant and the sample matrix. Other extraction methods such as boiling, grinding, or distilling the sample with appropriate solvents are used less frequently.

12.2.2.1   Blending

The use of an electric or air-driven blender is currently the most common method of extraction of biologic materials. The weighed sample is placed in a container, solvent is added, and the tissue is homogenized by motor-driven blades. Blending for 5 to 15 minutes followed by a repeat blending will extract most environmental toxicants. A homogenate in an organic solvent can be filtered through anhydrous sodium sulfate to remove water that might cause problems in the quantitation phase of the analysis. The use of sonication is a popular method for extracting tissue samples, particularly when the binding of toxicants to subcellular fractions is of interest. Sonicator probes rupture cells rapidly, thus allowing the solvent to come into intimate contact with all cell components. Differential centrifugation can then be used to isolate fractions of interest.

12.2.2.2 Shaking

Pollutants are generally extracted from water samples, and in some cases soil samples, by shaking with an appropriate solvent or solvent combination. Mechanical shakers are used to handle several water or soil samples at once. These devices allow the analyst to conduct long-term extractions (eg, 24 hr) if required. Two or more shakings normally are required for complete removal (ie, >98%) of the toxicant from the sample matrix.

12.2.2.3 Washing

A simple washing with water–detergent combinations or with solvents can be used to remove surface contamination from environmental samples such as fruits or plants or from a worker's hands, if dermal exposure from industrial chemicals or pesticides is suspected.

12.2.2.4 Continuous Extraction

The procedure called soxhlet extraction is performed on solid samples (eg, soil) and involves the use of an organic solvent or combination of solvents. The sample is weighed into a cup (thimble) of specialized porous material such as cellulose or fiberglass and placed in the apparatus. This consists of a boiling flask, in which the solvent is placed; an extractor, which holds the thimble; and a water-jacketed condenser. When heated to boiling, the solvent vaporizes, is condensed, and fills the extractor, thus bathing the sample and extracting the toxicant. A siphoning action drains the solvent back into the boiling flask, and the cycle begins again. Depending on the nature of the toxicant and sample matrix, the extraction can be completed in as little as 2 hr but may take as long as 3 to 4 days. Automated instruments have been introduced that perform the same operation in a shorter period of time (eg, 30 min) and use much less solvent (eg, 15–30 mL compared to 250 mL). They are expensive compared to the older method but are cost effective.

12.2.2.5 Supercritical Fluid Extraction

Conditions can be generated that allow materials to behave differently from their native state. For example, boiling points are defined as that temperature at which a liquid changes to a gas. If the liquid is contained and pressure exerted, the boiling point changes. For a particular liquid, a combination of pressure and temperature will be reached, called the critical point, at which the material is neither a liquid nor a gas. Above this point exists a region, called the supercritical region, at which increases in both pressure and temperature will have no effect on the material (ie, it will neither condense nor boil). This so-called supercritical fluid will exhibit properties of both a liquid and a gas. The supercritical fluid penetrates materials as if it were a gas and has solvent properties like a liquid.

Of all the materials available for use as a supercritical fluid, CO_2 has become the material of choice because of its chemical properties. Instruments have been developed to utilize the principles described to effect extractions of compounds from a

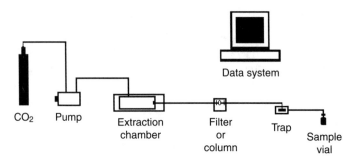

Figure 12.2. Schematic representation of a supercritical fluid extraction apparatus.

variety of sample matrices including asphalt, plant material, and soils (Fig. 12.2). The supercritical fluid is pumped through the sample, through a filter or column to a trap where the fluid vaporizes and solvent is added to transfer the analyses to a vial for analysis. More recent instruments combine the superfluid extraction system with a variety of columns and detectors to acquire data from complex samples.

12.2.3 Separation and Identification

During extraction processes, many undesirable components are released from the sample matrix that must be removed to obtain quantiative results from certain instruments. These components include plant and animal pigments, lipids, organic material from soil and water, and inorganic compounds. If not removed, the impurities decrease the sensitivity of the detectors and columns in the analytical instrument, mask peaks, or produce extraneous peaks on chromatograms. Although some more recently developed instruments automatically remove these substances and concentrate the samples to small volumes for quantitative analysis, they are expensive. Thus, most laboratories rely on other methods. These include adsorption chromatography, thin-layer chromatography (TLC), and solvent partitioning. Generally, adsorption chromatography is the method of choice to remove coextractives from the compound in question (Section 12.2.3.2c).

Because most techniques use large volumes of solvent, the solvent must be removed to obtain a working volume (eg, 5–10 mL) that is easy to manipulate by the analyst. This is accomplished by distillation, evaporation under a stream of air or an inert gas such as nitrogen, or evaporation under reduced pressure. Once the working volume is reached, extracts can be further purified by one or more procedures. In addition to the use of adsorbents, many organic toxicants will distribute between two immiscible solvents (eg, chloroform and water or hexane and acetonitrile). When shaken in a separatory funnel and then allowed to equilibrate into two original solvent layers, some of the toxicant will have transferred from the original extracting solvent into the other layer. With repeated additions (eg, 4 to 5 volumes), mixing, and removal, most or all of the compound of interest will have been transferred, leaving many interfering compounds in the original solvent. Regardless of the separation method or combination of methods used, the toxicant will be in a large volume of solvent in relation to its amount which is removed as described. Final volumes used to identify and quantitate compounds generally range from 250 µL to 10.0 mL.

Recent advances in circuit miniaturization and column technology, the development of microprocessors, and new concepts in instrument design have allowed sensitive measurement at the parts per billion and parts per trillion levels for many toxicants. This increased sensitivity has focused public attention on the extent of environmental pollution, because many toxic materials present in minute quantities could not be detected until technological advances reached the present state of the art. At present, most pollutants are identified and quantified by chromatography, spectroscopy, and bioassays.

Once the toxicant has been extracted and separated from extraneous materials, the actual identification procedure can begin, although it should be remembered that the purification procedures are themselves often used in identification (eg, peak position in gas–liquid chromatography [GLC] and high-performance liquid chromatography [HPLC]). Thus, no definite line can be drawn between the two procedures.

12.2.3.1 Chromatography

All chromatographic processes such as TLC, GLC, HPLC or capillary electrophoresis (CE) use a mobile and immobile phase to effect a separation of components. In TLC, the immobile phase is a thin layer of adsorbent placed on glass, resistant plastic, or fiberglass, and the mobile phase is the solvent. The mobile phase can be a liquid or gas, whereas the immobile phase can be a liquid or solid. Chromatographic separations are based on the interactions of these phases or surfaces. All chromatographic procedures use the differential distribution or partitioning of one or more components between the phases, based on the absorption, adsorption, ion-exchange, or size exclusion properties of one of the phases.

12.2.3.1a Paper

When the introduction of paper chromatography to common laboratory use occurred in the mid-1930s, it revolutionized experimental biochemistry and toxicology. This technique is still used in laboratories that lack the expensive instruments necessary for GLC or HPLC. The stationary phase is represented by the aqueous constituent of the solvent system, which is adsorbed onto the paper; the moving phase is the organic constituents. Separation is effected by partition between the two phases as the solvent system moves over the paper. Although many variations exist, including reverse-phase paper chromatography in which the paper is treated with a hydrophobic material, ion-exchange cellulose paper, and so on, all have been superseded by equivalent systems involving thin layers of adsorbents bonded to an inert backing.

12.2.3.1b   Thin-Layer Chromatogaphy

Many toxicants can be separated from interfering substances with TLC. In this form of chromatography, the adsorbent is spread as a thin layer (250–2000 μm) on glass, resistant plastic, or fiberglass backings. When the extract is placed near the bottom f the plate and the plate is placed in a tank containing a solvent system, the solvent migrates up the plate and the toxicant and other constituent move with the solvent; differential rates of movement result in separation. The compounds can be scraped from the plate and eluted from the adsorbent with suitable solvents. Recent developments in TLC adsorbents allow toxicants and other materials to be quantititated at the nanogram (10^{-9} g) and picogram (10^{-12} g) levels.

12.2.3.1c   Column: Adsorption, Hydrophobic, Ion Exchange

A large number of adsorbents are available to the analyst. The adsorbent can be activated charcoal, aluminum oxide, Florisil, silica, silicic acid, or mixed adsorbents. The characteristics of the toxicant determine the choice of adsorbent. When choosing an adsorbent, select conditions that either bind the coextractives to it, allowing the compound of interest to elute, or vice versa. The efficiency of separation depends on the flow rate of solvent through the column (cartridge) and the capacity of the adsorbent to handle the extract placed on it. This amount depends on the type and quantity of adsorbent, the capacity factor (k') and concentration of sample components, and the type and strength of the solvents used to elute the compound of interest. Many environmental samples contain a sufficient amount of interfering materials so that the analyst must prepare a column using a glass chromatography tube into which the adsorbent is added. In the most common sequence, the column is packed in an organic solvent of low polarity; the sample is added in the same solvent, and the column is then developed with a sequence of solvents or solvent mixtures of increasing polarity. Such a sequence might include (in order of increasing polarity) hexane, benzene, chloroform, acetone, and methanol. Once removed, the eluate containing the toxicant is reduced to a small volume for quantitation.

However, cartridge technologies are improving to allow similar concentrations of sample to be added that result in a less expensive and more rapid analysis. A number of miniaturized columns have been introduced since the early 1980s. Most contain 0.5 to 2.0 g of the adsorbent in a plastic tube with fitted ends. The columns can be attached to standard Luer Lock syringes. Other companies have designed vacuum manifolds that hold the collecting device. The column is placed on the apparatus, vacuum is applied, and the solvent is "pulled" through the column. Some advantages of these systems include preweighed amounts of adsorbent for uniformity, easy disposal of the coextractives remaining in the cartridge, no breakage, and decreased cost of the analysis because less solvent and adsorbent are used.

Other forms of column chromatography may be used. They include ion-exchange chromatography, permeation chromatography, and affinity chromatography. Ion-exchange chromatography depends on the attraction between charged molecules and opposite charges on the ion exchanger, usually a resin. Compounds so bound are eluted by changes in pH and, because the net charge depends on the relationship between pH of the solution and the isoelectric point of the compounds, compounds of different isoelectric point can be eluted sequentially. Both ionic and anionic exchangers are available. Permeation chromatography utilizes the molecular sieve properties of porous materials. Molecules large enough to be excluded from the pores of the porous material will move through the column faster than will smaller molecules not excluded, thus separating them. Cross-linked dextrans such as Sephadex or agarose (Sepharose) are commonly used materials. Affinity chromatography is a potent tool for biologically active macromolecules but is seldom used for purifying small molecules, such as most toxicants. It depends on the affinity of an enzyme for a substrate (or substrate analog) that has been incorporated into a column matrix or the affinity of a receptor for a ligand.

12.2.3.1d   *Gas–Liquid Chromatography*

GLC is used most commonly for the separation and quantitation of organic toxicants. This system consists of an injector port, oven, detector, amplifier (electrometer), and supporting electronics (Fig. 12.3). Current modern gas chromatographs use a capillary column to effect separation of complex mixtures of organic molecules and has replaced, to a large extent, the "packed" column. Instead of coating an inert support, the stationary phase is coated onto the inside of the column. The mobile phase is an inert gas (called the carrier gas), usually helium or nitrogen, that passes through the column.

When a sample is injected, the injector port is at a temperature sufficient to vaporize the sample components. Based on the solubility and volatility of these components with respect to the stationary phase, the components separate and are swept through the column by the carrier gas to a detector, which responds to the concentration of each component. The detector might not respond to all components. The

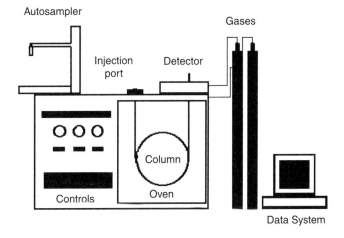

Figure 12.3. Schematic representation of a typical gas–liquid chromatograph.

electronic signal produced as the component passes through the detector is amplified by the electrometer, and the resulting signal is sent to a recorder, computer, or electronic data–collecting device for quantitation.

COLUMN TECHNOLOGY. Increased sensitivity and component resolution has resulted from advances in solid-state electronics and column and detector technologies. In the field of column technology, the capillary column has revolutionized toxicant detection in complex samples. This column generally is made of fused silica 5 to 60 m in length with a very narrow inner diameter (0.23–0.75 mm) to which a thin layer (eg, 1.0 µM) of polymer is bonded. The polymer acts as the immobile or stationary phase. The carrier gas flows through the column at flow rates of 1 to 2 mL/min.

Two types of capillary columns are used: the support-coated, open tubular (SCOT) column and the wall-coated, open tubular (WCOT) column. The SCOT column has a very fine layer of diatomaceous earth coated with liquid phase, which is deposited on the inside wall. The WCOT column is pretreated and then coated with a thin film of liquid phase. Of the two columns, the SCOT is claimed to be more universally applicable because of large sample capacity, simplicity in connecting it to the chromatograph, and lower cost. However, for difficult separations or highly complex mixtures, the WCOT is more efficient and is used to a much greater extent. Many older chromatographs are not designed to accommodate capillary columns, and because of these design restrictions, manufacturers offer the wide-bore capillary column along with the fittings and valving required to adapt the columns to older instruments. These columns also can be used on current instruments. With inner diameters of 0.55 to 0.75 mm, flow rates of 5.0 to 10.0 mL/min of carrier gas can be used to affect separations of components approaching that of the narrow-bore columns. Water samples chromatographed on capillary columns routinely separate 400 to 500 compounds, as compared with 90 to 120 resolved compounds from the packed column.

DETECTOR TECHNOLOGY. The second advance in GLC is detector technology. Five detectors are used widely in toxicant detection: the flame ionization (FID), flame photometric (FPD), electron capture (ECD), conductivity, and nitrogen–phosphorous detectors. Other detectors have application to toxicant analysis and include the Hall conductivity detector and the photoionization detector.

The FID operates on the principle of ion formation from compounds being burned in a hydrogen flame as they elute from a column. The concentrations of ions formed are several orders of magnitude greater than those formed in the uncontaminated flame. The ions cause a current to flow between two electrodes held at a constant potential, thus sending a signal to the electrometer.

The FPD is a specific detector in that it detects either phosphorous- or sulfur-containing compounds. When atoms of a given element are burned in a hydrogen-rich flame, the excitation energy supplied to these atoms produces a unique emission spectrum. The intensity of the wavelengths of light emitted by these atoms is directly proportional to the number of atoms excited. Larger concentrations cause a greater number of atoms to reach the excitation energy level, thus increasing the intensity of the emission spectrum. The change in intensity is detected by a photomultiplier, amplified by the electrometer, and recorded. Filters that allow only the emission wavelength of phosphorous (526 nm) or sulfur (394 nm) are inserted between the flame and the photomultiplier to give this detector its specificity.

The ECD is used to detect halogen-containing compounds, although it will produce a response to any electronegative compound. When a negative DC voltage is applied to a radioactive source (eg, ^{63}Ni, ^{3}H), low-energy ß particles are emitted, producing secondary electrons by ionizing the carrier gas as it passes through the detector. The secondary electron stream flows from the source (cathode) to a collector (anode), where the amount of current generated (called a standing current) is amplified and recorded. As electronegative compounds pass from the column into the detector, electrons are removed or "captured," and the standing current is reduced. The reduction is related to both the concentration and electronegativity of the compound passing through, and this produces a response that is recorded. The sensitivity of ECD is greater than that of any other detectors currently available.

Early electroyltic conductivity detectors operated on the principle of component combustion, which produced simple molecular species that readily ionized, thus altering the conductivity of deionized water. The changes were monitored by a DC bridge circuit and recorded. By varying the conditions, the detector could be made selective for different types of compounds (eg, chlorine-containing, nitrogen-containing).

The alkali flame detector can also be made selective. Enhanced response to compounds containing arsenic, boron, halogen, nitrogen, and phosphorous results when the collector (cathode) of an FID is coated with different alkali metal salts such as KBr, KCl, Na_2SO_4. As with conductivity detectors, by varying gas flow rates, types of salt, and electrode configuration, enhanced responses are obtained. The nitrogen–phosphorous alkali detector is used widely for analysis of herbicides. Alkali salts are embedded in a silica gel matrix and are heated electrically. The detector allows routine use of chlorinated solvents and derivatizing reagents that can be detrimental to other detectors.

The Hall electrolytic conductivity uses advanced designs in the conductivity cell, furnace, and an AC conductivity bridge to detect chlorine, nitrogen, and sulfur-containing compounds at sensitivities of 0.01 ng. It operates on the conductivity principle described previously. Another detector, the photoionization detector, uses an ultraviolet (UV) light source to ionize molecules by absorption of a photon of UV light. The ion formed has an energy greater than the ionization potential of the parent compound, and the formed ions are collected by an electrode. The current, which is proportional to concentration, is amplified and recorded. The detector can measure a number of organic and inorganic compounds in air, biologic fluids, and water. A number of instrument manufacturers have introduced portable GCs that can be transported for use on field sites.

12.2.3.1e *High-Performance Liquid Chromatography*

HPLC has become very popular in the field of analytical chemistry for the following reasons: It can be run at ambient temperatures; it is nondestructive to the compounds of interest, which can be collected intact; in many instances, derivatization

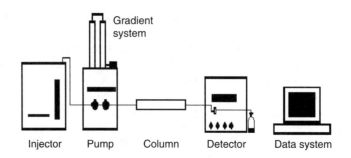

Figure 12.4. Schematic representation of a typical high performance liquid chromatograph.

is not necessary for response; and columns can be loaded with large quantities of the material for detection of low levels.

The instrument consists of a solvent reservoir, gradient-forming device, high-pressure pumping device, injector, column, and detector (Fig. 12.4). The principle of operation is very similar to that of GLC except that the mobile phase is a liquid instead of a gas. The composition of the mobile phase and its flow rate effect separations. The columns being developed for HPLC are too numerous to discuss in detail. Most use finely divided packing (3–10 μm in diameter), some have bonded phases, and others are alumina or silica. The columns normally are 15 to 25 cm in length, with small diameters (approximately 4.6 mm number diameter). A high-pressure pump is required to force the solvent through this type of column. The major detectors presently used for HPLC are UV or fluorescent spectrophotometers or differential refractometers.

12.2.3.1f   *Capillary Electrophoresis*

A relatively new analytical technique, CE is receiving considerable attention in the field of toxicology. Its uses appear endless and methods have been developed to analyze a diversity of compounds, including DNA adducts, drugs, small aromatic compounds, and pesticides. Commercial instruments are available that are composed of an autosampler, high voltage power supply, two buffer reservoirs, the capillary (approximately 70 cm × 75 μM in diameter) and a detector (Fig. 12.5). The versatility of the process lies in the ability to separate compounds of interest by a number of modes, including affinity, charge/mass ratios, chiral compounds, hydrophobicity, and size. The theory of operation is simple. Because the capillary is composed of silica, silanol groups are exposed in the internal surface, which can become ionized as the pH of the eluting buffer is increased. The ionization attracts cations to the silica surface, and when current is applied, these cations migrate toward the cathode, which causes a fluid migration through the capillary. This flow can be adjusted by changing the dielectric strength of the buffer, altering the pH, adjusting the voltage, or changing the viscosity.

Under these conditions both anions and cations are separated in a single separation, with cations eluting first. Neutral molecules (eg, pesticides) can be

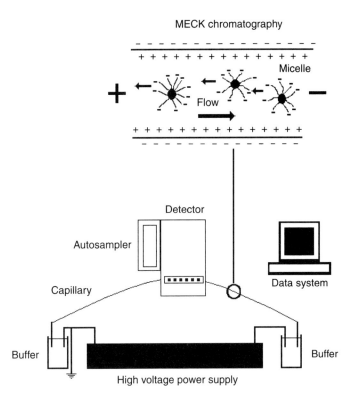

Figure 12.5. Schematic representation of a capillary electrophoresis chromatograph including a cross-section of the capillary during a micellar electrokinetic (MECK) analysis.

separated by adding a detergent (eg, sodium dodecyl sulfate) to the buffer, forming micelles into which neutral molecules will partition based on their hydrophobicity. Because the micelles are attracted to the anode, they move toward the cathode at a slower rate than does the remainder of fluid in the capillary, thus allowing separation. This process is called micellar electrokinetic capillary chromatography (MECK) (Fig. 12.5). Many of these analyses can be carried out in 5 to 10 min with sensitivities in the low parts per billion (ppb) range. A UV detector is usually used, but greatly sensitivities can be obtained using fluorescent-laser detectors.

12.2.3.2   Spectroscopy

In certain experiments involving radiation, observed results cannot be explained on the basis of the wave theory of radiation. It must be assumed that radiation comes in discrete units, called quanta. Each quantum of energy has a definite frequency v, and the quantum energy can be calculated by the equation $E = hv$, where h is

Planck's constant (6.6×10^{-27} erg-sec). Matter absorbs radiation one quantum at a time, and the energy of radiation absorbed becomes greater as either the frequency of radiation increases or the wavelength decreases. Therefore, radiation of shorter wavelength causes more drastic changes in a molecule than does that of longer wavelength. Spectroscopy is concerned with the changes in atoms and molecules when electromagnetic radiation is absorbed or emitted. Instruments have been designed to detect these changes, and these instruments are important to the field of toxicant analysis. Discussions of atomic absorption (AA) spectroscopy, mass spectroscopy (MS), infrared (IR), and UV spectroscopy follow. A summary of spectroscopic techniques is given in Table 12.2.

TABLE 12.2. CHARACTERISTICS OF SPECTROSCOPIC TECHNIQUES

Type	Principle	Uses
Visible and UV spectrometry	Energy transitions of bonding and nonbonding outer electrons of molecules, usually delocalized electrons	Routine qualitative and quantitative biochemical analysis including many colorinmetric assays. Enzyme assays, kinetic studies, and difference spectra
Spectrofluorimetry	Absorbed radiation emitted at longer wavelengths	Routine quantitative analysis, enzyme analysis and kinetics. More sensitive at lower concentrations than visible and UV absorption
Infrared and Raman spectroscopy	Atomic vibrations involving a change in dipole moment and a change in polarizability, respectively	Qualitative analysis and finger-printing of purified molecules of intermediate size
Flame spectrophotometry (emission and absorption)	Energy transitions of outer electrons of atoms after volatilization in a flame	Qualitative and quantitative analysis of metals; emission techniques; routine determination of alkali metals; absorption technique extends range of metals that may be determined and the sensitivity
Electron spin resonance spectrometry	Detection of magnetic moment associated with unpaired electrons	Research on metalloproteins, particularly enzymes and changes in the environment of free radicals introduced into biologic assemblies (eg, membranes)
Nuclear magnetic resonance spectrometry	Detection of magnetic moment associated with an odd number of protons in an atomic nucleus	Determination of structure of organic molecules of mol wt <20,000 daltons
Mass spectrometry	Determination of the abundance of positively ionized molecules and fragments	Qualitative analysis of small quantities of material (10^{-6}–10^{-9}g), particularly in conjunction with gas–liquid chromatography

Source: Modified from Williams BW, Wilson K, Principles amd Techniques of Practical Biochemistry. London: Edward Arnold, 1975.

12.2.3.2a   *Atomic Absorption Spectroscopy*

One of the more sensitive instruments used to detect metal-containing toxicants is the AA spectrophotometer. Samples are vaporized either by aspiration into an acetylene flame or by carbon rod atomization in a graphite cup or tube (flameless AA). The atomic vapor formed contains free atoms of an element in their ground state and, when illuminated by a light source that radiates light of a frequency characteristic of that element, the atom absorbs a photon of wavelength corresponding to its AA spectrum, thus exciting it. The amount of absorption is a function of concentration. The flameless instruments are much more sensitive than conventional flame AA. For example, arsenic can be detected at levels of 0.1 ng/mL and selenium at 0.2 mg/mL, which represent sensitivity three orders of magnitude greater than that of conventional flame AA.

12.2.3.2b   *Mass Spectroscopy*

The mass spectrometer is an outstanding instrument for the identification of compounds (Fig. 12.6). In toxicant analysis, MS is widely used as a highly sensitive detection method for GLC and is increasingly used with HPLC and CE because these instruments can be interfaced to the mass spectrometer. Chromatographic techniques (eg, GLC, CE, HPLC) are used to separate individual components as previ-

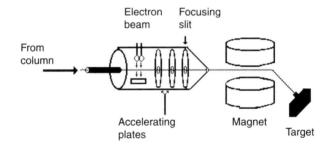

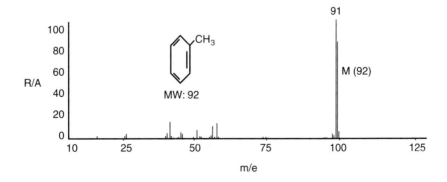

Figure 12.6. Schematic representation of a mass spectral detector and a mass spectrum of toluene.

ously described. A portion of the column effluent passes into the mass spectrometer, where it is bombarded by an electron beam. Electrons or negative groups are removed by this process, and the ions produced are accelerated. After acceleration
they pass through a magnetic field, where the ion species are separated by the different curvatures of their paths under gravity. The resulting pattern is characteristic
of the molecule under study. Two detectors are used primarily in pollutant analysis:
the quadripole and the ion trap. Both produce reliable and reproducible data, and if
routine maintenance is performed, both are reliable. Computer libraries of mass
spectral data continue to expand, and data are generated rapidly with current soft-
ware. Instrument costs have gone down, and tabletop instruments can be purchased
for $70,000 although research-grade instruments can cost several hundred thousand
dollars. By interfacing the detector with a computer system, data reduction, analysis, and quantitation are performed automatically.

12.2.3.2c Infrared Spectrophotometry

Atoms are in constant motion within molecules, and associated with these motions
are molecular energy levels that correspond to the energies of quanta of IR radiation.
These motions can be resolved into rotation of the whole molecule in space and into
motions corresponding to the vibration of atoms with respect to one another by bend-
ing or stretching covalent bonds. The vibrational motions are very useful in identifying complex molecules, because functional groups (eg, OH, C, O, SH) within the
molecule have characteristic absorption bands. The principle functional groups can
be determined and used to identify compounds in cases in which chemical evidence
permits relatively few possible structures. Standard IR spectrophotometers cover the
spectral range from 2.5 to 15.4 µm (wave number equivalent to 4000–650 cm^{-1}) and
use a source of radiation that passes through the sample and reference cells into a
monochrometer (a device to isolate spectral regions). The radiation is then collected,
amplified, and recorded. Current instruments use microprocessors, allowing a number of refinements that have increased the versatility of IR instruments so that more
precise qualitative and quantitative data can be obtained.

12.2.3.2d Ultraviolet/Visible Spectrophotometry

Transitions occurring between electronic levels of molecules produce absorptions
and emissions in the visible (VIS) and UV portions of the electromagnetic spectrum. Many inorganic and organic molecules show maximum absorption at specific
wavelengths in the UV/VIS range, and these can be used to identify and quantitate
compounds. Instruments designed to measure absorbance in the UV/VIS portions of
the spectrum (190–700 nm) have been used in many specific purposes, such as detectors in HPLC and CE. These detectors use small flow cells having short path-
lengths (approximately 10 mm) and hold small volumes (eg, 10.0 µL) through
which light at a specific wavelength passes. Basic spectrophotometers have the
same components as the IR instruments described previously, including a source
(usually a deuterium lamp) monochromator, beam splitter, sampler and reference
cells, and detector.

12.2.3.2e   *Nuclear Magnetic Resonance*

Nuclear magnetic resonance (NMR) detects atoms which have nuclei that possess a magnetic moment. These are usually atoms containing nuclei with an odd number of protons (charges). Such nuclei can exist in two states, a low energy state with the nuclear spin aligned parallel to the magnetic field and a high energy state with the spin perpendicular to the field. Basically, the instrument measures the absorption or radiowave necessary to change the nuclei from a low to a high energy state as the magnetic field is varied. It is used most commonly for hydrogen atoms, although ^{13}C and ^{31}P are also suitable. Because the field seen by a proton varies with its molecular environment, such molecular arrangements as CH_3, CH_2, CH, and so on, all give different signs, providing much information about the structure of the molecule in question.

12.2.3.2f   *Other Analytical Methods*

As previously mentioned, the instruments discussed earlier are the primary ones used in toxicant analysis, but an enormous number of analytical techniques are used in the field. Many of the instruments are expensive (eg, Raman spectrometer, x-ray emission spectrometer) and few laboratories possess them. Many other instruments are available, however, such as the specific-ion electrode, which is both sensitive and portable. Specific-ion electrodes have many other advantages in that sample color, suspended matter, turbidity, and viscosity do not interfere with analysis; therefore, many of the sample preparation steps are not required. Some of the species that can be detected at ppb levels are ammonia, carbon dioxide, chloride, cyanide, fluoride, lead, potassium, sulfide, and urea. Analytical pH meters or meters designed specifically for this application are used to calculate concentrations.

Finally, an increasing number of portable and direct reading instruments are now available to detect and quantitate environmental pollutants. Most of these measure airborne particulates and dissolved molecules and operate on such diverse principles as aerosol photometry, chemiluminescence, combustion, and polarography. Elemental analyzers have been developed for carbon, nitrogen, and sulfur using IR, chemiluminescence, and fluorescence, respectively. Analyses can be completed in about 1 min if the samples are gases, liquids, or small solids, and within 10 min if solid samples are larger. These devices are microprocessor controlled, contain built-in printers, and are used to analyze materials including gasolines, pesticides, protein solutions, and waste water.

12.3

BIOASSAY

The term bioassay is used in two distinct ways. First, the narrow definition is the use of a living organism in an assay designed to measure the amount of a toxicant present in the toxicity of a sample. This is done by comparing the toxic effect of the

TABLE 12.3. SOME ORGANISMS COMMONLY USED IN BIOASSAY PROCEDURES

Vertebrates
Fathead minnow, *Pimephales premelas*
Brook trout, *Solvelinus fontinalis*
Sheepshead minnow, *Cyprinodon variegatus*
Invertebrates
Water fleas, *Daphnia* spp
Grass shrimp, *Palaemonetes* spp
Shrimp, *Penaeus* spp
Algae
Green algae (Chlorophytes): *Selenastrum capricomutum*, *Chlorella* spp
Blue-green algae (Cyanophytes), *Anabaena flosaquae*
Red algae (Rhodophyta), *Porphyridium cruentum*

sample with the toxic effect of a graded series of known amount of a standard toxicant—that is, a standard curve. The second and less appropriate way is to use the word bioassay to include the use of animals to investigate the toxic effect of a toxicant. The latter is considered to be toxicity testing and is covered, in most of its many forms, in Chapter 11.

The bioassay technique has both advantages and disadvantages. It is the most nonspecific assay used for toxic chemicals because the endpoint most often used, the death of the organism, is common to many toxicants. However, it is rapid, inexpensive, and useful for obtaining an early indication of the equivalent toxicity of environmental samples. The effect of the environment on the toxicant can also be ascertained quickly.

The organisms most commonly used are aquatic and include plants as well as vertebrate and invertebrate animals. Some examples follow, and a list of species commonly used is shown in Table 12.3.

DAPHNIA. Several tests using the water flea *Daphnia* are conducted routinely. They include screening tests to obtain an index of the toxicity of pure or mixed compounds in water or waste treatment processes or to determine which of several processes may contribute to the eventual toxicity of plant effluents. A more standardized test is used for compliance with the National Pollution Discharge Elimination System, for which an index of the toxicity of effluents is required. The endpoint of the tests is acute lethality over a 24- to 48-hour period. The *Dalphnia* used are cultured and the culture conditions must be carefully controlled to assure reproducibility. Factors of importance are species selection (eg, *Daphnia magna, Daphnia pulex*), age, nutrition, osmotic and ionic balance of the medium, light, and temperature. A variety of chronic and multigeneration tests can also be carried out using *Daphnia*.

Grass shrimp (*Palaemonetes* spp) have been used in a variety of bioassays. They are used to identify toxic effluents and estimate pure compounds and to measure the toxic potential of dissolved pesticides, chlorine, metals, and industrial wastes. Several species have been used, but *Palaemonetes pugio* is used most commonly. Care must be taken with shipping and acclimatization to the medium. Mortality is usually the endpoint used with groups of 10 to 20 shrimp being exposed to each of the five or six concentrations of the test compound. A positive control is also conducted using a compound of known toxicity.

ALGAE. Algal cultures are exposed to a range of concentrations of the test chemical or effluent and the algal growth rates are determined over a 4- to 5-day period. Physical conditions and the composition of the medium must be controlled closely and some convenient method must be used to determine growth rate. Because growth rate is quite variable, not only a number of concentrations are used, but also enough replicates to permit statistical analysis. Negative controls (without test compound) and positive controls (with a compound of known toxicity to the species in question) are included routinely. Growth can be determined in one of many ways, including counting the cells manually under the light microscope, counting the cells in a cell counter, measuring chlorophyll fluorometrically, measuring adenosine triphosphate (ATP), or measuring the assimilation of a suitable ^{14}C-labeled precursor.

FISH. Fish are also used as bioassay organisms. Although these bioassays require more time and laboratory space than do algae or *Daphnia,* fish have the advantage of using a vertebrate organism, presumably closer to mammals in activation and detoxication pathways as well as in mode of toxic action. The most useful species among freshwater species is the fathead minnow, *Pimephales promelas*, and among saltwater species is the sheepshead minnow, *Cyprinodom variegatus.*

Suggested Further Reading

Buikema AL, Cairms J (eds.): *Aquatic Invertebrate Bioassays.* ASTM Special Technical Publication No.715. Philadelphia: American Society for Testing and Materials, 1980

Cairns J, Dickson KL: *Biological Methods for the Assessment of Water Quality.* ASTM Special Technical Publication 528. Philadelphia: American Society for Testing and Materials, 1973.

Ebing W (ed.): Analysis of Pesticides in Ground and Surface Water I and II. In *Chemistry of Plant Protection,* Vols. 11 and 12. Berlin, Germany: Springer-Verlag, 1995.

Everson RJ, Oehme FW: *Analytical Toxicology Manual.* Manhatten, KS: American College of Veterinary Toxicologists, 1981.

Frei RW, Hutzinger O (eds.): *Analytical Aspects of Mercury and Other Heavy Metals in the Environment.* New York: Gordon & Beach, 1975.

Glass GE: *Bioassay Techniques and Environmental Chemistry.* Ann Arbor, MI: Ann Arbor Science, 1973.

Howard PH: *Handbook of Environmental Fate and Exposure Data for Organic Chemicals.* Chelsea, MI: Lewis Publishers, Inc. (A 4-volume series that includes priority pollutants, solvents, and pesticides.) 1989–1993.

Laners JP (ed.): *Handbook of Capillary Electrophoresis.* Boca Raton, FL: CRC Press Inc., 1994.

National Academy of Sciences. *Decision Making for Regulatory Chemicals in the Environment.* Washington, DC: National Academy of Sciences, 1975.

Nelson AH: *Organic Chemicals in the Aquatic Environment.* Boca Raton, FL: CRC Press, Inc., 1994.

Pickering WF: *Pollution Evaluation: The Quantitative Aspects.* New York: Marcel Dekker, 1977.

Rand GM, Petrocelli SN: *Fundamentals of Aquatic Toxicology.* Washington, DC: Hemisphere, 1985.

Thoma JJ, Bond PB, Sunshine I (eds.): *Guidelines for Analytical Toxicology Programs,* Vols. 1 and 2. Cleveland: CRC Press Inc., 1977.

Ware GW (ed.): *Reviews of Environmental Contamination and Toxicology,* New York: Springer-Verlag. (This excellent series of review articles is approaching Vol. 150 and covers all aspects of toxicology.)

Zweig G (ed): *Analytical Methods for Pesticides and Plant Growth Regulators.* New York: Academic Press. (This was a multivolume series appearing between 1973 and 1989 that contains analytical methods for the analysis of food and food additives, fungicides, herbicides, nematocides, pheromones, rodenticides, and soil fumigants).

PREVENTION OF TOXICITY 13

ERNEST HODGSON

13.1

INTRODUCTION

Laws and regulations provide the framework for organized efforts to prevent toxicity, and sanctions are necessary to prevent those without social conscience from deliberately exposing their fellows to risks from toxic chemicals. This is not enough, however, because without a population educated to toxic hazards and their prevention, the laws could never be administered properly. Moreover, in many circumstances, and particularly in the home, wisdom dictates courses of action not necessarily prescribed by law. The key to toxicity prevention lies in information and education, with legislation, regulation, and penalties as final safeguards. In all probability, the better the general population is educated and informed, the less likely are laws to be necessary.

13.2

LEGISLATION AND REGULATION

In the best sense, legislation provides an enabling act describing the areas to be covered under the particular law and the general manner in which they are to be regulated, and designating an executive agency to write and enforce specific regulations within the intent of the legislative body. For example, the Toxic Substances Control Act (TSCA) was passed by Congress to regulate the introduction of chemicals into

commerce, to determine their hazards to the human population and the environment, and to regulate or ban those deemed hazardous. The task of writing and en-
forcing specific regulations was assigned to the Environmental Protection Agency
(EPA).

Legislative attempts to write specific regulations into laws usually fail. The resultant laws lack flexibility and, because they are written by lawyers rather than
toxicologists, seldom address the problem in a scientifically rigorous manner.

It should be borne in mind that legislation is a synthesis of science, politics,
and public and private pressure. It represents a society's best estimate, at that moment, of the risks it is prepared to take and those it wishes to avoid, as well as the
price it is prepared to pay. Such decisions properly include more than science. The
task of the toxicologist is to see that the science that is included is accurate and is
interpreted logically.

This section is based primarily on regulations in the United States, not because
these are the best but because, in toto, they are the most comprehensive. In many re-
spects, they are a complex mixture of overlapping laws and jurisdictions, providing
unnecessary work for the legal profession. At the same time, few if any toxic hazards in the home, workplace, or environment are not addressed.

13.2.1   Federal Government

Following is a summary of the most important federal statutes concerned in whole
or in part with the regulation of toxic substances.

CLEAN AIR ACT. The Clean Air Act is administered by the EPA. Although the principal
enforcement provisions are the responsibility of local governments, overall admin-
istrative responsibility rests with the EPA. This act requires criteria documents for
air pollutants and sets both national air quality standards and standards for sources
that create air pollutants, such as motor vehicles, power plants, and so on. Important
actions taken under this law include standards for a phased-out elimination of lead
in gasoline and the setting of sulfuric acid air emission guidelines for existing industrial plants.

CLEAN WATER ACT. The Clean Water Act, which amends the Federal Water Pollution
Control Act, is also administered by the EPA and provides for funding of municipal
sewage treatment plants. However, with respect to toxicity prevention, it is more
important that the act regulates emissions from municipal and industrial sources. It
has as its goal the elimination of discharges of pollutants and the protection of rivers
so that they are "swimmable and fishable" and applies to "waters of the United
States" subsequently defined to include all waters that reach navigable waters, wet-
lands, and intermittent streams. Some of the more important actions taken under
this statute include setting standards for emissions of inorganics from smelter operations and publishing priority lists of toxic pollutants. This act allows the federal
government to recover clean-up and other costs as damages from the polluting
agency, company, or individual.

SAFE DRINKING WATER ACT. Specifically applied to water supplied for human consumption, this act requires the EPA to set maximum levels for contaminants in water delivered to users of public water systems. Two criteria are extablished for a particular contaminant: the *maximum containment level goal (MCLG)* and the *maximum contaminant level (MCL)*. The former, the MCLG, is the level at which no known or anticipated adverse effects on the health of persons occur and that allows an adequate margin of safety. The latter, the MCL, is the maximum permissible level of a contaminant in water that is delivered to any user of a public water system. MCLs are expected to be as close to the MCLG as is feasible.

COMPREHENSIVE ENVIRONMENTAL RESPONSE, COMPENSATION AND LIABILITY ACT. This is an attempt to deal with the many waste sites that exist across the nation. It covers remedial action, including the establishment of a National Priorities List to identify those sites that should have a high priority for remediation.

CONSUMER PRODUCTS SAFETY ACT AND CONSUMER PRODUCTS SAFETY COMMISSION IMPROVEMENTS ACT. Administered by a Consumer Products Safety Commission, the Consumer Products Safety Act is designed to protect the public against risk of injury from consumer products and to set safety standards for such products.

CONTROLLED SUBSTANCES ACT. The Controlled Substances Act not only strengthens law enforcement in the field of drug abuse but also provides for research into the prevention and treatment of drug abuse.

FEDERAL FOOD, DRUG AND COSMETIC ACT. The Federal Food, Drug and Cosmetic Act is administered by the Food and Drug Administration (FDA). It establishes limits for food additives and cosmetic components, sets criteria for drug safety for both human and animal use, and requires the manufacturer to prove both safety and efficacy. The FDA is authorized to define the required toxicity testing for each product. This act contains the Delaney clause, which states that food additives that cause cancer in humans or animals at any level shall not be considered safe and are, therefore, prohibited from such use. This clause has recently been modified to permit the agency to use more flexible risk/benefit based guidelines. This law also empowers the FDA to establish and modify the generally recognized as safe (GRAS) list and to establish good laboratory practice (GLP) rules.

FEDERAL INSECTICIDE, FUNGICIDE AND RODENTICIDE ACT. Administered by the EPA, the Federal Insecticide, Fungicide and Rodenticide Act (FIFRA) regulates all pesticides and other agricultural chemicals, such as plant growth regulators, used in the United States. It includes registration requirements, with appropriate chemical and toxicological tests prescribed by the agency. This act also permits the agency to specify labels, to restrict application to certified applicators, and to deny, rescind, or modify registration. Under this act, the EPA also establishes tolerances for residues on raw agricultural products.

OCCUPATIONAL SAFETY AND HEALTH ACT. Administered by the Occupational Safety and Health Administration (OSHA), the Occupation Safety and Health Act concerns health and safety in the workplace. OSHA sets standards for worker exposure to specific chemicals, for air concentration values, and for monitoring procedures. Construction and environmental controls also come under this act. This act provides for research, information, education, and training in occupational safety and health. By establishing the National Institute for Occupational Safety and Health (NIOSH), the act provided for appropriate studies to be conducted so that regulatory decisions could be based on the best available information.

NATIONAL ENVIRONMENTAL POLICY ACT. The National Environmental Policy Act is an umbrella act covering all US government agencies, requiring them to prepare environmental impact statements for all federal actions affecting the quality of the human environment. Environmental impact statements must include not only an assessment of the effect of the proposed action on the environment, but also alternatives to the proposed action, the relationship between local short-term use and enhancements of long-term productivity, and a statement of irreversible commitment of resources. This act also created the Council on Environmental Quality, which acts in an advisory capacity to the president on matters affecting or promoting environmental quality.

RESOURCE CONSERVATION AND RECOVERY ACT. Also administered by the EPA, the Resource Conservation and Recovery Act (RCRA) is the most important act governing the disposal of hazardous wastes; it promulgates standards for identification of hazardous wastes, their transportation, and their disposal. Included in the latter are siting and construction criteria for landfills and other disposal facilities as well as the regulation of owners and operators of such facilities. The three principal areas covered are hazardous wastes, nonhazardous solid wastes, and underground storage tanks.

TOXIC SUBSTANCES CONTROL ACT. Administered by the EPA, the TSCA is mammoth, covering almost all chemicals manufactured in the United States for industrial and other purposes, excluding certain compounds covered under other laws such as FIFRA. The EPA may control or stop production of compounds deemed hazardous. Producers must give notice or intent to manufacture new chemicals or increase significantly the production of existing chemicals. They may be required to conduct toxicity and other tests. This law is as yet incompletely applied due to the enormous number of existing chemicals that must be evaluated. Once fully applied, it will be the most important statute affecting toxicology.

OTHER STATUTES WITH RELEVANCE TO THE PREVENTION OF TOXICITY. It should be noted that some of these statutes have been superseded by others, either in whole or in part.

- Comprehensive Employment and Training Act
- Dangerous Cargo Act
- Federal Coal Mine Health and Safety Act
- Federal Coal Mine Safety and Health Amendment Act
- Federal Caustic Poison Act

- Federal Railroad Safety Authorization Act
- Hazardous Materials Transport Act
- Lead-Based Paint Poison Prevention Act
- Marine Protection Research and Sanctuaries Act
- Poison Prevention Packaging Act
- Ports and Waterways Safety Act

13.2.2   State Governments

States are free to adopt legislation with toxicological significance although their jurisdiction does not extend beyond their geographic boundaries. In other cases, the states may enforce federal statutes under certain circumstances. For example, if state regulations concerning hazardous waste disposal is neither less comprehensive nor less rigorous than the federal statute, enforcement is delegated to the states. Similarly, certain aspects of FIFRA are enforced by individual states. In some cases (California is notable in this respect), states have passed laws considerably more comprehensive and more rigorous than the corresponding federal statute.

13.2.3   Legislation and Regulation in Other Countries

It would serve little purpose to enumerate all the laws affecting toxicology, toxicity testing, and the prevention of toxicity that have been promulgated in all countries that have such laws. Legislation in this area has been adopted in most countries of western Europe and in Japan. Although the laws in use in the United States are a complex mixture of overlapping statutes and enforcement agencies, they are probably the most comprehensive set of such laws in existence. Most other industrialized countries have legislation in the same areas, although the emphasis varies widely from one country to another. Many undeveloped countries, due to the lack of both trained manpower and financial resources, are unable to write and enforce their own code of regulations and instead adopt the regulatory decisions of either the United States or some other industrialized nation. For example, they will permit the use, in their own territory, of pesticides registered under FIFRA by the US EPA and will prohibit the use of pesticides not so registered.

13.3

PREVENTION IN DIFFERENT ENVIRONMENTS

Humans spend their time in many environments. Homes vary with climate, family income, and personal choice. The workplace varies from pristine mountains to industrial jungles, whereas the outdoor environment from which recreation, food, and water are derived varies through the same extremes. Each of these environments has its own specific complex of hazards, and thus requires its own set of rules and recommendations if these hazards are to be avoided.

13.3.1 Home

Approximately 50% of all accidental poisoning fatalities in the United States involve preschool children; thus prevention of toxicity is particularly important in homes with young children.

PRESCRIPTION DRUGS should always be kept in the original container (in the United States and some other countries, these are now required to have safety closures). They should be taken only by the persons for whom they were prescribed, and excess drugs should be discarded safely when the illness is resolved. When children are present, prescription drugs should be kept in a locked cabinet, because few cabinets are inaccessible to a determined child. Although nonprescription drugs are usually less hazardous, they are frequently flavored in an attractive way. Thus, it is prudent to follow the same rules as for prescription drugs.

HOUSEHOLD CHEMICALS such as lye, polishes, and kerosene should be kept in locked storage if possible; if not, they should be kept in as secure a place as possible, out of the reach of children. Such chemicals should never be stored in anything but the original containers. Certainly they should never be stored in beverage bottles, kitchen containers, and so on. Unnecessary materials should be disposed of safely in appropriate disposal sites.

CERTAIN HOUSEHOLD OPERATIONS such as interior painting, and so on, should be done only with adequate ventilation. Insecticide treatment should be done precisely in accordance with instructions on the label.

Increasing fuel costs have caused several changes in lifestyle, and some of these changes carry potential toxic hazards. They include more burning of wood and coal and the construction of heavily insulated houses with a concomitant reduction in ventilation. In the latter circumstances, improperly burning furnaces can generate high levels of CO and aromatic hydrocarbons, whereas even those burning properly may still generate oxides of nitrogen (NOx) at levels high enough to cause respiratory tract irritation in sensitive individuals. These effects can be avoided by ensuring that all heating equipment (eg, furnaces, wood stoves, heaters) is properly ventilated, maintained and checked regularly. In addition, some ventilation of the building itself should always be provided. Less ventilation is needed when the temperature is either excessively high or excessively low, and more is needed when the temperature is in the midrange, but under no circumstances should the homeowner strive for a completely sealed house.

13.3.2 Workplace

Exposure levels of hazardous chemicals in the air of work environments are mandated by OSHA as exposure limit values. The studies necessary to establish these limits are carried out by NIOSH. However, the more complete list of the better known threshold limit values (TLVs) is established by the American Conference of

Governmental Industrial Hygienists. Although TLVs are not binding in law, they are an excellent guide to the employer. In fact, they are often adopted by OSHA as exposure limit values. The concentrations thus expressed are the weighted average concentrations normally considered safe for an exposure of 8 h/day, 5 days/week. Absolute upper limits (excursion values) may also be included. Some exposure limits are shown in Table 13.1.

Concentrations at or lower than those normal or working exposures are usually maintained by environmental engineering controls. Operations that generate large amounts of dusts or vapors are conducted in enclosed spaces that are vented separately or under hoods. Other spaces are ventilated adequately, and temperature and humidity controls are installed where necessary.

Other precautions must be taken to prevent accidental or occasional increases in concentrations. Materials should be transported in "safe" containers, spilled material removed rapidly, and floor and wall materials selected to prevent contamination and allow easy cleaning.

Additional methods for the prevention of toxicity in the workplace include the use of personal safety equipment—protective clothing, gloves, and goggles are the most important. In particularly hazardous operations, closed-circuit air masks, gas masks, and so on, may also be necessary.

Preemployment instruction and preemployment physical examinations are of critical importance in most work situations involving hazardous chemicals. The former should make clear the hazards involved, the need to avoid exposure under normal working conditions, and the mechanisms by which exposure is limited. Furthermore, employees should understand how and when to contain spills and how and when to evacuate the area around the spill. Location and use of emergency equipment, showers, eye washes, and so on, should also be given, and the most important procedures should be posted in the work area.

TABLE 13.1. SOME SELECTED THRESHOLD LIMIT VALUES (1991)

Chemical	TLV–TWA[a] ppm	TLV–STEL[b] ppm	TLV–C[c] ppm
Acetaldehyde	100	150	—
Boron trifluoride	—	—	1
o-Dichlorobenzene	—	—	50
p-Dichlorobenzene	75	110	—
N-Ethylmorpholine	5	20	—
Fluorine	1	2	—
Phosgene	0.1	—	—
Trichloroethylene	50	200	—

[a]TLV–TWA, threshold limit value: time-weighted average concentration for a normal 8-hour workday and 40-hour workweek to which nearly all workers may be repeatedly exposed without adverse effect.
[b]TLV–STEL, threshold limit value: short-term exposure limit concentration. This time-weighted 15-minute average exposure should not be exceeded at any time during a workday even if the TLV–TWA is within limits. Intended as supplement to TLV–TWA.
[c]TLV–C, threshold limit value–ceiling, concentration that should not be exceeded at any time.

13.3.3 Pollution of Air, Water, and Land

The toxicological significance of pollution of the environment may be work related, as in the case of agricultural workers, or related to the outside environment encountered in daily life. In the case of agricultural workers, numerous precautions are necessary for the prevention of toxicity. For example:

• Pesticides and other agricultural chemicals should be kept only in the original container, carrying the label prescribed by EPA under FIFRA.
• Empty containers and excess chemicals should be disposed of properly in safe hazardous waste disposal sites, incinerated when possible or, in some cases, decontaminated.
• Workers should not reenter treated areas until the safe reentry period has elapsed.
• Certain workers such as applicators, those preparing tank mixes, and so on, should wear appropriate protective clothing, gloves, face masks, and so forth. The development of closed systems for mixing pesticides should help protect mixers and loaders of pesticides from exposure.
• Spraying operations should be carried out in such a way as to minimize drift, contamination of water, and so on.

Pesticides have caused a number of fatalities in the past. The current practice in some countries of restricting the most hazardous chemicals for use only by certified operators should greatly minimize pesticide poisoning in these locations.

Individuals can do little to protect themselves from poisoning by chemicals that pollute the air and water except to insist that discharge of toxicants into the environment be minimized. The exposure levels are low as compared with those in acute toxicity cases, and the effects may be indirect, as in the increase in preexisting respiratory irritation during smog. Thus, these effects can be determined only at the epidemiologic level. Because many persons are not affected or may not be affected for years, it is often argued that environmental contamination is not very important. However, a small percentage increase may represent a large number of people when the whole population is considered. Furthermore, chronic toxicity is not often reversible. Because in most industrialized countries laws already exist to control emission problems, if such problems exist in these countries they are usually problems of enforcement.

One of the most critical areas for the prevention of toxicity caused by environmental contamination is that of disposal of hazardous wastes. It is now apparent that past practices in many industrialized countries have created large numbers of waste sites in which the waste is often unidentified, improperly stored, and leaching into the environment. The task of rectifying these past errors is an enormous one just now being addressed.

The ideal situation for current and future practices is to reduce chemical waste to an irreducible minimum and then to place the remainder in secure storage. Waste reduction can be accomplished in many ways.

- Refine plant processes so that less waste is produced.
- Recycle waste into useful products.
- Concentrate wastes.
- Incinerate. The technology is available to incinerate essentially all waste to inorganic slag. Unfortunately, the technology is sophisticated and expensive. Inadequate incineration is itself a hazard because of the risk of generating dioxins and other toxicants and releasing them into the environment. Less complex and more easily maintained incinerators will be essential if this technology is to play a prominent role in waste reduction.

Safe storage for the remaining waste may be in dump sites or in above-ground storage. In either case, such storage ideally should be properly sited, constructed, maintained, and monitored.

Because of the nature of commerce, probably none of these measures will be successful unless the laws, penalties, and incentives are manipulated in such a way as to make safe disposal more attractive economically than unsafe disposal.

13.4

EDUCATION

Because chemicals, many of them hazardous, are an inevitable part of life in industrialized countries, education is probably the most important method for the prevention of toxicity. Unfortunately, it is also one of the most neglected. In a typical public debate concerning a possible chemical hazard, the principle protagonists tend to fall into two extreme groups. The "everything is OK" protagonists and the "ban it completely" protagonists. The media seldom seem to educate the public, usually serving only to add fuel to the flames.

The educational role of the toxicologist should be the voice of reason, presenting a balanced view of risks and benefits, and outlining alternatives whenever possible. The simple lesson that science deals not in certainty, but rather degrees of certitude, must be learned by all involved.

In terms of ongoing educational programs, there should be opportunities at all levels: elementary schools, high schools, university, adult education, and media education. Several approaches can be used to educate the general public in ideal situations:

- *Elementary schools*—Teach the rudiments of first aid and environmental concerns—proper disposal, etc.
- *High school*—Teach concepts of toxicology (dose response, etc.) and environmental toxicology (bioaccumulation, etc.). These concepts can be introduced into general science courses.

- *University*—In addition to toxicology degrees, general courses for nontoxicology and/or nonscience majors should stress a balanced approach, with both responsible use and toxicity prevention as desirable endpoints.
- *Media*—encourage a balanced approach to toxicity problems. Toxicologists should be available to media representatives and, where appropriate, should be involved directly.

Suggested Further Reading

American Conference of Governmental Industrial Hygienists: *TLVs—Threshold Limit Values for Chemical Substances and Physical Agents in the Work Environment with Intended Changes.* Cincinnati (published annually).

American Conference of Governmental Industrial Hygienists: *Documentation of the Threshold Limit Values for Substances in Workroom Air.* Cincinnati (published annually).

Doull J: Recommended limits for exposure to chemicals. In *Casarett & Doull's Toxicology, the Basic Science of Poisons,* 5th ed. Klaassen CD (ed.). New York: McGraw-Hill, 1996, pp 1025–1049.

Dreisbach RH: *Handbook of Poisoning: Prevention, Diagnosis and Treatment,* 11th ed. Los Altos, CA: Lange Medical, 1983.

Ellenhorn MJ, Barceloux DG: *Medical Toxicology: Diagnosis and Treatment of Human Poisoning.* New York: Elsevier Science Publishing Co., 1988.

Environmental Regulation: An International View. A series of papers on: I. Britain, TW Hall; II. European Economic Community, SP Johnson; III. The United States, JB Ritch, Jr; IV. An Industry View, RC Tineknell. *Chem Soc Rev* **5:**431–771, 1976.

Fan AM, Chang LW (eds.): *Toxicology and Risk Assessment: Principles, Methods and Applications.* New York: Marcel Dekker, Inc, 1996.

Merrill RA: Regulatory toxicology. In *Casarett & Doull's Toxicology, the Basic Science of Poisons,* 5th ed. Klaassen CD (ed.). New York: McGraw-Hill, 1996, pp 1011–1023.

Sandmeyer EE: Regulatory toxicology, Chapter 20. In *A Guide to General Toxicology.* Homberger F, Hayes JA, Pelikan EW (eds.). Basel: Karger, 1983.

DIAGNOSIS AND TREATMENT OF TOXICITY 14

ERNEST HODGSON

14.1

INTRODUCTION

It should be made clear at the outset that this chapter is not a manual on how to treat the poisoned individual. It is a brief summary without the necessary details even for adequate first aid and is designed only to introduce the student to the most important principles involved. Except for first aid, treatment of poisoning is the province of the medical practitioner, and even first aid is best rendered by those with specific training in the area, or at the very least those who have carefully reviewed such manuals as those written by Dreisbach or Ellenhorn and Barceloux (see Section 14.6). After removing the victim from contact with the suspected poison, the most useful action to be taken by someone without appropriate training is to call the nearest source of emergency medical care, emergency rescue squad, the local police, or the nearest hospital emergency room. Poison control centers are also available as sources of information and are invaluable as a backup for physician and emergency medical personnel.

Most of the material in this chapter is related to acute toxicity. Chronic toxicity rarely constitutes an immediately life-threatening crisis and is, in any case, less responsive to therapy.

14.2

DIAGNOSIS

14.2.1 Introduction

Following appropriate first aid (see Section 14.3.1), the removal of the poisoning victim from contact with the poison, and steps to prevent further absorption of the poison, the physician is required to make a diagnosis so that the treatment most appropriate to the specific compound can be initiated. Because the poisoning victim is frequently a child or, if an adult, may be comatose, it is often necessary to rely on parents, friends, eyewitnesses, or an examination of the scene (ie, containers, etc.) for useful background details. Relative to the toxicant involved, patients will fall into three classes.

In the *first class* of poisoning are those patients who have absorbed a known poison. The physician must initiate appropriate emergency treatment and estimate the quantity absorbed in order to approach further therapy with greater confidence. A maximum estimate can sometimes be determined from the amount missing from the container. Although fatal doses determined on experimental animals may not be similar to those for humans, they do give a rough idea of relative toxicity.

In the *second class* of poisoning, patients are known to be poisoned but the actual toxicant is unknown, usually because the poison is a complex mixture. The physician's task is to attempt to identify the toxicant, a task made difficult by the numerous trade names and proprietary mixtures. Some lists and reference sources are available, however (Table 14.1). In addition, the nearest poison control center is a source of in-

TABLE 14.1. SOME SOURCES OF INFORMATION ON THE IDENTITY OF TOXIC CHEMICALS

Published Works

General

Lewis RJ Sr: *Hazardous Chemicals Desk Reference.* New York: Van Nostrand Reinhold, 1991.

Likes KE (ed.). *Toxifile.* Chicago Micro Corporation (microfiche).

Rumack BH (ed.). *Poisindex.* Denver: National Center for Poison Information (microfiche).

————. *The Merck Index,* 12th ed. Rahway, NJ: Merck and Co, 1996.

Wexler P: Information *Resources in Toxicology* 2 ed. New York: Elsevier, 1988. Important guide to directories, reference works, data bases, organizations, etc.

Commercial and Industrial Chemicals

————. *Trades Names Index.* American Conference of Governmental Industrial Hygienists. Cincinnati, 1965, with annual supplements.

Gosselin RE, et al: *Clinical Toxicology of Comercial Products,* 4th ed. Baltimore: Williams & Wilkins, 1976.

Prescription Drugs

Wilson CO, Jones TE: *American Drug Index.* Philadelphia: Lippincott, published annually.

————. *Physicians Desk Reference.* Oradell, NJ: Medical Economics Data, published annually.

————. *Hospital Formulary.* Washington, DC: American Society of Hospital Pharmacists, published annually.

Non-Prescription Drugs

Griffenhagen GG (ed.). *Handbook of Non-Prescription Drugs.* Washington, DC: American Pharmaceutical Association, published annually.

Drugs of Abuse

Lowry WT, Gamiott JC: *Forensic Toxicology: Controlled Substances and Dangerous Drugs.* New York: Plenum Press, 1979.

Pesticides

Caswell RL (ed.). *Pesticide Handbook.* College Park, MD: Entomological Society of America, published annually.

Tomlin C (ed.). *The Pesticide Manual, Incorporating the Agrochemicals Handbook,* 10th ed. Surrey, UK, and The Royal Society of Chemistry, Cambridge, UK: Crop Protection Publications, British Crop Protection Council, 1994.

Computer Data Bases

Toxicology Data Base. Toxicology Information Science, Bethesda, MD: National Library of Medicine.

TOXLINE. Toxicology Information Science, Bethesda, MD: National Library of Medicine.

Telephone Sources

Poison Control Centers. See Directory of Poison Control Centers. Bulletin of National Clearinghouse for Poison Control Centers 24(8), 1980. Also Wexler, this table and local telephone directories, emergency listings

Chemical manufacturers

formation, as is the manufacturer. It is important that the first person on the scene or anyone rendering first aid to a poisoning victim sends the container, if available, with the patient when the patient is moved to the hospital or emergency center. Naturally, it should be resealed and properly packed to ensure that it does not cause further problems. Similarly, if the victim vomits, the vomitus should be collected and placed in a jar, and should accompany the patient. If the toxicant can be identified, appropriate therapy can be initiated; otherwise, the physician must rely on nonspecific life-support measures while the vomitus, urine, feces, or blood is analyzed.

In the *third class* of poisoning are those patients in whom the physician must carry out the differential diagnosis of a disease that may or may not be the result of poisoning. This consists of a complete case history, a complete physical examination, and appropriate laboratory tests.

14.2.2   Case History

The case history may be obtained from the victim or from parents, friends, neighbors, or eyewitnesses. The various individuals should be questioned separately to avoid overlooking important items. It is important to consider the occupation of the patient and whether the patient was at his normal job at the time of the poisoning. There are many known occupational hazards, including the following types of poisoning:

- *Carbon monoxide* (CO) poisoning may occur among blacksmiths, furnace or foundry workers, brick or cement makers, chimney cleaners, service-station attendants, parking attendants, garage workers, miners, refinery workers, plumbers, police officers, and sewer workers.
- Poisoning by *chlorinated hydrocarbons*, particularly solvents, may occur among rubber cement and plastic cement workers or users, leather workers, dry cleaners, painters, furniture finishers, cloth finishers, paint removers, and rubber workers.
- *Lead* poisoning can occur among welders, steamfitters, plumbers, painters, ceramic workers, battery makers, miners, pottery makers, electroplaters, printers, service-station attendants, and junk-metal refiners.
- *Methanol* poisoning can occur among bookbinders, bronzers, rubber and plastic cement users, dry cleaners, leather workers, printers, painters, and woodworkers.

Other types of poisoning are characteristic of particular tasks; those in the previous list are illustrative examples.

If the poisoning incident occurred in the home, the patient, the patient's home, and the immediate surroundings must be searched for poison containers. It is also important to check for possible ingestion of food, drink, and medicines; contact with insecticides or other agricultural chemicals; exposure to fumes, smoke, or gases; or skin contact with liquids such as insecticides or cleaning solvents.

14.2.3   Systemic Examination

The systemic examination covers various general aspects of function as well as observations that bear on particular organ systems. Although such examinations are useful and should always be performed, it should also be borne in mind that individual variation in humans is so great that in any particular case typical symptoms may not be present.

Blood pressure and *pulse rate* are often important general indicators. For example, blood pressure may be high in nicotine poisoning or low in poisoning by nitrites, arsenic, or fluorides. Similarly, a fast pulse may indicate poisoning by atropine, and a slow or irregular pulse may indicate poisoning by nitrites. *Weight loss, lethargy,* and *weakness* are often symptoms of chronic poisoning by such toxicants as lead and mercury, whereas an elevated *body temperature* is typical of poisoning with nitrophenols.

The *skin* is among the first tissues examined in a systemic examination. For example, cyanosis (a bluish color, especially of the lips) may indicate hypoxia or methemoglobinemia caused by nitrites, aniline, and so on, whereas redness or flushing may indicate poisoning by CO or cyanide. Jaundice, a yellow color visible in the skin and the eyes, may be due to quite different forms of poisoning—for example, liver injury caused by compounds such as carbon tetrachloride, and hemolysis, caused by compounds such as aniline or arsine. Overt damage to the skin, such as burns or corrosion, may be caused by acids, alkalis, or strong oxidizing agents such as permanganate or dichromate.

Effects on the *central nervous system* (CNS) may be indicated by a variety of physical, behavioral, or psychological symptoms. Muscular twitching and convulsions may be caused by a number of different insecticides, by nicotine, by amphetamines, or by many other toxicants. Headaches may be caused by poisoning with organophosphate insecticides, CO, and so on. Depression, drowsiness, and coma often follow barbiturate overdose or poisoning by ethanol, various industrial solvents, and many other chemicals. Delirium or hallucinations may follow ingestion of excessive alcohol, amphetamines, cocaine, or other chemicals. Metals such as thallium, lead, or mercury, as well as drugs such as antihistamines and barbiturates, may cause confusion or similar mental changes.

Examination of the head, including the eyes, ears, nose, and mouth may provide valuable clues as to the nature of the toxicant involved in poisoning cases, with the *eyes* being perhaps the most valuable diagnostic indicator. For example, blurred vision may result from poisoning with such chemicals as atropine, phosphate ester insecticides, cocaine, or methanol, whereas double vision can result from alcohol, barbiturates, nicotine, or phosphate ester insecticides. Dilated pupils can be caused by atropine and related drugs, cocaine, nicotine, solvents, and depressants. Contracted pupils can be due to morphine and related drugs, physostigmine and related drugs, or phosphate ester insecticides.

Indicators of toxicity problems related to the *ears* include tinnitus, deafness, or disturbances of equilibrium, any of which may be caused by compounds such as quinine or salicylates.

Examples of diagnostic features associated with the *mouth* include loosening of teeth and painful teeth due to heavy metal poisoning, dry mouth associated with atropine and related drugs, and excessive salivation due to poisoning by phosphate ester insecticides and heavy metals.

Symptoms related to the *cardiorespiratory system* are respiratory difficulty, including dyspnea on exertion; chest pain; and decreased vital capacity caused by a wide variety of toxicants, including salicylates, cyanide, CO, atropine, strychnine, and ethanol. Rapid respiration may be due to cyanide, atropine, cocaine, CO, salicylates, alcohol, or amphetamines. Slow respiration, however, may be due to such chemicals as barbiturates, morphine, or antihistamines and, paradoxically, may also be caused by cyanide, CO, and so on.

Although symptoms related to the *gastrointestinal* (GI) *system* may be valuable in diagnosis, some, such as vomiting, diarrhea, and abdominal pain, may be caused by almost any poison. A less common symptom, blood in the stool, may be caused by coumarin anticoagulants, thallium, iron, salicylates, and a number of corrosive materials.

Dysfunctions of the *urinary system* include anuria, the inability to excrete urine, which may result from poisoning with mercurials, carbon tetrachloride, formaldehyde, turpentine, oxalic acid, chlordane, castor beans, and many other compounds; proteinuria, the appearance of protein in the urine, may result from arsenic, mercury, or phosphorus poisoning, for example. Hematuria, hemoglobinuria, or myoglobinuria, the appearance of blood, hemoglobin, or myoglobin, respec-

TABLE 14.2. SUMMARY OF LABORATORY TESTS PERFORMED DURING SYSTEMIC EXAMINATION OF POISON VICTIMS

Test Type	Symptom	Example of Possible Causes
Blood, gross and microscopic	Leukopenia, agranulocytosis	Aminopyrine, phenylbutazone
	Anemia	Lead, naphthalene, chlorates, solanine, other plant poisons
	Cherry-red color	CO, cyanide
	Chocoloate color (methemoglobin)	Nitrates, nitrites, aniline dyes, chlorates
Blood, serum or plasma chemistry	Glucose (whole blood)	Increased after thiazide diuretics or or adrenal glucocorticoids; decreased after salicylates, lead, ethanol
	Uric acid (serum)	Increased after thiazide diuretics or ethanol
	Potassium (serum/plasma)	Increased after thiazide diuretics or ethanol
	Bromide	Serum chloride spuriously increased in bromism because standard tests measure total halides

Special chemical examinations: Analysis of lead or other heavy metals, insecticides, cholinesterase, barbiturates, alkaloids, etc., may be necessary in diagnosis of poisoning.
Source: Dreisback RH: Handbook of Poisoning, *11th ed. Los Altos, CA: Lange Medical, 1983.*

tively, in the urine, may also be indicative of particular poisons and, in some of these cases, the color of the urine may also be a useful indicator.

Effects on the *neuromuscular system* may often be difficult to distinguish from effects on the CNS, particularly muscular weakness or paralysis, which may be due to lead, arsenic, organic mercurials, thallium, triorthocresyl phosphate, carbon disulfide, and other compounds. Tremors, muscle stiffness, and muscle cramps may also be useful diagnostic indicators.

The laboratory examination is a critical part of the diagnostic process and deals primarily with the blood or other body fluids. A brief summary of the appropriate tests is shown in Table 14.2.

14.3

NONSPECIFIC THERAPY

Nonspecific therapy may be defined as therapy designed to maintain vital signs, decrease uptake, and increase elimination of the toxicant but which, at the same time, is not related directly to the specific mode of action of the toxicant.

14.3.1   First Aid and Emergency Management

Untrained people should rarely find it necessary to render first aid, but should never do so if the victim is either unconscious or is having convulsions. In any case of poisoning or suspected poisoning, professional help (the nearest poison control center, hospital emergency room, or emergency rescue squad) should be contacted immediately. With conscious patients, vomiting will then probably be induced, preferably with syrup of ipecac. This is never done, however, in cases of ingestion of acids, bases, or any petroleum product. In cases of inhaled toxicants, the victim is moved to fresh air. In cases of poisoning by dermal contamination, the skin is drenched with water; the clothing is removed from the affected area, after which the affected area is washed with soap and water. With eye contamination, the eye is washed with a gentle stream of water at a fountain or under a faucet.

In any poisoning case in which the patient's breathing is depressed, artificial respiration is given, preferably by direct inflation. If available, oxygen may be given. Chemical antidotes should not be given. In the case of an overdose of an injected drug, either prescription or drug of abuse, a tourniquet may be applied at the proximal side of the injection site.

In all poisoning cases, the patient should be kept warm, and either a physician should be brought to the site or transport of the patient to a treatment facility should be arranged. Because identification of the poison may be critical, anyone rendering first aid should be sure that the poison (in a properly sealed container) or vomited material is sent to the treatment facility with the patient. Any information as to what the victim was doing at the time of the poisoning, which chemicals are in use at the site, the physical characteristics and trade names of bulk chemicals at the site, and so on, should all be communicated to the treating physician.

14.3.2   Life Support

Further emergency treatment may be carried out at the treatment center and includes the following measures.

MAINTENANCE OF RESPIRATION AND CIRCULATION. Maintenance of respiration involves maintaning an adequate airway, if necessary by catheter, tracheostomy, or cricothyroid puncture, and also maintaining adequate pulmonary ventilation. This last may be by direct mouth-to-mouth inflation or by a portable resuscitator. Oxygen can be administered if available.

Circulatory failure is usually the result of shock; in this case, emergency therapy appropriate to shock is initiated immediately. The patient is placed in a supine position with lower limbs elevated, body warmth is maintained by blankets, an adequate airway is assured, and adequate circulating blood volume is restored and maintained. If the fall in blood pressure is severe, appropriate drug therapy is initiated along with plasma transfusion.

EMESIS. Emesis is best accomplished with syrup of ipecac but never after poisoning with corrosives (acids or bases) or petroleum derivatives. In the former case, the esophagus is subjected to further corrosive attack; in the latter, the risk of aspirating stomach contents into the airways is unacceptably high.

GASTRIC LAVAGE. In gastric lavage, special precautions are taken in the case of corrosives becuse the lavage tube may damage the esophagus or, in the case of petroleum derivatives, when the trachea should be intubated with a tube with an inflatable cuff. In convulsing patients, the convulsions should first be controlled. Materials used for gastric lavage include milk (for corrosives or to retard uptake), lemon juice (for alkali poisoning), activated charcoal suspension, saline, sodium bicarbonate, or milk of magnesia. Sodium bicarbonate is never given in the case of poisoning by acids, because the carbon dioxide (CO_2) generated may damage the stomach.

GASTROTOMY. Gastrotomy may be necessary if large quantities of solid matter (eg, tablets, capsules) are present that cannot be removed by lavage.

CATHARSIS OR INTESTINAL LAVAGE. Catharsis or intestinal lavage is not used in poisoning with corrosives, if electrolyte balance is disturbed, or if there is renal impairment.

14.3.3   Nonspecific Maintenance Therapy

Nonspecific maintenance therapy is largely a continuation of the procedures outlined above and is designed to maintain vital signs on a long-term basis. One should bear in mind that during this phase of the treatment good nutrition is important. This can be done intravenously (IV) or by stomach tube if necessary, but per os is preferable. In general, energy metabolism is most important, and excess fat and protein is avoided to reduce stress on the liver and kidneys. Pain can also contribute to functional difficulties, particularly in the case of shock. The treating physician may elect to relieve pain with meperidine (Demerol) because morphine is often counterindicated. This is particularly true in the case of CNS depression, respiratory difficulties, or liver involvement.

MAINTENANCE OF WATER AND ELECTROLYTE BALANCE. The means by which water and electrolytes are replaced are usually not critical in the absence of kidney impairment; however, they may become critical if renal function is impaired. Electrolytes and/or water are lost in urine, feces, expired air, sweat, and vomiting, and must be replaced either orally or IV. Simple calculations that indicate the necessary amount can be made based on body weight and serum ion analysis. Glucose may also be given to provide an energy source.

Acidosis may be due to the generation of an acidic metabolite such as formic acid from methanol, by loss of base, or by CO_2 retention. These problems are usually addressed by maintaining an adequate airway and giving artificial respiration to prevent CO_2 retention or by giving sodium bicarbonate either IV or orally.

MAINTENANCE OF NORMAL BODY TEMPERATURE. Neither hyperthermia nor hypothermia is desirable in the poisoned patient. The former increases metabolic rate and, hence, the O_2 requirement as well as the requirements for food and water. The latter, although reducing the metabolic rate, also reduces the rate of detoxication and the elimination of both the toxicant and its metabolites.

Because of the additional involvement of the detoxication system that would be entailed, chemical intervention in the case of hyperthermia is not recommended. The use of wet towels, cooling blankets, and air circulation is more appropriate. Similarly, in the case of hypothermia, total or partial immersion in warm water is recommended. Local heating is not appropriate because of the effect on skin capillaries.

CNS INVOLVEMENT. Toxic chemicals can cause convulsions by a number of mechanisms such as stimulation of peripheral receptors that affect the CNS by causing O_2 lack (hypoxia) or by inducing hypoglycemia. Because convulsions can be life threatening due to effects such as respiratory failure caused by spasms of the respiratory muscles or to postconvulsion depression, the treating physician will usually take emergency measures. Such measures may include artificial respiration in the postconvulsion period and restraint to prevent injury. The patient is kept in quiet surroundings and neither emesis nor gastric lavage is attempted unless failure to do so might cause death. Anticonvulsant drugs can be used but none which might cause either coma or respiratory depression. Fluid balance is maintained, an adequate airway is assured, and glucose is given to treat hypoglycemia.

Coma caused by poisons generally results from effects on brain cell function. Emergency measures include maintaining an adequate airway, aspirating mucus from the nose and mouth, giving artificial respiration, treating for shock, and giving gastric lavage with activated charcoal. These treatments are continued; attention is given to fluid balance, renal function and, eventually, if the coma persists, to tube feeding and to dialysis to eliminate the toxicant.

Hyperactivity and delirium occur with certain toxicants. Treatment is in part psychological and is designed to reduce tension. Hydrotherapy may be used for the same reason and, if absolutely necessary, drugs such as paraldehyde or scopolamine may be administered.

Hypoglycemic convulsions and coma are treated by administration of glucose, using the most appropriate route.

RESPIRATORY INVOLVEMENT. Many poisons affect respiration, either directly or indirectly. The effects include hypoxia, respiratory depression, and pulmonary edema. Several principles are involved in all respiratory problems, including maintaining an adequate airway, adequate pulmonary ventilation, and an adequate O_2 supply. Adequate airway is maintained either by the oropharyngeal method using a metal or plastic airway, or the tracheal method using a catheter, tracheostomy, or cricopharyngeal puncture (an opening in the cricopharyngeal cartilage), a procedure that can be done by a physician when other methods are not immediately possible. Adequate pulmonary ventilation can be assured by artificial respiration or a respirator, whereas O_2 can be administered directly. Pulmonary edema is first treated with morphine sulfate, oxygen, and aminophylline. Subsequently, diuretics and corticoid anti-inflammatory agents may be prescribed.

CIRCULATORY SYSTEM INVOLVEMENT. The treatment of one of the most common involvements, shock, has been mentioned. Congestive heart failure may result from poisons that cause myocardial damage. This is treated with rest, sodium restriction and, in serious cases, digitalis. Cardiac arrest may result from asphyxiation, CO, and so on. Emergency treatment consists of chest massage and artificial respiration. Subsequently, 0.9% saline is given IV, and epinephrine is injected and/or defibrillation is attempted. In short, all of the techniques available to the physician for the treatment of cardiac arrest, whatever the cause, may be attempted.

URINARY TRACT INVOLVEMENT. The principle problems in urinary tract involvement are renal failure and fluid retention. The former is treated by methods designed to restrict fluid retention until function can be restored. They include fluid restriction and oral administration of salts. If recovery does not occur within a few days or if blood creatine rises, dialysis should be carried out. Urine retention can be treated by catheterization.

INVOLVEMENT OF THE GI TRACT. Involvement of the GI tract can include vomiting, diarrhea, and distension of the abdomen. Although the first is often initially beneficial, vomiting eventually causes a loss of fluid balance. It can be treated by glucose administered IV in saline until vomiting stops, followed by dry foods in small quantity, followed by fluids. If drugs such as chlorpromazine or promethazine are not contraindicated by the nature of the poison or by other medical considerations, the treating physician may prescribe them to be given orally or in suppositories.

Similarly, diarrhea may affect fluid balance, which must also be corrected by IV glucose while food intake is restricted to liquids or low-residue foods. Drugs used include codeine or atropine; pectin kaolin mixtures may also be effective.

Distension of the abdomen is usually due to gas; it can be released by proper use of a rectal or colonic tube or intestinal intubation.

HEPATIC INVOLVEMENT. Liver damage can be acute, as is often the case with chloroform, carbon tetrachloride, and so on; or chronic, as may occur with ethanol. Characteristically, liver enzymes are found at elevated levels in the serum—for example, glutamic–oxalacetic transaminase, glutamic–pyruvic transaminase, lactic dehydrogenase, and alkaline phosphatase. In addition, the blood–bilirubin level is increased and bilirubin is also found in the urine. Urine urobilinogen is also increased. Usually, all drugs are discontinued and the patient is maintained under conditions of complete bed rest. Other symptoms such as vomiting are controlled; the diet, when eating can be resumed, is one with low protein, low fat, and high carbohydrate content.

BLOOD SYSTEM INVOLVEMENT. Methemoglobin formation is brought about by the oxidation of ferrous (Fe^{2+}) hemoglobin to ferric (Fe^{3+}) hemoglobin, usually as a result of such toxicants as nitrites, chlorates, and so on. The reaction can be reversed by methylene blue. On an emergency basis, O_2 is also administered. Hemolytic reactions may occur, particularly in persons with glucose-6-phosphate dehydrogenase deficiency. Urine flow must be maintained; if renal failure is imminent (high serum hemoglobin), an exchange transfusion may be necessary.

14.4

SPECIFIC THERAPY

When the toxicant can be identified with certainty, a specific antidote or combination of antidotes may be available. Such therapies, when available, are often rapid and reliable. Unfortunately, for many toxicants specific antidotes are not known; in many poisoning cases, it is not clear precisely which toxicant is involved or whether a mixture of toxicants is involved. Finally, even with known toxicants for which a specific antidote is available, the damage may have reached a point at which the antidote is no longer effective.

Specific therapy may be based on activation and detoxication reactions, mode of action, or elimination of the toxicant. Examples of the types of specific therapy are presented in Table 14.3. The examples in the following sections are chosen to illustrate the principles involved. In some cases, several antidotes, with different modes of action, are available for the same toxicant; this is also illustrated by the specific examples described later. The structures of the toxicants and antidotes used as examples in this section are shown in Fig. 14.1.

TABLE 14.3. EXAMPLES OF THERAPY RELATED TO MODE OF ACTION OF SPECIFIC TOXICANTS

Mechanism	Poison	Therapeutic Agent
Metabolism of toxicant		
Competition for activation reaction	Methanol	Ethanol
Stimulation of detoxication mechanism	Cyanide	Thiosulfate
Direct effect of toxicant		
Complexing agents	Lead	CaEDTA
Effects on receptor site		
Competition for receptor	CO	Oxygen
Receptor blocking	Carbaryl	Atropine
Repair mechanism		
Reversal of toxic effect	Parathion	2-PAM
	Nitrite	Methylene blue
Bypass of toxic effect	Methotrexate	Thymidine, adenine and glycine
Facilitation of excretion		
Administration of similar molecules	Bromide	Chloride

2-PAM, N-methypiridinium (2-pyridine-aldoxime methiodide).

14.4.1 Methanol

Methanol is a common cause of poisoning and results in a number of deaths annually. The acute effects appear to be due to the formation of formaldehyde by the action of alcohol dehydrogenase and subsequently formic acid by the action of aldehyde oxidase. Formaldehyde has been shown to affect the retina and is probably the cause of the blindness associated with methanol poisoning, whereas formic acid causes the acute acidosis associated with this toxicant. (See also Section 10.7.3 and Table 10.10.)

Various nonspecific treatments include induction of vomiting with syrup of ipecac and the use of gastric lavage; acidosis is countered by administration of sodium bicarbonate, and urine flow is maintained by oral or IV fluids. If the patient fails to respond to specific or nonspecific therapy, dialysis is performed.

The specific therapy for methanol poisoning is the administration of ethanol, initially orally and subsequently IV. The ethanol acts by competition for alcohol-metabolizing enzymes, thus permitting the excretion of methanol before it is activated to formaldehyde and formic acid. The toxicity of the acetaldehyde and acetic acid formed from ethanol is low as compared with that of formaldehyde and formic acid.

14.4.2 Cyanide

Hydrogen cyanide and its salts have a variety of uses, and cyanide ion may be released metabolically from a number of secondary plant chemicals. It acts primarily by inhibiting cytochrome oxidase, thus blocking cellular respiration (see Section 7.3.1 and Fig. 7.2). Other enzymes are also inhibited by cyanide, but the effects are

Toxicant	Antidote	
CH₃OH Methanol	C₂H₅OH Ethanol	
NaCN Sodium cyanide	NaNO₂ Sodium nitrite	Na₂S₂O₃ Sodium thiosulfate
Lead Mercury Arsenic		

$Toxicant$ column:
- CH₃OH — Methanol
- NaCN — Sodium cyanide
- Lead, Mercury, Arsenic
- CO — Carbon monoxide
- Parathion $(C_2H_5O)_2PO-\bigcirc-NO_2$
- Carbaryl
- Br⁻ — Bromide ion

Antidote column:
- C₂H₅OH — Ethanol
- NaNO₂ — Sodium nitrite; Na₂S₂O₃ — Sodium thiosulfate
- SH SH / CH₂CHCH₂OH — Dimercaprol (BAL); SH / (CH₃)₂CCH(NH₂)COOH — Penicillamine; (HOOCCH₂)₂NCH₂CH₂N(CH₂COOH)₂ — Ethylenediaminetetraacetic acid (EDTA)
- O₂ — Oxygen
- Atropine; 2-Pyridine-aldoxime methiodide (2-PAM)
- Atropine
- Cl⁺ — Chloride ion

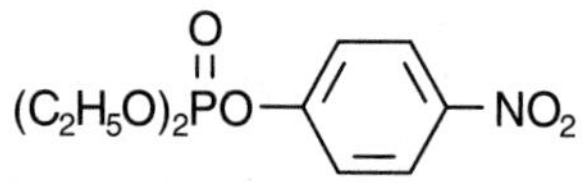

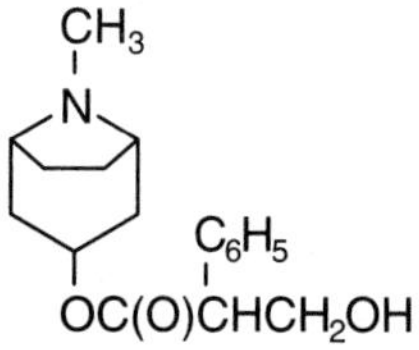

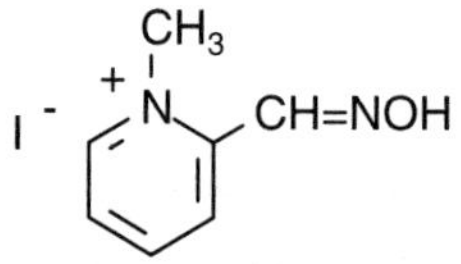

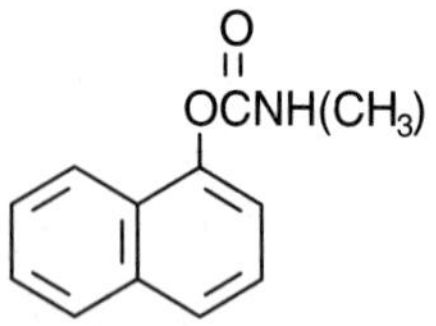

Figure 14.1. Toxicants and antidotes used in examples of specific therapy.

relatively unimportant as compared with those caused by the rapid, extensive, and high-affinity binding to cytochrome oxidase. Although the toxic dose is very small and the resultant poisoning is rapid and often fatal, chronic poisoning due to prolonged exposure to very small amounts is known.

Emergency measures for either inhaled or ingested cyanide include amyl nitrite, artificial respiration, and 100% O_2. In the case of ingestion, gastric lavage may also be used.

There are two forms of specific therapy. Sodium nitrite is administered to convert hemoglobin to methemoglobin. The latter then combines with cyanide to form cyanomethemoglobin. Although the affinity of cyanide for methemoglobin is less than its affinity for cytochrome oxidase, the large amount of hemoglobin available makes this a useful therapy. Methemoglobinemia itself is hazardous, however, and the nitrite dose must be calculated so as to cause no more than 25% to 40% conversion of hemoglobin. In the second form of specific therapy, thiosulfate is administered to provide a sulfur donor for the reaction, catalyzed by the enzyme cyanide–thiosulfate sulfur transferase, which converts cyanide to thiocyanate (CN^- to SCN^-). Thus, the two specific therapies represent one case in which there is removal from the site of action by competition with another binding site, and one in which a detoxication mechanism is stimulated by providing a reactant that is normally rate-limiting in vivo. When these two specific antidotes are assessed in an experimental setting (eg, by their effect on the LD50 for cyanide) they are clearly synergistic, being much more than additive in their effect.

14.4.3   Lead and Mercury

Although chronic lead poisoning is thought of as the most common and dangerous form, particularly among children, acute lead poisoning is also a hazard. In acute lead poisoning, the unabsorbed lead compound must be removed either by gastric lavage with dilute magnesium or sodium sulfate solution or by emesis. Subsequently, urine flow must be maintained, and chelation therapy must be started. Dimercaprol and CaEDTA both function by chelating the lead and rendering it excretable. These two drugs are given by injection; subsequently, penicillamine can be given orally. The treatment is monitored by following blood and urine lead concentrations.

Inorganic mercury, particularly in the form of mercuric salts, can be acutely toxic or can give rise to chronic toxicity. In acute poisoning, gastric lavage or emesis is used to remove unabsorbed material. Subsequently, dimercaprol is used to complex the mercury and render it excretable. Dialysis can be used to speed elimination if necessary. Dimercaprol is also used to treat chronic mercury poisoning.

Organic compounds of heavy metals, such as tetraethyl lead and methyl mercury, can also cause serious poisoning. They differ from the inorganic ions in uptake, toxicokinetics, mode of action, and therapy and should be treated separately. (See also Section 10.6 for a discussion of toxic effects of lead, mercury, and other metals.)

14.4.4   Carbon Monoxide

CO is a common cause of poisoning, both deliberate, as in suicide attempts, and accidental. CO is produced by the incomplete combustion of fossil fuels, in automobiles, in industrial machinery, in home furnaces, and so on, and exerts its toxic effects by binding reversibly, but with high affinity, to hemoglobin. It not only forms carboxyhemoglobin, thus occupying sites normally occupied by O_2, but also increases the affinity of unbound sites for O_2, thus impairing the release of O_2 to the tissues. Because the affinity of CO is 250 times that of O_2, it is imperative to remove the victim from the source of CO. The patient is kept at rest to reduce O_2 demand. The specific therapy involves competition for the receptor, hemoglobin, by the physiological ligand, O_2. Respiration is maintained artificially, and either O_2 or, preferably, a mixture of 95% O_2 and 5% CO_2 is administered. Because the affinity of CO is high, the use of high O_2 concentration is critical.

Although not often available, the use of a compression chamber at about 2 atmospheres is extremely helpful. Not only is more O_2 available to compete for hemoglobin, but the increased solubility also allows some transport by the plasma.

14.4.5   Organophosphorus Cholinesterase Inhibitors

Organophosphorus (OP) cholinesterase inhibitors are compounds that exert their toxic effects by phosphorylating cholinesterase, thus bringing about its inhibition and preventing the breakdown of acetylcholine, giving rise to a situation in which the acetylcholine receptors remain occupied (see Section 7.2.1 and Fig. 7.1). Because death is the result of respiratory failure, the maintenance of an adequate airway and artificial respiration are of critical importance. Two forms of specific therapy are available. Atropine is used immediately because it competes with acetylcholine for the receptor site, thus preventing the toxic effects of an excess of this neurotransmitter. Subsequently, N-methylpyridinium 2-aldoxime (2-PAM) is used in conjunction with atropine because it reacts with the phosphorylated cholinesterase and removes the phosphorylating group, thus restoring the enzyme to normal activity. One should bear in mind that the use of two antidotes with different modes of action can be synergistic. In this case, the combination of 2-PAM and atropine can be 50 times as effective as might be expected from a simple additive effect.

14.4.6   Carbamate Cholinesterase Inhibitors

Although the overall mode of action is the same as that of OP compounds as noted in the previous section, the carbamylated cholinesterase is less stable than the phosphorylated enzyme, and its regeneration cannot be accelerated by 2-PAM. Thus, although the nonspecific therapy is the same, only atropine is used as a specific antidote, 2-PAM being without effect.

14.4.7   Bromide

Bromide ion is toxic, and its excretion can be stimulated by administering excess chloride. Excess chloride is normally excreted by the kidney, and the active transport mechanism cannot distinguish between the two ions. This is not a particularly rapid method, but fortunately bromide ion is neither particularly toxic nor particularly fast acting.

14.5

CHRONIC TOXICITY

Chronic toxicity caused by chemicals frequently is not reversible, nor is it susceptible to specific antidotes. Cancer, for example, requires surgical intervention or the use of relatively nonspecific cellular poisons or radiation therapy. Certain forms of chronic toxicity involving the accumulation of chemicals that are not readily eliminated may be alleviated by therapy designed to facilitate excretion of the toxicant.

Treatment of neoplastic diseases depends on total destruction of the tumor cell type: if by surgery, all of the tumor must be removed; if by chemotherapy, all of the tumor cells must be killed, unlike in bacterial and viral diseases, in which a significant reduction in the causative organism permits the immune system to reassert its normal function. Thus, surgery alone is successful only when the tumor is discrete and readily removed in toto. Most chemotherapeutic drugs are cytotoxic but have been shown to affect tumor cells somewhat more readily than other cells. Toxic side effects are common, and the toxic dose is often close to the therapeutic one. Only the great benefit involved (ie, saving life) justifies the risk. These chemotherapeutic agents include alkylating agents such as cyclophosphamide and antimetabolites such as methotrexate, as well as alkaloids, antibiotics, enzymes, and metal coordination complexes (ie, vincristine, asparaginase, and cisplatin, respectively). All appear to act at one or more points in the nucleic acid replication/protein synthesis cycles.

The use of chelation therapy as described for acute lead poisoning can also be used to facilitate excretion of accumulated lead in chronic lead poisoning. A dramatic example of the treatment of chronic toxicity by the facilitation of excretion is that developed for kepone (chlordecone) poisoning. Although the compound is readily excreted through the bile, it is reabsorbed from the intestine (enterohepatic circulation). Feeding cholestyramine, an ion-exchange resin that can bind kepone, interrupts the cycle and permits the excretion of kepone at a rate some sevenfold higher than in the untreated patient.

Suggested Further Reading

Dreisbach RH: *Handbook of Poisoning,* 11th ed. Los Altos, CA: Lange Medical, 1983.
Ellenhorn MJ, Barceloux DG: *Medical Toxicology: Diagnosis and Treatment of Human Poisoning.* New York: Elsevier Science Publishing Co., 1988.

Goldsten A, Aronow L, Kalman SM: *Principles of Drug Action: The Basis of Pharmacology.* New York: Wiley, 1974. (See Chapter 5, Drug toxicity.)

Guzelian PS: Chlordecone poisoning: a case study in approaches for detoxification of humans exposed to environmental chemicals. *Drug Metab Rev* **13:**663–679, 1982.

Haddad LM, Winchester JF: *Clinical Management of Poisoning and Drug Overdose.* Philadelphia: WB Saunders, 1983.

Loomis TA, Hayes AW: *Essentials of Toxicology,* 4th ed. San Diego, CA: Academic Press, 1996 (See Chapter 11, The basis of antidotal therapy, and Chapter 14, Clinical toxicology.)

Snodgrass WR: Clinical toxicology. In *Casarett & Doull's Toxicology: The Basic Science of Poisons,* 5th ed. Klaassen CD (ed.). New York: McGraw Hill, 1996, pp 969–987.

BASICS OF ENVIRONMENTAL TOXICOLOGY

15

GERALD A. LEBLANC

15.1

INTRODUCTION

Industrial endeavors are intimately associated with the extensive use of a wide array of chemicals. Similarly, pesticides and other agricultural chemicals have revolutionized farm and forest productivity. Historically, chemical wastes generated through industrial processes were disposed of through flagrant release into the environment. Gasses quickly dispersed into the atmosphere, and liquids were diluted into receiving waters, where they were transported efficiently away from the site of generation. Potential adverse effects of the application of such chemicals to the environment were viewed as insignificant relative to the benefits bestowed by such practices. Then in 1962, a science writer for the US Fish and Wildlife Service, Rachel Carson, published a book that began by describing a world devoid of birds and from that the title *Silent Spring* was inspired. In her book, Ms. Carson described graphically incidents of massive fish and bird kills resulting from insecticide use in areas ranging from national forests to residential areas. Furthermore, she implied that such pollutant effects on wildlife may be heralding similar incipient effects on human health.

The resulting awakening of the general public to the hazards of chemicals in the environment spurred several landmark activities related to environmental protection, including Earth Day, organization of the US Environmental Protection Agency (EPA), and the enactment of several pieces of legislation aimed at regulating and limiting the release of chemicals into the environment. Appropriate regulation of the release of chemicals into the environment without applying unnecessarily stringent limitations on industry and agriculture requires a comprehensive understanding of the toxicological properties and consequences of release of the chemicals into the environment. It was from this need that modern environmental toxicology evolved.

Environmental toxicology is defined as *the study of the fate and effects of chemicals in the environment.* Although this definition would encompass toxic chemicals found naturally in the environment (ie, animal venoms, microbial and plant toxins), environmental toxicology typically is associated with the study of environmental chemicals of anthropogenic origin. Environmental toxicology can be divided into two subcategories: environmental health toxicology and ecotoxicology. Environmental health toxicology is *the study of the adverse effects of environmental chemicals on human health,* whereas ecotoxicology focuses on *the effects of environmental contaminants on ecosystems and constituents thereof* (eg, fish, wildlife). Assessing the toxic effects of chemicals on humans involves the use of standard animal models (ie, mice, rats) as well as epidemiologic evaluations of exposed human populations (eg, farmers, factory workers). In contrast, ecotoxicology involves the study of the adverse effects of toxicants on a myriad of organisms that compose ecosystems, ranging from microorganisms to top predators. Furthermore, comprehensive insight into the effects of chemicals in the environment requires assessments ancillary to toxicology, such as the fate of the chemical in the environment (Chapter 16) and toxicant interactions with abiotic (nonliving) components of ecosystems. Comprehensive assessments of the adverse effects of environmental chemicals thus utilize expertise from many scientific disciplines, with the ultimate goal of elucidating the adverse effects of chemicals that are present in the environment (retrospective hazard assessment) and predicting any adverse effects of chemicals before they are discharged into the environment (prospective hazard assessment). The ecological hazard assessment process is discussed in Chapter 17.

Historically, chemicals that have posed major environmental hazards tend to share three insidious characteristics: environmental persistence, bioaccumulation (the propensity to accumulate in living things), and high toxicity.

15.2

ENVIRONMENTAL PERSISTENCE

Many abiotic and biotic processes exist in nature that function in concert to eliminate (ie, degrade) toxic chemicals. Accordingly, many chemicals released into the environment pose minimal hazard simply because of their limited life span in the environment. Chemicals that have historically posed environmental hazard (eg, DDT, PCBs, TCDD) resist degradative processes and accordingly persist in the environment for extremely long periods of time (Table 15.1). Continued disposal of persistent chemicals into the environment can result in their accumulation to environmental levels sufficient to pose toxicity. Such chemicals can continue to pose a hazard long after their disposal into the environment has ceased. For example, significant contamination of Lake Ontario by the pesticide mirex occurred from the 1950s through the 1970s. Mass balance studies performed in the 1990s revealed that 80% of the mirex deposited into the lake persisted. One decade following the conta-

TABLE 15.1. ENVIRONMENTAL HALF-LIFE OF SOME CHEMICAL CONTAMINANTS

Contaminant	Half-life	Media
DDT	10 years	Soil
TCDD	9 years	Soil
Atrazine	25 months	Water (pH 7.0)
Benzoperylene (PAH)	14 months	Soil
Phenanthrene (PAH)	138 days	Soil
Carbofuran	45 days	Water (pH 7.0)

mination in 1980 of Lake Apopka, Florida, with pesticides including DDT and dicofol, populations of alligators continued to experience severe reproductive impairment. Both biotic and abiotic processes contribute to the degradation of chemicals.

15.2.1   Abiotic Degradation

A plethora of environmental forces compromise the structural integrity of chemicals in the environment. Many prominent abiotic degradative processes occur due to the influences of light (photolysis) and water (hydrolysis).

PHOTOLYSIS. Light, primarily in the ultraviolet (UV) range, has the potential to break chemical bonds and thus can contribute significantly to the degradation of some chemicals. Photolysis is most likely to occur in the atmosphere or in surface waters, where light intensity is greatest. Photolysis is dependent on both the intensity of the light and the capacity of the pollutant molecules to absorb the light. Unsaturated aromatic compounds such as the polycyclic aromatic hydrocarbons tend to be highly susceptible to photolysis due to their high capacity to absorb light energy. Light energy can also facilitate the oxygenation of environmental contaminants via hydrolytic or oxidative processes. The photooxidation of the organophosphorus (OP) pesticide parathion is depicted in Fig. 15.1.

HYDROLYSIS. Water, often in combination with light energy or heat, can break chemical bonds. Hydrolytic reactions commonly result in the insertion of an oxygen atom into the molecule with the commensurate loss of some component of the molecule. Ester bonds, such as those found in (OP) pesticides (eg, parathion, Fig. 15.1), are highly susceptible to hydrolysis, which dramatically lowers the environmental half-lives of these chemicals. Hydrolytic rates of chemicals are influenced by the temperature and pH of the aqueous media. Rates of hydrolysis increase with increasing temperature and with extremes in pH.

15.2.2   Biotic Degradation

Although many environmental contaminants are susceptible to abiotic degradative processes, such processes often occur at extremely slow rates. Environmental degradation of chemical contaminants can occur at greatly accelerated rates through the action of microorganisms. Microorganisms (primarily bacteria and fungi) de-

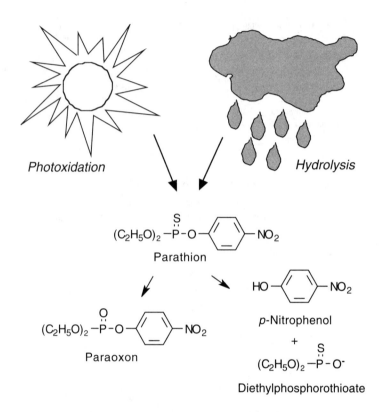

Figure 15.1. The effect of sunlight (photooxidation) and precipitation (hydrolysis) on the degradation of parathion.

grade chemicals in an effort to derive energy from these sources. These biotic degradative processes are enzyme-mediated, and thus typically occur at rates that far exceed abiotic degradation. Biotic degradative processes can lead to complete mineralization of chemicals to water, carbon dioxide (CO_2), and basic inorganic constituents. Biotic degradation includes those processes associated with abiotic degradation (ie, hydrolysis, oxidation, photolysis) and processes such as the removal of chlorine atoms (dehalogenation), the scission of ringed structures (ring cleavage), and the removal of carbon chains (dealkylation).

15.2.3 Nondegradative Elimination Processes

Many processes are operative in the environment that contribute to the regional elimination of a contaminant by altering its distribution. Contaminants with sufficiently high vapor pressure can evaporate from contaminated terrestrial or aquatic compartments and be transferred through the atmosphere to new locations. Such processes of global distillation are considered largely responsible for the worldwide distribution of relatively volatile organochlorine pesticides such as lindane and hexachlorobenzene. Entrainment by wind and upper atmospheric currents of contaminant particles or dust onto which the contaminants are sorbed also contribute to contaminant redistribution. Sorption of contaminant to suspended solids in an aquatic environment with commensurate sedimentation can result with the removal of contaminants from the water column and its redistribution into bottom sediments. Sediment sorption of contaminants greatly reduces bioavailability because the propensity of a lipophilic chemical to partition from sediments to organisms is significantly less than its propensity to partition from water to organism. More highly water soluble contaminants can be removed and redistributed through runoff and soil percolation. For example, the herbicide atrazine is one of the most abundantly used pesticides in the United States. It is used to control broadleaf and weed grasses in both agriculture and landscaping. Atrazine is ubiquitous in surface waters due to its extensive use. A study of midwestern states revealed that atrazine was detectable in 92% of the reservoirs assayed. In addition, atrazine has the propensity to migrate into groundwater because of its relatively high water solubility and low predilection to sorb to soil particles. Indeed, field studies have shown that surface application of atrazine typically results in the contamination of the aquifer below the application site. A more detailed account of the fate of chemicals in the environment is presented in Chapter 16.

15.3

BIOACCUMULATION

Environmental persistence alone does not render a chemical problematic in the environment. If the chemical cannot enter the body of organisms, then it would pose no threat of toxicity (see Chapter 2). Once absorbed, the chemical must accumulate in the body to sufficient levels to elicit toxicity. Bioaccumulation is defined as *the process by which organisms accumulate chemicals both directly from the abiotic environment (ie, water, air, soil) and from dietary sources (trophic transfer).* Environmental chemicals are taken up by organisms largely by passive diffusion. Primary sites of uptake include membranes of the lungs, gills, and gastrointestinal (GI) tract. Although integument (skin) and associated structures (eg, scales, feathers, fur) provide a protective barrier against many environmental insults, significant dermal uptake of some chemicals can occur. Because the chemicals must traverse the lipid bilayer of membranes to enter the body, bioaccumulation potential of chemicals is positively correlated with their lipophilicity (lipid solubility) (Fig. 15.2).

The aquatic environment is the major site at which lipophilic chemicals traverse the barrier between the abiotic environment and the biota. This is because: (1) lakes, rivers, and oceans serve as sinks for these chemicals, and (2) aquatic organisms pass tremendous quantities of water across their respiratory membranes (ie, gills), allowing for the efficient extraction of the chemicals from the water. Aquatic

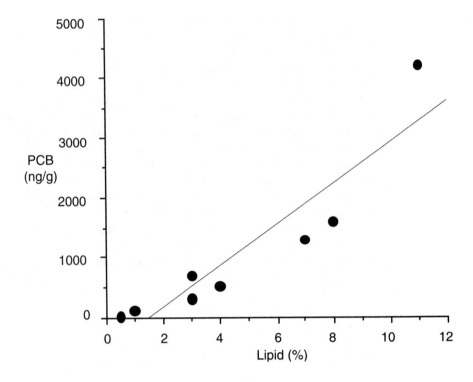

Figure 15.2. Relationship between lipid content of various organisms sampled from Lake Ontario and whole body PCB concentration. (*Data derived from Oliver BG, Niimi AJ:* Environ Sci Technol *22:388–397, 1988.*)

organisms can bioaccumulate lipophilic chemicals and attain body concentrations that are several orders of magnitude greater than the concentration of the chemical found in the environment (Table 15.2). The degree to which aquatic organisms accumulate xenobiotics from the environment is largely dependent upon the lipid content of the organism, since body lipids serve as the primary site of retention of the chemicals (Fig. 15.2).

TABLE 15.2. BIOACCUMULATION OF SOME ENVIRONMENTAL CONTAMINANTS BY FISH

Chemical	Bioaccumulation Factor[a]
DDT	127,000
TCDD	39,000
Endrin	6,800
Pentachlorobenzene	5,000
Leptophos	750
Trichlorobenzene	183

[a]Bioaccumulation factor is defined as the ratio of the chemical concentration in the fish and in the water at steady-state equilibrium.
Source: Data derived from: LeBlanc, GA. Trophic-level differences in the bioconcentration of chemicals: implications in assessing environmental biomagnification. Environ Sci Technol **28:**154–160, 1995.

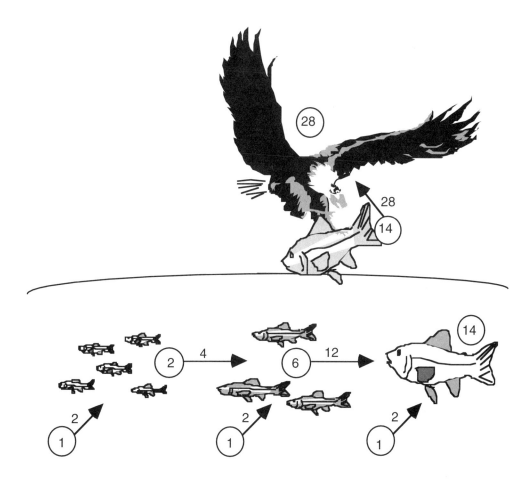

Figure 15.3. Bioaccumulation of a chemical along a generic food chain. In this simplistic paradigm, the amount of the chemical in the water is assigned an arbitrary concentration of 1 and it is assumed that the chemical will bioaccumulate either from the water to the fish or from one trophic level to another by a factor of 2. Circled numbers represent the concentration of chemical in the respective compartment. Numbers associated with arrows represent the concentration of chemical transferred from one compartment to another.

Chemicals can also be transferred along food chains from prey organism to predator (trophic transfer). For highly lipophilic chemicals, this transfer can result in increasing concentrations of the chemical with each progressive link in the food chain (biomagnification). As depicted in Fig. 15.3, a chemical that bioaccumulates by a factor of 2, regardless of whether the source of the contaminant is the water or food, would have the potential to magnify at each trophic level leading to high levels in the birds of prey relative to that found in the abiotic environment. The food chain transfer of DDT was responsible for the decline in many bird-eating raptor populations that contributed to the decision to ban the use of this pesticide in the United States.

Bioaccumulation can lead to a delayed onset of toxicity because the toxicant may initially be sequestered in lipid deposits, but is mobilized to target sites of toxicity when these lipid stores are utilized. For example, lipid stores are often mobilized in preparation for reproduction. The loss of the lipid can result in the release of lipophilic toxicants rendering them available for toxic action. Such effects can result in mortality of adult organisms as they approach reproductive maturity. Lipophilic chemicals can also be transferred to offspring in lipids associated with the yolk of oviparous organisms or the milk of mammals, resulting in toxicity to offspring that was not evident in the parental organisms.

15.3.1 Factors That Influence Bioaccumulation

The propensity for an environmental contaminant to bioaccumulate is influenced by several factors. The first consideration is environmental persistence. The degree to which a chemical bioaccumulates is dictated by the concentration present in the environment. Contaminants that are readily eliminated from the environment will generally not be available to bioaccumulate. An exception would be instances in which the contaminant is introduced continuously into the environment (eg, receiving water of an effluent discharge).

As discussed previously, lipophilicity is a major determinant of the bioaccumulation potential of a chemical. However, lipophilic chemicals also have greater propensity to sorb to sediments, thus rendering them less available to bioaccumulate. For example, sorption of benzo(*a*)pyrene to humic acids reduced its propensity to bioaccumulate in sunfish by a factor of 3. Fish from oligotrophic lakes, having low suspended solid levels, have been shown to accumulate more DDT than do fish from eutrophic lakes that have high suspended solid contents.

Once absorbed by the organism, the fate of the contaminant will influence its bioaccumulation. Chemicals that are readily biotransformed (Chapter 3) are rendered more water soluble and less lipid soluble. The biotransformed chemical is thus less likely to be sequestered in lipid compartments and more likely to be eliminated from the body. As depicted in Table 15.3, chemicals that are suscepti-

TABLE 15.3. MEASURED AND PREDICTED BIOACCUMULATION FACTORS OF CHEMICALS THAT DIFFER IN SUSCEPTIBILITY TO BIOTRANSFORMATION IN FISH [a]

Chemical	Susceptibility to Biotransformation	Bioaccumulation Factor	
		Predicted	*Measured*
Chlordane	Low	47,900	38,000
PCB	Low	36,300	42,600
Mirex	Low	21,900	18,200
Pentachlorophenol	High	4,900	780
Tris(2,3-dibromo-propyl)phosphate	High	4,570	3

[a] Predicted bioaccumulation factors were based on their relative lipophilicity as described by Mackay, D: Correlation of bioaccumulation factors. *Environ Sci Technol* **16**:274-278, 1982.

ble to biotransformation bioaccumulate much less than would be predicted based on lipophilicity. Conjugation of xenobiotics to glutathione and glucuronic acid (Chapter 3) can target the xenobiotic for biliary elimination through active transport processes, thus greatly increasing the rate of elimination (Chapter 5). Differences in chemical elimination rates contribute to species differences in bioaccumulation.

15.4

TOXICITY

15.4.1 Acute Toxicity

Acute toxicity is defined as *toxicity elicited as a result of short-term exposure to a toxicant.* Incidents of acute toxicity in the environment are commonly associated with accidents (eg, derailment of a train resulting in leakage of a chemical into a river) or the imprudent use of chemicals (eg, aerial drift of a pesticide to nontarget areas). Discharge limits placed on industrial and municipal wastes, when adhered to, have generally been successful in protecting against acute toxicity to organisms in waste-receiving areas. As discussed in Chapter 11, the acute toxicity of a chemical is commonly quantified as the LC50 or LD50. Although these measures do not provide any insight into the environmentally acceptable levels of contaminants (a concentration that kills 50% of the exposed organisms is hardly tolerable), LC50 and LD50 values do provide statistically sound and reproducible measures of the relative acute toxicity of chemicals. LC50 and LD50 ranges for aquatic and terrestrial wildlife, respectively, and their interpretations are presented in Table 15.4.

Acute toxicity of environmental chemicals is determined experimentally with select species that serve as representatives of particular levels of trophic organization within an ecosystem (ie, mammal, bird, fish, invertebrate, vascular plant, algae). For example, the EPA requires acute toxicity tests with representatives of at least eight different species of freshwater and marine organisms (16 tests) that include fish, invertebrates, and plants when establishing water quality criteria for a chemical. Attempts are often made to rank classes of organisms with respect to toxicant sensitivity; however, no organism is consistently more or less susceptible to

TABLE 15.4. RANKING SCHEME FOR ASSESSING THE ACUTE TOXICITY OF CHEMICALS TO FISH AND WILDLIFE

Fish LC50 (mg/L)	Avian/Mammalian LD50 (mg/kg)	Toxicity Rank	Example of Contaminant
>100	>5000	Relatively nontoxic	Barium
10–100	500–5000	Moderately toxic	Cadmium
1–10	50–500	Very toxic	1,4-Dichlorobenzene
<1	<50	Extremely toxic	Aldrin

the acute toxicity of chemicals. Furthermore, the use of standard species in toxicity assessment presumes that these species are "representative" of the sensitivity of other members of that level of ecological organization. Such presumptions, however, are often incorrect.

15.4.2   Mechanisms of Acute Toxicity

Environmental chemicals can elicit acute toxicity by many mechanisms. Following are example mechanisms that are particularly relevant to the types of chemicals that are more commonly responsible for acute toxicity in the environment at the present time.

CHOLINESTERASE INHIBITION. The inhibition of cholinesterase activity is characteristic of acute toxicity associated with OP and carbamate pesticides (see Chapter 7, Section 7.2.1 and Fig. 7.1 for more detail on cholinesterase inhibition). Typically, 40% to 80% inhibition of brain cholinesterase activity is reported in lethally poisoned fish. Acute toxicity resulting from cholinesterase inhibition is relatively common among fish and birds as a result of the high volume usage of OP and carbamate insecticides in applications such as lawn care, agriculture, and golf course maintenance. Cholinesterase inhibition in fish commonly occurs following heavy rains in aquatic habitats adjacent to areas treated with the pesticides and subject to runoff from these areas. Acute toxicity in birds commonly occurs in birds that feed in areas that have recently had pesticides aplied to them.

NARCOSIS. A common means by which industrial chemicals elicit acute toxicity, particularly to aquatic organisms, is through narcosis. Narcosis occurs when a chemical accumulates, in a nonspecific manner, in cellular membranes and interfers with the normal function of the membranes. Typical narcosis responses are decreased activity, reduced reaction to external stimuli, and increased pigmentation (in fish). The effects are reversible, and an organism typically returns to normal activity once the chemical is removed from the organism's environment. Prolonged narcosis can result in death. Approximately 60% of industrial chemicals that enter the aquatic environment elicit acute toxicity through narcosis. Chemicals that elicit toxicity by means of narcosis typically do not elicit toxicity at specific target sites and are sufficiently lipophilic to accumulate in the lipid phase or the lipid–aqueous interface of membranes to sufficient levels to disrupt membrane function. Chemicals that induce narcosis include alcohols, ketones, benzenes, ethers, and aldehydes.

PHYSICAL EFFECTS. Perhaps most graphic among recent incidents of environmental acute toxicity are the physical effects of petroleum following oil spills. Slicks of oil on the surface of contaminated waters result in the coating of animals, such as birds and marine mammals, that frequent the air–water interface. Such a spill of unprecedented magnitude and consequence in the United States occurred on March 24, 1989, when the hull of the Exxon *Valdez* was ruptured on Bligh Reef in Prince William Sound, Alaska. Nearly 11 million gallons of crude oil spilled onto the nearshore waters, killing more wildlife than any prior oil spill in history. Thousands of sea birds and mammals succumbed to the acute effects of the oil.

Hypothermia is considered a major cause of death of oiled marine birds and mammals. These organisms insulate themselves from the frigid waters by maintaining a layer of air among the spaces within their coat of fur or feathers. The oil penetrates the fur/feather barrier and purges the insulating air. As a result, the animals rapidly succumb to hypothermia. In addition to hypothermia, these animals can also experience oil toxicosis. Inhalation of oil, as well as ingestion through feeding and preening, can result in the accumulation of hydrocarbons to toxic levels. Toxicity to sea otters has been correlated to degree of oiling and is characterized by pulmonary emphysema (bubbles of air within the connective tissue of the lungs), gastric hemorrhages, and liver damage.

15.4.3   Chronic Toxicity

Chronic toxicity is defined as *toxicity elicited as a result of long-term exposure to a toxicant.* Sublethal indices are generally associated with chronic toxicity. These include reproductive, immune, endocrine, and developmental dysfunction. However, chronic exposure also can result in direct mortality not observed during acute exposure. For example, chronic exposure of highly lipophilic chemicals can result in the eventual bioaccumulation of the chemical to concentrations that are lethal to the organisms. Alternatively, as discussed previously, mobilization of lipophilic toxicants from lipid compartments during reproduction may result in lethality. It is important to recognize that although theoretically all chemicals elicit acute toxicity at a sufficiently high dose, all chemicals are not chronically toxic. Chronic toxicity is measured by endpoints such as the highest level of the chemical that does not elicit toxicity during continuous, prolonged exposure (no observed effect level [NOEL]), the lowest level of the chemical that elicits toxicity during continuous, prolonged exposure (lowest observed effect level [LOEL]), or the chronic value (CV), which is the geometric mean of the NOEL and the LOEL. Chronic toxicity of a chemical is often judged by the acute:chronic ratio (ACR), which is calculated by dividing the acute LC50 value by the CV. Chemicals that have an ACR of less than 10 typically have low-to-no chronic toxicity associated with them (Table 15.5).

TABLE 15.5. ACUTE AND CHRONIC TOXICITY OF PESTICIDES MEASURED FROM LABORATORY EXPOSURES OF FISH SPECIES

Pesticide	LC50 (µg/L)	Acute Toxicity	Chronic Value (µg/L)	ACR	Chronic Toxicity
Endosulfan	166	Extremely toxic	4.3	39	Yes
Chlordecone	10	Extremely toxic	0.3	33	Yes
Malathion	3,000	Very toxic	340	8.8	No
Carbaryl	15,000	Moderately toxic	378	40	Yes

The following must always be considered when assessing the chronic toxicity of a chemical:

1. Simple numerical interpretations of chronic toxicity based on ACRs serve only as gross indicators of the potential chronic toxicity of the chemical. Laboratory exposure designed to establish chronic values most often focuses on a few general endpoints such as survival, growth, and reproductive capacity. Examination of more subtle endpoints of chronic toxicity may reveal significantly different chronic values.

2. Laboratory exposures are conducted with a few test species that are amenable to laboratory manipulation. The establishment of chronic and ACR values with these species should not be considered absolute. Toxicants may elicit chronic toxicity in some species and not in others.

3. Interactions among abiotic and biotic components of the environment may contribute to the chronic toxicity of chemicals; such interactions, however, may not occur in laboratory assessments of direct chemical toxicity.

These considerations are exemplified in the following incidents of chronic toxicity of chemicals in the environment.

15.4.4 Species–Specific Chronic Toxicity

TRIBUTYLTIN-INDUCED IMPOSEX IN NEOGASTROPODS. In the early 1970s, scientists noted that dogwhelks inhabiting the coast of England exhibited a hermaphroditic-like condition, whereby females possessed a penis in addition to normal female genitalia. Although hermaphrodism is a reproductive strategy utilized by some molluscan species, dogwhelks are dioecious. This pseudohermaphroditic condition, called imposex, has since been documented worldwide in more than 40 species of neogastropods. Imposex has been implicated in reduced fecundity of neogastropod populations, population declines, and local extinction of affected populations.

The observation that imposex occurred primarily in marinas suggested causality with some contaminant originating from such facilities. Field experiments demonstrated that neogastropods transferred from pristine sites to marinas often developed imposex. Laboratory studies eventually implicated tributyltin, a biocide used in marine paints, as the cause of imposex. Tributyltin is toxic to most marine species evaluated in the laboratory at low parts-per-billion (ppb) concentrations (Table 15.6). Exposure of neogastropods, however, to low parts-per-trillion (ppt) concentrations can cause imposex (Table 15.6). Thus, neogastropods are uniquely sensitive to the toxicity of tributyltin with effects produced that were not evident in standard laboratory toxicity characterizations.

15.4.5 Abiotic and Biotic Interactions

CHLOROFLUOROCARBONS-OZONE-UV-B RADIATION–AMPHIBIAN INTERACTIONS. The atmospheric release of chlorofluorocarbons (CFCs) has been implicated in the depletion of the Earth's stratospheric ozone layer, which serves as a filter against harmful UV radiation.

TABLE 15.6 TOXICITY OF TRIBUTYLTIN TO AQUATIC ORGANISMS

Species	Acute Toxicity (LC50, µg/L)	Chronic Toxicity (LOEL, µg/L)	Imposex (µg/L)
Daphnid	1.7	—	—
Polychaete worm	—	0.10	—
Copepod	1.0	0.023	—
Oyster	1.3	0.25	—
Dogwhelk	—	—	≤0.0010

Temporal increases in UV-B radiation have been documented and pose increasing risks of a variety of maladies to both plant and animal life.

Commensurate with the increase in UV-B radiation levels at the Earth's surface has been the decline in many amphibian populations. Multiple causes may be responsible for these declines, including loss of habitat, pollutants, and increased incidence of disease; however, recent studies suggest that increases in UV-B radiation may be a major contributor to the decline in some populations. Field surveys in the Cascade Mountains in Oregon revealed a high incidence of mortality among embryos of the Cascades frog and western toad. Incubation of eggs, deposited in the environment, in the laboratory along with the pond water in which the eggs were collected resulted in low mortality, suggesting that contaminants in the water were not directly responsible for the mortality. Experiments conducted to assess the role of ambient levels of UV-B radiation on embryo mortality demonstrated that the placement of UV-B filters over the embryos significantly increased viability of the embryos.

Several amphibian species were examined for photolyase activity. This enzyme is responsible for the repair of DNA damage caused by UV-B radiation. A greater than 80-fold difference in photolyase activity was observed among the species examined. Photolyase activity was appreciably lower in species known to be experiencing population decline as compared to species showing stable population levels. Recent studies have also suggested that ambient UV-B radiation levels can enhance the susceptibility of amphibian embryos to mortality originating from fungal infection.

These observations suggest that CFCs may be contributing to the decline in amphibian populations. However, this toxicological effect is the result of abiotic interactions (eg, chlorofluorocarbon affecting ozone affecting UV-B radiation) (Fig. 15.4). In addition, abiotic (UV-B) and biotic (fungus) interactions may also be contributing to the toxicity. Such effects would not be predicted from direct laboratory assessments of the toxicity of CFCs to amphibians and highlight the necessity of considering possible indirect toxicity associated with environmental contaminants.

MASCULINIZATION OF FISH DUE TO MICROBIAL INTERACTIONS WITH KRAFT PULPMILL EFFLUENT. Field surveys of mosquito fish populations in the state of Florida revealed populations containing females that exhibited male traits, such as male-type mating behavior and the modi-

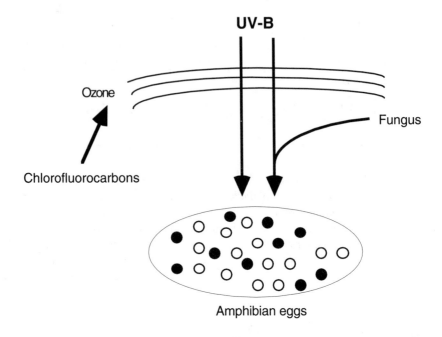

Figure 15.4. Abiotic and biotic interactions leading to the indirect toxicity of chlorofluorocarbons (CFCs) to amphibians. Atmospheric release of CFCs causes the depletion of the stratospheric ozone layer (abiotic–abiotic interaction). Depleted ozone allows for increased penetration of UV-B radiation (abiotic–abiotic interaction). UV-B radiation alone and in combination with fungus (abiotic–biotic interaction) causes increased mortality of amphibian embryos.

fication of the anal fin to resemble the sperm-transmitting gonopodium of males. Masculinized females were found to occur downstream of kraft pulpmill effluents, suggesting that components of the effluent were responsible for the masculinizing effect. Direct toxicity assays performed with the effluent did not produce such effects. However, the inclusion of microorganisms along with the effluent resulted in masculinization. Further studies revealed that phytosterols present in the kraft pulpmill effluent can be converted to androgenic C19 steroids by microorganisms, and these steroids are capable of masculinizing female fish (Fig. 15.5). Thus abiotic (phytosterols):biotic (microorganisms) interactions in the environment must occur before this occult toxicity associated with the kraft pulpmill effluent is unveiled.

ENVIRONMENTAL CONTAMINANTS AND DISEASE AMONG MARINE MAMMALS. Massive mortality has occurred in recent years among populations of harbor seals, bottlenose dolphins, and other marine mammals worldwide. In many instances this mortality has been attributed to disease. For example, nearly 18,000 harbor seals died in the North, Irish, and Baltic seas in the late 1980s as a result of the phocine distemper virus. Incidence of the disease outbreak was highest in areas containing high levels of pollutants, and seals that succumbed to the disease were found to have high tissue levels of poly-

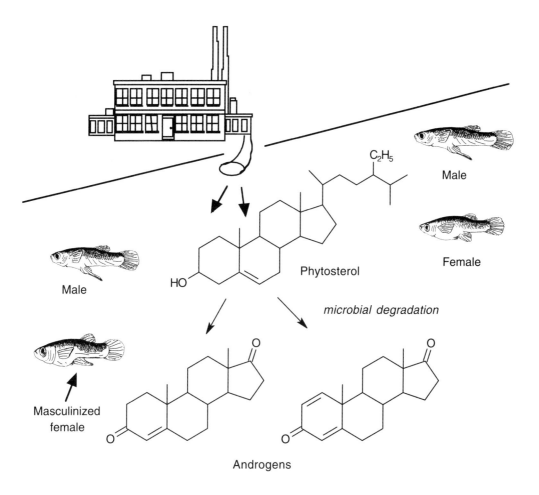

Figure 15.5. Indirect toxicity of kraft pulpmill effluent to mosquito fish. Phytosterols in the mill effluent are converted to C19 steroidal androgens through the action of microorganisms in the environment. These androgens masculinize both anatomy and behavior of female mosquito fish. An arrow identifies the modified anal fin on the masculinized female.

chlorinated biphenyls (PCBs). PCBs and other organochlorine chemicals such as DDT, hexachlorobenzene, and dieldrin have been shown to immunosuppress laboratory animals. Thus, accumulation of these chemicals by the seals may have increased their susceptibility to the virus. This hypothesis was tested by feeding seals herring caught either from a relatively pristine area or from a polluted coastal area for 93 weeks, then assessing the integrity of the immune system in the seals. Seals fed the contaminated fish did indeed have impaired immune responses, lending credence to the hypothesis that organochlorine contaminants in the marine environment are rendering some species immunodeficient. Mortality occured, not as a direct result of chemical toxicity, but as a result of increased susceptibility to pathogens.

15.5

CONCLUSION

Environmental toxicologists have learned a great deal about the effects of chemicals in the environment and the characteristics of chemicals that are responsible for the hazards they pose. Much of the information gained has resulted from retrospective analyses of the environmental consequences of the deposition of chemicals into the environment. Such analyses have resulted in curtailing the release of demonstrated hazardous chemicals into the environment and have provided benchmark information on which the regulation of chemicals proposed for release into the environment can be based. The recognition that environmentally hazardous chemicals commonly share characteristics of persistence, potential to bioaccumulate, and high toxicity has resulted in development and use of chemicals that lack one or more of these characteristics yet fulfill societal needs previously served by hazardous chemicals. For example, recognition that persistence and propensity to bioaccumulate were largely responsible for the environmental hazards posed by many organochlorine pesticides led to the development and use of alternative classes of chemicals such as organophosphorus, carbamate, and pyrethroid pesticides. Although these chemicals all possess the toxicity necessary to function as pesticides, their lack of persistence and reduced propensity to bioaccumulate makes them more suitable for use in the environment.

Such advances in our understanding of the fate and effects of chemicals in the environment does not imply that the role of environmental toxicologists in the twenty-first century will diminish. A dearth of information persists in areas vital to continued protection of natural resources against chemical insult. These include understanding: (1) the unique susceptibilities of key species to the toxicity of different classes of chemicals, (2) the interactions of chemical contaminants with abiotic components of the environment that lead to increased toxicity or hazard, and (3) the consequences of toxicant effects on individuals with respect to ecosystem viability. In addition, continued research is needed on developing molecular and cellular biomarkers of toxicant exposure and effect that could be used to predict dire consequences to the ecosystem before such effects are manifested at higher levels of biologic organization. The role of the environmental toxicologist no doubt will increase in prospective activities aimed at reducing the risk associated with chemical contaminants in the environments before problems arise and, it is hoped, will decrease with respect to assessing damage caused by such environmental contaminants.

Suggested Further Reading

Persistence

Burns LA, Baughman GL: Fate modeling. In *Fundamentals of Aquatic Toxicology*, Rand GM, Petrocelli SR (eds.). New York: Hemisphere, 1985, pp 558–586.

Dauterman WC, Hodgson E: Chemical transformations and interactions. In *Introduction to Environmental Toxicology*, Guthrie FE, Perry JJ (eds.). New York: Elsevier, 1980, pp 358–374.

Larson RA, Weber EJ: *Reaction Mechanisms in Environmental Organic Chemistry*. Boca Raton, FL: Lewis Publishers, 1994.

Bioaccumulation

Banerjee S, Baughman GA: Bioconcentration factors and lipid solubility. *Environ Sci Technol* **25:**536–539, 1991.

Barron, MG: Bioconcentration. *Environ Sci Technol* **24:**1612–1618, 1990.

Barron MG: Bioaccumulation and bioconcentration in aquatic organisms. In *Handbook of Ecotoxicology*, Hoffman DJ, Rattner BA, Burton GA Jr, Cairns J Jr (eds.). Boca Raton, FL: Lewis Publishers, 1995, pp 652–666.

LeBlanc GA: Trophic-level differences in the bioconcentration of chemicals: implications in assessing environmental biomagnification. *Environ Sci Technol* **28:**154–160, 1995.

Mackay D: Correlation of bioconcentration factors. *Environ Sci Technol* **16:**274–278, 1982.

Acute Toxicity

Kelso DD, Kendziorek M: Alaska's response to the Exxon *Valdez* oil spill. *Environ Sci Technol* **25:**183–190, 1991.

LeBlanc GA: Interspecies relationships in acute toxicity of chemicals to aquatic organimsms. *Environ Toxicol Chem* **3:**47–60, 1984.

Parrish PR: Acute toxicity tests. In *Fundamentals of Aquatic Toxicology*, Rand GM, Petrocelli SR (eds.). New York: Hemisphere, 1985, 31–57.

Stansley W: Field results using cholinesterase reactivation techniques to diagnose acute anticholinesterase poisoning in birds and fish. *Arch Environ Contam Toxicol* **25:**315–321, 1993.

van Wezel AP, Opperhuizen A: Narcosis due to environmental pollutants in aquatic organisms: residue-based toxicity, mechanisms, and membrane burdens. *Crit Rev Toxicol* **25:**255–279, 1995.

Chronic Toxicity

Adams WJ: Aquatic toxicology testing methods. In *Handbook of Ecotoxicology*, Hoffman DJ, Rattner BA, Burton GA Jr, Cairns J Jr, (eds.). Boca Raton, FL: Lewis Publishers, 1995, pp 25–46.

Blaustein AR, Hoffman PD, Hokit DG, Kiesecker JM, Walls SC, Hays JB: UV repair and resistance to solar UV-B in amphibian eggs: a link to population declines? *Proc Natl Acad Sci USA* **91:**1791–1795, 1994.

Colborn T, Clement C (eds.): *Chemically-Induced Alterations in Sexual and Functional Development: The Wildlife/Human Connection*. Princeton, N.J: Princeton Scientific, 1992.

Gibbs PE, Pascoe PL, Bryan GW: Tributyltin-induced imposex in stenoglossan gastropods: pathological effects on the female reproductive system. *Comp Biochem Physiol* **100C:** 231–235, 1991.

LeBlanc GA: Are environmental sentinels signaling? *Environ Health Perspect* **103:**888–890, 1995.

LeBlanc GA, Bain LF: Chronic toxicity of environmental contaminants: sentinels and biomarkers. *Environ Health Perspect* 1997. In press.

Petrocelli SR: Chronic toxicity tests. In *Fundamentals of Aquatic Toxicology,* Rand GM, Petrocelli SR (eds.). New York: Hemisphere, 1985, pp 96–109.

Rand GM, Petrocelli SR: Introduction. In *Fundamentals of Aquatic Toxicology*, Rand GM, Petrocelli SR (eds.). New York: Hemisphere, 1985, pp 1–30.

TRANSPORT AND FATE OF TOXICANTS IN THE ENVIRONMENT

16

DAMIAN SHEA

16.1

INTRODUCTION

More than 100,000 chemicals are released into the global environment every year through normal production, use, and disposal. To understand and predict the potential risk that this environmental contamination poses to humans and wildlife, knowledge concerning the toxicity of a chemical must be coupled to knowledge on how chemicals enter into and behave in the environment. The simple box model shown in Fig. 16.1 illustrates the relationship between a toxicant source, its fate in the environment, its effective exposure or dose, and resulting biologic effects. A *prospective* or *predictive* assessment of a chemical hazard would begin by characterizing the source of contamination, modeling the chemical's fate to predict exposure, and using exposure–dose response functions to predict effects (moving from left to right in Fig. 16.1). A common application would be to assess the potential effects of a new waste discharge. A *retrospective* assessment would proceed in the opposite direction starting with some observed effect and reconstructing events to find a probable cause. Assuming that there is a reliable dose–exposure response function, the key to successful use of this simple relationship is to develop a qualitative description and quantitative model of the sources and fate of toxicants in the environment.

Toxicants are released into the environment in many ways and can travel along many pathways during their lifetime. A toxicant present in the environment at a given point in time and space can experience three possible outcomes: It can be *stationary* and add to the toxicant inventory and exposure at that location; it can be *transported* to another location; or it can be *transformed* into another chemical

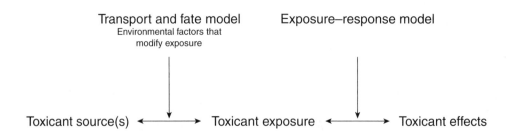

Figure 16.1. Environmental fate models are used to help determine how the environment modifies exposure resulting from various sources of toxicants.

species. Environmental contamination and exposure resulting from the use of a chemical is modified by the transport and transformation of the chemical in the environment. Dilution and degradation can attenuate the source emission, whereas processes that focus and accumulate the chemical can magnify the source emission. The actual fate of a chemical depends on the chemical's use pattern and physical–chemical properties, combined with the characteristics of the environment into which it is released.

Conceptually and mathematically, the transport and fate of a toxicant in the environment is very similar to that in a living organism. Toxicants can enter an organism or environmental system by many routes (ie, dermal, oral, and inhalation versus smoke stack, discharge pipe, or surface runoff). Toxicants are redistributed from their point of entry by fluid dynamics (blood flow versus water or air movement) and intermedia transport processes such as partitioning (blood–lipid partitioning versus water–soil partitioning) and complexation (protein binding versus binding to natural organic matter). Toxicants are transformed in both humans and the environment to other chemicals by reactions such as hydrolysis, oxidation, and reduction. Many enzymatic processes that detoxify and activate chemicals in humans are very similar to microbial biotransformation pathways in the environment.

In fact, physiologically based pharmacokinetic models are similar to environmental fate models. In both cases a complicated system is divided into simpler compartments, the rate of transfer between the compartments is estimated, and the rate of transformation within each compartment also is estimated. The obvious difference is that environmental systems are inherently much more complex because they have more routes of entry, more compartments, more variables (each with a greater range of values), and a lack of control over these variables for systematic study. The discussion that follows is a general overview of the transport and transformation of toxicants in the environment in the context of developing qualitative and quantitative models of these processes.

16.2

SOURCES OF TOXICANTS TO THE ENVIRONMENT

Environmental sources of toxicants can be categorized as either *point sources* or *nonpoint sources* (Fig. 16.2). Point sources are discrete discharges of chemicals that are usually identifiable and measurable, such as industrial or municipal effluent outfalls, chemical or petroleum spills and dumps, smokestacks, and other stationary atmospheric discharges. Nonpoint sources are more diffuse inputs over large areas with no identifiable single point of entry, such as agrochemical (pesticide and fertilizer) runoff, mobile sources emissions (automobiles), atmospheric deposition, desorption or leaching from very large areas (contaminated sediments or mine tailings), and groundwater inflow. Nonpoint sources often include multiple smaller point sources, such as septic tanks or automobiles, that are impractical to consider on an individual basis. Thus, the identification and characterization of a source is relative to the environmental compartment or system being considered. For example, there may be dozens of important toxicant sources to a river, and each must be considered when assessing the hazards of toxicants to aquatic life in the river or to humans who might drink the water or consume the fish and shellfish. However, these toxicant sources can be mixed well in the river, resulting in a rather homogenous and large point source to a downstream lake or estuary (Fig. 16.2).

The rate (units of g/h) at which a toxicant is emitted by a source (*mass emission rate*) can be estimated from the product of the toxicant concentration in the medium (g/m^3) and the flow rate of the medium (m^3/h). This would appear to be relatively simple for point sources, particularly point sources that are monitored routinely to meet environmental regulations. However, the measurement of trace concentrations of chemicals in complex effluent matrices is not a trivial task (see Chapter 12). Often the analytical methods prescribed for monitoring by environmental agencies are not sensitive enough or selective enough to measure important toxicants or their reactive metabolites. Estimating the mass emission rates for nonpoint sources usually is very difficult. For example, the atmospheric deposition of toxicants to a body of water can be highly dependent on both space and time, and high annual loads can result from continuous deposition of trace concentrations that are difficult to measure. The loading of pesticides from an agricultural field to an adjacent body of water also varies with time and space, as shown in Fig. 16.3 for the herbicide atrazine. Rainfall following the application of atrazine results in drainage-ditch loadings more than 100-fold higher than just 2 weeks following the rain. A much smaller but longer lasting increase in atrazine loading occurs at the edge of the field following the rain. Again, the need to define the spatial scale of concern when identifying and characterizing a source is shown. If there is concern with the fate of atrazine within a field, the source is defined by the application rate. If there is concern with the fate and exposure of atrazine in an adjacent body of water, the source may be defined as the drainage ditch and/or as runoff from the edge of field. In the latter case, either appropriate measurements must be taken in the field or the transport of atrazine from the field must be modeled.

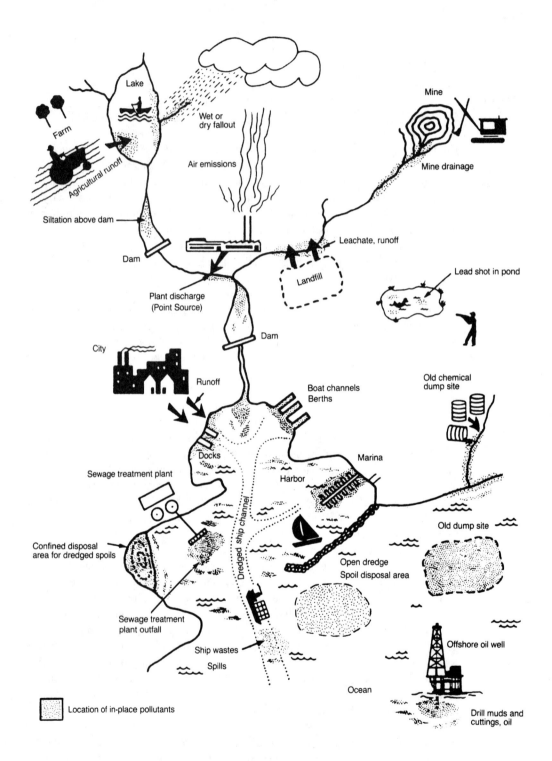

Labels in figure:

Lake
Farm
Agricultural runoff
Wet or dry fallout
Air emissions
Mine
Mine drainage
Siltation above dam
Dam
Leachate, runoff
Landfill
Lead shot in pond
Plant discharge (Point Source)
Dam
City
Runoff
Boat channels
Berths
Old chemical dump site
Docks
Marina
Sewage treatment plant
Harbor
Old dump site
Confined disposal area for dredged spoils
Dredged ship channel
Open dredge Spoil disposal area
Sewage treatment plant outfall
Ship wastes
Spills
Offshore oil well
Ocean
Drill muds and cuttings, oil

Location of in-place pollutants

Figure 16.2. Toxicants enter the environment through many point and nonpoint sources. Reproduced with permission from Arthur D. Little, Inc.

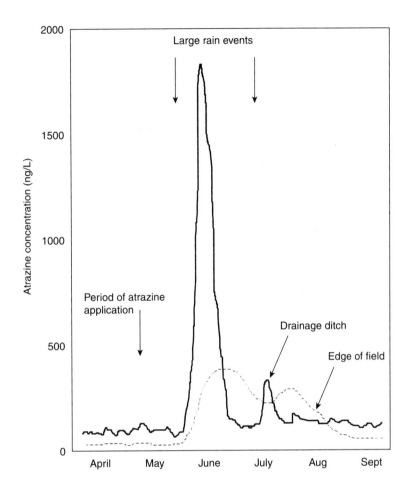

Figure 16.3. The loading of atrazine from an agricultural field to an adjacent body of water is highly dependent on rainfall and the presence of drainage ditches that collect the chemical and focus its movement in the environment.

16.3

TRANSPORT PROCESSES

Following the release of a toxicant into an environmental compartment, transport processes will determine its spatial and temporal distribution in the environment. The transport medium (or fluid) is usually either air or water, whereas the toxicant may be in dissolved, gaseous, condensed, or particulate phases. Physical transport can be categorized as either *advection* or *diffusion*.

16.3.1 Advection

Advection is the passive movement of a chemical in bulk transport media either within the same medium (intraphase or homogeneous transport) or between different media (interphase or heterogeneous transport). Examples of homogeneous advection include transport of a chemical in air on a windy day, or a chemical dissolved in water moving in a flowing stream, in surface runoff (nonpoint source), or in a discharge effluent (point source). Examples of heterogeneous advection include the deposition of a toxicant sorbed to a suspended particle that settles to bottom sediments, atmospheric deposition to soil or water, and even ingestion of contaminated particles or food by an organism (ie, bioaccumulation). Advection takes place independently from the presence of a chemical; the chemical is simply going along for the ride. Advection is not influenced by diffusion and can transport a chemical either in the same or opposite direction as diffusion. Thus, advection is often called *nondiffusive transport*.

16.3.1.1 Homogeneous Advection

The homogeneous advective transport rate (N, g/h) is simply described in mathematical terms by the product of the chemical concentration in the advecting medium (C, g/m^3) and the flow rate of the medium (G, m^3/h):

$$N = GC$$

For example, if the flow of water out of a lake is 1000 m^3/h and the concentration of the toxicant is 1 µg/m^3, then the toxicant is being advected from the lake at a rate of 1000 µg/h (or 1 mg/h). The emission rates for many toxicant sources can be calculated in the same way.

As with source emissions, advection of air and water can vary substantially with time and space within a given environmental compartment. Advection in a stream reach might be several orders of magnitude higher during a large rain event compared to a prolonged dry period, while at one point in time, advection within a stagnant pool might be several orders of magnitude lower than a connected stream. Thus, as with source characterization we must match our estimates of advective transport to the spatial and temporal scales of interest. Again, a good example is the movement of atrazine from an agricultural field (Fig. 16.3). Peak flow advective rates that follow the rain might be appropriate for assessing acute toxicity during peak flow periods, but not for estimating exposure at other times of the year. Conversely, an annual mean advective rate would underestimate exposure during peak flow, but would be more appropriate for assessing chronic toxicity.

In surface waters advective currents often dominate the transport of toxicants, and they can be estimated from hydrodynamic models or current measurements. In many cases, advective flow can be approximated by the volume of water exchanged per unit time by assuming conservation of mass and measuring flow into or out of the system. This works only for well-mixed systems that have no or only small volumes of stagnant water. In bodies of water that experience density stratification (ie, thermocline), separate advective models or residence times can be used for each layer of water. In air, advection also dominates the transport of chemicals, with air currents being driven by pressure gradients. The direction and magnitude of air velocities are recorded continuously in many areas, and daily, seasonal, or annual means can be used to estimate advective air flow.

Advective air and water currents are much smaller in soil systems, but they still influence the movement of chemicals that reside in soil. Advection of water in the saturated zone is usually solved numerically from hydrodynamic models. Advection of air and water in the unsaturated zone is complicated by the heterogeneity of these soil systems. Models are usually developed for specific soil property classes, and measurements of these soil properties are made at a specific site to determine which soil-model layers to link together.

16.3.1.2 Heterogeneous Advection

Heterogeneous advective transport involves a secondary phase within the bulk advective phase, such as when a particle in air or water acts as a carrier of a chemical. In many cases, heterogeneous advection can be treated the same as homogeneous advection if the flowrate of the secondary phase and the concentration of chemical in the secondary phase are known. Using the lake example, if the volume fraction of suspended particles in the lake water is 10^{-5}, the flowrate of suspended particles is 0.01 m^3/h, and the concentration of the toxicant in the solid particles is 100 mg/m^3, then the advective flow of the toxicant on suspended particles would be 1 mg/h, or the same as the homogeneous advection via water. Although the flowrate of particles is much lower than that of water, the concentration of the toxicant is much higher in the suspended particles than when dissolved in the water. This is typical of a hydrophobic toxicant such as DDT or benzo(a)pyrene. In soil and sedimentary systems, colloidal particles (often macromolecular detritus) can play a very important role in heterogeneous advective transport, because they have greater mobility than larger particles and they often have greater capacity to sorb many toxicants because of their higher organic carbon content and higher surface area–mass ratio. In highly contaminated sites, organic cosolvents can be present in the water (usually groundwater) and act as a high capacity and high efficiency carrier of toxicants through heterogeneous advection in the water.

Unfortunately, the dynamics of heterogeneous transport are rarely simple, particularly over shorter scales of time and space. In addition to advection of particles with flowing water, aqueous phase heterogeneous transport also includes particle settling, resuspension, burial in bottom sediments, and mixing of bottom sediments. Particle settling can be an important mechanism for transporting hydrophobic toxicants from the water to the bottom sediments. Modeling this process can be as simple as using an overall mass transfer coefficient or can include rigorous modeling of particles with different size, density, and organic carbon content. Estimates of particle settling are usually obtained through the use of laboratory settling chambers, in situ sediment traps, or by calculation using Stoke's Law. Resuspension of bottom sediments occurs when sufficient energy is transferred to the sediment bed from advecting water, internal waves, boats, dredging, fishing, and the movement of sediment-dwelling organisms (ie, bioturbation). Resuspension rates are difficult to measure and are often highly variable in both time and space. Much as the annual runoff of pesticides from an agricultural field may be dominated by a few rain events, annual resuspension rates can be dominated by a major storm, and in smaller areas by a single boat or school of bottom fish. Resuspension rates can be estimated from sediment traps deployed just above the sediment surface or from the difference between particle settling and permanent burial or sedimentation. Sedimentation is the net result of particle settling and resuspension and can be measured using radionuclide dating methods (eg, ^{210}Pb). Sediment dating itself becomes difficult when there is significant mixing of the surface sediments (eg, through bioturbation). Thus, the heterogeneous transport of toxicants on aqueous particles can be rather complicated, although many aquatic systems have been modeled reasonably well.

Heterogeneous advective transport in the air occurs primarily through the absorption of chemicals into falling water droplets (wet deposition) or the sorption of chemicals into solid particles that fall to the earth's surface (dry deposition). Under certain conditions, both processes can be treated as simple first-order advective transport using a flowrate and concentration in the advecting medium. For example, wet deposition is usually characterized by a washout coefficient that is proportional to rainfall intensity.

16.3.2 Diffusion

Diffusion is the transport of a chemical by random motion due to a state of disequilibrium. For example, diffusion causes the movement of a chemical within a phase (eg, water) from a location of relatively high concentration to a place of lower concentration until the chemical is homogeneously distributed throughout the phase. Likewise, diffusive transport will drive a chemical between media (eg, water and air) until their equilibrium concentrations are reached, and thus the chemical potentials or fugacities are equal in each phase.

16.3.2.1 Diffusion Within a Phase

Diffusional transport within a phase can result from random (thermal) motion of the chemical (molecular diffusion), the random turbulent mixing of the transport medium (turbulent diffusion), or a combination of both. Turbulent diffusion usually dominates the diffusive (but not necessarily the advective) chemical transport in air and water due to the turbulent motions or eddies that are common in nature. In porous media (sediment and soil), the water velocities are typically too low to create eddies, but random mixing still occurs as water tortuously flows around particles. This mechanical diffusion is often called dispersion by hydrologists, and dispersion on larger scales, such as when groundwater detours around large areas of less permeable soil, is called macrodispersion. Note, however, that the term dispersion is often used by meteorologists and engineers to describe any turbulent diffusion.

Although different physical mechanisms can cause diffusive mixing, they all cause a net transport of a chemical from areas of higher concentration to areas of lower concentration. All diffusive processes are also referred to as *Fickian transport* because they all can be described mathematically by Fick's First Law, which states that the flow (or flux) of a chemical (N, g/h) is proportional to its concentration gradient (dC/dx):

$$N = -DA \left(\frac{dC}{dx} \right)$$

where D is the diffusivity or mass transfer coefficient (m^2/h), A is the area through which the chemical is passing (m^2), C is the concentration of the diffusing chemical (g/m^3), and x is the distance being considered (m). The negative sign is simply the convention that the direction of diffusion is from high to low concentration (diffusion is positive when dC/dx is negative). Note that many scientists and texts define diffusion as an area-specific process with units of g/m^2h, and thus the area term (A) is not included in the diffusion equation. This is simply an alternative designation that describes transport as a flux density (g/m^2h) rather than as a flow (g/h). In either case, the diffusion equation can be integrated numerically and even expressed in three dimensions using vector notation. However, for most environmental situations there is usually no accurate estimate of D or dx, so we combine the two into a one-dimensional mass transfer coefficient (k_M) with units of velocity (m/h). The chemical flux is then the product of this velocity, area, and concentration:

$$N = -k_M A C$$

Mass transfer coefficients can be estimated from laboratory, mesocosm, and field studies and are widely used in environmental fate models. Mass transfer coefficients can be derived separately for molecular diffusion, turbulent diffusion, and dispersion in porous media and all three terms can be added to the chemical flux equation. Usually, this is not necessary because one term often dominates the transport in specific environmental regions. Consider the vertical diffusion of methane gas generated by methanogenic bacteria in deep sediments. Molecular diffusion dominates in the highly compacted and low porosity deeper sediments. Dispersion becomes important as methane approaches the more porous surface sediments. Following methane gas ebulation from the sediment porewater, turbulent diffusion will dominate transport in a well-mixed water column (ie, not a stagnant pool or beneath a thermocline, where molecular diffusion will dominate). At the water surface, eddies tend to be damped and molecular diffusion may again dominate transport. Under stagnant atmospheric conditions (ie, a temperature inversion), molecular diffusion will continue to dominate, but will yield to more rapid mixing when typical turbulent conditions are reached. The magnitude and variability of the transport rate generally increase as the methane moves vertically through the environment, except when very stagnant conditions are encountered in the water or air. Modeling the transport of a chemical in air is particularly difficult because of the high spatial and temporal variability of air movement. Note also that advective processes in water or air usually transport chemicals at a faster rate than either molecular or turbulent diffusion.

16.3.2.2   Diffusion Between Phases

The transport of a chemical between phases is sometimes treated as a third category of transport processes or even as a transformation reaction. Interphase or intermedia transport is not a transformation reaction because the chemical is moving only between phases; it is not reacting with anything or changing its chemical structure. Instead, intermedia transport is simply driven by diffusion between two phases. When a chemical reaches an interface such as air–water, particle–water, or (biologic) membrane–water, two diffusive regions are created at either side of the interface. The classic description of this process is the Whitman two-film or two-resistance mass transfer theory, in which chemicals pass through two stagnant boundary layers by molecular diffusion, while the two bulk phases are assumed to be mixed homogeneously. This allows the use of a first-order function of the concentration gradient in the two phases, in which the mass transfer coefficient will depend only on the molecular diffusivity of the chemical in each phase and the thickness of the boundary layers. This is fairly straightforward for transfer at the air–water interface (and often at the membrane–water interface), but not for the particle–water or particle–air interfaces.

Diffusive transport between phases can be described mathematically as the product of the departure from equilibrium and a kinetic term:

$$N = kA\,(C_1 - C_2 K_{12})$$

where N is the transport rate (g/h), k is a transport rate coefficient (m/h), A is the interfacial area (m^2), C_1 and C_2 are the concentrations in the two phases, and K_{12} is the equilibrium partition coefficient. At equilibrium, K_{12} equals C_1/C_2, so the term describing the departure from equilibrium $(C_1 - C_2 K_{12})$ becomes zero, and thus the net rate of transfer is also zero. The partition coefficients are readily obtained from thermodynamic data and equilibrium partitioning experiments. The transport rate coefficients are usually estimated from the transport rate equation itself by measuring intermedia transport rates (N) under controlled laboratory conditions (ie, temperature, wind and water velocities) at known values of A, C_1, C_2, and K_{12}. These measurements must then be extrapolated to the field, sometimes with great uncertainty. This uncertainty, along with the knowledge that many interfacial regions have reached or are near equilibrium, has led many to assume simply that equilibrium exists at the interface. Thus, the net transport rate is zero and the phase distribution of a chemical is simply described by its equilibrium partition coefficient.

16.4

EQUILIBRIUM PARTITIONING

When a small amount of a chemical is added to two immiscible phases and then shaken, the phases will eventually separate and the chemical will partition between the two phases according to its solubility in each phase. The concentration ratio at equilibrium is the partition coefficient:

$$\frac{C_1}{C_2} = K_{12}$$

In the laboratory, K_{12} is usually determined from the slope of C_1 versus C_2 over a range of concentrations. Partition coefficients can be measured for essentially any two-phase system: air–water, octanol–water, lipid–water, particle–water, and so on. In situ partition coefficients also can be measured where site-specific environmental conditions might influence the equilibrium phase distribution.

16.4.1 Air–Water Partitioning

Air–water partition coefficients ($K_{air-water}$) are essentially Henry's Law constants (H):

$$K_{air-water} = H = \frac{C_{air}}{C_{water}}$$

where H can be expressed in dimensionless form (same units for air and water) or in units of pressure divided by concentration (eg, Pa m^3/mol). The latter is usually written as

$$H' = \frac{P_{air}}{C_{water}}$$

where P_{air} is the partial vapor pressure of the chemical. When H is not measured directly, it can be estimated from the ratio of the chemical's vapor pressure and aqueous solubility, although care must be exercised about using vapor pressures and solubilities that apply to the same temperature and phase. Chemicals with high Henry's Law constants (such as alkanes and many chlorinated solvents) have a tendency to escape from water to air and typically have high vapor pressures, low aqueous solubilities, and low boiling points. Chemicals with low Henry's Law constants (such as alcohols, chlorinated phenols, larger polycyclic aromatic hydrocarbons, lindane, and atrazine) tend to have high water solubility and/or very low vapor pressure. Note that some chemicals that are considered to be "nonvolatile," such as DDT, are often assumed to have low Henry's Law constants. However, DDT also has a very low water solubility, yielding a rather high Henry's Law constant. Thus, DDT readily partitions into the atmosphere, as is now apparent from the global distribution of DDT.

16.4.2 Octanol–Water Partitioning

For many decades, chemists have been measuring the octanol–water partition coefficient (K_{ow}) as a descriptor of hydrophobicity, or how much a chemical "hates" to be in water. It is now one of the most important and frequently used physicochemical properties in toxicology and environmental chemistry. In fact, toxicologists often simply use the symbol P, for partition coefficient, as if no other partition coefficient is important. Strong correlations exist between K_{ow} and many biochemical and toxicological properties. Octanol has a similar carbon:oxygen ratio as lipids and the K_{ow} correlates particularly well with lipid–water partition coefficients. This has led many to use K_{ow} as a measure of lipophilicity, or how much a chemical "loves" lipids. This really is not the case because most chemicals have an equal affinity for octanol and other lipids (within about a factor of 10), but their affinity for water varies by many orders of magnitude. Thus, it is largely aqueous solubility that determines K_{ow}, not octanol or lipid solubility. Generally, K_{ow} is expressed as log K_{ow} because K_{ow} values range from less than 1 (alcohols) to more than 1 billion (larger alkanes and alkyl benzenes).

16.4.3 Lipid–Water Partitioning

In most cases, it can be assumed that the equilibrium distribution and partitioning of organic chemicals in both mammalian and nonmammalian systems is a function of lipid content in the animal and that the lipid–water partition coefficient (K_{LW}) is equal to K_{OW}. Instances in which this is not the case include specific binding sites (eg, kepone in the liver) and nonequilibrium conditions caused by slow elimination rates of higher level organisms or structured lipid phases that sterically hinder accumulation of very hydrophobic chemicals. For aquatic organisms in constant contact with water, the bioconcentration factor, or fish–water partition coefficient (K_{FW}) is simply:

$$K_{FW} = f_{lipid}\, K_{OW}$$

where f_{lipid} is the mass fraction of lipid in the fish (g lipid/g fish). Several studies have shown that this relationship works well for many fish and shellfish species, and an aggregate plot of K_{FW} versus K_{OW} for many different fish species yields a slope of 0.048, which is about the average lipid concentration of fish (5%). Again, nonequilibrium conditions will cause deviation from this equation. Such deviations are found at both the top and bottom of the aquatic food chain. Phytoplankton can have higher apparent lipid–water partition coefficients because their large surface area:volume ratios increase the relative importance of surface sorption. Top predators such as marine mammals also have high apparent lipid–water partition coefficients because of very slow elimination rates. Thus, the deviations occur not because "there is something wrong with the equation," but because the underlying assumption of equilibrium is not appropriate in these cases.

16.4.4   Particle–Water Partitioning

It has been known for several decades that many chemicals preferentially associate with soil and sediment particles rather than the aqueous phase. The particle-water partition coefficient (K_P) describing this phenomenon is:

$$K_P = \frac{C_S}{C_W}$$

where C_S is the concentration of chemical in the soil or sediment (mg/kg dry weight) and C_W is the concentration in water (mg/L). Using this form, K_P has units of L/kg, or reciprocal density. Dimensionless partition coefficients are sometimes used where K_P is multiplied by the particle density (in kg/L). It has also been observed, first by pesticide chemists in soil systems and later by environmental engineers and chemists in sewage effluent and sediment systems, that nonionic organic chemicals were primarily associated with the organic carbon phase(s) of particles. A plot of K_P versus the mass fraction of organic carbon in the soil (f_{OC}, g/g) is linear, with a near-zero intercept yielding the simple relationship:

$$K_P = f_{OC} K_{OC}$$

where K_{OC} is the organic carbon–water partition coefficient (L/kg). Studies with many chemicals and many sediment/soil systems have demonstrated the utility of this equation when the fraction of organic carbon is about 0.5% or greater. At lower organic carbon fractions, interaction with the mineral phase becomes relatively more important (although highly variable), resulting in a small positive intercept of K_P versus f_{OC}. The strongest interaction between organic chemicals and mineral phases appears to be with dry clays. Thus, K_P will likely change substantially as a function of water content in low organic carbon, clay soils.

Measurements of K_{OC} have been taken directly from partitioning experiments in sediment– and soil–water systems over a range of environmental conditions in both the laboratory and the field. Not surprisingly, the K_{OC} values for many organic chemicals are highly correlated with their K_{OW} values. Plots of the two partition coefficients for hundreds of chemicals with widely ranging K_{OW} values yield slopes from about 0.3 to 1, depending on the classes of compounds and the particular methods included. Most fate modelers continue to use a slope of 0.41, which was reported by the first definitive study on the subject in the early 1980s. Thus, we now have a means of estimating the partitioning of a chemical between a particle and water by using the K_{OW} and f_{OC}:

$$K_P = f_{OC} K_{OC} = f_{OC} 0.41 K_{OW}$$

This relationship is commonly used in environmental fate models to predict aqueous concentrations from sediment measurements by substituting the equilibrium expression for K_P and rearranging to solve for C_W:

$$K_P = \frac{C_S}{C_W} = f_{OC}\ 0.41\ K_{OW}$$

$$C_W = \frac{C_S}{f_{OC}\ 0.41\ K_{OW}}$$

This last equation forms the basis for the Environmental Protection Agency's (EPA's) sediment quality criteria, which is to be used to assess the potential toxicity of contaminated sediments. The idea is to simply measure C_S and f_{OC}, look up K_{OW} in a table, compute the predicted C_W, and compare this result to established water quality criteria for the protection of aquatic life or human life (eg, carcinogenicity risk factors). The use of this simple equilibrium partitioning expression for this purpose currently is the subject of much debate among both scientists and policy makers.

16.5

TRANSFORMATION PROCESSES

The potential environmental hazard associated with the use of a chemical is directly related to its persistence in the environment (see Chapter 15), which in turn depends on the rates of chemical transformation reactions. Transformation reactions can be divided into two classes: reversible reactions that involve continuous exchange among chemical states (ionization, complexation), and irreversible reactions that permanently transform a parent chemical into a daughter or reaction product (photolysis, hydrolysis, and many redox reactions). Reversible reactions are usually abiotic, although biologic processes can still exert great influence over them (eg, via production of complexing agents or a change in pH). Irreversible reactions can be abiotic or mediated directly by biota, particularly bacteria.

16.5.1 Reversible Reactions

16.5.1.1 Ionization

Ionization refers to the dissociation of a neutral chemical into charged species. The most common form of neutral toxicant dissociation is acid–base equilibria. The hypothetical monoprotic acid, HA, will dissociate in water to form the conjugate acid–base pair (H^+, A^-) usually written as:

$$HA + H_2O = H_3O^+ + A^-$$

The equilibrium constant for this reaction, the acidity constant (K_a) is defined by the law of mass action, and is given by:

$$K_a = \frac{[H_3O^+][A^-]}{[HA]}$$

For convenience, equilibrium constants are often expressed as the negative logarithm, or pK, value. Thus, the relative proportion of the neutral and charged species will be a function of the pK_a and solution pH. When the pH is equal to pK_a, equal concentrations of the neutral and ionized forms will be present. When pH is less than the pK_a, the neutral species will be predominant; when pH is greater than pK_a, the ionized species will be in excess. The exact equilibrium distribution can be calculated from the equilibrium expression discussed earlier and the law of mass conservation.

The fate of a chemical is often a function of the relative abundance of a particular chemical species as well as the total concentration. For example, the neutral chemical might partition into biologic lipids or organic carbon in soil to a greater extent than the ionized form. Many acidic toxicants (pentachlorophenol) exhibit higher toxicities to aquatic organisms at lower pH, where the neutral species predominates. However, specific ionic interactions will take place only with the ionized species. A classic example of how pH influences the fate and effects of a toxicant is with hydrogen cyanide (HCN). The pK_a of HCN is about 9 and the toxicity of CN^- is much higher than that of HCN for many aquatic organisms. Thus, the discharge of a basic (high pH) industrial effluent containing cyanide would pose a greater hazard to fish than a lower pH effluent (everything else being equal). The effluent could be treated to reduce the pH well below the pK_a according to the reaction:

$$CN^- + H^+ = HCN_{(aq)}$$

thus reducing the hazard to the fish. However, HCN has a rather high Henry's Law constant and will partition into the atmosphere:

$$HCN_{(aq)} = HCN_{(air)}$$

This may be fine for the fish, but birds in the area and humans working at the industrial plant will now have a much greater exposure to HCN. Thus, both the fate and toxicity of a chemical can be influenced by simple ionization reactions.

16.5.1.2   Precipitation and Dissolution

A special case of ionization is the dissolution of a neutral solid phase into soluble species. For example, the binary solid metal sulfide CuS dissolves in water according to:

$$CuS(s) + H^+ = Cu^{2+} + HS^-$$

The equilibrium constant for this reaction, the solubility product (K_{sp}), is given by:

$$K_{sp} = \frac{[Cu^{2+}][HS^-]}{[H^+]}$$

The solubility product for CuS is very low ($K_{sp} = 10^{-19}$ as written) so that the presence of sulfide in water acts to immobilize Cu (and many other metals) and reduce effective exposure. The formation of metal sulfides is important in anaerobic soil and sediment, stagnant ponds and basins, and many industrial and domestic sewage treatment plants and discharges. Coprecipitation of metals also can be a very important removal process in natural waters. In aerobic systems, the precipitation of hydrous oxides of manganese and iron often incorporate other metals as impurities. In anaerobic systems, the precipitation of iron sulfides can include other metals as well. These coprecipitates are usually not thermodynamically stable, but their conversion to stable mineral phases often takes place on geologic time scales.

16.5.1.3 Complexation and Chemical Speciation

Natural systems contain many chemicals that undergo ionic or covalent interactions with toxicants to change toxicant speciation, and chemical speciation can have a profound effect on both fate and toxicity. Again, using copper as an example, inorganic ions (Cl^-, OH^-) and organic detritus (humic acids, peptides) will react with dissolved Cu^{2+} to form various metal–ligand complexes. Molecular diffusivities of complexed copper will be lower than uncomplexed (hydrated) copper and will generally decrease with the size and number of ligands. The toxicity of free, uncomplexed Cu^{2+} to many aquatic organisms is much higher than Cu^{2+} that is complexed to chelating agents such as EDTA or glutathione. Many transition metal toxicants, such as Cu, Pb, Cd, and Hg, have high binding constants with compounds that contain amine, sulfhydryl, and carboxylic acid groups. These groups are quite common in natural organic matter. Even inorganic complexes of OH^- and Cl^- reduce Cu^{2+} toxicity. In systems in which a mineral phase is controlling Cu^{2+} solubility, the addition of these complexing agents will shift the solubility equilibrium according to LeChatelier's Principle as shown here for CuS and OH^-, Cl^-, and GSH (glutathione):

$$CuS(s) + H^+ = Cu^{2+} + HS^- \qquad K_{sp}$$
$$Cu^{2+} + OH^- = CuOH^+ \qquad K_{CuOH}$$
$$Cu^{2+} + Cl^- = CuCl^+ \qquad K_{CuCl}$$
$$Cu^{2+} + GSH = CuGS^+ + H^+ \qquad K_{CuGS}$$

Each successive complexation reaction "leaches" Cu^{2+} from the solid mineral phase, thereby increasing the total copper in the water but not affecting the concentration of (or exposure to) Cu^{2+}. These equilibria can be combined into one reaction:

$$4\,CuS(s) + 3H^+ + OH^- + Cl^- + GSH = Cu^{2+} + 4HS^- + CuOH^+ + CuCl^+ + CuGS^+$$

and the overall equilibrium constant derived as shown:

$$K_{overall} = (4) \, K_{sp} \times K_{CuOH} \times K_{CuCl} \times K_{CuGS}$$

$$= \frac{[Cu^{2+}][CuOH^+][CuCl^+][CuGS^+][HS^-]^4}{[H^+][OH^-][Cl^-][GS^-]}$$

A series of simultaneous equations can be derived for these reactions to compute the concentration of individual copper species and the total concentration of copper, $[Cu]_T$, would be given by:

$$[Cu]_T = [Cu^{2+}] + [CuOH^+] + [CuCl^+] + [CuGS^+]$$

Thus the total copper added to a toxicity test or measured as the exposure (eg, by atomic absorption spectroscopy) may be much greater than that which is available to an organism to induce toxicological effects.

Literally hundreds of complex equilibria like this can be combined to model what happens to metals in aqueous systems. Numerous speciation models exist for this application that include all of the necessary equilibrium constants. Several of these models include surface complexation reactions that take place at the particle–water interface. Unlike the partitioning of hydrophobic organic contaminants into organic carbon, metals actually form ionic and covalent bonds with surface ligands, such as sulfhydryl groups on metal sulfides and oxide groups on the hydrous oxides of manganese and iron. Metals also can be biotransformed to more toxic species (eg, conversion of elemental mercury to methyl mercury by anaerobic bacteria), less toxic species (oxidation of tributyl tin to elemental tin), or temporarily immobilized (eg, via microbial reduction of sulfate to sulfide, which then precipitates as an insoluble metal sulfide mineral).

16.5.2 Irreversible Reactions

The reversible transformation reactions discussed previously alter the fate and toxicity of chemicals, but do not change irreversibly the structure or properties of the chemical. An acid can be neutralized to its conjugate base and vice versa. Copper can precipitate as a metal sulfide, dissolve and form a complex with numerous ligands, and later reprecipitate as a metal sulfide. Irreversible transformation reactions alter the structure and properties of a chemical forever.

16.5.2.1 Hydrolysis

Hydrolysis is the cleavage of organic molecules by reaction with water with a net displacement of a leaving group (X) with OH^-:

$$RX + H_2O = ROH + HX$$

Hydrolysis is part of the larger class of chemical reactions called nucleophilic displacement reactions, in which a nucleophile (electron-rich species with an unshared pair of electrons) attacks an electrophile (electron deficient) cleaving one covalent bond to form a new one. Hydrolysis is usually associated with surface waters but also takes place in the atmosphere (fogs and clouds), groundwater, at the particle–water interface of soils and sediments, and in living organisms.

Hydrolysis can proceed through numerous mechanisms via attack by H_2O (neutral hydrolysis) or by acid (H^+) or base (OH^-) catalysis. Acid- and base-catalyzed reactions proceed via alternative mechanisms that require less energy than neutral hydrolysis. The combined hydrolysis rate term is a sum of these three constituent reactions and is given by:

$$\frac{d\,[RX]}{dt} = k_{obs}[RX] = k_a[H^+][RX] + k_n[RX] + k_b[OH^-][RX]$$

where [RX] is the concentration of the hydrolyzable chemical, k_{obs} is the macroscopic observed hydrolysis rate constant, and k_a, k_n, and k_b are the rate constants for the acid-catalyzed, neutral, and base-catalyzed hydrolysis. If we assume that the hydrolysis can be approximated by first-order kinetics with respect to RX (which is usually true), the rate term is reduced to:

$$k_{obs} = k_a[H^+] + k_n + k_b[OH^-]$$

Neutral hydrolysis is dependent only on water, which is present in excess, so k_n is a simple pseudo–first-order rate constant (with units t^{-1}). The acid- and base-catalyzed hydrolysis depend on the molar quantities of [H^+] and [OH^-], respectively, so k_a and k_b have units of $M^{-1}t^{-1}$. The observed or apparent hydrolysis half-life at a fixed pH is then given by:

$$t_{1/2} = \frac{\ln 2}{k_{obs}}$$

Compilations of hydrolysis half-lives at pH and temperature ranges encountered in nature can be found in many sources. Reported hydrolysis half-lives for organic compounds at pH 7 and 298K range at least 13 orders of magnitude. Many esters hydrolyze within hours or days, whereas some organic chemicals will never hydrolyze. For halogenated methanes, which are common groundwater contaminants, half-lives range from about 1 y for CH_3Cl to about 7000 y for CCl_4. The half-lives of halomethanes follow the strength of the carbon–halogen bond, with half-lives decreasing in the order F>Cl>Br. Small structural changes can alter hydrolysis rates dramatically. An example is the difference between tetrachloroethane ($Cl_2HC–CHCl_2$) and tetrachloroethene ($Cl_2C=CCl_2$), which have hydrolysis half-lives of about 0.5 y and 10^9 y, respectively. In this case, the hydrolysis rate is affected by the C–Cl bond strength and the steric bulk at the site of nucleophilic substitution.

The apparent rate of hydrolysis and the relative abundance of reaction products is often a function of pH because alternative reaction pathways are preferred at different pH. Using halogenated hydrocarbons as an example, base-catalyzed hydrolysis will result in elimination reactions, whereas neutral hydrolysis will take place via nucleophilic displacement reactions. An example of the pH dependence of hydrolysis is illustrated by the base-catalyzed hydrolysis of the structurally similar insecticides DDT and methoxychlor. Under a common range of natural pH (5 to 8), the hydrolysis rate of methoxychlor is invariant whereas the hydrolysis of DDT is about 15-fold faster at pH 8 compared to pH 5. Only at higher pH (>8) does the hydrolysis rate of methoxychlor increase. In addition, the major product of DDT hydrolysis throughout this pH range is the same (DDE), whereas the methoxychlor hydrolysis product shifts from the alcohol at pH 5 to 8 (nucleophilic substitution) to the dehydrochlorinated DMDE at pH above 8 (elimination). This illustrates the necessity to conduct detailed mechanistic experiments as a function of pH for hydrolytic reactions.

16.5.2.2   Photolysis

Photolysis of a chemical can proceed by either direct absorption of light (direct photolysis) or reaction with another chemical species that has been produced or excited by light (indirect photolysis). In either case, photochemical transformations such as bond cleavage, isomerization, intramolecular rearrangement, and various intermolecular reactions can result. Photolysis can take place wherever sufficient light energy exists, including the atmosphere (in the gas phase and in aerosols and fog/cloud droplets), surface waters (in the dissolved phase or at the particle–water interface), and in the terrestrial environment (on plant and soil/mineral surfaces).

Photolysis dominates the fate of many chemicals in the atmosphere because of the high solar irradiance. Near the Earth's surface, chromophores such as nitrogen oxides, carbonyls, and aromatic hydrocarbons play a large role in contaminant fate in urban areas. In the stratosphere, light is absorbed by ozone, oxygen, organohalogens, and hydrocarbons with global environmental implications. The rate of photolysis in surface waters depends on light intensity at the air–water interface, the transmittance through this interface, and the attenuation through the water column. Open ocean waters ("blue water") can transmit blue light to depths of 150 m, whereas highly eutrophic or turbid waters might absorb all light within 1 cm of the surface.

16.5.2.3   Oxidation–Reduction Reactions

Although many redox reactions are reversible, they are included here because many of the redox reactions that influence the fate of toxicants are irreversible on the temporal and spatial scales that are important to toxicity.

Oxidation is simply defined as a loss of electrons. Oxidizing agents are electrophiles and thus gain electrons on reaction. Oxidations can result in the increase in the oxidation state of the chemical, as in the oxidation of metals or oxidation can incorporate oxygen into the molecule. Typical organic chemical oxidative reactions include dealkylation, epoxidation, aromatic ring cleavage, and hydroxylation. The term autooxidation or weathering is commonly used to describe the general oxidative degradation of a chemical (or chemical mixture such as petroleum) on exposure to air. Chemicals can react abiotically in both water and air with oxygen, ozone, peroxides, free radicals, and singlet oxygen. The last two are common intermediate reactants in indirect photolysis. Mineral surfaces are known to catalyze many oxidative reactions. Clays and oxides of silicon, aluminum, iron, and manganese can provide surface active sites that increase rates of oxidation. There are a variety of complex mechanisms associated with this catalysis so it is difficult to predict the catalytic activity of soils and sediment in nature.

Reduction of a chemical species takes place when an electron donor (reductant) transfers electrons to an electron acceptor (oxidant). Organic chemicals typically act as the oxidant, whereas abiotic reductants include sulfide minerals, reduced metals or sulfur compounds, and natural organic matter. There are also extracellular biochemical reducing agents such as porphyrins, corrinoids, and metal-containing coenzymes. Most of these reducing agents are present only in anaerobic environments in which anaerobic bacteria themselves are busy reducing chemicals. Thus, it is usually very difficult to distinguish biotic and abiotic reductive processes in nature. Well-controlled and sterile laboratory studies are required to measure abiotic rates of reduction. These studies indicate that many abiotic reductive transformations could be important in the environment, including dehalogenation; dealkylation; and the reduction of quinones, nitrosamines, azoaromatics, nitroaromatics, and sulfoxides. Functional groups that are resistant to reduction include aldehydes, ketones, carboxylic acids (and esters), amides, alkenes, and aromatic hydrocarbons.

16.5.2.4   Biotransformations

As shown throughout much of this textbook, vertebrates have developed the capacity to transform many toxicants into other chemicals, sometimes detoxifying the chemical and sometimes activating it. The same or similar biochemical processes that hydrolyze, oxidize, and reduce toxicants in vertebrates also take place in many lower organisms. In particular, bacteria, protozoans, and fungi provide a significant capacity to biotransform toxicants in the environment. Although many vertebrates can metabolize toxicants faster than these lower forms of life, the aggregate capacity of vertebrates to biotransform toxicants (based on total biomass and exposure) is insignificant to the overall fate of a toxicant in the environment. In this section, the term *biotransformation* is used to include all forms of direct biologic transformation reactions.

Biotransformations follow a complex series of chemical reactions that are enzymatically mediated and are usually irreversible reactions that are energetically favorable, resulting in a decrease in the Gibbs free energy of the system. Thus, the potential for biotransformation of a chemical depends on the reduction in free energy that results from reacting the chemical with other chemicals in its environment (eg, oxygen). As with inorganic catalysts, microbes simply use enzymes to lower the activation energy of the reaction and increase the rate of the transformation. Each successive chemical reaction further degrades the chemical, eventually mineralizing it to inorganic compounds (eg, CO_2, H_2O, inorganic salts) and continuing the carbon and hydrologic cycles on Earth.

Usually, microbial growth is stimulated because the microbes capture the energy released from the biotransformation reaction. As the microbial population expands, overall biotransformation rates increase, even though the rate for each individual microbe may be constant or even decrease. This complicates the modeling and prediction of biotransformation rates in nature. When the toxicant concentration (and potential energy) is small relative to other substrates or when the microbes cannot capture the energy efficiently from the biotransformation, microbial growth is not stimulated, but biotransformation often still proceeds inadvertently through cometabolism.

Biotransformation can be modeled using simple Michaelis–Menten enzyme kinetics, Monod microbial growth kinetics, or more complex numerical models that incorporate various environmental parameters and even the formation of microbial mats or slime that affects diffusion of the chemical and nutrients to the microbial population. Microbial ecology involves a complex web of interaction among numerous environmental processes and parameters. The viability of microbial populations and the rates of biotransformation depend on many factors such as genetic adaptation, moisture, nutrients, oxygen, pH, and temperature. Although a single factor may limit biotransformation rates at a particular time and location, generalizations cannot be made concerning what limits biotransformation rates in the environment. Biotransformation rates often increase with temperature (according to the Arrhenius Law) within the optimum range that supports the microbes, but many exceptions exist for certain organisms and chemicals. The availability of oxygen and various nutrients (eg, C, N, P, Fe, Si) often limits microbial growth, but the limiting nutrient often changes with space (eg, down river) and time (seasonally and even diurnally).

Long-term exposure of microbial populations to certain toxicants often is necessary for adaptation of enzymatic systems capable of degrading those toxicants. This was the case with the Exxon *Valdez* oil spill in Alaska in 1989. Natural microbial populations in Prince William Sound, Alaska, had developed enzyme systems that oxidize petroleum hydrocarbons because of long-term exposure to natural oil seeps and to hydrocarbons that leached from the pine forests in the area. Growth of these natural microbial populations was nutrient limited during the summer. Thus, the application of nutrient formulations to the rocky beaches of Prince William Sound stimulated microbial growth and helped to degrade the spilled oil.

In terrestrial systems with high nutrient and oxygen content, low moisture and high organic carbon can control biotransformation by limiting microbial growth and the availability of the toxicant to the microbes. For example, biotransformation rates of certain pesticides have been shown to vary two orders of magnitude in two separate agricultural fields that were both well aerated and nutrient rich, but spanned the common range of moisture and organic carbon content.

16.6

ENVIRONMENTAL FATE MODELS

The previouos discussion provides a brief qualitative introduction to the transport and fate of chemicals in the environment. The goal of most fate chemists and engineers is to translate this qualitative picture into a conceptual model and ultimately into a quantitative description that can be used to predict or reconstruct the fate of a chemical in the environment (Fig. 16.1). This quantitative description usually takes the form of a mass balance model. The idea is to compartmentalize the environment into defined units (control volumes) and to write a mathematical expression for the mass balance within the compartment. As with pharmacokinetic models, transfer between compartments can be included as the complexity of the model increases.

There is a great deal of subjectivity to assembling a mass balance model. However, each decision to include or exclude a process or compartment is based on one or more assumptions—most of which can be tested at some level. Over time, the applicability of various assumptions for particular chemicals and environmental conditions become known and model standardization becomes possible.

The construction of a mass balance model follows the general outline of this chapter.

1. Define the spatial and temporal scales to be considered and establish the environmental compartments or control volumes.
2. Identify and quantify the source emissions.
3. Write the mathematical expressions for advective and diffusive transport processes.
4. Quantify the chemical transformation processes.

This model-building process is illustrated in Fig. 16.4. In this example, simply equate the change in chemical inventory (total mass in the system) with the differ-

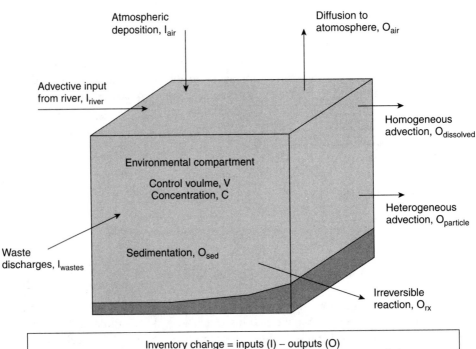

Figure 16.4. Constructing a simple chemical mass balance model.

ence between chemical inputs and outputs to the system. The inputs could include numerous point and nonpoint sources or could be a single estimate of total chemical load to the system. The outputs include all of the loss mechanisms: transport out of the compartment and irreversible transformation reactions. If steady state can be assumed (ie, the chemical's concentration in the compartment is not changing over the time scale of the model), the inventory change is zero and a simple mass balance equation is left to solve. Unsteady-state conditions would require a numerical solution to the differential equations.

There are many tricks and shortcuts to this process. For example, rather than compiling all of the transformation rate equations (or conducting the actual kinetic experiments), there are many sources of typical chemical half-lives based on pseudo–first-order rate expressions. It is usually prudent to begin with these "best estimates" of half-lives in air, water, soil, and sediment and perform a sensitivity analysis with the model to determine which processes are most important. The most important processes can be reassessed to ascertain whether more detailed rate expressions are necessary. An illustration of this mass balance approach is given in

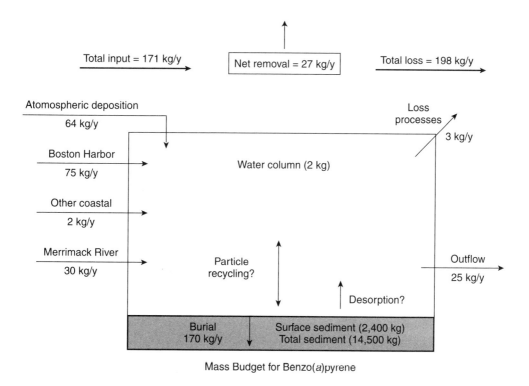

Mass Budget for Benzo(a)pyrene

Figure 16.5. The information provided by a chemical mass balance model. The annual mass budget of benzo(a)pyrene in Massachusetts Bay is shown.

Fig. 16.5 for benzo(*a*)pyrene. This approach allows a first-order evaluation of how chemicals enter the environment, what happens to them in the environment, and what the exposure concentrations will be in various environmental media. Thus, the chemical mass balance provides information relevant to toxicant exposure to both humans and wildlife.

Suggested Further Reading

Transport and Fate Processes

Burns LA, Baughman GL: *Fate Modeling*. In Rand GM, Petrocelli SR (eds.). *Fundamentals of Aquatic Toxicology*. New York: Hemisphere, 1985.

Hemond HF, Fechner EJ: *Chemical Fate and Transport in the Environment*. New York: Academic Press, 1994, p 338.

Larson RA, Weber EJ: *Reaction Mechanisms in Environmental Organic Chemistry*. Boca Raton, FL: Lewis Publishers, 1994, p 433.

Mackay D: *Multimedia Environmental Models: The Fugacity Approach*. Chelsea, MI: Lewis Publishers, 1991, p 257.

Sherwood TK, Pigford RL, Wilke CR: *Mass Transfer*. New York: McGraw-Hill, 1975, p 212.

Compilations of Environmental Fate Data

Howard PH: *Handbook of Environmental Fate and Exposure Data for Organic Chemicals* (several volumes). Chelsea, MI: Lewis Publishers, 1989.

Hutzinger O (ed.): *The Handbooks of Environmental Chemistry* (several volumes and years). Berlin: Springer-Verlag.

Mackay D, Shiu WY, Ma KC: *Illustrated Handbook of Physical–Chemical Properties and Environmental Fate for Organic Chemicals* (several volumes). Chelsea, MI: Lewis Publishers, 1993.

ECOLOGICAL RISK ASSESSMENT

17

DAMIAN SHEA

17.1

INTRODUCTION

Risk assessment is the process of assigning magnitudes and probabilities to adverse effects associated with an event. The development of risk assessment methodology has focused on accidental events (eg, an airplane crash) and specific environmental stresses to humans (eg, the exposure of humans to chemicals), and thus most risk assessment is characterized by discrete events or stresses affecting well-defined endpoints (eg, the incidence of human death or cancer). This *single stress–single endpoint* relationship allows the use of relatively simple statistical and mechanistic models to estimate risk and is widely used in human health risk assessment. However, this simple paradigm has only partial applicability to ecological risk assessment because of the inherent complexity of ecological systems and the exposure to numerous physical, chemical, and biologic stresses that have both direct and indirect effects on a diversity of ecological components, processes, and endpoints. Thus, the roots of ecological risk assessment can be found in human health risk assessment, but the methodology for ecological risk assessment is not well developed and the estimated risks are highly uncertain. In spite of these limitations, resource managers and regulators are looking to ecological risk assessment to provide a scientific basis for prioritizing problems that pose the greatest ecological risk and to focus research efforts in areas that will yield the greatest reduction in uncertainty.

To this end, the US Environmental Protection Agency (EPA) has issued guidelines for planning and conducting ecological risk assessments. Because of the complexity and uncertainty associated with ecological risk assessment, the EPA guidelines provide only a loose framework for organizing and analyzing data, assumptions, and uncertainties to evaluate the likelihood of adverse ecological effects. However, the guidelines represent a broad consensus of the present scientific knowledge and ex-

431

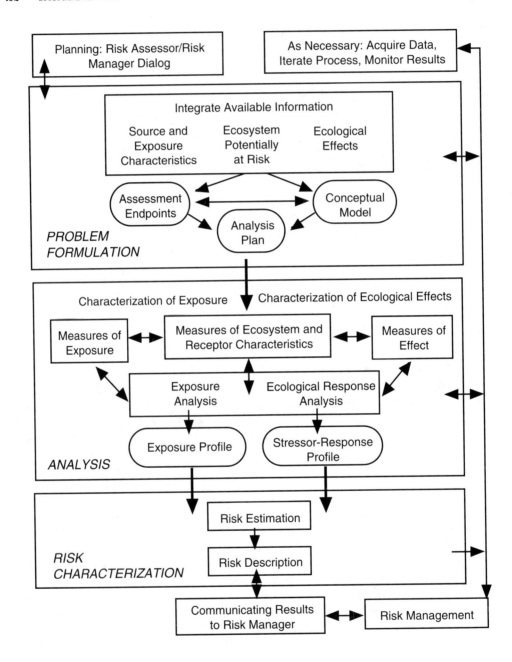

Figure 17.1. The ecological risk assessment framework as set forth by the US Environmental Protection Agency.

perience on ecological risk assessment. This chapter presents a brief overview of the ecological risk assessment process as presently described by the EPA.

Ecological risk assessment can be defined as *the process that evaluates the likelihood that adverse ecological effects may occur or are occurring as a result of exposure to one or more stressors*. Estimating the *likelihood* can range from qualitative judgments to quantitative probabilities, although quantitative risk estimates are still rare in ecological risk assessment. The *adverse ecological effects* are changes that are considered undesirable because they alter valued structural or functional characteristics of ecological systems and usually include the type, intensity, and scale of the effect as well as the potential for recovery. The statement that effects *may occur or are occurring* refers to the dual *prospective* and *retrospective* nature of ecological risk assessment. The inclusion of *one or more stressors* is a recognition that ecological risk assessments may address single or multiple chemical, physical, and/or biologic stressors. Because risk assessments are conducted to provide input to management decisions, most risk assessments focus on stressors generated or influenced by anthropogenic activity. However, natural phenomena also will induce stress that results in adverse ecological effects and cannot be ignored.

The overall ecological risk assessment process is shown in Fig. 17.1 and includes three primary phases: (1) problem formulation, (2) analysis, and (3) risk characterization. Problem formulation includes the development of a conceptual model of stressor–ecosystem interactions and the identification of risk assessment endpoints. The analysis phase involves evaluating exposure to stressors and the relationship between stressor characteristics and ecological effects. Risk characterization includes estimating risk through integration of exposure and stressor–response profiles, describing risk by establishing lines of evidence and determining ecological effects, and communicating this description to risk managers. Although discussions between risk assessors and risk managers are emphasized at both risk assessment initiation (planning) and completion (communicating results), usually a clear distinction is drawn between risk assessment and risk management. Risk assessment focuses on evaluating the likelihood of adverse effects scientifically, and risk management involves the selection of a course of action in response to an identified risk that is based on many factors (eg, social, legal, economic) in addition to the risk assessment results. Monitoring and other data acquisition are often necessary during any phase of the risk assessment process and the entire process is typically iterative rather than linear. The evaluation of new data or information may require revisiting a part of the process or conducting a new assessment.

17.2

FORMULATING THE PROBLEM

Problem formulation is a process for generating and evaluating preliminary hypotheses about why ecological effects have occurred, or may occur, because of human activities. During problem formulation, management goals are evaluated to help establish objectives for the risk assessment, the ecological problem is defined, and the plan for analyzing data and characterizing risk is developed. The objective of this process is to develop (1) assessment endpoints that adequately reflect management goals and the ecosystem they represent, and (2) conceptual models that describe critical relationships between a stressor and assessment endpoint or among several stressors and assessment endpoints. The assessment endpoints and the conceptual models are then integrated to develop a plan or proposal for risk analysis.

17.2.1 Selecting Assessment Endpoints

Assessment endpoints are *explicit expressions of the actual environmental value that is to be protected* and they link the risk assessment to management concerns. Assessment endpoints include both a valued or key ecological entity and an attribute of that entity that is important to protect and that is potentially at risk. The scientific basis for a risk assessment is enhanced when assessment endpoints are both ecologically relevant and susceptible to the stressors of concern. Assessment endpoints that also logically represent societal values and management goals increase the likelihood that the risk assessment will be understood and used in management decisions.

17.2.1.1 Ecological Relevance

Ecologically relevant endpoints reflect important attributes of the ecosystem and can be related functionally to other components of the ecosystem; they help sustain the structure, function, and biodiversity of an ecosystem. For example, ecologically relevant endpoints might contribute to the food base (eg, primary production), provide habitat, promote regeneration of critical resources (eg, nutrient cycling), or reflect the structure of the community, ecosystem, or landscape (eg, species diversity). Ecological relevance becomes most useful when it is possible to identify the potential cascade of adverse effects that could result from a critical initiating effect such as a change in ecosystem function. The selection of assessment endpoints that address both specific organisms of concern and landscape-level ecosystem processes becomes increasingly important (and more difficult) in landscape-level risk assessments. In these cases, it may be possible to select one or more species and an ecosystem process to represent larger functional community or ecosystem processes. Extrapolations like these must be explicitly described in the conceptual model (see Section 17.2.2).

17.2.1.2 Susceptibility to Stressors

Ecological resources or entities are considered susceptible if they are sensitive to a human-induced stressor to which they are exposed. *Sensitivity* represents how readily an ecological entity responds to a particular stressor. Measures of sensitivity may include mortality or decreased growth or fecundity resulting from exposure to a toxicant, or behavioral abnormalities such as avoidance of food-source areas or nesting sites because of the proximity of stressors such as noise or habitat alteration. Sensitivity is directly related to the mode of action of the stressors. For example, chemical sensitivity is influenced by individual physiology, genetics, and metabolism. Sensitivity also is influenced by individual and community life-history characteristics. For example, species with long life cycles and low reproductive rates are more vulnerable to extinction from increases in mortality than are species with short life cycles and high reproductive rates. Species with large home ranges may be more sensitive to habitat fragmentation compared to those species with smaller home ranges within a fragment. Sensitivity may be related to the life stage of an organism when exposed to a stressor. Young animals often are more sensitive to stressors than are adults. In addition, events like migration and molting often increase sensitivity because they require significant energy expenditure that make these organisms more vulnerable to stressors. Sensitivity also may be increased by the presence of other stressors or natural disturbances.

Exposure is the other key determinant in susceptibility. In ecological terms, exposure can mean co-occurrence, contact, or the absence of contact, depending on the stressor and assessment endpoint. The characteristics and conditions of exposure influence how an ecological entity responds to a stressor and thus determine what ecological entities might be susceptible. Therefore, one must consider information on the proximity of an ecological entity to the stressor along with the timing (eg, frequency and duration relative to sensitive life stages) and intensity of exposure. Note that adverse effects may be observed even at very low stressor exposures if a necessary resource is limited during a critical life stage. For example, if fish are unable to find suitable nesting sites during their reproductive phase, risk is significant even when water quality is high and food sources are abundant.

Exposure may take place at one point in space and time, but effects may not arise until another place or time. Both life history characteristics and the circumstances of exposure influence susceptibility in this case. For example, exposure of a population to endocrine modulating chemicals can affect the sex ratio of offspring, but the population impacts of this exposure may not become apparent until years later, when the cohort of affected animals begins to reproduce. Delayed effects and multiple stressor exposures add complexity to evaluations of susceptibility. For example, although toxicity tests may determine receptor sensitivity to one stressor, the degree of susceptibility may depend on the co-occurrence of another stressor that alters receptor response significantly. Again, conceptual models need to reflect these additional factors.

17.2.1.3 Defining Assessment Endpoints

Assessment endpoints provide a transition between management goals and the specific measures used in an assessment by helping to identify measurable attributes to quantify and model. However, in contrast to management goals, no intrinsic value is assigned to the endpoint so it does not contain words such as *protect* or *maintain,* and it does not indicate a desirable direction for change. Two aspects are required to define an assessment endpoint. The first is the valued ecological entity such as a species, a functional group of species, an ecosystem function or characteristic, or a specific valued habitat. The second is the characteristic about the entity of concern that is important to protect and potentially at risk.

Expert judgment and an understanding of the characteristics and function of an ecosystem are important for translating general goals into usable assessment endpoints. Endpoints that are too broad and vague (ecological health) cannot be linked to specific measurements. Endpoints that are too narrowly defined (hatching success of bald eagles) may overlook important characteristics of the ecosystem and fail to include critical variables. Clearly defined assessment endpoints provide both direction and boundaries for the risk assessment.

Assessment endpoints directly influence the type, characteristics, and interpretation of data and information used for analysis and the scale and character of the assessment. For example, an assessment endpoint such as "fecundity of bivalves" defines local population characteristics and requires very different types of data and ecosystem characterization compared with "aquatic community structure and function." When concerns are on a local scale, the assessment endpoints should not focus on landscape concerns. However, if ecosystem processes and landscape patterns are being considered, survival of a single species would provide inadequate representation of this larger scale.

The presence of multiple stressors also influences the selection of assessment endpoints. When it is possible to select one assessment endpoint that is sensitive to many of the identified stressors, yet responds in different ways to different stressors, it is possible to consider the combined effects of multiple stressors while still discriminating among effects. For example, if recruitment of a fish population is the assessment endpoint, it is important to recognize that recruitment may be adversely affected at several life stages, in different habitats, through different ways, by different stressors. The measures of effect, exposure, and ecosystem and receptor characteristics chosen to evaluate recruitment provide a basis for discriminating among different stressors, individual effects, and their combined effect.

Although many potential assessment endpoints may be identified, practical considerations often drive their selection. For example, assessment endpoints usually must reflect environmental values that are protected by law or that environmental managers and the general public recognize as a critical resource, or an ecological function that would be significantly impaired if the resource were altered. Another example of a practical consideration is the extrapolation across scales of time, space, or level of biologic organization. When the attributes of an assessment endpoint can be measured directly, extrapolation is unnecessary and this uncertainty is avoided. Assessment endpoints that cannot be linked with measurable attributes are not appropriate for a risk assessment. However, assessment endpoints that cannot be measured directly but can be represented by surrogate measures that are easily monitored and modeled can still provide a good foundation for the risk assessment.

17.2.2   Developing Conceptual Models

Conceptual models link anthropogenic activities with stressors and evaluate the relationships among exposure pathways, ecological effects, and ecological receptors. The models also may describe natural processes that influence these relationships.

Conceptual models include a set of risk hypotheses that describe predicted relationships between stressor, exposure, and assessment endpoint response, along with the rationale for their selection. Risk hypotheses are hypotheses in the broad scientific sense; they do not necessarily involve statistical testing of null and alternative hypotheses or any particular analytical approach. Risk hypotheses may predict the effects of a stressor or they may postulate what stressors may have caused observed ecological effects.

Diagrams can be used to illustrate the relationships described by the conceptual model and risk hypotheses. Conceptual model diagrams are useful tools for communicating important pathways and for identifying major sources of uncertainty. These diagrams and risk hypotheses can be used to identify the most important pathways and relationships to consider in the analysis phase. The hypotheses considered most likely to contribute to risk are identified for subsequent evaluation in the risk assessment.

The complexity of the conceptual model depends on the complexity of the problem, number of stressors and assessment endpoints being considered, nature of effects, and characteristics of the ecosystem. For single stressors and single assessment endpoints, conceptual models can be relatively simple relationships. In cases in which conceptual models describe both the pathways of individual stressors and assessment endpoints and the interaction of multiple and diverse stressors and assessment endpoints, several submodels would be required to describe individual pathways. Other models may then be used to explore how these individual pathways interact. An example of a conceptual model for a watershed in shown in Fig. 17.2.

17.2.3   Selecting Measures

The last step in the problem formulation phase is the development of an analysis plan or proposal that identifies measures to evaluate each risk hypothesis and that describes the assessment design, data needs, assumptions, extrapolations, and specific methods for conducting the analysis. There are three categories of measures that can be selected. *Measures of effect* (also called *measurement endpoints*) are measures used to evaluate the response of the assessment endpoint when exposed to a stressor. *Measures of exposure* are measures of how exposure may be occurring, including how a stressor moves through the environment and how it may co-occur with the assessment endpoint. *Measures of ecosystem and receptor characteristics* include ecosystem characteristics that influence the behavior and location of assessment endpoints, the distribution of a stressor, and life history characteristics of the assessment endpoint that may affect exposure or response to the stressor. These diverse measures increase in importance as the complexity of the assessment increases.

An important consideration in the identification of these measures is their response sensitivity and ecosystem relevance. Response sensitivity is usually highest with measures at the lower levels of biologic organization, but the ecosystem rele-

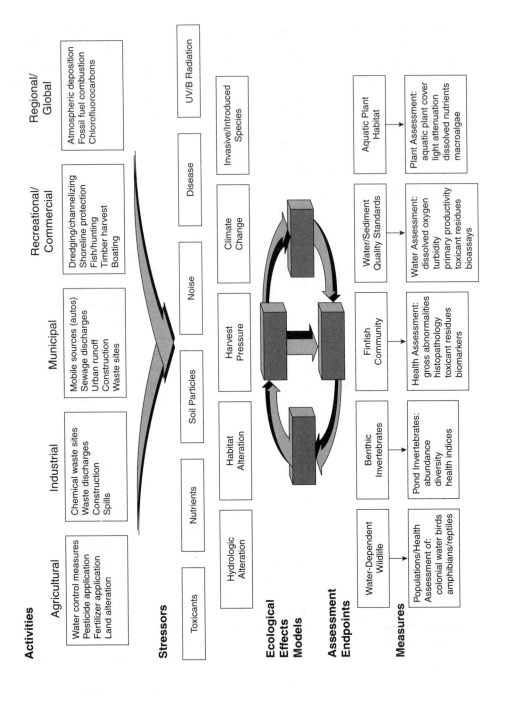

Figure 17.2. An example of a conceptual model for a watershed. Human activities, shown at the top of diagram, result in various stressors that induce ecological effects. Assessment endpoints and related measures that are associated with these effects are shown at the bottom of the diagram.

438

vance is highest at the higher levels of biologic organization. This dichotomy is illustrated in Fig. 17.3. In general, the time required to ellicit a response also increases with the level of biologic organization. Note that toxicologists focus on measures at lower levels of biologic organization, relying on an extrapolation based on the tenet that effects of toxicants on populations and communities are initiated at the molecular–cellular level, and if this insult is not corrected for or adapted to, then effects on physiological systems and individual organisms result. For certain toxic modes of action (eg, reproductive toxicity), this could result in effects at the population and community levels. In contrast, ecologists focus on measures at the popula-

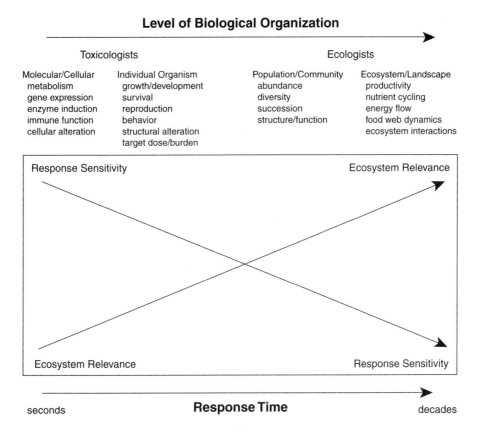

Figure 17.3. The response time and sensitivity of an ecological receptor is a function of the level of biologic organization. Higher levels of organization have greater ecosystem relevance. However, as the level of biologic organization increases, response time increases, sensitivity decreases, and causal relationships become more uncertain. Ecological risk assessments must balance the need for sensitive, timely, and well-established responses with ecological relevance.

tion level or higher for obvious reasons of ecological relevance. Often, a combination of measures is necessary to provide reasonable sensitivity, ecosystem relevance, and causal relationships.

17.3
ANALYZING EXPOSURE AND EFFECTS INFORMATION

The second phase of ecological risk assessment, the analysis phase, includes two principal activities: characterization of exposure and characterization of ecological effects (Fig. 17.1).

17.3.1 Characterizing Exposure

In exposure characterization, credible and relevant data are analyzed to describe the source(s) of stressors, the distribution of stressors in the environment, and the contact or co-occurrence of stressors with ecological receptors. An exposure profile is developed that identifies receptors and exposure pathways, describes the intensity and spatial and temporal extent of exposure, describes the impact of variability and uncertainty on exposure estimates, and presents a conclusion about the likelihood that exposure will occur.

A source description identifies where the stressor originates, describes what stressors are generated, and considers other sources of the stressor. Exposure analysis may start with the source when it is known, but some analyses may begin with known exposures and attempt to link them to sources, whereas other analyses may start with known stressors and attempt to identify sources and quantify contact or co-occurrence. The source description includes what is known about the intensity, timing, and location of the stressor and whether other constituents emitted by the source influence transport, transformation, or bioavailability of the stressor of interest.

Many stressors have natural counterparts and/or multiple sources that must be considered. For example, many chemicals occur naturally (eg, most metals), are generally widespread due to multiple sources (eg, polycyclic aromatic hydrocarbons), or may have significant sources outside the boundaries of the current assessment (eg, regional atmospheric deposition of PCBs). Many physical stressors also have natural counterparts such as sedimentation from construction activities versus natural erosion. In addition, human activities may change the magnitude or frequency of natural disturbance cycles, such as the frequency and severity of flooding. Source characterization can be particularly important for new biologic stressors (eg, invasive species), because many of the strategies for reducing risks focus on preventing entry in the first place. Once the source is identified, the likelihood of entry may be characterized qualitatively.

Because exposure occurs where receptors co-occur with or contact stressors in the environment, characterizing the spatial and temporal distribution of a stressor is a necessary precursor to estimating exposure. The stressor's spatial and temporal distribution in the environment is described by evaluating the pathways that stressors take from the source as well as the formation and subsequent distribution of secondary stressors. For chemical stressors, the evaluation of pathways usually follows the type of transport and fate modeling described in Chapter 16. Some physical stressors such as sedimentation also can be modeled, but other physical stressors require no modeling because they eliminate entire ecosystems or portions of them, such as when a wetland is filled, a resource is harvested, or an area is flooded.

The movement of biologic stressors has been described as diffusion and/ or jump-dispersal processes. Diffusion involves a gradual spread from the site of introduction and is a function primarily of reproductive rates and motility. Jump-dispersal involves erratic spreads over periods of time, usually by means of a vector. The gypsy moth and zebra mussel have spread in this manner—the gypsy moth via egg masses on vehicles and the zebra mussel via boat ballast water. Biologic stressors can use both diffusion and jump-dispersal strategies, which makes it difficult to predict dispersal rates. An additional complication is that biologic stressors are influenced by their own survival and reproduction.

The creation of secondary stressors can greatly alter risk. Secondary stressors can be formed through biotic or abiotic transformation processes and may be of greater or lesser concern than the primary stressor. Physical disturbances can generate secondary stressors, such as when the removal of riparian vegetation results in increased nutrients, sedimentation, and altered stream flow. For chemicals, the evaluation of secondary stressors usually focuses on metabolites or degradation products. In addition, secondary stressors can be formed through ecosystem processes. For example, nutrient inputs into an estuary can decrease dissolved oxygen concentrations because they increase primary production and subsequent decomposition. A changeover from an aerobic to an anaerobic environment often is accompanied by the production of sulfide via sulfate reducing bacteria. Sulfide can act as a secondary stressor to oxygen-dependent organisms, but it also can reduce exposure to metals through the precipitation of metal sulfides (see Chapter 16).

The distribution of stressors in the environment can be described using measurements or models or a combination of the two. If stressors have already been released, direct measurements of environmental media or a combination of modeling and measurement is preferred. However, a modeling approach may be necessary if the assessment is intended to predict future scenarios or if measurements are not possible or practicable.

17.3.2   Characterizing Ecological Effects

In ecological effects characterization, relevant data are analyzed to evaluate stressor–response relationships and/or to provide evidence that exposure to a stressor causes an observed response. The characterization describes the effects that are elicited by a stressor, links these effects with the assessment endpoints, and evaluates how the effects change with varying stressor levels. The conclusions of the ecological effects characterization are summarized in a stressor–response profile.

17.3.2.1   Analyzing Ecological Response

Ecological response analysis has three primary components: determining the relationship between stressor exposure and ecological effects, evaluating the plausibility that effects may occur or are occurring as a result of the exposure, and linking measurable ecological effects with the assessment endpoints.

Evaluating ecological risks requires an understanding of the relationships between stressor exposure and resulting ecological responses. The stressor–response relationships used in a particular assessment depend on the scope and nature of the ecological risk assessment as defined in problem formulation and reflected in the analysis plan. For example, a point estimate of an effect (such as an LC50) might be compared with point estimates from other stressors. The stressor–response function (eg, shape of the curve) may be critical for determining the presence or absence of an effects threshold or for evaluating incremental risks, or stressor–response functions may be used as input for ecological effects models. If sufficient data are available, cumulative distribution functions can be constructed using multiple point estimates of effects. Process models that already incorporate empirically derived stressor–response functions also can be used. However, many stressor–response relationships are very complex, and ecological systems frequently show responses to stressors that involve abrupt shifts to new community or system types.

In simple cases, the response will be one variable (eg, mortality) and quantitative univariate analysis can be used. If the response of interest is composed of many individual variables (eg, species abundances in an aquatic community), multivariate statistical techniques must be used. Multivariate techniques (eg, factor and cluster analysis) have a long history of use in ecology but have not yet been applied extensively in risk assessment. Stressor–response relationships can be described using any of the dimensions of exposure (ie, intensity, time, or space). Intensity is probably the most familiar dimension and is often used for chemicals (eg, dose, concentration). The duration of exposure also can be used for chemical stressor–response relationships; for example, median acute effects levels are always associated with a time parameter (eg, 24 hr, 48 hr, 96 hr). Both the time and spatial dimensions of exposure can be important for physical disturbances such as flooding. Single-point estimates and stressor–response curves can be generated for some biologic stressors. For pathogens such as bacteria and fungi, inoculum levels may be related to the level of symptoms in a host or actual signs of the pathogen. For other biological stressors such as introduced species, developing simple stressor–response relationships may be inappropriate.

Causality is the relationship between cause (one or more stressors) and effect (assessment endpoint response to one or more stressors). Without a sound basis for linking cause and effect, uncertainty in the conclusions of an ecological risk assessment will be high. Developing causal relationships is especially important for risk assessments driven by observed adverse ecological effects such as fish kills or long-term declines in a population. Criteria need to be established for evaluating causality. For chemicals, ecotoxicologists have slightly modified Koch's postulates to provide evidence of causality:

1. The injury, dysfunction, or other putative effect of the toxicant must be regularly associated with exposure to the toxicant and any contributory causal factors.
2. Indicators of exposure to the toxicant must be found in the affected organisms.
3. The toxic effects must be seen when normal organisms or communities are exposed to the toxicant under controlled conditions, and any contributory factors should be manifested in the same way during controlled exposures.
4. The same indicators of exposure and effects must be identified in the controlled exposures as in the field.

Although useful as an ideal, this approach may not be practical if resources for experimentation are not available or if an adverse effect may be occurring over such a wide spatial extent that experimentation and correlation may prove difficult or yield equivocal results. In most cases, extrapolation will be necessary to evaluate causality. The scope of the risk assessment also influences extrapolation through the nature of the assessment endpoint. Preliminary assessments that evaluate risks to general trophic levels, such as fish and birds, may extrapolate among different genera or families to obtain a range of sensitivity to the stressor. However, assessments concerned with management strategies for a particular species may employ population models.

Whatever methods are employed to link assessment endpoints with measures of effect, it is important to apply the methods in a manner consistent with sound ecological and toxicological principles. For example, it is inappropriate to use structure–activity relationships to predict toxicity from chemical structure unless the chemical under consideration has a similar mode of toxic action to the reference chemicals. Similarly, extrapolations from upland avian species to waterfowl may be more credible if factors such as differences in food preferences, physiology, and seasonal behavior (eg, mating and migration habits) are considered.

Finally, many extrapolation methods are limited by the availability of suitable databases. Although these databases are generally largest for chemical stressors and aquatic species, even in these cases data do not exist for all taxa or effects. Chemical effects databases for mammals, amphibians, or reptiles are extremely limited, and there is even less information on most biologic and physical stressors. Extrapolations and models are only as useful as the data on which they are based and should recognize the great uncertainties associated with extrapolations that lack an adequate empirical or process-based rationale.

17.3.2.2 Developing a Stressor–Response Profile

The final activity of the ecological response analysis is developing a stressor–response profile to evaluate single species, populations, general trophic levels, communities, ecosystems, or landscapes—whatever is appropriate for the defined assessment endpoints. For example, if a single species is affected, effects should represent appropriate parameters such as effects on mortality, growth, and reproduction, whereas at the community level, effects may be summarized in terms of structure or function depending on the assessment endpoint. At the landscape level, there may be a suite of assessment endpoints and each should be addressed separately. The stressor–response profile summarizes the nature and intensity of effect(s), the time scale for recovery (where appropriate), causal information linking the stressor with observed effects, and uncertainties associated with the analysis.

17.4

CHARACTERIZING RISK

Risk characterization is the final phase of an ecological risk assessment (Fig. 17.1). During risk characterization, risks are estimated and interpreted and the strengths, limitations, assumptions, and major uncertainties are summarized. Risks are estimated by integrating exposure and stressor–response profiles using a wide range of techniques such as comparisons of point estimates or distributions of exposure and effects data, process models, or empirical approaches such as field observational data. Risks are described by evaluating the evidence supporting or refuting the risk estimate(s) and interpreting the adverse effects on the assessment endpoint. Criteria for evaluating adversity include the nature and intensity of effects, spatial and temporal scales, and the potential for recovery. Agreement among different lines of evidence of risk increases confidence in the conclusions of a risk assessment.

17.4.1   Estimating Risk

Risk estimation determines the likelihood of adverse effects to assessment endpoints by integrating exposure and effects data and evaluating any associated uncertainties. The process uses the exposure and stressor–response profiles. Risks can be estimated by one or more of the following approaches: (1) estimates based on best professional judgment and expressed as qualitative categories such as low, medium, or high; (2) estimates comparing single-point estimates of exposure and effects such as a simple ratio of exposure concentration to effects concentration (quotient method); (3) estimates incorporating the entire stressor–response relationship often as a nonlinear function of exposure; (4) estimates incorporating variability in exposure and effects estimates providing the capability to predict changes in the magnitude and likelihood of effects at different exposure scenarios; (5) estimates based on process models that rely partially or entirely on theoretical approximations of exposure and effects; and (6) estimates based on empirical approaches, including field observational data. An example of the first approach, using qualitative categorization, is shown in Fig. 17.4

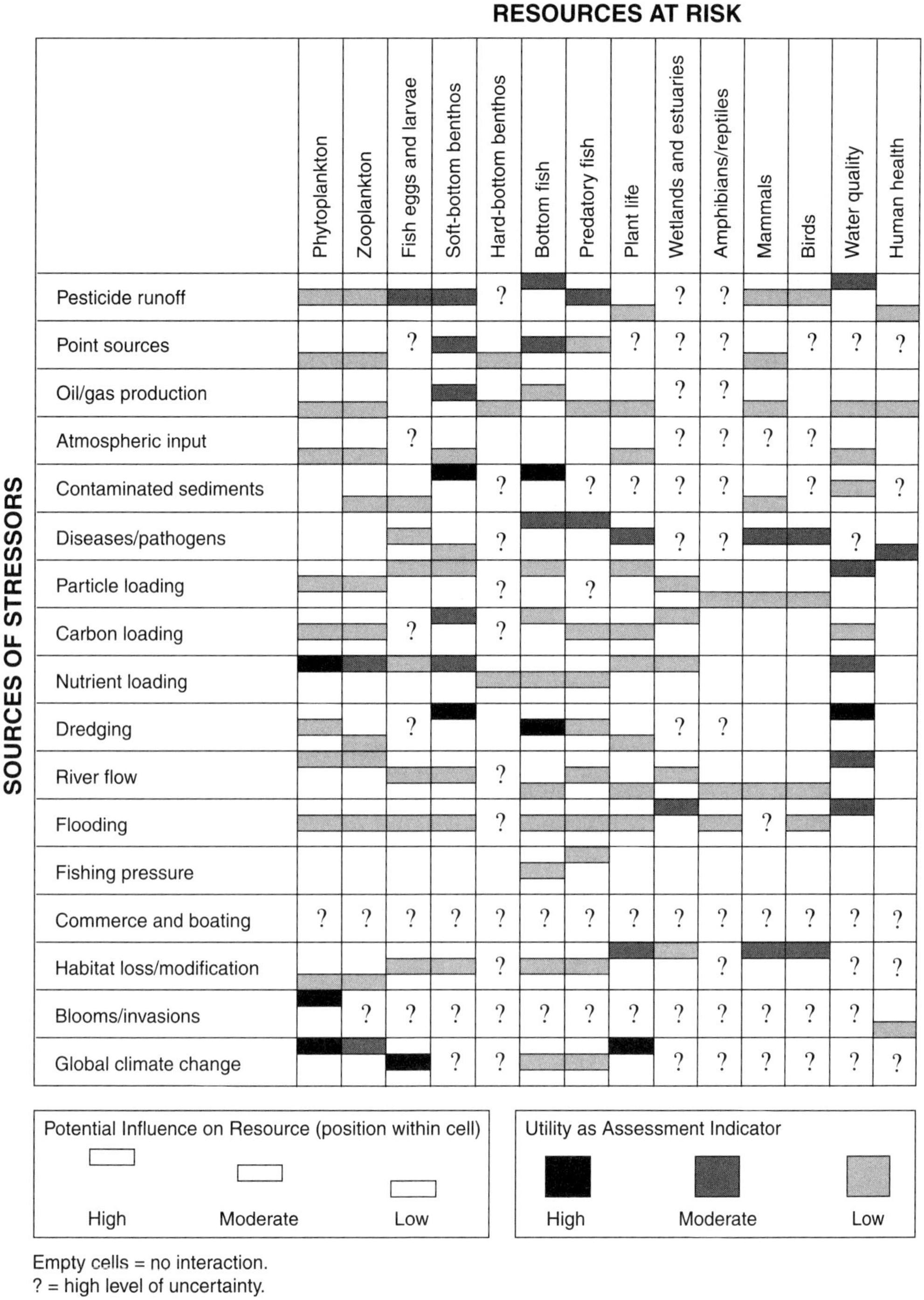

Figure 17.4. An example of a qualitative categorization of ecological risk for a hypothetical matrix of stressors and resources at risk.

17.4.2   Describing Risk

After risks have been estimated, available information must be integrated and inter-preted to form conclusions about risks to the assessment endpoints. Risk descrip-tions include an evaluation of the lines of evidence supporting or refuting the risk estimate(s) and an interpretation of the adverse effects on the assessment endpoint. Confidence in the conclusions of a risk assessment may be increased by using sev-eral lines of evidence to interpret and compare risk estimates. These lines of evi-dence may be derived from different sources or by different techniques relevant to adverse effects on the assessment endpoints, such as quotient estimates, modeling results, field experiments, or field observations. Some of the factors to consider when evaluating separate lines of evidence are

- The relevance of evidence to the assessment endpoints
- The relevance of evidence to the conceptual model
- The sufficiency and quality of data and experimental designs used in sup-porting studies
- The strength of cause–effect relationships
- The relative uncertainties of each line of evidence and their direction

At this point in risk characterization, the changes expected in the assessment endpoints have been estimated and described. The next step is to interpret whether these changes are considered adverse and meaningful. Meaningful adverse changes are defined by ecological and/or social concerns and, thus, usually depend on the best professional judgment of the risk assessor. Five criteria have been proposed by the EPA for evaluating adverse changes in assessment endpoints and are as follows:

1. Nature of effects
2. Intensity of effects
3. Spatial scale
4. Temporal scale
5. Potential for recovery

The extent to which the five criteria are evaluated depends on the scope and com-plexity of the ecological risk assessment. However, understanding the underlying assumptions and science policy judgments is important even in simple cases. For example, when exceedance of a previously established decision rule such as a benchmark stressor level or water quality criteria is used as evidence of adversity, the reasons why exceedences of the benchmark are considered adverse should be understood clearly.

To distinguish ecological changes that are adverse from those ecological events that are within the normal pattern of ecosystem variability or result in little or no meaningful alteration of biota, it is important to consider the nature and intensity of effects. For example, an assessment endpoint involving survival, growth, and re-production of a species must consider whether predicted effects involve survival and reproduction or only growth; or, if survival of offspring are affected, the relative loss must be considered.

It is important to consider both the ecological and statistical contexts of an effect when evaluating intensity. For example, a statistically significant 1% decrease in fish growth may not be relevant to an assessment endpoint of fish population viability, and a 10% decline in reproduction may be worse for a population of slowly reproducing marine mammals than for rapidly reproducing planktonic algae.

Natural ecosystem variation can make it very difficult to observe (detect) stressor-related perturbations. For example, natural fluctuations in marine fish populations, often very large and cyclic events (eg, fish migration), are very important in natural systems. Predicting the effects of anthropogenic stressors against this background of variation can be very difficult. Thus, a lack of statistically significant effects in a field study does not automatically mean that adverse ecological effects are absent. Rather, factors such as statistical power to detect differences, natural variability, and other lines of evidence must be considered in reaching conclusions about risk.

Spatial and temporal scales also need to be considered in assessing the adversity of the effects. The spatial dimension encompasses both the extent and pattern of effect, as well as the context of the effect within the landscape. Factors to consider include the absolute area affected, the extent of critical habitats affected compared with a larger area of interest, and the role or use of the affected area within the landscape. Adverse effects to assessment endpoints vary with the absolute area of the effect. A larger affected area may be (1) subject to a greater number of other stressors, increasing the complications from stressor interactions; (2) more likely to contain sensitive species or habitats; or (3) more susceptible to landscape-level changes because many ecosystems may be altered by the stressors.

Nevertheless, a smaller area of effect is not always associated with lower risk. The function of an area within the landscape may be more important than the absolute area. Destruction of small but unique areas, such as submerged vegetation at the land–water margin, may have important effects on local wildlife populations. Also, in river systems, both riffle and pool areas provide important microhabitats that maintain the structure and function of the total river ecosystem. Stressors acting on some of these microhabitats may present a significant risk to the entire system. Spatial factors also are important for many species because of the linkages between ecological landscapes and population dynamics. Linkages between one or more landscapes can provide refuge for affected populations, and species may require adequate corridors between habitat patches for successful migration.

The temporal scale for ecosystems can vary from seconds (photosynthesis, prokaryotic reproduction) to centuries (global climate change). Changes within a forest ecosystem can occur gradually over decades or centuries and may be affected by slowly changing external factors such as climate. The time scale of stressor-induced changes operates within the context of multiple natural time scales. In addition, temporal responses for ecosystems may involve intrinsic time lags, so that responses from a stressor may be delayed. Thus, it is important to distinguish the long-term impacts of a stressor from the immediately visible effects. For example, visible changes resulting from eutrophication of aquatic systems (eg, turbidity, excessive macrophyte growth, population decline) may not become evident for many years after initial increases in nutrient levels.

Considering the temporal scale of adverse effects leads us to a consideration of recovery. Recovery is the rate and extent of return of a population or community to a condition that existed before the introduction of a stressor. Because ecosystems are dynamic and even under natural conditions are constantly changing in response to changes in the physical environment (weather, natural catastrophes, etc.) or other factors, it is unrealistic to expect that a system will remain static at some level or return to exactly the same state that it was before it was disturbed. Thus, the attributes of a "recovered" system must be defined carefully. Examples might include productivity declines in an eutrophic system, reestablishment of a species at a particular density, species recolonization of a damaged habitat, or the restoration of health of diseased organisms.

Recovery can be evaluated in spite of the difficulty in predicting events in ecological systems. For example, it is possible to distinguish changes that are usually reversible (eg, recovery of a stream from sewage effluent discharge), frequently irreversible (eg, establishment of introduced species), and always irreversible (eg, species extinction). It is important to consider whether significant structural or functional changes have occurred in a system that might render changes irreversible. For example, physical alterations such as deforestation can change soil structure and seed sources such that forests cannot grow again easily.

Natural disturbance patterns can be very important when evaluating the likelihood of recovery from anthropogenic stressors. Ecosystems that have been subjected to repeated natural disturbances may be more vulnerable to anthropogenic stressors (eg, overfishing). Alternatively, if an ecosystem has become adapted to a disturbance pattern, it may be affected when the disturbance is removed (eg, fire-maintained grasslands). The lack of natural analogues makes it difficult to predict recovery from novel anthropogenic stressors such as exposure to synthetic chemicals.

The relative rate of recovery also can be estimated. For example, fish populations in a stream are likely to recover much faster from exposure to a degradable chemical than from habitat alterations resulting from stream channelization. It is critical to use knowledge of factors such as the temporal scales of organisms' life histories, the availability of adequate stock for recruitment, and the interspecific and trophic dynamics of the populations in evaluating the relative rates of recovery. A fisheries stock or forest might recover in several decades, a benthic infaunal community in years, and a planktonic community in weeks to months.

17.5

MANAGING RISK

When risk characterization is complete, a description of the risk assessment is communicated to the risk manager (Fig. 17.1) to support a risk management decision. This communication is usually a report and might include:

- A description of risk assessor–risk manager planning results
- A review of the conceptual model and the assessment endpoints
- A discussion of the major data sources and analytical procedures used
- A review of the stressor–response and exposure profiles
- A description of risks to the assessment endpoints, including risk estimates and adversity evaluations
- A summary of major areas of uncertainty and the approaches used to address them
- A discussion of science policy judgments or default assumptions used to bridge information gaps, and the basis for these assumptions

After the risk assessment is completed, risk managers may consider whether additional follow-up activities are required. Depending on the importance of the assessment, confidence level in the assessment results, and available resources, it may be advisable to conduct another iteration of the risk assessment in order to facilitate a final management decision. Ecological risk assessments frequently are designed in sequential tiers that proceed from simple and relatively inexpensive evaluations to more costly and complex assessments. Initial tiers are based on conservative assumptions, such as maximum exposure and ecological sensitivity. When an early tier cannot define risk sufficiently to support a management decision, a higher assessment tier that may require either additional data or applying more refined analysis techniques to available data may be needed. Higher tiers provide more ecologically realistic assessments while making less conservative assumptions about exposure and effects.

Another option is to proceed with a management decision based on the risk assessment and develop a monitoring plan to evaluate the results of the decision. For example, if the decision was to mitigate risks through exposure reduction, monitoring could help determine whether the desired reduction in exposure (and effects) was achieved. Monitoring is also critical for determining the extent and nature of any ecological recovery that may be occurring.

Ecological risk assessment is important for environmental decision making because of the high cost of eliminating environmental risks associated with human activities and the necessity of making regulatory decisions in the face of uncertainty. Ecological risk assessment provides only a portion of the information required to make risk management decisions, but this information is critical to scientifically defensible risk management. Thus, ecological risk assessments should provide input to a diverse set of environmental decision making processes, such as the regulation of hazardous waste sites, industrial chemicals, and pesticides, or the management of watersheds affected by multiple nonchemical and chemical stressors.

Suggested Further Reading

Bartell SM, Gardner RH, O'Neill RV: *Ecological Risk Estimation.* Boca Raton, FL: Lewis Publishers, 1992.

Cardwell RD, Parkhurst BR, Warren-Hicks W, Volosin JS: Aquatic ecological risk. *Water Environ Technol* **5:**47–51, 1993.

Harwell MA, Cooper W, Flaak R: Prioritizing ecological and human welfare risks from environmental stresses. *Environ Manag* **16**:451–464, 1993.

Kendall RJ, Lacher TE, Bunck C, Daniel B, Driver C, Grue CE, Leighton F, Stansley W, Watanabe PG, Whitworth M: An ecological risk assessment of lead shot exposure in non-waterfowl avian species: upland game birds and raptors. *Environ Toxicol Chem* **15**:4–20, 1996.

National Research Council: A paradigm for ecological risk assessment. In *Issues in Risk Assessment.* Washington, DC: National Academy Press, 1993

National Research Council: *Science and judgment in risk assessment.* Washington, DC: National Academy Press, 1994.

National Research Council: *Understanding risk: informing decisions in a democratic society.* Washington, DC: National Academy Press, 1996.

Ruckelshaus WD: Science, risk, and public policy. *Science* **221**:1026–1028, 1983.

Solomon KR, Baker DB, Richards RP, Dixon KR, Klaine SJ, La Point TW, Kendall RJ, Weisskopf CP, Giddings JM, Geisy JP, Hall LW, Williams WM: Ecological risk assessment of atrazine in North American surface waters. *Environ Toxicol Chem* **15**(1):31–76, 1996.

Suter GW II: Endpoints for regional ecological risk assessments. *Environ Manag* **14**:19–23, 1990.

Suter GW II: *Ecological risk assessment.* Boca Raton, FL: Lewis Publishers, 1993.

Suter GW II: A critique of ecosystem health concepts and indexes. *Environ Toxicol Chem* **12**:1533–1539, 1993.

US Environmental Protection Agency: Summary report on issues in ecological risk assessment. Washington, DC: Risk Assessment Forum, US Environmental Protection Agency. EPA/625/3-91/018, 1991.

US Environmental Protection Agency: Framework for ecological risk assessment. Washington, DC: Risk Assessment Forum, US Environmental Protection Agency. EPA/630/R-92/001, 1992.

US Environmental Protection Agency: Peer review workshop report on a framework for ecological risk assessment. Washington, DC: Risk Assessment Forum, US Environmental Protection Agency. EPA/625/3-91/022, 1992.

US Environmental Protection Agency: A review of ecological assessment case studies from a risk assessment perspective. Washington, DC: Risk Assessment Forum, US Environmental Protection Agency. EPA/630/R-92/005, 1993.

US Environmental Protection Agency: Ecological risk assessment issue papers. Washington, DC: Risk Assessment Forum, US Environmental Protection Agency. EPA/630/R-94/009, 1994.

US Environmental Protection Agency: Proposed Guidelines for ecological risk assessment. Washington, DC: Risk Assessment Forum, US Environmental Protection Agency. EPA/630/R-95/002B, 1996.

FUTURE CONSIDERATIONS FOR ENVIRONMENTAL AND HUMAN HEALTH

18

ERNEST HODGSON

18.1

INTRODUCTION

Speculation concerning future developments in toxicology can be made only against an assessment of where the science has come from and its current status. Toxicology, in spite of its use of many state-of-the-art techniques and exploration of the most fundamental molecular mechanisms of toxic action, is, at its heart, an applied science serving the needs of society. Society is served in two principal ways: the protection of human health and the protection of the environment. In both of these aspects two avenues are explored: studies of chemicals in use and the development of new chemicals that are both safe and effective. These studies range from studies of the mechanisms of toxic action to in vivo toxicity testing, but the ultimate goal is a meaningful assessment of risk resulting from exposure to the chemicals in question.

The vast increase in public awareness of the potential of chemicals to cause harmful effects and the propensity of the print and electronic media to fan the flames of controversy in this area make certain the continued need for toxicologists. We need to ask what they will be doing during the next few decades compared to what they have been doing in the immediate past.

Through the 1950s and 1960s, toxicology tended to be a largely descriptive science, relating the results of in vivo dosing to a variety of toxic endpoints, in many cases little more than the median lethal dose (LD50) or median lethal concentration (LC50). However, ongoing studies of xenobiotic-metabolizing enzymes were attracting more attention and techniques for chemical analysis of toxicants were starting to undergo a remarkable metamorphosis. The 1970s were most remarkable for developments in metabolism and the beginnings of a boom in mode of toxic action studies, whereas the 1980s and the 1990s have seen the incorporation of the techniques of molecular biology

451

into many aspects of toxicology, but perhaps to greatest effect in studies of the mechanisms of chemical carcinogenesis and the induction of xenobiotic-metabolizing enzymes. It should be emphasized that all of these activities proceed simultaneously, and that increased emphasis and interest in any particular area is often preceded by the development of new techniques—for example, the tremendous increase in specificity and sensitivity of chemical methods has proceeded simultaneously with the introduction of molecular biologic techniques into studies of mechanisms of toxic action.

The future, both immediate and long term, will provide important information on all aspects of toxic action and the role of toxicology in public life will mature as the importance of toxicology is perceived by the population in general, first in developed countries and ultimately around the world. The fundamental role of the toxicologist, namely the acquisition and dissemination of information about all aspects of the deleterious effects of chemicals on living organisms, will not change; however, the manner in which it is carried out will almost certainly change. The next several decades will be exciting times for toxicologists, and those in training at this time have much to anticipate.

Change can be expected in almost every aspect of both the applied and the fundamental aspects of toxicology: risk communication, risk assessment, hazard and exposure assessment, in vivo toxicity, development of selective chemicals, in vitro toxicology, and biochemical and molecular toxicology will all change, as will the integration of all of these areas into new paradigms of risk assessment and of the ways in which chemicals affect human health and the environment.

18.2

RISK MANAGEMENT

Public decisions concerning the use of chemicals will continue to be a blend of science, politics, and law, with the media spotlight continuing to shine on the most contentious aspects: The role of the trained toxicologist to serve as the source of scientifically sound information and as the voice of reason will be even more critical. As the chemist extends our ability to detect smaller and smaller amounts of toxicants in food, air, and water, the concept that science, including toxicology, does not deal in certainty but only in degrees of certitude must be made clear to all. Although this concept is easy for most scientists to grasp, it appears difficult, even arcane, to the general public and almost impossible to the average attorney or politician.

18.3

RISK ASSESSMENT

In the past, risk assessment has consisted largely of computer-based models written to start from hazard assessment assays, such as chronic toxicity assays on rodents, encompass the necessary extrapolations between species and between high and low doses, and then produce a numerical assessment of the risk to human health. Although the hazard assessment tests and the toxic endpoints are different, an analogous situation exists in environmental risk assessment. Although many of these risk-assessment programs were statistically sophisticated, they frequently did not rise above the level of number crunching, and more often than not, different risk assessment programs, starting with the same experimental values, produced very different numerical assessments of risk to human health or to the environment. The need to incorporate mechanistic data, including mode of action studies and physiologically based pharmacokinetics, has already been realized. The immediate future in risk assessment will focus on the difficult but necessary task of integrating experimental data from all levels into the risk-assessment process. A continuing challenge to toxicologists engaged in hazard or risk assessment is that of risk from chemical mixtures. Neither human beings nor ecosystems are exposed to chemicals one at a time, yet logic dictates that the initial assessment of toxicity start with individual chemicals. The resolution of this problem will require considerable work at all levels, in vivo and in vitro, into the implications of chemical interactions for the expression of toxicity, particularly chronic toxicity.

18.4

HAZARD AND EXPOSURE ASSESSMENT

The enormous cost of multispecies, multidose, lifetime evaluations of chronic effects has already made the task of carrying out hazard assessments of all chemicals in commercial use impossible. At the same time, quantative structure activity relationships (QSAR) studies are not yet predictive enough to indicate which chemicals should be so tested and which chemicals need not be tested. In exposure assessment, continued development of analytical methods will permit ever more sensitive and selective determinations of toxicants in food and the environment; values at the femtomole level are likely to become commonplace. Emphasis must be placed on the significance of such minute exposures on human health and the environment, as well as the effects of chemical mixtures and the potential for interactions that affect the ultimate expression of toxicity. Developments in QSAR, in short-term tests based on the expected mechanism of toxic action and simplification of chronic testing procedures, will all be necessary if the chemicals to which the public and the environment are exposed are to be assessed adequately for their potential to cause harm.

18.5

IN VIVO TOXICITY

Although developments continue in elucidating the mechanisms of chemical carcinogenicity much remains to be done with regard to this and other chronic endpoints, particularly developmental and reproductive toxicity, chronic neurotoxicity, and immunotoxicity. The further utilization of the methods of molecular biology should bring rapid advances in all of these areas. It will be a challenge to integrate all of this information into useful paradigms for responsible and meaningful risk assessments.

18.6

IN VITRO TOXICITY

In vitro studies of toxic mechanisms will depend heavily on developments in molecular biology, and great advances can be expected. Many of the ethical problems associated with carrying out studies on the effects of toxicants on humans will be circumvented at the in vitro level by the use of cloned and expressed human enzymes, receptors, ans so on, although the integration of these data into intact organism models will still require experimental animals.

18.7

BIOCHEMICAL AND MOLECULAR TOXICOLOGY

As indicated previously, contributions to all aspects of the mechanistic study of toxic action from the use of biochemical and molecular techniques can be expected. No doubt new techniques will be developed, answers will be found to many questions that did not yield to earlier techniques and new questions will be raised. The challenge, as always, will be to integrate the results from these studies—studies that will reach new levels of sophistication—into useful and productive approaches to reduce chemical effects on human health and the environment.

18.8

DEVELOPMENT OF SELECTIVE TOXICANTS

Almost all aspects of contemporary human society depend on the use of numerous chemicals. Except in the unlikely event that society decides to return to a more simplistic and, in fact, more primitive, more unhealthy, and more demanding lifestyle, the challenge is in learning how to live with anthropomorphic chemicals, not in learning how to live without them. In many aspects, such as the production of food and fiber and the maintenance of human health, the development of selective pesticides, drugs, and so on is needed. New techniques in molecular biology, in particularly the availability of cloned and expressed human enzymes and receptors and new knowledge of human polymorphisms, will make this task easier, as will similar knowledge of target species, including microorganisms causing human disease, and insects and weeds affecting the production of food and fiber, and so on.

GLOSSARY

....

acetylation. The addition of an acetyl group from acetyl coenzyme A to a xenobiotic or xenobiotic metabolite by the enzyme N-acetyltransferase. Polymorphisms in this enzyme can be important in the expression of toxicity in humans.

acetylator phenotype. Variation in the expression of N-acetyltransferase isoforms in humans gives rise to two subpopulations—fast and slow acetylators. Slow acetylators are more susceptible to the toxic effects of toxicants that are detoxified by acetylation.

acid deposition. Wet and dry air pollutants that lower the pH of deposition and subsequently the pH of the environment. Acid rain with a pH of 4 or lower refers to the wet components. Normal rain has a pH of about 5.6. Sulfuric acid from sulfur and nitric acid from nitrogen oxides are the major contributors. In lakes in which the buffering capacity is low, the pH becomes acidic enough to cause fish kills, and the lakes cannot support fish populations. A contributing factor is the fact that acidic conditions concurrently release toxic metals, such as aluminum, into the water.

activation (bioactivation). In toxicology, this term is used to describe metabolic reactions of a xenobiotic in which the product is more toxic than is the substrate. Such reactions are most commonly monooxygenations, the products of which are electrophiles that, if not detoxified by phase-two (conjugation) reactions, may react with nucleophilic groups on cellular macromolecules such as proteins and DNA.

active oxygen. Used to describe various short-lived highly reactive intermediates in the reduction of oxygen. Active oxygen species such as superoxide anion and hydroxyl radical are known or believed to be involved in several toxic actions. Superoxide anion is detoxified by superoxide dismutase.

acute toxicity tests. The most common tests for acute toxicity are the LC50 and LD50 tests which are designed to measure mortality in response to an acute toxic insult. Other tests for acute toxicity include dermal irritation tests, dermal sensitization tests, eye irritation tests, photoallergy tests, and phototoxicity tests. *See also* Eye Irritation Tests; LC50; and LD50.

acute toxicity. Refers to adverse effects on, or mortality of, organisms following soon after a brief exposure to a chemical agent. Either a single exposure or multiple exposures within a short time period may be involved, and an acute effect is generally regarded as an effect that occurs within the first few days after exposure, usually less than 2 weeks.

adaptation to toxicants. Refers to the ability of an organism to show insensitivity or decreased sensitivity to a chemical that normally causes deleterious effects. The terms resistance and tolerance are closely related and have been used in several different ways. However, a concensus is emerging to use the term *resistance* to mean that situation in which a change in the genetic constitution of a population in response to the stressor chemical enables a greater number of individuals to resist the toxic action than were able to resist it in the previous unexposed population. Thus, an essential feature of resistance is selection and then inheritance by subsequent generations. In microorganisms, this frequently involves mutations and induction of enzymes by the toxicant; in higher organisms, it usually involves selection for genes already present in the population at low frequency. The term *tolerance* is then reserved for situations in which individual organisms acquire the ability to resist the effect of a toxicant, usually as a result of prior exposure.

Ah locus. A gene(s) controlling the trait of responsiveness for induction of enzymes by aromatic hydrocarbons. In addition to aromatic hydrocarbons such as the polycyclics, the chlorinated dibenzo-*p*-dioxins, dibenzofurans, and biphenyls, as well as the brominated biphenyls, are also involved. This trait, originally defined by studies of induction of hepatic aryl hydrocarbon hydroxylase activity following 3-methylcholanthrene treatment, is inherited by simple autosomal dominance in crosses and backcrosses between C57BL/6 (Ah-responsive) and DBA/2 (Ah-nonresponsive) mice.

Ah receptor (AHR). A protein coded for by a gene of the Ah locus. The initial location of the Ah receptor is believed to be in the cytosol and, after binding to a ligand such as TCDD, is transported to the nucleus. Binding of aromatic hydrocarbons to the Ah receptor of mice is a prerequisite for the induction of many xenobiotic metabolizing enzymes, as well as for two responses to TCDD: epidermal hyperplasia and thymic atrophy. Ah responsive mice have a high-affinity receptor, whereas the Ah-nonresponsive mice have a low-affinity receptor.

air pollution. In general, the principal air pollutants are carbon monoxide, oxides of nitrogen, oxides of sulfur, hydrocarbons, and particulates. The principal sources are transportation, industrial processes, electric power generation, and the heating of buildings. Hydrocarbons such as benzo(*a*)pyrene are produced by incomplete combustion and are associated primarily with the automobile. They are usually not present at levels high enough to cause direct toxic effects but are important in the formation of photochemical air pollution, formed as a result of interactions between oxides of nitrogen and hydrocarbons in the presence of ultraviolet light, giving rise to lung irritants such as peroxyacetyl nitrate, acrolein, and formaldehyde. Particulates are a heterogeneous group of particles, often seen as smoke, that are important as carriers of absorbed hydrocarbons and as irritants to the respiratory system.

alkylating agents. These are chemicals that can add alkyl groups to DNA, a reaction that can result either in mispairing of bases or in chromosome breaks. The mechanism of the reaction involves the formation of a reactive carbonium ion that combines with electron rich bases in DNA. Thus alkylating agents such as dimethylnitrosomine are frequently carcinogens and/or mutagens.

Ames test. An in vitro test for mutagenicity utilizing mutant strains of the bacterium *Salmonella typhimurium*, which is used as a preliminary screen of chemicals for assessing potential carcinogenicity. Several strains are available that cannot grow in the absence of histidine because of metabolic defects in histidine biosynthesis. Mutagens and presumed carcinogens can cause mutations that enable the strains to regain their ability to grow in a histidine deficient medium. The test can be performed in the presence of the S-9 fraction from rat liver to allow metabolic activation of promutagens. There is a high correlation between bacterial mutagenicity and carcinogenicity of chemicals.

antagonism. In toxicology, antagonism is usually defined as that situation in which the toxicity of two or more compounds administered together is less than that expected from consideration of their toxicities when administered alone. Although this includes lowered toxicity resulting from induction of detoxifying enzymes, this is frequently considered separately because of the time that must elapse between treatment with the inducer and subsequent treatment with the toxicant. Antagonism not involving induction is often at a marginal level of detection and is consequently difficult to explain. Such antagonism may involve competition for receptor sites or nonenzymatic combination of one toxicant with another to reduce the toxic effect. Physiological antagonism, in which two agonists act on the same physiological system but produce opposite effects, may also occur.

antibody. A large protein first expressed on the surface of the B cells of the immune system, followed by a series of events resulting in a clone of plasma cells that secrete the antibody into body fluids. Antibodies bind to the substance (generally a protein) that stimulated their production but may cross react with related proteins. The natural function is to bind foreign substances such as microbes or microbial products but, because of their specificity, antibodies are used extensively in research and in diagnostic and therapeutic proceedures.

antidote. A compound administered in order to reverse the harmful effect(s) of a toxicant. They may be toxic mechanism specific, as in the case of 2-pyridine aldoxime (2-PAM) and organophosphate poisoning, or nonspecific, as in the case of syrup of ipecac, used to induce vomiting and, thereby, elimination of toxicants from the stomach.

behavioral toxicity. Behavior may be defined as an organism's motor or glandular response to changes in its internal or external environment. Such changes may be simple or highly complex, innate or learned, but in any event represent one of the final integrated expressions of nervous function. Behavioral toxicity is adverse or potentially adverse effects on such expression brought about by exogenous chemicals.

binding, covalent. *See* **covalent binding.**

bioaccumulation. The accumulation of a chemical either from the medium (usually water) directly or from consumption of food containing the chemical. Biomagnification is often used as a synonym for bioaccumulation, but is more correctly used to describe an increase in concentration of a chemical as it passes from organisms at one trophic level to organisms at higher trophic levels.

bioactivation. *See* **activation.**

bioassay. This term is used in two distinct ways. The first and most appropriate is the use of a living organism to measure the amount of a toxicant present in a sample or the toxicity of a sample. This is done by comparing the toxic effect of the sample with that of a graded series of a known standard. The second and less appropriate meaning is the use of animals to investigate the toxic effects of chemicals as in chronic toxicity tests.

biomagnification. *See* **bioaccumulation**

carcinogen. Any chemical or process involving chemicals that induces neoplasms that are not usually observed, the earlier induction of neoplasms than are commonly observed, and/or the induction of more neoplasms than are usually found.

carcinogen, epigenetic. Cancer-causing agents that exert their carcinogenic effect by mechanisms other than genetic, such as by immunosuppression, hormonal imbalance, or cytotoxicity. They may act as cocarcinogens or promoters. Epigenetic carcinogenesis is not as well understood a phenomenon as is genotoxic carcinogenesis.

carcinogen, genotoxic. Cancer-causing agents that exert their carcinogenic effect by a series of events that is initiated by an interaction with DNA, either directly or through an electrophilic metabolite.

carcinogen, proximate. *See* carcinogen, ultimate.

carcinogen, ultimate. Many, if not most, chemical carcinogens are not intrinsically carcinogenic but require metabolic activation to express their carcinogenic potential. The term *precarcinogen* describes the initial reactive compound, the term *proximate carcinogen* describes its more active products, and the term *ultimate carcinogen* describes the product that is actually responsible for carcinogenesis by its interaction with DNA.

carcinogenesis. This is the process encompassing the conversion of normal cells to neoplastic cells and the further development of these neoplastic cells into a tumor. This process results from the action of specific chemicals, certain viruses, or radiation. Chemical carcinogens have been classified into those that are genotoxic and those that are epigenetic (ie, not genotoxic).

chronic toxicity. This term is used to describe adverse effects manifested after a long time period of uptake of small quantities of the toxicant in question. The dose is small enough so that no acute effects are manifested, and the time period is frequently a significant part of the expected normal lifetime of the organism. The most serious manifestation of chronic toxicity is carcinogenesis, but other types of chronic toxicity are also known (eg, reproductive effects, behavioral effects).

chronic toxicity tests. Chronic tests are those conducted over the greater part of the lifespan of the test species or, in some cases, more than one generation. The most important tests are carcinogenicity tests, and the most common test species are rats and mice.

cocarcinogenesis. Cocarcinogenesis is the enhancement of the conversion of normal cells to neoplastic cells. This process is manifested by enhancement of carcinogenesis when the agent is administered either before or together with a carcinogen. Cocarcinogenesis should be distinguished from promotion as, in the latter case, the promoter must be administered after the initiating carcinogen.

comparative toxicology. The study of the variation in the expression of the toxicity of exogenous chemicals toward organisms of different taxonomic groups or of different genetic strains.

compartment. In pharmaco(toxico)kinetics, a compartment is a hypothetical volume of an animal system wherein a chemical acts homogeneously in transport and transformation. A single mathematical compartment may be one, two, or more physiological tissues or entities. Compartmental models are mathematical depictions of physiological reality. Transport into, out of, or between compartments is described by rate constants, which are used in models of the intact animal.

conjugation reactions. *See* **phase-two reactions.**

covalent binding. This involves the covalent bond or "shared electron pair" bond. Each covalent bond consists of a pair of electrons shared between two atoms and occupying two stable orbitals, one of each atom. Although this is distinguished from the ionic bond or ionic valence, in fact chemical bonds may show both covalent and ionic character. In toxicology, the term *covalent binding* is used less precisely to refer to the binding of toxicants or their reactive metabolites to endogenous molecules (usually macromolecules) to produce stable adducts resistant to rigorous extraction procedures. A covalent bond between ligand and macromolecule is generally assumed. Many forms of chronic toxicity involve covalent binding of the toxicant to DNA or protein molecules within the cell.

cross resistance, cross tolerance. These terms describe the situation in which either resistance or tolerance to a particular toxicant (as defined under adaptation to toxicants) is induced by exposure to a different toxicant. This is commonly seen in resistance of insects to insecticides in which selection with one insecticide brings about a broad spectrum of resistance to insecticides of the same or different chemical classes. Such cross resistance is usually caused by the inheritance of a high level of nonspecific xenobiotic-metabolizing enzymes.

cytotoxicity. Cellular injury or death brought about by chemicals external to the cell. Such chemicals may be soluble mediators produced by the immune system or they may be chemicals (toxicants) to which the organism has been exposed.

Delaney Amendment. *See* **Food, Drug and Cosmetics Act.**

detoxication. A metabolic reaction or sequence of reactions that reduces the potential for adverse effect of a xenobiotic. Such sequences normally involve an increase in water solubility that facilitates excretion and/or the reaction of a reactive product with an endogenous substrate (conjugation), thereby not only increasing water solubility but also reducing the possibility of interaction with cellular macromolecules. Not to be confused with detoxification. *See also* Detoxification.

detoxification. Treatment by which toxicants are removed from intoxicated patients or a course of treatment during which dependence on alcohol or other drugs of abuse is reduced or eliminated. Not to be confused with detoxication. *See also* Detoxication.

distribution. The term *distribution* refers both to the movement of a toxicant from the portal of entry to the tissue and also to the description of the different concentrations reached in different locations. The first involves the study of transport mechanisms primarily in the blood, and both are subject to mathematical analysis in toxicokinetic studies.

dosage. The amount of a toxicant drug or other chemical administered or taken expressed as some function of the organism, (eg, mg/kg body weight/day).

dose. The total amount of a toxicant, drug, or other chemical administered or taken by the organism.

dose response. In toxicology, the quantitative relationship between the amount of a toxicant administered or taken and the incidence or extent of the adverse effect.

dose–response assessment. A step in the risk-assessment process to characterize the relationship between the dose of a chemical administered to a population of test animals and the incidence of a given adverse effect. It involves mathematical modeling techniques to extrapolate from the high-dose effects observed in test animals to estimate the effects expected from exposure to the typically low doses that may be encountered by humans.

Draize Test. *See* **eye irritation test**.

drugs of abuse. Although all drugs may have deleterious effects on humans, drugs of abuse either have no medicinal function or are taken at higher than therapeutic doses. Some drugs of abuse may affect only higher nervous functions (ie, mood, reaction time, and coordination), but many produce physical dependence and have serious physical effects, with fatal overdose being a common occurrence. The drugs of abuse include central nervous system (CNS) depressants such as ethanol, methaqualone (Quaalude), and secobarbital; CNS stimulants such as cocaine, methamphetamine (speed), caffeine, and nicotine; opioids such as heroin and morphine; hallucinogens such as lysergic acid diethylamide (LSD), phencyclidine (PCP), and tetrahydrocannabinol (THC), the most important active principle of marijuana,

drugs, therapeutic. All therapeutic drugs can be toxic at some dose. The danger to the patient is dependent on the nature of the toxic response, the dose necessary to produce the toxic response, and the relationship between the therapeutic and the toxic dose. Drug toxicity is affected by all of those factors that affect the toxicity of xenobiotics, including (genetic) variation, diet, age, and the presence of other exogenous chemicals. The risk of toxic side effects from a particular drug must be weighed against the expected benefits; the use of a quite dangerous drug with only a narrow tolerance between the therapeutic and toxic doses might well be justified if it is the sole treatment for an otherwise fatal disease. For example, cytotoxic agents used in the treatment of cancer are known carcinogens.

ecotoxicology. *See* **environmental toxicology**.

electron transport system (ETS). This term is often restricted to the mitochondrial system, although it applies equally well to other systems, including that of microsomes and chloroplasts. The mitochondrial ETS (also termed *respiratory chain* or *cytochrome chain*) consists of a series of cytochromes and other electron carriers arranged in the inner mitochondrial membrane. These components transfer the electrons from NADH or FADH$_2$ generated in metabolic oxidations to oxygen, the final electron acceptor, through a series of alternate oxidations and reductions. The energy that these electrons lose during these transfers is used to pump H$^+$ from the matrix into the intermembrane space, creating an electrochemical proton gradient that drives oxidative phosphorylation. The energy is conserved as adenosine triphosphate (ATP).

electron transport system (ETS) inhibitors. The three major respiratory enzyme complexes of the mitochondrial electron transport system can all be blocked by inhibitors. For example, rotenone inhibits the NADH dehydrogenase complex, antimycin A inhibits the b–c complex, and cyanide and carbon monoxide inhibit the cytochrome oxidase complex. Although oxidative phosphorylation inhibitors prevent phosphorylation while allowing electron transfers to proceed, ETS inhibitors prevent both electron transport and ATP production.

electrophilic. Electrophiles are chemicals that are attracted to and react with electron-rich centers in other molecules in reactions known as electrophilic reactions. Many activation reactions produce electrophilic intermediates such as epoxides, which exert their toxic action by forming covalent bonds with nucleophilic centers in cellular macromolecules such as DNA or proteins.

endoplasmic reticulum. The endoplasmic reticulum (ER) is an extensive branching and anastomosing double membrane distributed in the cytoplasm of eucaryotic cells. The ER is of two types: Rough ER (RER) contains attached ribosomes on the cytosolic surface and smooth ER (SER) is devoid of ribosomes are involved in protein biosynthesis, and RER is abundant in cells specialized for protein synthesis. Many xenobiotic-metabolizing enzymes are integral components of both SER and RER, such as the cytochrome P450–dependent monooxygenase system and the flavin-containing monooxygenase, although the specific content is usually higher in SER. When tissue or cells are disrupted by homogenization, the ER is fragmented into many smaller (c. 100 nm diameter) closed vesicles called microsomes, which can be isolated by differential centrifugation.

enterohepatic circulation. This term describes the excretion of a compound into the bile and its subsequent reabsorption from the small intestine and transport back to the liver, where it is available again for biliary excretion. The most important mechanism is conjugation in the liver, followed by excretion into the bile. In the small intestine the conjugation product is hydrolyzed, either nonenzymatically or by the microflora, and the compound is reabsorbed to become a substrate for conjugation and reexcretion into the bile.

environmental toxicology. This is concerned with the movement of toxicants and their metabolites in the environment and in food chains and the effect of such toxicants on populations of organisms.

epigenetic carcinogen. *See* **carcinogen, epigenetic.**

exposure assessment. A component of risk assessment. The number of individuals likely to be exposed to a chemical in the environment or in the workplace is assessed, and the intensity, frequency, and duration of human exposure are estimated.

eye irritation test (Draize Test). Eye irritation tests measure irritancy of compounds applied topically to the eye. These tests are variations of the Draize test, and the experimental animal used is the albino rabbit. The test consists of adding the material to be tested directly into the conjunctival sac of one eye of each of several albino rabbits, the other eye serving as the control. This test is probably the most controversial of all toxicity tests, being criticized primarily on the grounds that it is inhumane. Moreover, because both concentrations and volumes used are high and show high variability, it has been suggested that these tests cannot be extrapolated to humans. However, because visual impairment is a critical toxic endpoint, tests for ocular toxicity are essential. Attempts to solve the dilemma have taken two forms: to find substitute in vitro tests and to modify the Draize test so that it becomes not only more humane, but also more predictive for humans.

Federal Insecticide, Fungicide and Rodenticide Act (FIFRA). This law is the basic US law under which pesticides and other agricultural chemicals distributed in interstate commerce are registered and regulated. First enacted in 1947, FIFRA placed the regulation of agrochemicals under control of the US Department of Agriculture. In 1970, this responsibility was transferred to the newly created Environmental Protection Agency (EPA). Subsequently, FIFRA has been revised extensively by the Federal Environmental Pesticide Control Act (FEPCA) of 1972 and by the FIFRA amendments of 1975, 1978, and 1980. Under FIFRA, all new pesticide products used in the United States must be registered with the EPA. This requires the registrant to submit information on the composition, intended use, and efficacy of the product, along with a comprehensive database establishing that the material can be used without causing unreasonable adverse effects on humans or on the environment.

fetal alcohol syndrome (FAS). FAS refers to a pattern of defects in children born to alcoholic mothers. Three criteria for FAS are: prenatal or postnatal growth retardation; characteristic facial anomalies such as microcephaly, small eye opening, and thinned upper lip; and central nervous system dysfunction, such as mental retardation and developmental delays.

food additives. Chemicals may be added to food as preservatives (either antibacterial or antifungal compounds or antioxidants) to change the physical characteristics, for processing, or to change the taste or odor. Although most food additives are safe and without chronic toxicity, many were introduced when toxicity testing was relatively unsophisticated and some have been shown subsequently to be toxic. The most important inorganic additives are nitrate and nitrite. Well-known examples of food additives include the antioxidant butylatedhydroxyanisole (BHA), fungistatic agents such as methyl *p*-benzoic acid, the emulsifier propylene glycol, sweeteners such as saccharin and aspartame, and dyes such as tartrazine and Sunset Yellow.

food contaminants (food pollutants). Food contaminants, as opposed to food additives, are those compounds included inadvertantly in foods, that are raw, cooked, or processed. They include bacterial toxins such as the exotoxin of *Clostridium botulinum*, mycotoxins such as aflatoxins from *Aspergillus flavus*, plant alkaloids, animal toxins, pesticide residues, residues of animal food additives such as diethylstilbestrol (DES) and antibiotics, and a variety of industrial chemicals such as polychlorinated biphenyls (PCBs) and polybrominated biphenyls (PBBs).

Food, Drug and Cosmetics Act. The Federal Food, Drug and Cosmetic Act is administered by the Food and Drug Administration (FDA). It establishes limits for food additives, sets criteria for drug safety for both human and animal use, and requires proof of both safety and efficacy. This act contains the Delaney Amendment, which states that food additives that cause cancer in humans or animals at any level shall not be considered safe and are, therefore, prohibited. The Delaney Amendment has been modified to permit more flexible use of mechanistic and cost–benefit data. This law also empowers the FDA to establish and modify the "Generally Recognized as Safe" (GRAS) list and to establish Good Laboratory Practice (GLP) rules.

forensic toxicology. Forensic toxicology is concerned with the medicolegal aspects of the adverse effects of chemicals on humans and animals. Although primarily devoted to the identification of the cause and circumstances of death and the legal issues arising therefrom, forensic toxicologists also deal with sublethal poisoning cases.

free radicals. Molecules that have unpaired electrons. Free radicals may be produced metabolically from xenobiotics and, because they are extremely reactive, may be involved in interactions with cellular macromolecules, giving rise to adverse effects. Examples include the trichloromethyl radical produced from carbon tetrachloride or the carbene radical produced by oxidation of the acetal carbon of methylenedioxyphenyl synergists.

genotoxic carcinogen. *See* **carcinogen, genotoxic.**

genotoxicity. Genotoxicity is an adverse effect on the genetic material (DNA) of living cells that, on the replication of the cells, is expressed as a mutagenic or a carcinogenic event. Genotoxicity results from a reaction with DNA that can be measured either biochemically or in short-term tests with endpoints that reflect DNA damage.

Good Laboratory Practice (GLP). In the United States, this is a code of laboratory procedures laid down under federal law and to be followed by laboratories undertaking toxicity tests, the results of which will be used for regulatory or legal purposes.

generally regarded as safe (GRAS) list. *See* **Food, Drug and Cosmetics Act.**

hazard identification. Considered the final step in risk assessment, hazard identification involves the qualitative determination of whether exposure to a chemical causes an increased incidence of an adverse effect, such as cancer or birth defects, in a population of test animals and an evaluation of the relevance of this information to the potential for causing similar effects in humans.

hepatotoxicity. Hepatotoxicants are those chemicals causing adverse effects on the liver. The liver may be particularly susceptible to chemical injury because of its anatomic relationship to the most important portal of entry, the gastrointestinal (GI) tract, and its high concentration of xenobiotic-metabolizing enzymes. Many of these enzymes, particularly cytochrome P450, metabolize xenobiotics to produce reactive intermediates that can react with endogenous macromolecules such as proteins and DNA to produce adverse effects.

immunotoxicity. This term can be used in either of two ways. The first refers to toxic effects mediated by the immune system, such as dermal sensitivity reactions to compounds like 2,4-dinitrochlorobenzene. The second and currently most acceptable definition refers to toxic effects that impair the functioning of the immune system—for example, the ability of a toxicant to impair resistance to infection.

in vitro tests. Literally, these are tests conducted outside of the body of the organism. In toxicity testing they would include studies using isolated enzymes, subcellular organelles, or cultured cells. Although technically the term would not include tests involving intact eukaryotes (eg, the Ames test), it frequently is used by toxicologists to include all short-term tests for mutagenicity that are normally used as indicators of potential carcinogenicity.

in vivo tests. Tests carried out on the intact organism, although the evaluation of the toxic endpoint almost always requires pathological or biochemical examination of the test organism's tissues. They may be acute, subchronic, or chronic. The best known are the lifetime carcinogenesis tests carried out on rodents.

induction. The process of causing a quantitative increase in an enzyme as a result of de novo protein synthesis following exposure to an inducing agent. This can occur either by a decrease in the degradation rate or an increase in the synthesis rate or both. Increasing the synthesis rate is the most common mechanism for induction by xenobiotics. Coordinate (pleiotypic) induction is the induction of multiple enzymes by a single inducing agent. For example, phenobarbital can induce isozymes of both cytochrome P450 and glutathione *S*-transferase.

industrial toxicology. A specific area of environmental toxicology dealing with the work environment; it includes risk assessment, establishment of permissible levels of exposure, and worker protection.

inhibition. In its most general sense, inhibition means a restraining or a holding back. In biochemistry and biochemical toxicology, inhibition is a reduction in the rate of an enzymatic reaction, and an inhibitor is any compound causing such a reduction. Inhibition of enzymes important in normal metabolism is a significant mechanism of toxic action of xenobiotics, whereas inhibition of xenobiotic-metabolizing enzymes can have important consequences in the ultimate toxicity of their substrates. Inhibition is sometimes used in toxicology in a more general and rather ill-defined way to refer to the reduction of an overall process of toxicity, as in the inhibition of carcinogenesis by a particular chemical.

initiation. The initial step in the carcinogenic process involving the conversion of a normal cell to a neoplastic cell. Initiation is considered to be a rapid and essentially irreversible change involving the interaction of the ultimate carcinogen with DNA; this change primes the cell for subsequent neoplastic development via the promotion process.

intoxication. In the general sense, this term refers primarily to inebriation with ethyl alcohol, secondarily to excitement or delirium caused by other means, including other chemicals. In the clinical sense it refers to poisoning or becoming poisoned. In toxicology, it is sometimes used as a synonym for activation—that is, the production of a more toxic metabolite from a less toxic parent compound. This latter use of intoxication is ambiguous and should be abandoned in favor of the aforementioned general meanings, and activation or bioactivation used instead.

isozymes (isoenzymes). Isozymes are multiple forms of a given enzyme that occur within a single species or even a single cell and that catalyze the same general reaction but are coded for by different genes. Different isozymes may occur at different life stages and/or in different organs and tissues, or they may coexist within the same cell. The first well-characterized isozymes were those of lactic dehydrogenase. Several xenobiotic-metabolizing enzymes exist in multiple isozymes, including cytochrome P450 and glucuronosyltransferase.

LC50 (median lethal concentration). The concentration of a test chemical that, when a population of test organisms is exposed to it, is estimated to be fatal to 50% of the organisms under the stated conditions of the test. Normally used in lieu of the LD50 test in aquatic toxicology and inhalation toxicology.

LD50 (median lethal dose). The quantity of a chemical compound that, when applied directly to test organisms, is estimated to be fatal to 50% of those organisms under the stated conditions of the test. The LD50 value is the standard for comparison of acute toxicity between toxicants and between species. Because the results of LD50 determinations may vary widely, it is important that both biological and physical conditions be narrowly defined (eg, strain, sex, and age of test organism; time and route of exposure; environmental conditions). The value may be determined graphically from a plot of log dose against mortality expressed in probability units (probits) or, more recently, by using one of several computer programs available.

lethal synthesis. This term is used to describe the process by which a toxicant, similar in structure to an endogenous substrate, is incorporated into the same metabolic pathway as the endogenous substrate, ultimately being transformed into a toxic or lethal product. For example, fluroacetate simulates acetate in intermediary metabolism, being transformed via the tricarboxylic acid cycle to fluorocitrate, which then inhibits aconitase, resulting in disruption of the TCA cycle and energy metabolism.

lipophilic. The physical property of chemical compounds that causes them to be soluble in nonpolar solvents (eg, chloroform and benzene) and, generally, relatively insoluble in polar solvents such as water. This property is important toxicologically because lipophilic compounds tend to enter the body easily and to be excretable only when they have been rendered less lipophilic by metabolic action.

maximum tolerated dose (MTD). The MTD has been defined for testing purposes by the US Environmental Protection Agency as the highest dose that causes no more than a 10% weight decrement, as compared to the appropriate control groups, and does not produce mortality, clinical signs of toxicity, or pathologic lesions (other than those that may be related to a neoplastic response) that would be predicted to shorten the animals' natural life span. It is an important concept in chronic toxicity testing; however, the relevance of results produced by such large doses has become a matter of controversy.

membranes. Membranes of tissues, cells, and cell organelles are all basically similar in structure. They appear to be bimolecular lipid leaflets with proteins embedded in the matrix and also arranged on the outer polar surfaces. This basic plan is present in spite of many variations, and it is important in toxicological studies of uptake of toxicants by passive diffusion and active transport.

microsomes. Microsomes are small closed vesicles (c. 100 nm diameter) that represent membrane fragments formed from the endoplasmic reticulum when cells are disrupted by homogenization. Microsomes are separated from other cell organelles by differential centrifugation. The cell homogenate contains rough microsomes that are studded with ribosomes and are derived from rough endoplasmic reticulum, and smooth microsomes that are devoid of ribosomes and are derived from smooth endoplasmic reticulum. Microsomes are important preparations for studying the many processes carried out by the endoplasmic reticulum, such as protein biosynthesis and xenobiotic metabolism.

mode of action (mode of toxic action). Terms used to describe the mechanism(s) that enables a toxicant to exert its toxic effect. The term(s) may be narrowly used to describe only those events at the site of action or more broadly, to describe the sequence of events from uptake from the environment, through metabolism, distribution, and so on, up to and including events at the site of action.

monooxygenase (mixed-function oxidase). An enzyme for which the cosubstrates are an organic compound and molecular oxygen. In reactions catalyzed by these enzymes, one atom of a molecule of oxygen is incorporated into the substrate whereas the other atom is reduced to water. Monooxygenases of importance in toxicology include cytochrome P450 and the flavin-containing monooxygenase, both of which initiate the metabolism of lipophilic xenobiotics by the introduction of a reactive polar group into the molecule. Such reactions may represent detoxication or may generate reactive intermediates of importance in toxic action. The term *mixed-function oxidase* is now considered obsolete and should not be used. The term *multifunction oxidase* was never widely adopted and also should not be used.

mutagenicity. Mutations are heritable changes produced in the genetic information stored in the DNA of living cells. Chemicals capable of causing such changes are known as *mutagens* and the process is known as *mutagenesis.*

mycotoxins. Toxins produced by fungi. Many, such as aflatoxins, are particularly important in toxicology.

nephrotoxicity. A pathologic state that can be induced by chemicals (nephrotoxicants) and in which the normal homeostatic functioning of the kidney is impaired. It is often associated with necrosis of the proximal tubule and may involve either the excretion of large volumes of very dilute urine or excretion of minimal amounts of urine.

neurotoxicity. This is a general term referring to all toxic effects on the nervous system, including toxic effects measured as behavioral abnormalities. Because the nervous system is complex, both structurally and functionally, and has considerable functional reserve, the study of neurotoxicity is a many-faceted branch of toxicology. It involves electrophysiology, receptor function, pathology, behavior, and other aspects.

no observed effect level (NOEL). This is the highest dose level of a chemical that, in a given toxicity test, causes no observable effect in the test animals. The NOEL for a given chemical varies with the route and duration of exposure and the nature of the adverse effect (ie, the indicator of toxicity). The NOEL for the most sensitive test species and the most sensitive indicator of toxicity is usually employed for regulatory purposes. Effects considered are usually adverse effects, and this value may be called the *no observed adverse effects level* (NOAEL).

Occupational Safety and Health Administration (OSHA). In the United States, OSHA is the government agency concerned with health and safety in the workplace. Through the administration of the Occupational Safety and Health Act, OSHA sets the standards for worker exposure to specific chemicals, for air concentration values, and for monitoring procedures. OSHA is also concerned with research (through the National Institute for Occupational Safety and Health [NIOSH]), information, education, and training in occupational safety and health.

oncogenes. Oncogenes are genes that, when activated in cells, can transform the cells from normal to neoplastic. Sometimes oncogenes are carried into normal cells by infecting viruses, particularly RNA viruses or retroviruses. In some cases, however, the oncogene is already present in the normal human cell, and it needs only a mutation or other activating event to change it from a harmless and possible essential gene, called a *proto-oncogene,* into a cancer-producing gene. More than 30 oncogenes have been identified in humans.

oxidative phosphorylation. The conservation of chemical energy extracted from fuel oxidations by the phosphorylation of adenosine diphosphate (ADP) by inorganic phosphate to form adenosine triphosphate (ATP) is accomplished in several ways. The majority of ATP is formed by respiratory chain–linked oxidative phosphorylation associated with the electron transport system in the mitochondrial inner membrane. The oxidations are tightly coupled to phosphorylations through a chemiosmotic mechanism in which H^+ are pumped across the inner mitochondrial membrane. Uncouplers of oxidative phosphorylation serve as H^+ ionophores to dissipate the H^+ gradient, and thus uncouple the phosphorylations from the oxidations.

oxidative stress. Damage to cells and cellular constituents and processes by reactive oxygen species generated in situ. Oxidative stress may be involved in such toxic interactions as DNA damage, lipid peroxidation, and pulmonary and cardiac toxicity. Because of the transitory nature of most reactive oxygen species, although oxidative stress is often invoked as a mechanism of toxicity, rigorous proof may be lacking.

partition coefficient. This is a measure of the relative lipid solubility of a chemical and is determined by measuring the partitioning of the compound between a lipid phase and an aqueous phase (eg, octanol and water). The partition coefficient is important in studies of the uptake of toxicants because compounds with high co-efficients (lipophilic compounds) are usually taken up more readily by organisms and tissues.

pharmacokinetics. The study of the quantitative relationship between absorption, distribution, and excretion of chemicals and their metabolites. It involves deriva-tion of rate constants for each of these processes and their integration into mathe-matical models that can predict the distribution of the chemical throughout the body compartments at any point in time after administration. Pharmacokinetics has been carried out most extensively in the case of clinical drugs. When applied specifically to toxicants, the term *toxicokinetics* is often used.

phase-one reactions. These reactions introduce a reactive polar group into lipo-philic xenobiotics. In most cases this group becomes the site for conjugation dur-ing phase-two reactions. Such reactions include microsomal monooxygenations, cytosolic and mitochondrial oxidations, cooxidations in the prostaglandin syn-thetase reaction, reductions, hydrolyses, and epoxide hydrolases. The products of phase-one reactions may be potent electrophiles that can be conjugated and detoxified in phase-two reactions or that may react with nucleophilic groups on cellular constituents, thereby causing toxicity.

phase-two reactions. Reactions involving the conjugation with endogenous sub-strates of phase-one products and other xenobiotics that contain functional groups such as hydroxyl, amino, carboxyl, epoxide, or halogen. The endogenous metabolites include sugars, amino acids, glutathione, and sulfate. The conjuga-tion products, with rare exceptions, are more polar, less toxic, and more readily excreted than are their parent compounds. There are two general types of conju-gations: type I (eg, glycoside and sulfate formation), in which an activated conju-gating agent combines with the substrate to yield the conjugated product; and type II (eg, amino acid conjugation), in which the substrate is activated and then combines with an amino acid to yield a conjugated product.

poison (toxicant). A poison (toxicant) is any substance that causes a harmful effect when administered to a living organism. Due to a popular connotation that poi-sons are, by definition, fatal in their effects and that their administration is usu-ally involved with attempted homicide or suicide, most toxicologists prefer the less prejudicial term toxicant. Poison is a quantitative concept. Almost any sub-stance is harmful at some dose and, at the same time, is harmless at a very low dose. There is a range of possible effects, from subtle long-term chronic toxicity to immediate lethality.

pollution. This is contamination of soil, water, food, or the atmosphere by the discharge or admixture of noxious materials. A *pollutant* is any chemical or substance contaminating the environment and contributing to pollution.

portals of entry. The sites at which xenobiotics enter the body. They include the skin, the gastrointestinal (GI) tract, and the respiratory system.

potentiation. *See* **synergism and potentiation.**

precarcinogen. *See* **carcinogen, ultimate.**

promotion. The facilitation of the growth and development of neoplastic cells into a tumor. This process is manifested by enhancement of carcinogenesis when the agent is given after a carcinogen.

pulmonary toxicity. This term refers to the effects of compounds that exert their toxic effects on the respiratory system, primarily the lungs.

quantitative structure activity relationships (QSAR). The relationship between the physical and/or chemical properties of chemicals and their ability to cause a particular effect, enter into particular reactions, and so on. The goal of QSAR studies in toxicology is to develop procedures whereby the toxicity of a compound can be predicted from its chemical structure by analogy with the properties of other toxicants of known structure and toxic properties.

reactive intermediates (reactive metabolites). Chemical compounds, produced during the metabolism of xenobiotics, that are more chemically reactive than is the parent compound. Although they are susceptible to detoxication by conjugation reactions, these metabolites, as a consequence of their increased reactivity, have a greater potential for adverse effects than does the parent compound. A well-known example is the metabolism of benzo(*a*)pyrene to its carcinogenic dihydrodiol epoxide derivative as a result of metabolism by cytochrome P450 and epoxide hydrolase. Reactive intermediates involved in toxic effects include epoxides, quinones, free radicals, reactive oxygen species, and a small number of unstable conjugation products.

resistance. *See* **adaptation to toxicants.**

Resource Conservation and Recovery Act (RCRA). Administered by the EPA, the RCRA is the most important act governing the disposal of hazardous wastes in the United States; it promulgates standards for identification of hazardous wastes, their transportation, and their disposal. Included in the last are siting and construction criteria for landfills and other disposal facilities as well as the regulation of owners and operators of such facilities.

risk assessment (risk analysis). The process by which the potential adverse health effects of human exposure to chemicals are characterized; it includes the development of both qualitative and quantitative expressions of risk. The process of risk assessment may be divided into four major components: hazard identification, dose–response assessment (high-dose to low-dose extrapolation), exposure assessment, and risk characterization.

risk, toxicologic. The probability that some adverse effect will result from a given exposure to a chemical is known as the *risk*. It is the estimated frequency of occurrence of an event in a population and may be expressed in absolute terms (eg, 1 in 1 million) or in terms of relative risk, (ie, the ratio of the risk in question to that in an equivalent unexposed population).

safety factor (uncertainty factor). A number by which the no observed effect level (NOEL) is divided to obtain the acceptable daily intake (ADI) of a chemical for regulatory purposes. The safety factor is intended to account for the uncertainties inherent in estimating the potential effects of a chemical on humans from results obtained with test species. The safety factor allows for possible differences in sensitivity between the test species and humans, as well as for variations in the sensitivity within the human population. The size of safety factor (eg, 100–1000) varies with confidence in the database and the nature of the adverse effect. Small safety factors indicate a high degree of confidence in the data, an extensive database, and/or the availability of human data. Large safety factors are indicative of an inadequate and uncertain database and/or the severity of the unexpected toxic effect. The use of safety factors is restricted to noncarcinogenic toxicants.

selectivity (selective toxicity). A characteristic of the relationship between toxic chemicals and living organisms whereby a particular chemical may be highly toxic to one species but relatively innocuous to another. The search for and study of selective toxicants is an important aspect of comparative toxicology because chemicals toxic to target species but innocuous to nontarget species are extremely valuable in agriculture and medicine. The mechanisms involved vary from differential penetration rates through different metabolic pathways to differences in receptor molecules at the site of toxic action.

solvents. In toxicology this term usually refers to industrial solvents. These belong to many different chemical classes and a number of these are known to cause problems of toxicity to humans. They include aliphatic hydrocarbons (eg, hexane), halogenated aliphatic hydrogens (eg, methylene chloride), aliphatic alcohols (eg, methanol), glycols and glycol ethers (eg, propylene and propylene glycol), and aromatic hydrocarbons (eg, toluene).

subchronic toxicity. Toxicity due to chronic exposure to quantities of a toxicant that do not cause any evident acute toxicity for a time period that is extended but is not so long as to constitute a significant part of the lifespan of the species in question. In subchronic toxicity tests using mammals, a 30- to 90-day period is considered appropriate.

synergism and potentiation. The terms synergism and potentiation have been variously used and defined but in any case involve a toxicity that is greater when two compounds are given simultaneously or sequentially than would be expected from a consideration of the toxicities of the compounds given alone. In an attempt to make the use of these terms uniform, it is suggested that, insofar as toxic effects are concerned, they be used as defined as follows: Both involve toxicity greater than would be expected from the toxicities of the compounds administered separately, but in the case of *synergism* one compound has little or no intrinsic toxicity administered alone, whereas in the case of *potentiation* both compounds have appreciable toxicity when administered alone.

teratogenesis. This term refers to the production of defects in the reproduction process resulting in either reduced productivity due to fetal or embryonic mortality or the birth of offspring with physical, mental, behavioral, or developmental defects. Compounds causing such defects are known as *teratogens*.

therapy. Poisoning therapy may be nonspecific or specific. Nonspecific therapy is treatment for poisoning that is not related to the mode of action of the particular toxicant. It is designed to prevent further uptake of the toxicant and to maintain vital signs. Specific therapy, however, is therapy related to the mode of action of the toxicant and not simply to the maintenance of vital signs by treatment of symptoms. Specific therapy may be based on activation and detoxication reactions, on mode of action, or on elimination of the toxicant. In some cases more than one antidote, with different modes of action, is available for the same toxicant.

threshold dose. The dose of a toxicant below which no adverse effect occurs. The existence of such a threshold is based on the fundamental tenet of toxicology that, for any chemical, there exists a range of doses over which the severity of the observed effect is directly related to the dose, the threshold level representing the lower limit of this dose range. Although practical thresholds are considered to exist for most noncarcinogenic adverse effects, it has been argued that there is no threshold dose for carcinogens.

threshold limit value (TLV). Upper permissive limits of airborne concentrations of substances. They represent conditions under which it is believed that nearly all workers may be exposed repeatedly, day after day, without adverse effect. Threshold limits are based on the best available information from industrial experience, from experimental human and animal studies, and, when possible, from a combination of the three.

threshold limit value—ceiling (TLV—C). This is the concentration that should not be exceeded even momentarily. For some substances (eg, irritant gases) only one TLV category, the TLV—C, may be relevant. For other substances, two or three TLV categories may need to be considered.

threshold limit value—short-term exposure limit (TLV—STEL). This is the maximal concentration to which workers can be exposed for a period up to 15 min continuously without suffering from (1) irritation, (2) chronic or irreversible tissue change, or (3) narcosis of sufficient degree to increase accident proneness, impair self-rescue, or materially reduce work efficiency, provided that no more than four excursions per day are permitted, that at least 60 min elapse between exposure periods, and provided that the daily TLV—TWA is not exceeded.

threshold limit value—time weighted average (TLV—TWA). This is the TWA concentration for a normal 8-hr workday or 40-hr workweek to which nearly all workers may be exposed repeatedly day after day, without adverse effect. Time-weighted averages allow certain permissible excursions above the limit, provided they are compensated by equivalent excursions below the limit during the workday. In some instances, the average concentration is calculated for a workweek rather than for a workday.

tolerance. *See* **adaptation toxicants.**

Toxic Substances Control Act (TSCA). Enacted in 1976, the TSCA provides the EPA with the authority to require testing and to regulate chemicals, both old and new, entering the environment. It was intended to supplement sections of the Clean Air Act, the Clean Water Act, and the Occupational Safety and Health Act that already provide for regulation of chemicals. Manufacturers are required to submit information to allow the EPA to identify and evaluate the potential hazards of a chemical prior to its introduction into commerce. The act also provides for the regulation of production, use, distribution, and disposal of chemicals.

toxicant. *See* **poison.**

toxicokinetics. *See* **pharmacokinetics.**

toxicology. Toxicology is defined as that branch of science that deals with poisons (toxicants) and their effects; a poison is defined as any substance that causes a harmful effect when administered, either by accident or design, to a living organism. There are difficulties in bringing a more precise definition to the meaning of poison and in the definition and measurement of toxic effect. The range of deleterious effects is wide and varies with species, sex, developmental stage, and so on, whereas while the effects of toxicants are always dose dependent.

toxin. A *toxin* is a toxicant produced by a living organism. Toxin should never be used as a synonym for toxicant.

transport. In toxicology this term refers to the mechanisms that bring about movement of toxicants and their metabolites from one site in the organism to another. *Transport* usually involves binding to either blood albumins or blood lipoproteins.

ultimate carcinogen *See* **carcinogen, ultimate.**

venom. A venom is a toxin produced by an animal specifically for the poisoning of other species via a mechanism designed to deliver the toxin to its prey. Examples include the venom of bees and wasps, delivered by a sting, and the venom of snakes, delivered by fangs.

water pollution. Water pollution is of concern in both industrialized and nonindustrialized nations. Chemical contamination is most common in industrialized nations, whereas microbial contamination is more important in nonindustrialized areas. Surface water contamination has been the primary cause for concern but, since the discovery of insecticides in groundwater, contamination of water from this source is also a problem. Water pollution may arise from runoff of agricultural chemicals, from sewage, or from specific industrial sources. Agricultural chemicals found in water include insecticides, herbicides, fungicides, and nematocides; fertilizers, although less of a toxic hazard, contribute to such environmental problems as eutrophication. Other chemicals of concern include low-molecular-weight halogenated hydrocarbons such as chloroform, dichloroethane, and carbon tetrachloride; polychlorinated biphenyls (PCBs); chlorophenols; 2,3,7,8-tetrachlorodibenzo-*p*-dioxin (TCDD); phthalate ester plasticizers; detergents; and a number of toxic inorganics.

xenobiotic. A general term used to describe any chemical interacting with an organism that does not occur in the normal metabolic pathways of that organism. The use of this term in lieu of "foreign compound," among others, is gaining wide acceptance.

INDEX

Note: Page numbers in bold refer to chemical structures; page numbers followed by f or t refer to figures or tables.